DANIELS AND WORTHINGHAM'S

Muscle Testing

Techniques of Manual Examination and Performance Testing

DANIELS AND WORTHINGHAM'S

Muscle Testing

Techniques of Manual Examination and Performance Testing

NINTH EDITION

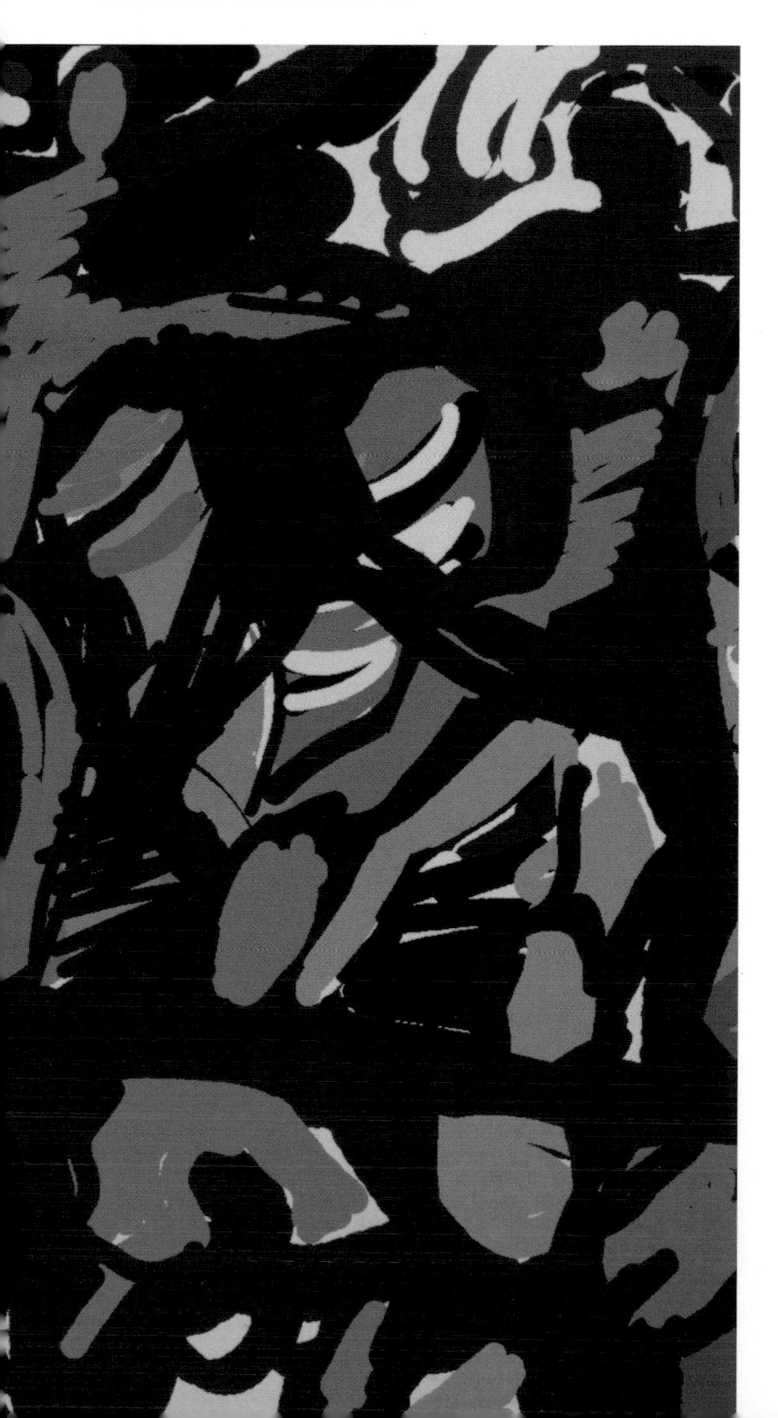

HELEN J. HISLOP, PhD, ScD, FAPTA
Professor Emerita
Department of Biokinesiology and Physical Therapy
University of Southern California
Los Angeles, California

DALE AVERS, DPT, PhD
Associate Professor
Department of Physical Therapy Education
College of Health Professions
SUNY Upstate Medical University
Syracuse, New York

MARYBETH BROWN, PT, PhD, FAPTA
Professor
Physical Therapy Program, Biomedical Sciences
University of Missouri
Columbia, Missouri

ELSEVIER

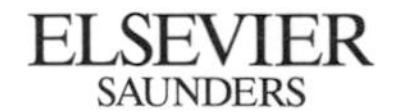

3251 Riverport Lane
St. Louis, Missouri 63043

DANIELS AND WORTHINGHAM'S MUSCLE TESTING: TECHNIQUES OF MANUAL EXAMINATION AND PERFORMANCE TESTING, NINTH EDITION

ISBN: 978-1-4557-0615-0

Notices

Knowledge and best practice in this field are constantly changing. As new research and experience broaden our understanding, changes in research methods, professional practices, or medical treatment may become necessary.
Practitioners and researchers must always rely on their own experience and knowledge in evaluating and using any information, methods, compounds, or experiments described herein. In using such information or methods they should be mindful of their own safety and the safety of others, including parties for whom they have a professional responsibility.
With respect to any drug or pharmaceutical products identified, readers are advised to check the most current information provided (i) on procedures featured or (ii) by the manufacturer of each product to be administered, to verify the recommended dose or formula, the method and duration of administration, and contraindications. It is the responsibility of practitioners, relying on their own experience and knowledge of their patients, to make diagnoses, to determine dosages and the best treatment for each individual patient, and to take all appropriate safety precautions.
To the fullest extent of the law, neither the Publisher nor the authors, contributors, or editors, assume any liability for any injury and/or damage to persons or property as a matter of products liability, negligence or otherwise, or from any use or operation of any methods, products, instructions, or ideas contained in the material herein.

Library of Congress Cataloging-in-Publication Data

Hislop, Helen J.
Daniels and Worthingham's muscle testing : techniques of manual examination and performance testing. —9th ed. / Helen J. Hislop, Dale Avers, Marybeth Brown.
p. ; cm.
Muscle testing
Includes bibliographical references and index.

ISBN 978-1-4557-0615-0 (hardcover : alk. paper)

I. Avers, Dale. II. Brown, Marybeth. III. Daniels, Lucille. Muscle testing. IV. Title. V. Title: Muscle testing.
[DNLM: 1. Muscles—physiology. 2. Physical Examination—methods. WE 500]
616.7'40754—dc23

2012037279

Vice President and Publisher: Linda Duncan
Content Strategist: Jolynn Gower
Senior Content Development Specialist: Christie M. Hart
Publishing Services Manager: Catherine Jackson
Senior Project Manager: Mary Pohlman
Designer: Brian Salisbury

Printed in China

Last digit is the print number: 9 8 7 6 5 4 3 2

Dedication

I would like to dedicate this book to Dorothy R. Hewitt, PT, MA, FAPTA, in recognition of her long and successful career and her many contributions to the development of physical therapy.

In addition to being a highly esteemed clinician, Ms. Hewitt's 70-year-long career included several chair positions, beginning at the University of Pennsylvania, where she was department chair and founding director of the renowned Physical Therapy Program. In addition, she served as Director of Education and Recruitment for the American Physical Therapy Association (APTA) and acted as a liaison between the APTA and the American Medical Association—helping to resolve differences and bridge the gap between the two fields.

Ms. Hewitt later served as Director of Los Angeles Orthopedic Hospital and combined clinical work with volunteer teaching at the University of Southern California and other local schools where faculty were in short supply. During this same period she was elected as Second Vice President of the APTA Board of Directors and was appointed to the Editorial Board of the APTA journal.

After a long tenure at Orthopedic Hospital, Ms. Hewitt changed her focus and opened a private practice, which she maintained successfully for some 20 years along with continuing activities for the APTA. When family obligations called for her return to New York, she was appointed Chair of the Physical Therapy Education Program at SUNY Upstate Medical University, a position she held until her retirement.

Sadly, Dorothy Hewitt died on November 9, 2011, at the age of 93, just as this book was being finalized. Her knowledge and experience greatly influenced this and previous editions, and her lifelong efforts helped bring us to where we are today—a successful, effective, and independent profession.

Helen J. Hislop

In grateful appreciation to all my students and colleagues who continue to challenge me to think differently about our practice of physical therapy.

Dale Avers

I would like to dedicate this book to my students—past, present, and future—for these are the men and women who have made and continue to make my days tremendously fun and totally worthwhile. This book is also dedicated to my wonderful colleagues who are the true backbone of our profession.

Marybeth Brown

CONTRIBUTOR

Jacqueline Montgomery, MA, PT
Former Director of Physical Therapy
Rancho Los Amigos National Rehabilitation Center
Downey, California;
Former Clinical Professor
Department of Biokinesiology and Physical Therapy
University of Southern California
Los Angeles, California

PREFACE

For nearly 70 years, *Daniels and Worthingham's Muscle Testing* has been informing students and practitioners about the art and science of manual muscle testing. Over the past seven decades there have been nine editions of the text, including this current edition.

The last three editions of the book included a chapter on functional (developmental) muscle testing of the child. However, we have elected to remove the chapter from the current edition owing to the explosion of new material available to the pediatric therapist, which is far more detailed and comprehensive than anything we could provide in an entry-level text. We have also removed the chapter on upright motor control. In the past decade clinical specialists have developed evidence-based assessment tools that are more comprehensive than those covered in our original chapter—hence the decision to omit it from the new edition.

What is most noteworthy about the ninth edition is the inclusion of four new chapters. Clinical practice has changed considerably over the years and the original basis for muscle testing, to identify the ravages of polio, no longer drives current clinical decision-making. Two-thirds of the patients we now see in clinic are older than 60 years of age and what is required for much of our assessment of older clientele are functional tests. Thus, Chapter 9 is devoted to functional testing that is appropriate for older patients (including the very old) as well as for men and women of all ages who are deconditioned and/or obese. These functional tests identify deficits in strength, balance, and range of motion and determine if muscle performance is adequate for the maintenance of independence.

Chapter 8 presents alternatives to manual muscle testing such as 1-repetition maximum testing and other equipment-based methods for strength and power testing. This new chapter also includes the rationale for when to use various tests. All of the suggested performance and strength tests have demonstrated reliability and validity, with reasonable sensitivity and specificity as well. A third new chapter, Chapter 2, delineates the relevance and limitations of manual and other forms of testing. The final new chapter, Chapter 10, features case studies that illustrate the need for multiple approaches to the assessment of muscle strength and offers interpretations of the use of muscle testing in various practice settings using an evidence-based approach. Also new to this edition are muscle tests that have emerged in the literature in recent years that have become mainstream for treating patients with shoulder and back impairments. All of the new tests and chapters are heavily referenced, providing a rich resource for practitioners with various levels of skill, and are accompanied by original and new drawings. Thus, much like our field, the *Muscle Testing* book has evolved, reflecting changes that are typical of a vibrant and viable clinical profession.

It is important to remind the reader that mastery of muscle testing, whether performed manually or using a strength-testing device, requires substantial practice. The only way to acquire proficiency in clinical evaluation procedures is to practice over and over again. As experience with patients matures over time, the nuances that can never be fully described for the wide variety of patients encountered by the clinician will become as much intuition as science. The master clinician will include muscle testing as part and parcel of every patient evaluation, regardless whether a formal detailed document is completed or whether the test is used as a prelude to treatment planning. Muscle testing continues to be among the most fundamental skills of the physical therapist and others who are concerned with abnormalities of human motion.

Because proficiency in muscle testing can only be achieved if the practitioner has a thorough understanding of anatomy, anatomical drawings are presented throughout the book, many in cross-section format, and descriptions of origins and insertions and functions are also provided. Study them well.

We are enormously grateful to our forebears for the work that went into the creation of this text. We are grateful as well to the individuals who helped in the creation of the book, particularly our developmental editor, Linda Wood; Yoshi Miyake for the new artwork; Judith Burnfield for the muscle test videos; Mary Pohlman and Christie Hart, and the rest of the team at Elsevier. Special thanks go to the individuals who contributed to and reviewed sections of the book during its development. We thank Richard Bohannan, Susan George, Sue Miller, Christopher Neville, Kevin Neville, and Patrick VanBeveren for their valuable insights. Finally, we thank Marianne Munson and Jillian Johnson for assistance in preparation of the manuscript.

Helen J. Hislop, PhD, ScD, FAPTA
Dale Avers, DPT, PhD
Marybeth Brown, PT, PhD, FAPTA

CONTENTS

Chapter 10
Case Studies 405

Chapter 11
Ready Reference Anatomy 413

INTRODUCTION

This book presents manual muscle testing within the context of strength testing. Classic muscle testing is a fundamental skill of every physical therapist and is essential to the diagnosis and assessment of movement impairments. However, as manual muscle testing has come under scientific scrutiny, it is obvious that its use to evaluate and assess strength as a component of functional movement patterns and tasks is inadequate. Therefore, in addition to the classic presentation of manual muscle testing, this edition presents methods of strength testing that are valid, objective, and applicable across various settings. Chapter 8 presents a variety of strength testing methods using common equipment. If normative values are available, these are included. Chapter 9 describes functional tests that have a significant strength component. Age-based norms are included when available. Chapter 10 describes patient scenarios that describe various uses of strength testing.

Muscle strength is a critical component of functional movement. Assessment must include accurate measurement of the quantity of strength within the context of functional tasks and movement. Especially for the lower extremities, methods that allow the expansion of the findings of manual muscle testing from an impairment to a function level are needed. Quantitative assessment promotes accurate assessment of progress and patient performance within the context of age-based normative values. Although few "hard numbers" of threshold strength levels exist for specific functional movements, we have identified the known muscles that have been correlated with a specific task and, in some cases, have suggested values that may serve as a target for the identification of strength as a factor of a specific functional task.

The manual muscle testing portion of this book, as in its previous editions, directs its focus on manual procedures. Joint motions (e.g., hip flexion) rather than individual muscles (e.g., iliopsoas) are the focus of this text because of the contributions of more than one muscle to a movement. Although prime movers of a movement can be identified, secondary or accessory movers may be equally important and should not be overlooked or underestimated. Rarely is a prime mover the only active muscle, and rarely is it used under isolated control for a given movement. For example, knee extension is the prerogative of the five muscles of the quadriceps femoris, yet none of the five extend the knee in isolation from its synergists. Regardless, definitive activity of any muscle in a given movement can be precisely detected by kinesiology electromyography, and such studies, although numerous, remain incomplete.

Range of motion in this book is presented only to illustrate the range required to test a movement correctly. A consensus of typical ranges is presented with each test, but the techniques of measurement used are not within the scope of this text.

BRIEF HISTORY OF MUSCLE TESTING

Wilhelmine Wright and Robert W. Lovett, MD, Professor of Orthopedic Surgery at Harvard University Medical School, were the originators of the muscle testing system that incorporated the effect of gravity.[1,2] Janet Merrill, PT, Director of Physical Therapeutics at Children's Hospital and the Harvard Infantile Paralysis Commission in Boston, an early colleague of Dr. Lovett, stated that the tests were used first by Wright in Lovett's office gymnasium in 1912.[3] The seminal description of the tests used largely today was written by Wright and published in 1912[1]; this was followed by an article by Lovett and Martin in 1916[4] and by Wright's book in 1928.[5] Miss Wright was a precursor of the physical therapist of today, there being no educational programs in physical therapy in her time, but she headed Lovett's physical therapeutic clinic. Lovett credits her fully in his 1917 book, *Treatment of Infantile Paralysis*,[6] with developing the testing for polio. In Lovett's book, muscles were tested using a resistance-gravity system and graded on a scale of 0 to 6. Another early numerical scale in muscle testing was described by Charles L. Lowman, MD, founder and medical director of Orthopedic Hospital, Los Angeles.[7] Lowman's system (1927) covered the effects of gravity and the full range of movement on all joints and was particularly helpful for assessing extreme weakness. Lowman further described muscle testing procedures in the Physiotherapy Review in 1940.[8]

H.S. Stewart, a physician, published a description of muscle testing in 1925 that was very brief and was not anatomically or procedurally consistent with what is done today.[9] His descriptions included a resistance-based grading system not substantially different from that in use today: maximal resistance for a normal muscle; completion of the motion against gravity with no other resistance for a grade of fair, and so forth. At about the time of Lowman's book, Arthur Legg, MD, and Janet Merrill, PT, wrote a valuable small book on poliomyelitis in 1932. This book, which offered a comprehensive system of muscle testing, was used extensively in physical therapy educational programs during the early 1940s; muscles were graded on a scale of 0 to 5, and a plus or minus designation was added to all grades except 1 and zero.[10]

Among the earliest clinicians to organize muscle testing and support such testing with sound and documented kinesiologic procedures in the way they are used today were Henry and Florence Kendall. Their earliest published documents on comprehensive manual muscle testing became available in 1936 and 1938.[11,12] The 1938 monograph on muscle testing was published and distributed to all Army hospitals in the United States by the U.S. Public Health Service. Another early contribution came from Signe Brunnstrom and Marjorie Dennen in 1931; their syllabus described a system of grading movement rather than individual muscles as a modification of Lovett's work with gravity and resistance.[13]

In this same time period, Elizabeth Kenny came to the United States from Australia, where she had had unique experiences treating polio victims in the Australian back country. Kenny made no contributions to muscle testing, and in her own book and speeches she was clearly against such an evaluative procedure, which she deemed to be harmful.[14] Her one contribution was to heighten the awareness of organized medicine to the dangers of prolonged and injudicious immobilization of the polio patient, something that physical therapists in the United States had been saying for some time but were not widely heeded at the time.[12,13,15,16] Kenny also advocated the early use of "hot fomentations" (hot packs) in the acute phase of the disease.[14] Kenny vociferously maintained that poliomyelitis was not a central nervous system disease resulting in flaccid paresis or paralysis but rather "mental alienation" of muscles from the brain.[15,16] In her system, "deformities never occurred"[14]; however, she never presented data on muscular strength or imbalance in her patients at any point in the course of their disease.[15,16]

The first comprehensive text on muscle testing still in print (which went through five editions) was written by Lucille Daniels, MA, PT; Marian Williams, PhD, PT; and Catherine Worthingham, PhD, PT, and was published in 1946.[17] These three authors prepared a comprehensive handbook on the subject of manual testing procedures that was concise and easy to use. It remains one of the most used texts the world over at the present time and is the predecessor for all subsequent editions of *Daniels and Worthingham's Muscle Testing* including this edition.

The Kendalls (together and then Florence alone after Henry's death in 1979) developed and published work on muscle testing and related subjects for more than 6 decades, certainly one of the more remarkable sagas in physical therapy or even medical history.[18-20] Their first edition of *Muscles: Testing and Function* appeared in 1949.[18] Earlier, the Kendalls had developed a percentage system ranging from 0 to 100 to express muscle grades as a reflection of normal; they reduced the emphasis on this scale, only to return to it in the latest edition (1993), in which Florence again advocated the 0 to 10 scale.[20] The contributions of the Kendalls should not be considered as limited to grading scales, however. Their integration of muscle function with posture and pain in two separate books[18,19] and then in one book[20] is a unique and extremely valuable contribution to the clinical science of physical therapy.

Muscle testing procedures used in national field trials that examined the use of gamma globulin in the prevention of paralytic poliomyelitis were described by Carmella Gonnella, Georgianna Harmon, and Miriam Jacobs, all physical therapists.[21] The later field trials for the Salk vaccine also used muscle testing procedures.[22] The epidemiology teams at the Centers for Disease Control were charged with assessing the validity and reliability of the vaccine. Because there was no other method of accurately "measuring" the presence or absence of muscular weakness, manual muscle testing techniques were used.

A group from the D.T. Watson School of Physiatrics near Pittsburgh, which included Jesse Wright, MD; Mary Elizabeth Kolb, PT; and Miriam Jacobs, PT, PhD, devised a test procedure that eventually was used in the field trials.[23] The test was an abridged version of the complete test procedure but did test key muscles in each functional group and body part. It used numerical values that were assigned grades, and each muscle or muscle group also had an arbitrary assigned factor that corresponded (as closely as possible) to the bulk of the tissue. The bulk factor multiplied by the test grade resulted in an "index of involvement" expressed as a ratio.

Before the trials, Kolb and Jacobs were sent to Atlanta to train physicians to conduct the muscle tests, but it was decided that experienced physical therapists would be preferable to maintain the reliability of the test scores.[23] Lucy Blair, then the Poliomyelitis Consultant in the American Physical Therapy Association, was asked by Catherine Worthingham of the National Foundation for Infantile Paralysis to assemble a team of experienced physical therapists to conduct the muscle tests for the field trials. Kolb and Jacobs trained a group of 67 therapists in the use of the abridged muscle test.[23] A partial list of participants was appended to the Lilienfeld paper in the Physical Therapy Review in 1954.[22] This approach and the evaluations by the physical therapists of the presence or absence of weakness and paralysis in the field trial samples eventually resulted in resounding approval of the Salk vaccine.

Since the polio vaccine field trials, sporadic research in manual muscle testing has occurred as well as continued challenges of its worth as a valid clinical assessment tool. Iddings and colleagues noted that intertester reliability among practitioners varied by about 4%, which compares favorably with the 3% variation among the carefully trained therapists who participated in the vaccine field trials.[24]

There is growing interest in establishing norms of muscular strength and function. Early efforts in this direction were begun by Willis Beasley[25] (although his earliest work was presented only at scientific meetings) and continued by Marian Williams[26] and Helen J. Hislop,[27,28] which set the stage for objective measures by Bohannon[29] and others. The literature on objective measurement increases yearly, an effort that is long overdue. The data from these studies must be applied to manual testing so that correlations between instrumented muscle assessment and manual assessment can ensue.

In the meantime, until instrumented methods become affordable for every clinic, manual techniques of muscle testing will remain in use. The skill of manual muscle testing is a critical clinical tool that every physical therapist must not only learn but also master. A physical therapist who aspires to recognition as a master clinician will not achieve that status without acquiring exquisite skills in manual muscle testing and precise assessment of muscle performance.

HOW TO USE THIS BOOK

The general principles that govern manual muscle testing are described in Chapter 1. A new Chapter 2 describes the purposes and limitations of manual muscle testing, placing manual muscle testing in the context of strength testing across settings. Chapters 3 through 7 present the techniques for testing motions of skeletal muscle groups in the body region covered by that chapter. Chapter 4 reflects changes to practice through the expansion of the trunk muscle strength testing section, the addition of pelvic floor muscle testing, and the expansion of the respiratory muscle section. Chapters 8 and 9 are new chapters that describe methods of strength testing using equipment and instruments (Chapter 8) and through functional tests (Chapter 9). Students should learn manual muscle testing within the context of strength testing to avoid some of the limitations described in Chapter 2. Chapter 10 uses cases to describe different methods of strength testing in various patient populations and settings.

For instant access to anatomical information without carrying a large anatomy text to a muscle testing session, a Ready Reference Anatomy section is given in Chapter 11. This chapter is a synopsis of muscle anatomy, muscles as part of motions, muscle innervations, and myotomes.

To assist readers, each muscle has been assigned an identification number based on a regional sequence, beginning with the head and face and proceeding through the neck, thorax, abdomen, perineum, upper extremity, and lower extremity. This reference number is retained throughout the text for cross-referencing purposes. Two lists of muscles with their reference numbers are presented, one alphabetical and one by region, to assist readers in finding muscles in the Ready Reference section.

NAMES OF THE MUSCLES

Muscle names have conventions of usage. The most formal usage (and the correct form for many journal manuscripts) is the terminology established by the International Anatomical Nomenclature Committee and approved or revised in 1955, 1960, and 1965.[30] However, common usage often neglects these prescribed names in favor of shorter or more readily pronounced names. The authors of this text make no apologies for not keeping strictly to formal usage. Most of the muscles cited do follow the Nomina Anatomica. Others are listed by the names in most common use. The alphabetical list of muscles (see Chapter 11) gives the name used in this text and the correct Nomina Anatomica term, when it differs, in parentheses.

ANATOMICAL AUTHORITIES

The authors of this book relied on both the American and British versions of Gray's Anatomy as principal references for anatomical information; the British edition (Williams et al) was always the final arbiter because of its finer detail and precision.

THE CONVENTION OF ARROWS IN THE TEXT

Red arrows in the text denote the direction of movement of a body part, either actively by the patient or passively by the examiner. The length and direction of the arrow indicates the relative excursion of the part.

Examples:

  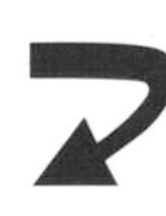 

Black arrows in the text denote resistance by the examiner. The arrow indicates distance, and the width gives some relative idea of whether resistance is large or small.

Examples:

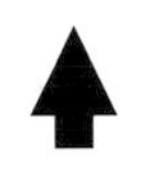  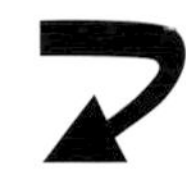 

REFERENCES

Cited References

1. Wright WG. Muscle training in the treatment of infantile paralysis. Boston Med Surg J. 1912;167:567–574.
2. Lovett RW. Treatment of infantile paralysis. Preliminary report. JAMA. 1915;64:2118.
3. Merrill J. Personal letter to Lucille Daniels dated January 5, 1945.
4. Lovett RW, Martin EG. Certain aspects of infantile paralysis and a description of a method of muscle testing. JAMA. 1916;66:729–733.
5. Wright WG. Muscle Function. New York: Paul B. Hoeber; 1928.
6. Lovett RW. Treatment of Infantile Paralysis. 2nd ed. Philadelphia: Blakiston's Son & Co.; 1917.
7. Lowman CL. A method of recording muscle tests. Am J Surg. 1927;3:586–591.
8. Lowman CL. Muscle strength testing. Physiother Rev. 1940;20:69–71.
9. Stewart HS. Physiotherapy: Theory and Clinical Application. New York: Paul B. Hoeber; 1925.
10. Legg AT, Merrill J. Physical therapy in infantile paralysis. In: Mock. Principles and Practice of Physical Therapy. Vol 2. Hagerstown, MD: W.F. Prior; 1932.
11. Kendall HO. Some interesting observations about the after care of infantile paralysis patients. J Excep Child. 1936;3:107.
12. Kendall HO, Kendall FP. Care during the recovery period of paralytic poliomyelitis. U.S. Public Health Bulletin No. 242. Washington, D.C.: U.S. Government Printing Office; 1938.

13. Brunnstrom S, Dennen M. Round table on muscle testing. New York: Annual Conference of the American Physical Therapy Association, Federation of Crippled and Disabled, Inc. (mimeographed); 1931.
14. Kenny E. Paper read at Northwestern Pediatric Conference at St. Paul University Club, November 14, 1940.
15. Plastridge AL. Personal report to the National Foundation for Infantile Paralysis after a trip to observe work of Sister Kenny, 1941.
16. Kendall HO, Kendall FP. Report on the Sister Kenny Method of Treatment in Anterior Poliomyelitis made to the National Foundation for Infantile Paralysis. New York, March 10, 1941.
17. Daniels L, Williams M, Worthingham CA. Muscle Testing: Techniques of Manual Examination. Philadelphia: W.B. Saunders; 1946.
18. Kendall HO, Kendall FP. Muscles: Testing and Function. Baltimore: Williams & Wilkins; 1949.
19. Kendall HO, Kendall FP. Posture and Pain. Baltimore: Williams & Wilkins; 1952.
20. Kendall FP, McCreary EK, Provance PG. Muscles: Testing and Function. 4th ed. Baltimore: Williams & Wilkins; 1993.
21. Gonella C, Harmon G, Jacobs M. The role of the physical therapist in the gamma globulin poliomyelitis prevention study. Phys Ther Rev. 1953;33:337–345.
22. Lilienfeld AM, Jacobs M, Willis M. Study of the reproducibility of muscle testing and certain other aspects of muscle scoring. Phys Ther Rev. 1954;34:279–289.
23. Kolb ME. Personal communication, October 1993.
24. Iddings DM, Smith LK, Spencer WA. Muscle testing. Part 2: Reliability in clinical use. Phys Ther Rev. 1961;41: 249–256.
25. Beasley W. Quantitative muscle testing: Principles and applications to research and clinical services. Arch Phys Med Rehabil. 1961;42:398–425.
26. Williams M, Stutzman L. Strength variation through the range of joint motion. Phys Ther Rev. 1959;39:145–152.
27. Hislop HJ. Quantitative changes in human muscular strength during isometric exercise. Phys Ther. 1963;43: 21–36.
28. Hislop HJ, Perrine JJ. Isokinetic concept of exercise. Phys Ther. 1967;47:114–117.
29. Bohannon RW. Manual muscle test scores and dynamometer test scores of knee extension strength. Arch Phys Med Rehabil. 1986;67:204.
30. International Anatomical Nomenclature Committee. Nomina Anatomica. Amsterdam: Excerpta Medica Foundation; 1965.

Other Readings

Bailey JC. Manual muscle testing in industry. Phys Ther Rev. 1961;41:165–169.

Bennett RL. Muscle testing: A discussion of the importance of accurate muscle testing. Phys Ther Rev. 1947;27: 242–243.

Borden R, Colachis S. Quantitative measurement of the Good and Normal ranges in muscle testing. Phys Ther. 1968;48: 839–843.

Brunnstrom S. Muscle group testing. Physiother Rev. 1941;21: 3–21.

Currier DP. Maximal isometric tension of the elbow extensors at varied positions. Phys Ther. 1972;52:52.

Downer AH. Strength of the elbow flexor muscles. Phys Ther Rev. 1953;33:68–70.

Fisher FJ, Houtz SJ. Evaluation of the function of the gluteus maximus muscle. Am J Phys Med. 1968;47:182–191.

Frese E, Brown M, Norton BJ. Clinical reliability of manual muscle testing: Middle trapezius and gluteus medius muscles. Phys Ther. 1987;67:1072–1076.

Gonnella C. The manual muscle test in the patient's evaluation and program for treatment. Phys Ther Rev. 1954;34: 16–18.

Granger CV. The clinical discernment of muscle weakness. Arch Phys Med. 1963;44:430–438.

Hoppenfeld S. Physical Examination of the Spine and Extremities. New York: Appleton-Century-Crofts; 1976.

Janda V. Muscle Function Testing. Boston: Butterworths; 1983.

Jarvis DK. Relative strength of hip rotator muscle groups. Phys Ther Rev. 1952;32:500–503.

Kendall FP. Testing the muscles of the abdomen. Phys Ther Rev. 1941;21:22–24.

Lovett RW. Treatment of infantile paralysis: Preliminary report. JAMA. 1915;64:2118.

Palmer ML, Epler ME. Clinical Assessment Procedures in Physical Therapy. Philadelphia: J.B. Lippincott; 1990.

Salter N, Darcus HD. Effect of the degree of elbow flexion on the maximum torque developed in pronation and supination of the right hand. J Anat. 1952;86B:197.

Smidt GL, Rogers MW. Factors contributing to the regulation and clinical assessment of muscular strength. Phys Ther. 1982;62:1283–1289.

Wadsworth CT, Krishnan R, Sear M, et al. Intrarater reliability of manual muscle testing and hand held dynametric testing. Phys Ther. 1987;67:1342–1347.

Wintz M. Variations in current muscle testing. Phys Ther Rev. 1959;39:466–475.

Zimny N, Kirk C. Comparison of methods of manual muscle testing. Clin Manag. 1987;7:6–11.

CHAPTER 1

Principles of Manual Muscle Testing

THE GRADING SYSTEM

Grades for a manual muscle test are recorded as numerical scores ranging from zero (0), which represents no activity, to five (5), which represents a "normal" or best-possible response to the test or as great a response as can be evaluated by a manual muscle test. Because this text is based on tests of motions rather than tests of individual muscles, the grade represents the performance of all muscles in that motion. The numerical 5 to 0 system of grading is the most commonly used convention across health care professions.

Each numerical grade can be paired with a word that describes the test performance in qualitative, but not quantitative, terms. These qualitative terms, when written, are capitalized to indicate that they too represent a score. Qualitative test grades are not quantitative in any manner.

Numerical Score	Qualitative Score
5	Normal (N)
4	Good (G)
3	Fair (F)
2	Poor (P)
1	Trace activity (T)
0	Zero (no activity) (0)

These grades are based on several factors of testing and response that will be elaborated in this chapter.

OVERVIEW OF TEST PROCEDURES

The Break Test

Manual resistance is applied to a limb or other body part after it has completed its range of motion or after it has been placed at end range by the therapist. The term *resistance* is always used to denote a concentric force that acts in opposition to a contracting muscle. Manual resistance should always be applied in the direction of the "line of pull" of the participating muscle or muscles. At the end of the available range, or at a point in the range where the muscle is most challenged, the patient is asked to hold the part at that point and not allow the therapist to "break" the hold with manual resistance. For example, a seated patient is asked to flex the elbow to its end range; when that position is reached, the therapist applies resistance at the wrist, trying to force the muscle to "break" its hold and thus move the forearm downward into extension. This is called a break test, and it is the procedure most commonly used in manual muscle testing today.

As a recommended alternative procedure, the therapist may choose to place the muscle or muscle group to be tested in the end or test position rather than have the patient actively move it there. In this procedure the therapist ensures correct positioning and stabilization for the test.

Active Resistance Test

An alternative to the break test is the application of manual resistance against an actively contracting muscle or muscle group (i.e., against the direction of the movement as if to prevent that movement). This may be called an "active resistance" test. During the motion, the therapist gradually increases the amount of manual resistance until it reaches the maximal level the patient can tolerate and motion ceases. This kind of manual muscle test requires considerable skill and experience to perform and is so often equivocal that its use is not recommended.

Application of Resistance

The principles of manual muscle testing presented here and in all published sources since 1921 follow the basic tenets of muscle length–tension relationships as well as those of joint mechanics.[1,2] In the case of the biceps brachii, for example, when the elbow is straight, the biceps lever is short; leverage increases as the elbow flexes and becomes maximal (most efficient) at 90°, but as flexion continues beyond that point, the lever arm again decreases in length and efficiency.

In manual muscle testing, external force (resistance) is applied at the end of the range in one-joint muscles to allow for consistency of procedure. Two-joint muscles are typically tested in mid-range where length-tension is more favorable. Ideally, all muscles and muscle groups should be tested at optimal length-tension, but there are many occasions in manual muscle testing where the therapist is not able to distinguish between Grade 5 and 4 without putting the patient at a mechanical disadvantage. Thus, the one-joint brachialis, hip abductors, and quadriceps muscles are tested at end range and the two-joint hamstrings and gastrocnemius muscles are tested in mid-range.

The point on an extremity, or part, where the therapist should apply resistance is near the distal end of the segment to which the muscle attaches. There are two common exceptions to this rule: the hip abductors and the scapular muscles. In the patient who has an unstable knee, resistance to the hip abductors should be applied at the distal femur just above the knee. When using the short lever, hip abductor strength must be graded no better than Grade 4 even when the muscle takes maximal resistance. However, in testing a patient with Grade 5 knee strength and joint integrity, the therapist should apply resistance at the ankle; the longer lever provided by resistance at the ankle is a greater challenge for the hip abductors and is more indicative of the functional demands required in gait. It follows that when a patient cannot tolerate maximal resistance at the ankle, the muscle cannot be considered Grade 5.

An example of testing with a short lever occurs in the patient with an above-knee amputation, where the grade awarded, even when the patient can hold against maximal resistance, is Grade 4. Because the weight of the leg is so reduced and the therapist's lever arm for resistance application is so short, patients can easily give the impression of a false Grade 5 yet may struggle with the force demands of a prosthesis in the real world. The muscular force available should not be overestimated in predicting a patient's functional ability in any circumstances such as age or disability.

In testing the vertebroscapular muscles (e.g., rhomboids), the preferred point of resistance is on the arm rather than on the scapula where these muscles insert. The longer lever more closely reflects the functional demands that incorporate the weight of the arm. Other exceptions to the general rule of applying distal resistance include a painful condition to be avoided or a healing wound in a place where resistance might otherwise be given.

The application of manual resistance should never be sudden or uneven (jerky). The therapist should apply resistance with full patient awareness in a somewhat slow and gradual manner, slightly exceeding the muscle's force as it builds over 2-3 seconds to achieve the maximum tolerable force intensity. Applying resistance that slightly exceeds the muscle's force generation will more likely encourage a maximum effort and an accurate break test. Critical to the accuracy of a manual muscle test is the location of the resistance and the consistency of application across all patients. (The therapist should make a note of the point of resistance, if a variation is used, to ensure consistency in testing).

The application of resistance permits an assessment of muscular strength when it is applied in the direction opposite the muscular force or torque. The therapist also should understand that the weight of the limb plus the influence of gravity is part of test response. When the muscle contracts in a parallel direction to the line of gravity, it is noted as "gravity minimal." It is suggested that the commonly used term "gravity eliminated" be avoided because, of course, that can never occur except in a zero-gravity environment. Thus, weakened muscles are tested in a plane horizontal to the direction of gravity; the body part is supported on a smooth, flat surface in such a way that friction force is minimal (Grades 2, 1, and 0). A powder board may be used to minimize friction. For stronger muscles that can complete a full range of motion in a direction against the pull of gravity (Grade 3), resistance is applied perpendicular to the line of gravity (Grades 4 and 5). Acceptable variations to antigravity and gravity-minimal positions are discussed in individual test sections.

CRITERIA FOR ASSIGNING A MUSCLE TEST GRADE

The grade given on a manual muscle test comprises both subjective and objective factors. Subjective factors include the therapist's impression of the amount of resistance to give before the actual test and then the amount of resistance the patient actually tolerates during the test. Objective factors include the ability of the patient to complete a full range of motion or to hold the position once placed there, the ability to move the part against gravity, or an inability to move a part at all. All these factors require clinical judgment, which makes manual muscle testing an exquisite skill that requires considerable practice and experience to master. An accurate test grade is important not only to establish a functional diagnosis but also to assess the patient's longitudinal progress during the period of recovery and treatment.

The Grade 5 (Normal) Muscle

The wide range of "normal" muscle performance leads to a considerable underestimation of a muscle's capability. If the therapist has no experience in examining persons who are free of disease or injury, it is unlikely that there will be any realistic judgment of what is Grade 5 and how much normality can vary. Generally, a student learns manual muscle testing by practicing on classmates, but this provides only minimal experience compared to what is needed to master the skill. It should be recognized, for example, that the average therapist cannot "break" knee extension in a reasonably fit young man, even by doing a handstand on his leg!

The therapist should test "normal" muscles at every opportunity, especially when testing the contralateral limb in a patient with a unilateral problem. In almost every instance when the therapist cannot break the patient's hold position when applying maximum resistance, a grade of 5 is assigned. A grade of 5 must be accompanied by the ability to complete full range of motion or maintain end-point range against maximal resistance.

The Grade 4 (Good) Muscle

The grade of 4 represents the true weakness in manual muscle testing procedures (pun intended). Sharrard counted remaining alpha motor neurons in the spinal cords of individuals with poliomyelitis at the time of autopsy.[3] He correlated the manual muscle test grades in the patient's chart with the number of motor neurons remaining in the anterior horns. His data revealed that more than 50% of motor neurons of a muscle group were gone when the muscle test grade was 4. Thus, when the muscle could withstand considerable but less than "normal" resistance, it had already been deprived of at least half of its innervation.

Grade 4 is used to designate a muscle group that is able to complete a full range of motion against gravity but that is not able to hold the test position against maximum resistance. The Grade 4 muscle "gives" or "yields" to some extent at the end of its range with maximal resistance. When maximal resistance clearly breaks, irrespective of age or disability, the muscle is assigned a grade of 4. However, if pain limits the ability to maximally resist the force applied by the therapist, evaluation of actual strength may not be realistic and should be documented as such. An example might be, "Elbow flexion appeared strong but painful."

The Grade 3 (Fair) Muscle

The Grade 3 muscle test is based on an objective measure. The muscle or muscle group can complete a full range of motion against only the resistance of gravity. If a tested muscle can move through the full range against gravity but additional resistance, however mild, causes the motion to break, the muscle is assigned a grade of 3.

Sharrard cited a residual autopsy motor neuron count of 15% in polio-paretic muscles that had been assessed as Grade 3, meaning that 85% of the innervating neurons had been destroyed.[3] These findings suggest that, in most instances, we markedly overestimate the strength of muscles even at the Grade 3 level.

Direct force measurements have demonstrated that the force level of the Grade 3 muscle usually is low, so that a much greater span of functional loss exists between Grades 3 and 5 than between Grades 3 and 1. Beasley, in a study of children ages 10 to 12 years, reported the Grade 3 in 36 muscle tests as no greater than 40% of normal (one motion), the rest being 30% or below normal "strength" with the majority falling between 5% and 20% of a Grade 5.[4] A grade of 3 may represent a *functional threshold* for many movements tested, indicating that the muscle or muscles can achieve the minimal task of moving the part upward against gravity through its range of motion such as when dressing. Although this ability is significant for the upper extremity, it falls far short of the functional requirements of many lower extremity muscles used in walking, particularly such groups as the hip abductors and the plantar flexors. The therapist must be sure that muscles given a grade of 3 are not in the joint "locked" position during the test (e.g., locked elbow when testing elbow extension).

The Grade 2 (Poor) Muscle

The Grade 2 muscle is one that can complete the full range of motion in a position that minimizes the force of gravity. This position often is described as the horizontal plane of motion. Eliminating friction of the testing surface may be required to assure an accurate strength assessment. Use of a powder board or other such friction-eliminating surface is helpful.

The Grade 1 (Trace) Muscle

The Grade 1 muscle means that the therapist can detect visually or by palpation some contractile activity in one or more of the muscles that participate in the movement being tested (provided that the muscle is superficial enough to be palpated). The therapist also may be able to see or feel a tendon pop up or tense as the patient tries to perform the movement. There is, however, no movement of the part as a result of this contractile activity.

A Grade 1 muscle can be detected with the patient in almost any position. When a Grade 1 muscle is suspected, the therapist should passively move the part into the test position and ask the patient to hold the position and then relax; this will enable the therapist to palpate the muscle or tendon, or both, during the patient's attempts to contract the muscle and also during relaxation. Care should be taken to avoid substitution of other muscles.

The Grade 0 (Zero) Muscle

The Grade 0 muscle is completely inert on palpation or visual inspection.

Plus (+) and Minus (−) Grades

Use of a plus (+) or minus (−) addition to a manual muscle test grade is usually discouraged but there are two exceptions noted in the next section. Avoiding the use of plus or minus signs restricts manual muscle test grades to those that are meaningful, defendable, and reliable. The use of pluses and minuses adds a level of subjectivity that lacks reliability.

The Grade 2+ is given when assessing the strength of the plantar flexors when either of the following two conditions exist. The first is when the patient, while weight bearing, can complete a partial heel rise using correct form (see test for plantar flexion in Chapter 6). The second condition is when the plantar flexion test is performed in supine position (not recommended) and the patient takes maximum resistance and completes full available range. The 2+ Grade is clearly distinguished from Grade 2, which indicates that full range is completed with no resistance. A grade of 3 or better can be given to the plantar flexors only when the patient is weight bearing.

The Grade 2− muscle can complete partial range of motion in the horizontal plane, the gravity-minimized position. The difference between Grade 2 and Grade 1 muscles represents such a broad functional difference that a minus sign is important in assessing even minor improvements in return of function. For example, the patient with Guillain-Barré syndrome who moves from muscle Grade 1 to Grade 2− demonstrates a quantum leap forward in terms of recovery and prognosis.

The Grade 4 (Good) Muscle Revisited

Historically, manual muscle testing has employed two grading systems, one using numbers (5–0) and the other using descriptors (Normal to Zero). Although both systems convey the same information, the authors favor the numerical system because it avoids use of the vague and subjective term "good." As noted previously, there is no other term in muscle testing that is more problematic. Too often clinical practitioners, including therapists and physicians, construe the term in the literal sense, interpreting "good" to mean totally adequate. The assumption is that if strength is adequate, then the patient is not in need of rehabilitation.

However, an abundance of evidence demonstrates unequivocally that once the therapist discerns that strength is no longer normal, but "good" instead, the muscle being tested has already lost approximately half its strength. Evidence of this has already been presented.[5] More recently, Bohannon found that force values for muscles that were graded as "normal" ranged from 80 to 625 Newtons,[6] an astronomical difference, further demonstrating how difficult it is to distinguish a "good" muscle from a "normal" muscle.

It is unclear how a grade of "good" became synonymous with achievement of a satisfactory end point of treatment. Certainly, the pressure from third-party payers to discharge patients as soon as possible does not help the therapist fulfill the minimum goal of reaching "prior level of function." Nonetheless, the opportunity for patients to recover muscle forces to the fullest extent possible is a primary goal of an intervention. If this goal is not met, patients (especially aging individuals) may lose their independence or find themselves incapable of returning to a desired sport or activity because their weak muscles fatigue too quickly. Athletes who have not fully recovered their strength before returning to a sport are far more likely to suffer a reinjury, potentially harming themselves further.

There are numerous examples of instances in which a "good" muscle cannot meet its functional demands. When the gluteus medius is "good," a patient will display a positive Trendelenburg's sign. When the soleus is "good," heel rise fails to occur during the latter portion of the stance phase of gait, which reduces gait speed.[7] When the abdominals are "good," there is difficulty stabilizing the pelvis while arising from bed or when sitting up, and this often results in back pain. "Good" simply is not good enough.

Repeatedly there is a disconnect between what patients can functionally accomplish and the manual muscle strength grade the therapist assigns, particularly in older adults. By the time a person reaches the age of 80 years, approximately 50% of their muscle mass and strength is lost due to natural decline[8] and yet, how many therapists assign a manual muscle test grade of "normal" to an 80-year-old, even though the individual's strength is half of what it used to be? Functionally, these same older adults with "normal strength" cannot get out of a chair without pushing on the arms or ascend stairs without pulling on the railing. Muscle grades that are inaccurate based on the patient's age, gender, and presumed strength or because the therapist cannot apply adequate resistance must be avoided.

In summary, a "good" muscle isn't always "good." Everything must be done to ensure accuracy in manual muscle test grading and to provide the intervention necessary to fully restore strength and function to "normal." Substituting the numerical system of 5–0 for the subjective terms "good" or "normal" in manual muscle testing assessment is a start in the right direction.

Available Range of Motion

When a contracture or fixed joint limitation (e.g., total knee replacement) limits joint range of motion, the patient performs only within the range available. In this circumstance, the *available range* is the full range of motion for that patient at that time, even though it is not "normal." This is the range used to assign a muscle testing grade. For example, the normal knee extension range is 135° to 0°. A patient with a 20° knee flexion contracture is tested for knee extension strength at the end of available range or –20°. If this range (in sitting) can be completed with maximal resistance, the grade assigned would be a 5. If the patient cannot complete that range, the grade assigned MUST be less than 3. The patient then should be repositioned in the side-lying position to ascertain the correct grade.

SCREENING TESTS

In the interests of time and cost-efficient care, it is rarely necessary to perform a muscle test on each muscle of the body. Two exceptions among several are patients with Guillain-Barré syndrome and those with incomplete spinal cord injuries. To screen for muscles that need definitive testing, the therapist can use a number of maneuvers to rule out movements that do not need testing. Observation of the patient before the examination will provide valuable clues to muscular weakness and performance deficits. For example, the therapist can do the following:

- Observe the patient as he or she enters the treatment area to detect gross abnormalities of gait.
- Observe the patient sit and rise from a chair, fill out admission or history forms, or remove street clothing.
- Ask the patient to walk on the toes and then on the heels.
- Ask the patient to grip the therapist's hand.
- Perform gross checks of bilateral muscle groups: reaching toward the floor, overhead, and behind the back.

If evidence from the above "quick checks" suggests a deficit in movement, manual muscle testing can quickly be isolated to the region observed to be weak, in the interest of time and to optimize the patient's clinic visit.

PREPARING FOR THE MUSCLE TEST

The therapist and the patient must work in harmony if the test session is to be successful. This means that some basic principles and inviolable procedures should be second nature to the therapist.

1. The patient should be as free as possible from discomfort or pain for the duration of each test. It may be necessary to allow some patients to move or be positioned differently between tests.
2. The environment for testing should be quiet and nondistracting. The temperature should be comfortable for the partially disrobed patient.
3. The plinth or mat table for testing must be firm to help stabilize the part being tested. The ideal is a hard surface, minimally padded or not padded at all. The hard surface will not allow the trunk or limbs to "sink in." Friction of the surface material should be kept to a minimum. When the patient is reasonably mobile a plinth is fine, but its width should not be so narrow that the patient is afraid of falling or sliding off. Sometimes a low mat table is the more practical choice. The height of the table should be adjustable to allow the therapist to use proper leverage and body mechanics.
4. Patient position should be carefully organized so that position changes in a test sequence are minimized. The patient's position must permit adequate stabilization of the part or parts being tested by virtue of body weight or with help provided by the therapist.
5. All materials needed for the test must be at hand. This is particularly important when the patient is anxious for any reason or is too weak to be safely left unattended.

Materials needed include the following:

- Manual muscle test documentation forms (Figure 1-1)
- Pen, pencil, or computer terminal
- Pillows, towels, pads, and wedges for positioning
- Sheets or other draping linen
- Goniometer
- Stopwatch
- Specific equipment for specific functional tests
- Test forms for functional tests
- Interpreter (if needed)
- Assistance for turning, moving, or stabilizing the patient
- Emergency call system (if no assistant is available)
- Reference material

SUMMARY

From the foregoing discussion, it should be clear that manual muscle testing is an exacting clinical skill. Practice, practice, and more practice create the experience essential to building the skill to an acceptable level of clinical proficiency, to say nothing of clinical mastery.

DOCUMENTATION OF MANUAL MUSCLE EXAMINATION

LEFT				RIGHT		
3	2	1	Date of Examination / Examiner's Name	1	2	3
			NECK			
			Capital extension			
			Cervical extension			
			Combined extension (capital plus cervical)			
			Capital flexion			
			Cervical flexion			
			Combined flexion (capital plus cervical)			
			Combined flexion and rotation (Sternocleidomastoid)			
			Cervical rotation			
			TRUNK			
			Extension—Lumbar			
			Extension—Thoracic			
			Pelvic elevation			
			Flexion			
			Rotation			
			Diaphragm strength			
			Maximal inspiration less full expiration (indirect intercostal test) (inches)			
			Cough (indirect forced expiration) (F, WF, NF, 0)			
			UPPER EXTREMITY			
			Scapular abduction and upward rotation			
			Scapular elevation			
			Scapular adduction			
			Scapular adduction and down-ward rotation			
			Shoulder flexion			
			Shoulder extension			
			Shoulder scaption			
			Shoulder abduction			
			Shoulder horizontal abduction			
			Shoulder horizontal adduction			
			Shoulder external rotation			
			Shoulder internal rotation			
			Elbow flexion			
			Elbow extension			
			Forearm supination			
			Forearm pronation			
			Wrist flexion			
			Wrist extension			
			Finger metacarpophalangeal flexion			
			Finger proximal interphalangeal flexion			
			Finger distal interphalangeal flexion			
			Finger metacarpophalangeal extension			
			Finger abduction			
			Finger adduction			
			Thumb metacarpophalangeal flexion			
			Thumb interphalangeal flexion			

FIGURE 1-1 Documentation of manual muscle examination. F, functional (only slight impairment); WF, weak functional (moderate impairment); NF, nonfunctional (severe impairment); 0, cough is absent.

MANUAL MUSCLE EXAMINATION - Page 2

LEFT 3	LEFT 2	LEFT 1		RIGHT 1	RIGHT 2	RIGHT 3
			Thumb metacarpophalangeal extension (motion superior to plane of metacarpals)			
			Thumb interphalangeal extension			
			Thumb carpometacarpal abduction (motion perpendicular to plane of palm)			
			Thumb carpometacarpal abduction and extension (motion parallel to plane of palm)			
			Thumb adduction			
			Thumb opposition			
			Little finger opposition			
			LOWER EXTREMITY			
			Hip flexion			
			Hip flexion, abduction, and external rotation with knee flexion (Sartorius)			
			Hip extension			
			Hip extension (Gluteus maximus)			
			Hip abduction			
			Hip abduction and flexion			
			Hip adduction			
			Hip external rotation			
			Hip internal rotation			
			Knee flexion			
			Knee flexion with leg external rotation			
			Knee flexion with leg internal rotation			
			Knee extension			
			Ankle plantar flexion			
			Ankle plantar flexion (Soleus)			
			Foot dorsiflexion and inversion			
			Foot inversion			
			Foot eversion with plantar flexion			
			Foot eversion with dorsiflexion			
			Great toe metatarsophalangeal flexion			
			Toe metatarsophalangeal flexion			
			Great toe interphalangeal flexion			
			Toe interphalangeal flexion			
			Great toe metatarsophalangeal extension			
			Toe metatarsophalangeal extension			
			Great toe interphalangeal extension			
			Toe interphalangeal extension			

Comments: ____________________

Diagnosis ____________ Onset ____________ Age ________ Birth date ________

Patient Name ______________________________
last first middle ID number

FIGURE 1-1, cont'd

Cited References

1. LeVeau BF. Williams and Lissner's Biomechanics of Human Motion. 3rd ed. Philadelphia: WB Saunders; 1992.
2. Soderberg GL. Kinesiology: Application to Pathological Motion. Baltimore: Williams & Wilkins; 1997.
3. Sharrard WJW. Muscle recovery in poliomyelitis. J Bone Joint Surg Br. 1955;37:63-69.
4. Beasley WC. Normal and fair muscle systems: Quantitative standards for children 10 to 12 years of age. Presented at 39th Scientific Session of the American Congress of Rehabilitative Medicine, Cleveland, Ohio; August 1961.
5. Beasley WC. Influence of method on estimates of normal knee extensor force among normal and post-polio children. Phys Ther Rev. 1956;36:21-41.
6. Bohannon RW, Corrigan D. A broad range of forces is encompassed by the maximum manual muscle test grade of five. Percept Mot Skills. 2000;90(3 Pt 1):747-750.
7. Perry J. Gait Analysis: Normal and Pathological Function. 2nd ed. Thorofare, NJ: Slack, Inc.; 2010.
8. Piering AW, Janowski AP, Moore MT, et al. Electromyographic analysis of four popular abdominal exercises. J Athl Train. 1993;28:120-126.

Other Readings

Bohannon RW. Internal consistency of manual muscle testing scores. Percep Mot Skills. 1997;85:736-738.

Bohannon RW. Measuring knee extensor muscle strength. Am J Phys Med Rehabil. 2001;80:13-18.

Bohannon RW. Manual muscle testing: does it meet the standards of an adequate screening test? Clin Rehabil. 2005;19:662-667.

Corrigan D, Bohannon RW. Relationship between knee extension force and stand-up performance in community-dwelling elderly women. Arch Phys Med Rehabil. 2001;82(12): 1666-1672.

Dvir Z. Grade 4 in manual muscle testing: the problem with submaximal strength assessment. Clin Rehabil. 1997;11: 36-41.

Great Lakes ALS Study Group. A comparison of muscle strength testing techniques in amyotrophic lateral sclerosis. Neurology. 2003;61:1503-1507.

Jepsen J, Lawson L, Larsen A, et al. Manual strength testing in 14 upper limb muscles: a study of inter-rater reliability. Acta Orthop Scand. 2004;75:442-448.

Li RC, Jasiewicz JM, Middleton J, et al. The development, validity, and reliability of a manual muscle testing device with integrated limb position sensors. Arch Phys Med Rehabil. 2006;87:411-417.

Mulroy SJ, Lassen KD, Chambers SH, et al. The ability of male and female clinicians to effectively test knee extension strength using manual muscle testing. J Orthop Sports Phys Ther. 1997;26:192-199.

Phillips BA, Lo SK, Mastaglia FL. Muscle force using "break" testing with a hand-held myometer in normal patients aged 20 to 69 years. Arch Phys Med Rehabil. 2000;81: 653-661.

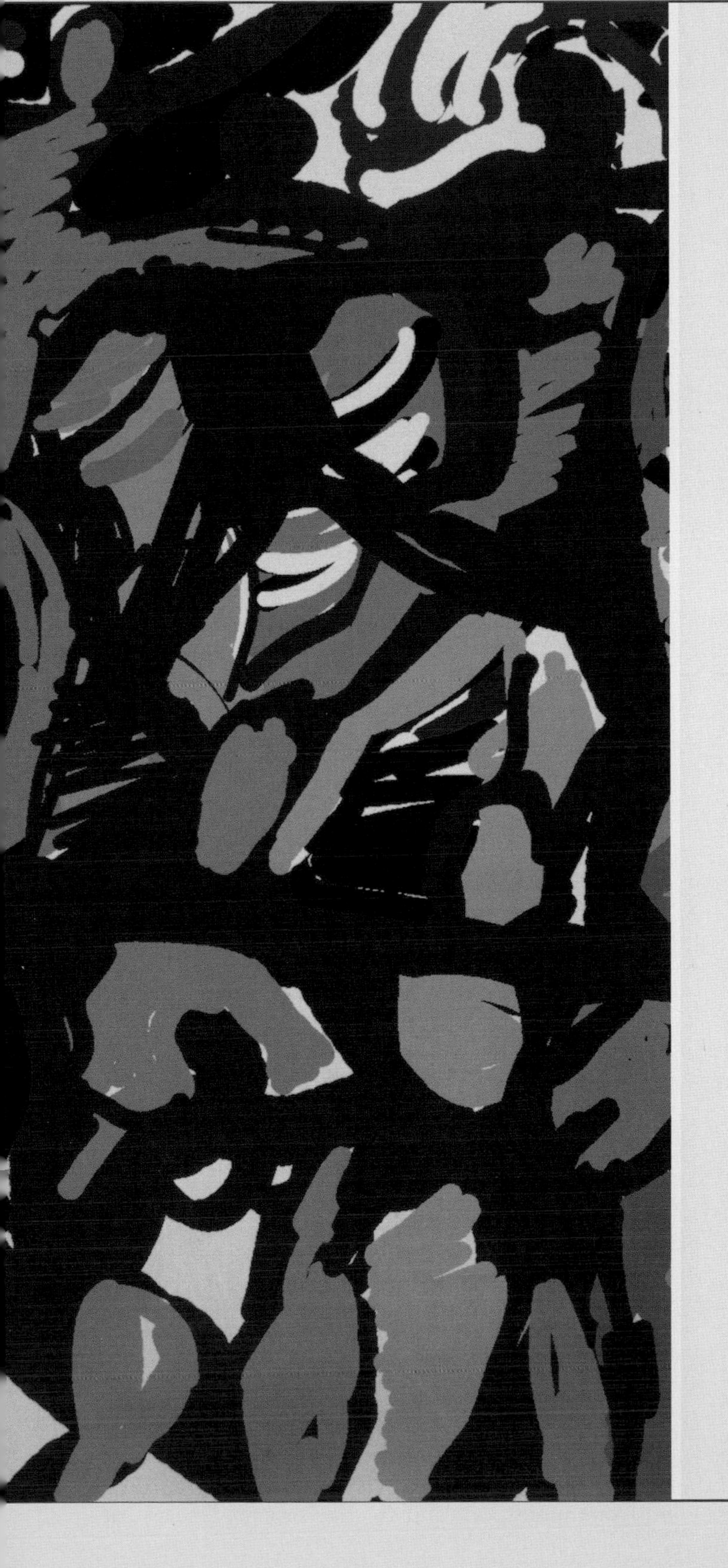

CHAPTER 2

Relevance and Limitations of Manual Muscle Testing

INTRODUCTION

Manual muscle testing (MMT) is well recognized as the most common strength testing technique in physical therapy and other health professions, having first appeared during the poliomyelitis epidemic in New England before World War I. (See "Brief History of Muscle Testing" in the Introduction). Manual muscle testing serves unique purposes that can vary according to the setting in which it is practiced. Although manual muscle testing is an essential and foundational skill in a therapist's examination techniques, it also has its limitations. Appreciating these limitations and learning how to compensate for them helps make MMT as relevant today as it was when first conceptualized in the polio era.

THE EXAMINER AND THE VALUE OF THE MUSCLE TEST

The knowledge and skill of the examiner determine the accuracy and defensibility of a manual muscle test. Specific aspects of these qualities include the following:

- Knowledge of the location and anatomical features of the muscles in a test. In addition to knowing the muscle attachments, the examiner should be able to visualize the location of the tendon and its muscle in relationship to other tendons and muscles and other structures in the same area (e.g., the tendon of the extensor carpi radialis longus lies on the radial side of the tendon of the extensor carpi radialis brevis at the wrist).
- Knowledge of the direction of muscle fibers and their "line of pull" in each muscle.
- Knowledge of the function of the participating muscles (e.g., synergist, prime mover, agonist, and antagonist).
- Consistent use of a standardized method for each different test.
- Consistent use of proper positioning and stabilization techniques for each test procedure. Stabilization of the proximal segment of the joint being tested is achieved in several ways. These ways include patient position (via body weight), the use of a firm surface for testing, patient muscle activation, and manual fixation by the examiner.
- Ability to identify patterns of substitution in a given test and how they can be detected based on a knowledge of which other muscles can be substituted for the one(s) being tested.
- Ability to detect contractile activity during both contraction and relaxation, especially in minimally active muscle.
- Sensitivity to differences in contour and bulk of the muscles being tested in contrast to the contralateral side or to normal expectations based on such things as body size, occupation, or leisure work.
- Awareness of any deviation from normal values for range of motion and the presence of any joint laxity or deformity.
- Understanding that the muscle belly must not be grasped at any time during a manual muscle test except specifically to assess muscle mass.
- Ability to identify muscles with the same innervation that will ensure a comprehensive muscle evaluation and accurate interpretation of test results (because weakness of one muscle in a myotome should require examination of all).
- Relating the diagnosis to the sequence and extent of the test (e.g., the patient with C7 complete tetraplegia will require definitive muscle testing of the upper extremity but only confirmatory tests in the lower extremities).
- Ability to modify test procedures when necessary while not compromising the test result and understanding the influence of the modification on the result.
- Knowledge of fatigue on the test results, especially muscles tested late in a long testing session, and a sensitivity to fatigue in certain diagnostic conditions such as myasthenia gravis or multiple sclerosis.
- Understanding of the effect of sensory and perceptual loss on movement.

The examiner also may inadvertently *influence* the test results and should be especially alert when testing in the following situations:

- The patient with open wounds or other conditions requiring gloves, which may blunt palpation skills.
- The patient who must be evaluated under difficult conditions such as in an intensive care unit with multiple tubes and monitors or immediately after surgery, the patient in traction, the patient for whom turning is contraindicated, the patient on a ventilator, and the patient in shackles or restraints.
- The patient cannot assume test positions, such as the prone position.
- The therapist must avoid the temptation to use shortcuts or "tricks of the trade" before mastering the basic procedures lest such shortcuts become an inexact personal standard. One such pitfall for the novice tester is to inaccurately assign a muscle grade from one test position that the patient could not perform successfully to a lower grade without actually testing in the position required for the lower grade.

For example, when testing trunk flexion, a patient just partially clears the scapula from the surface with the hands behind the head (the position for the Grade 5 test). The temptation may exist to assign a grade of 4 to this test, but this may "overrate" the true strength of trunk flexion unless the patient is actually tested with the arms across the chest to confirm Grade 4.

The good clinician never ignores a patient's comments and must be a good listener, not just to the patient's questions but also to the words the patient uses and their meaning. This quality is the first essential of good communication and is the primary means of

Early Kendall Examination

Accuracy in giving examinations depends primarily on the examiner's knowledge of the isolated and combined actions of muscles in individuals with normal muscles as well as in those with weak or paralyzed muscles.

The fact that muscles act in combination permits substitution of a strong muscle for a weaker one. For accurate muscle examinations, no substitutions should be permitted; that is, the movement described as a test movement should be done without shifting the body or turning the part to allow other muscles to perform the movement for the weak or paralyzed group. The only way to recognize substitution is to know normal function, and realize the ease with which a normal muscle performs the exact test movement.

KENDALL HO, KENDALL FP

From Care During the Recovery Period in Paralytic Poliomyelitis. Public Health Bulletin No. 242. Washington, DC: U.S. Government Printing Office; 1939: 26.

encouraging understanding and respect between therapist and patient. The patient is the best guide to a successful muscle test.

INFLUENCE OF THE PATIENT ON THE TEST

The intrusion of a living, breathing, feeling person into the testing situation may distort scoring for the unwary examiner. The following circumstances should be recognized:

- There may be variation in the assessment of the true effort expended by a patient in a given test (reflecting the patient's desire to do well or to seem more impaired than is actually the case).
- The patient's willingness to endure discomfort or pain may vary (e.g., the stoic, the complainer, the high competitor).
- The patient's ability to understand the test requirements may be limited in some cases because of comprehension and language barriers.
- The motor skills required for the test may be beyond those possessed by some patients, making it impossible for them to perform as requested.
- Lassitude and depression may cause the patient to be indifferent to the test and the examiner.
- Cultural, social, and gender issues may be associated with palpation and exposure of a body part for testing.
- The size and noncompatibility between big and small muscles can cause considerable differences in grading, though not an individual variation (e.g., the gluteus medius versus a finger extensor). There is a huge variability in maximum torque between such muscles, and the examiner must use care not to assign a grade that is inconsistent with muscle size and architecture.

USE OF MANUAL MUSCLE TESTING IN VARIOUS CLINICAL SETTINGS

Manual muscle testing is used in many different types of health care settings. In this section, we will discuss some of the more common applications of MMT in various clinical and therapeutic settings, with emphasis on the specific challenges often seen in each. The reader should be aware that the examples provided here are not limited to these settings only.

Acute Care Facilities

Often patients seen in acute care facilities are either acutely ill or are postoperative patients. In the acutely ill patient, manual muscle testing may be used to assess the patient's mobility status in order to inform a discharge plan. A manual strength exam performed as part of a general assessment may provide information concerning the amount of assistance the patient requires and whether the patient will need an assistive device. Assessing the patient's strength to help ensure safe transfers from bed to chair, to a standing position, or on and off the toilet is an essential part of the acute-care patient management process. A strength assessment may also inform the therapist of the patient's ability to follow directions and/or to verbalize concerns such as following a stroke or in the presence of delirium or other cognitive loss.[1,2]

Strength assessment may also indicate the presence of pain before full-body movements such as transfers. Strength assessment could take the form of active movement followed by resistance, such as in a manual muscle test or in a 10-repetition maximum such as in a seated shoulder dip.

Strength assessment in the postoperative patient informs the therapist of the integrity of the patient's nervous system. The therapist may be the first person requiring the patient to move actively after surgery, and thus may be the first one to observe the patient's ability to contract a muscle. Although this scenario is rare, clearly the consequences of assuming an attitude of "all is well" and finding out during a transfer that the patient cannot use part of an extremity would have avoidable consequences. Strength testing in this scenario might take the form of isometric contractions, especially if there are contraindications to joint movement, suspected postsurgical pain as in a newly repaired fractured hip, or in restricted range of motion such as in a total hip arthroplasty. If testing is done in a manner that differs from the published directions, documentation should describe how the test was performed. For example, if isometric testing was done at the hip because the patient was not permitted to move the hip through full range after a hip arthroplasty, the therapist should document the test accordingly: "Patient's strength at the hip appeared to be under volitional control, but pain and postsurgical precautions prevented thorough assessment."

Key movements that should be assessed for viability and for the strength necessary to perform transfers or gait include elbow extension, grip, shoulder depression, knee extension, hip abduction, ankle plantar, and dorsiflexion. Functional tests that might be useful in assessing the patient include gait speed, chair stand, timed transfer, or the timed up-and-go test (see Chapter 9).

Special considerations for the acute care setting may include the patient's rapid fluctuations in response to medications, illness, or pain. Reassessment may be necessary when any changes in strength are documented along with therapist's insights into why the changes are occurring. Clearly, strength gains are not possible in the short time a typical patient is in acute care, but rather should be attributed to increased confidence in moving, less pain, better understanding of the movement to be performed, motor learning, and so forth.

Acute Rehabilitation Facilities

Strength assessment in the acute rehabilitation setting may be performed as a baseline assessment to determine progress over time and to identify key impairments that affect the patient's mobility-related and other functional goals. Knowledge of community-based norms for mobility such as chair stands, distance walked, stair climbing speed, floor transfer ability, and gait speed will inform the therapist's clinical decision-making. (See Chapter 9 for a more complete description of these tests.) A standard manual muscle test and/or a 10-repetition maximum (10-RM) strength assessment are other methods used to assess relevant strength abilities.

As in the acute care setting, assessment of strength for mobility tasks is critical in the acute rehabilitation setting. Recognition of key muscle groups in specific mobility tasks, such as the plantar-flexors in gait speed, is key to informed clinical decision-making.

Special considerations for the acute rehabilitation setting often include rapid change over a short period. Positive changes may be attributed to increased comfort and less pain, less apprehension, neuroplasticity, and a change in medications. Negative changes may be attributed to a decline in medical status, pain, or depression, for example. Muscle fatigue resulting from poor fitness and excessive sedentary behavior or general body fatigue related to frailty or post–acute care implications may affect the perception of strength. The patient may not be able to assume a proper test position because of postsurgical restrictions or a lack of range of motion, requiring the therapist to do a strength-screen rather than a strength test. This screen cannot serve as an accurate baseline because of the lack of standardization. Functional testing may be more informative and accurate in these situations. The therapist should take special care to document any deviations from the standardized manual muscle test.

Long-term Care Facilities

Strength testing and assessment approaches used in long-term care settings are similar to those used in acute rehabilitation. Strength assessment can serve as a baseline to identify key impairments that impact a patient's fall-risk, mobility, and other functional goals as well as to determine the patient's progress over time. Strength screening can be part of a required annual assessment for long-term residents. Strength in the form of a chair-stand test or grip strength is a key component of the diagnosis of frailty and therefore can inform prognosis.[3]

Frailty is a common geriatric syndrome, characterized by decreased reserve and increased vulnerability to adverse outcomes including falls, hospitalization, institutionalization, and death.[4] The majority of residents in long-term care are considered frail.[5] Lack of strength is a significant cause of frailty and serves as a diagnostic criterion. Box 2-1 lists the diagnostic criteria for frailty. Based on these criteria, strength assessment and functional testing can be valuable in the intervention of nursing home residents.[4]

Box 2-1 Diagnostic Criteria for Frailty

Diagnostic criteria for frailty include the presence of three or more of the following:[4,10]

1. Unintentional weight loss (>10 lb in past year)
2. General feeling of exhaustion on 3 or more days/week (self-report)
3. Weakness (grip strength in lowest 20%; <23 lb for women; <32 lb for men)
4. Slow walking speed (lowest 20% = <0.8 m/s)
5. Low levels of physical activity (in kcal/week lowest 20%; = 270 kcal/week for women; 383 kcal/week for men—equivalent to sitting quietly and/or lying down for the vast majority of the day)

The presence of one or two of these characteristics indicates prefrailty.

Although a natural consequence of aging is a gradual loss of strength and power, it should not be assumed that older adults are functionally weaker than younger adults.[6-8] Because manual muscle testing has a ceiling effect, the therapist should not have lower expectations or overestimate strength in frail older adults. *Criteria for grading remain the same for people of all ages and conditions.* Because the ceiling effect of a manual muscle test can be so profound, especially in regard to function, functional testing is a better option for strength testing and assessment in the long-term care setting.[9] Community criterion reference values exist that guide the long-term care therapist in establishing appropriate goals and expectations (Box 2-2). Older adults might be better served with strength training options such as a leg press or latissimus pull down rather than the cuff weights or a recumbent cross-trainer such as NuStep so often seen in long-term care settings. The reader is referred to Chapter 8 for strength measurement options.

The Home Health Setting

Strength testing and assessment of home health patients for the purpose of comparison with community-based norms and for identification of impairments related to function are the primary purposes of manual muscle testing and alternative strength-testing methods in the home health setting. Returning a patient to community-based mobility may prevent frailty and increase the patient's quality of life. Lower-extremity strength is a primary component of these goals. Box 2-2 lists community mobility requirements that can be used as outcome goals for home health patients and serve to guide strength testing. Additionally, for a homebound patient to receive home health services, the Centers for Medicare and Medicaid Services require patients to demonstrate "considerable and taxing effort in leaving the home," a criterion that has strength implications.[11]

Outpatient Clinics

Strength testing and assessment in outpatient clinics provide essential information such as the: (1) origin of the patient's pain, (2) quality of the contraction, (3) symmetry between sides and between the primary mover (agonist) and opposing muscles (antagonist), and (4) weakness within a kinetic chain (body segments linked by a series of joints).[15] This information aids in making a diagnosis. It can also provide a baseline assessment for changes over time such as in the case of sciatica-induced weakness.[16] Challenges of manual muscle testing in the outpatient setting can include the presence of pain that prohibits a full, voluntary contraction and limitations of range of motion such as with retraction and upward rotation of the scapula at the shoulder. Although a weak and painful or strong and painful contraction can be diagnostic criteria, it can preclude the assessment of quantitative strength.[17] The ceiling effect of manual muscle testing often prevents an accurate assessment of strength quantity. Therefore, we recommend that quantitative strength be assessed through a 1-RM or 10-RM strength assessment when pain permits (see Chapter 8). It is useful to assess the noninvolved side to ascertain asymmetry.

Careful differentiation is required to use strength assessment and testing for diagnostic (as opposed to quantification) purposes. For example, the Cyriax method (see Chapter 8) of maintaining the joint in a neutral, relaxed position while assessing the muscle's contraction in various directions can reveal the presence of a contractile lesion if pain is produced during a contraction, while keeping noncontractile (e.g., connective tissues) elements on slack.[17] Alternatively, if the contraction is not painful while the joint is in a neutral position, an inert lesion, such as a bone spur or capsular inflammation, may be implicated.

The presence of pain, joint restriction, or muscle tightness may prevent the patient from assuming the correct testing position for accurate assessment of muscle testing. While this text advocates testing the muscle in a pain-free position, substitution patterns are more difficult to discern; thus specific muscle strength quantification may not be possible. However, the therapist can document asymmetrical differences, points in the range where pain exists or does not exist, and the nature of the pain that aid the therapist in making an accurate diagnosis.

Another challenge for therapists in outpatient settings is the variety of patients seen in a given day. For example, a therapist may see a college or professional athlete in the same afternoon as a frail older adult. Careful discernment of appropriate strength testing is critical to avoid over or underestimation of strength limitations. Using alternative

Box 2-2 Community Mobility Requirements

To be considered mobile, an individual should be able to:

Walk 300 m minimum per errand[12]
Run multiple errands during one trip outside the home[13]
Carry a package weighing 7.5 lb[13]
Change direction while walking[14]
Step onto and off of a curb without support
Achieve a gait speed of >0.8 m/s
Make postural transitions including stooping, lifting, reaching, and reorientation of head—independent of change in direction
Climb stairs
Navigate slopes and uneven surfaces
Step over objects

muscle strength assessments as described in Chapters 8 and 9 may be useful.

Wellness Clinics

Muscle screening provides feedback to participants regarding their abilities relative to age-matched normative samples that may impact functional abilities such as gait speed and chair stands. Although individual manual muscle testing is not routinely done as part of a wellness screening, functional movements such as floor transfers, 30-second sit to stands, or hand grip tests are useful to ascertain individual fitness levels and risk of disability. [4,10] The information gleaned from a wellness assessment may indicate the need for an individualized physical therapy assessment of strength.[18,19]

Summary

Manual muscle testing has utility in all clinical settings. It is incumbent on the therapist, however, to judiciously use manual muscle testing when and if appropriate and to choose alternative forms of testing (e.g., functional and instrumented tests) when the information obtained from manual muscle testing is inadequate.

Even though muscle testing has tremendous value, there are situations in which it is not particularly informative, nor even accurate. Some of the clinical scenarios in which muscle testing is not optimal have already been discussed (for example, in the presence of pain), but more detail will be presented in the next section.

LIMITATIONS OF MANUAL MUSCLE TESTING

Manual muscle testing has significant limitations. When it was first developed, the majority of patients seen by physical therapists were patients with polio. Today's patient population has changed enormously and therapists now see hundreds of patient types ranging in age from infancy to 100-plus years. Muscle examination has changed concomitantly to more accurately reflect the needs of clients, and manual muscle testing is only one approach among many. Each form of testing has its advantages and disadvantages, as will be noted in this chapter and elsewhere in this book. The major limitations of manual testing are discussed in the following section.

Population Variation

Many articles that report manual muscle testing results are based on studies of normal adults or specific subpopulations such as athletes, sedentary, and aged adults. Children occupy a separate category. Additionally, results of muscle testing values are reported in individuals with a wide variety of pathologies including Parkinson's disease, cerebral palsy, and muscular dystrophy. Because of this wide variation, it is necessary to modify grading procedures but not testing technique. Thus, test grades are not consistent from one patient population to another. Some testers also erroneously believe that the assigned grade should be modified based on age or ability, which should not be the case. Rather, manual muscle testing interpretation requires knowledge of the strength requirements of the task.

Objectivity

Manual muscle testing, as originally described, suffers from a lack of objectivity, when objectivity is defined as a test not dependent primarily on the judgment of the examiner.[20,21] It is described in terms of an ordinal scale using terms such as Good and Fair, further reducing its objectivity.

Validity and Reliability

Reliability in manual muscle testing varies considerably according to the muscle tested, the experience of the examiner, the age of the patient, and the particular condition being tested. For example, in a study of 102 boys ages 5 to15 years with Duchenne's muscular dystrophy, intra-rater reliability ranged from 0.65 to .93 with the proximal muscles having the higher reliability values.[22] The muscles with gravity minimized also had higher reliability values. In another study of physical therapists comparing manual muscle testing to hand-held muscle dynamometry in 11 patients, reliability was high and differentiated between grades at all levels.[23] Frese and colleagues performed a reliability study among therapists on the middle trapezius and gluteus medius muscles and found 28% to 45% agreement for the same grade and 89% to 92% agreement within one grade.[24] They found the reliability to be poor, as measured by Cohen's weighted Kappa. In muscles with grades below 3 (Fair) reliability declines.[24-27] Reliability also decreases in the muscles of the lower extremity.[27]

Clearly, the reliability of manual muscle testing is of concern, and yet it remains an important screening and diagnostic tool. Therapists, especially novices, must be cautious about their test procedures and make vigorous attempts to standardize their methods. Reliability is increased by adhering to the same procedure for each test (for one or several examiners), by providing clear instructions to the subject, and by having a quiet and comfortable environment for the test. To further enhance the reliability of the manual muscle test, the following steps should be taken:[28-30]

- Proper positioning so the test muscle is the prime mover
- Adequate stabilization of regional anatomy

- Observation of the manner in which the patient or subject assumes and maintains the test position
- Consistent timing, pressure, and position
- Avoidance of preconceived impressions regarding the test outcome
- Nonpainful contacts—nonpainful execution of the test

Sensitivity

Manual muscle testing also lacks sensitivity. Years ago, Beasley reported that patients with various neurological disorders who had Grade 4 (Good) knee extension force were only about 43% of normal, rather than the traditionally defined 75% of normal.[25] The Fair (3) group actually had force generation that was only 9% of Normal, rather than 50% of Normal usually assigned with MMT.[25] Similar sensitivity was reported for detecting muscle force deficits relative to normal.[26]

Because manual muscle testing as originally described is subjective, the historical and conventional acceptability for reliability is that among examiners and in successive tests with the same examiner, the results should be within one-half of a grade (or within a plus or minus of the base grade).[29] Others maintain that within the same grade is acceptable, pluses and minuses notwithstanding.[30] However, even if this historical convention is used, therapists are unreliable in differentiating between the grades of 4 (Good) and 5 (Normal).[9,26]

Diagnostic Validity

Manual muscle testing is useful in the assessment of weakness of muscles directly involved with pain, injury and neuromusculoskeletal disorders.[28] In a study to detect differences between sides using manual muscle testing, sensitivity ranged from 62.9 to 72.3%, increasing with more pronounced strength differences.[28]

Ceiling Effect

Manual muscle testing has wide variability in the range of forces reported for a given grade, especially in the upper range of the scale, further reducing its sensitivity. For example, in a subset of 4 studies, men with a manual muscle testing grade of 5 (Normal, by a negative break test) for knee extension and tested with hand-held muscle dynamometry concurrently demonstrated values of 85.4 to 650.0 Newtons.[9] Additionally, the four studies analyzed represented all settings with a variety of patient types. The Grade 5 (Normal) represented 86% of the range of measureable forces. Bohannon reports that knee extension forces of more than 800 Newtons are not unusual for young men.[28] Thus, manual muscle testing suffers from a profound ceiling effect. Many patients may be classified as having Grade 5 (Normal) strength when they may have strength deficits only appreciated through more objective means. This ceiling effect may mask changes in strength that have functional and prognostic consequences. Thus, it is not recommended that manual muscle testing be used as a measure of progress over the grade of 3 (Fair).

Another concern of the applicability of manual muscle testing is its lack of accuracy to identity impairments related to function, secondary to the curvilinear relationship. The curvilinear relationship suggests that above a relative threshold, strength gains are not as apparent, because the threshold for a functional task has been exceeded. Traditional manual muscle testing may not reflect the amount of strength needed to perform functional tasks such as getting up from the floor or throwing a baseball. When a basic manual muscle test screen reveals test grades that are above Grade 3 and in particular, where there are side-to-side differences, the therapist should rely on instrumented or functional testing to further clarify deficiencies and to differentiate between Grades 4 and 5 (see Chapters 8 and 9).

Tester Strength

A break test in manual muscle testing requires the tester to exert greater force than the patient in any given muscle. When testing a very strong individual, such as a weight-lifter or football player, a great amount of force on the part of the tester is required. Women traditionally have less upper body strength than men, and differences have been recorded in manual muscle testing forces between female and male testers, leading to an underestimation of the patient's quadriceps strength.[26,31] For example, Beasley found in a sample of female therapists testing the quadriceps in patients with polio that of those graded a 5, the mean force was only 53% of normal subjects.[25] Examiner strength has been found to limit testing accuracy of hand-held dynamometry, an objective measure of the force generated in manual muscle testing.[23,32-35] Mulroy and colleagues also found that female therapists overgraded the strength of the quadriceps in 14 of 19 patients, in part because of greater patient strength.[31] Male therapists assigned too high a grade in 2 of 19 patients.[31] Tester strength seems to be a factor in hand-held dynamometry when the subject's muscle strength exceeds 120 Newtons.[35]

Summary

Manual muscle testing appears to be both reliable and valid in the presence of profound weakness such as that seen in neuromuscular diseases. However, when used in individuals with near normal levels of strength, it is recommended that manual muscle testing be used as a screening tool that informs alternative forms of strength testing such as those described in Chapters 8 and 9. There does not seem to be evidence for the use of manual muscle testing to measure progress such as in strengthening activities, particularly for Grade 3 and above.

REFERENCES

Cited References

1. Bittner EA, Martyn JA, George E, et al. Measurement of muscle strength in the intensive care unit. Crit Care Med. 2009;37:S321-S330.
2. Andrews AW, Bohannon RW. Short-term recovery of limb muscle strength after acute stroke. Arch Phys Med Rehabil. 2003;84:125-130.
3. Vermeulen J, Neyens JC, van Rossum E, et al. Predicting ADL disability in community-dwelling elderly people using physical frailty indicators: a systematic review. BMC Geriatr. 2011;11:33.
4. Fried LP, Tangen CM, Walston J, et al. Frailty in older adults: evidence for a phenotype. J Gerontol Med Sci. 2001;56A:M146-M156.
5. Fried TR, Mor V. Frailty and hospitalization of long-term stay nursing home residents. J Am Geriatr Soc. 1997; 45:265-269.
6. Bortz WM. A conceptual framework of frailty: a review. J Gerontol. 2002;57A:M283-M288.
7. Visser M, Kritchevsky SB, Goodpaster B, et al. Leg muscle mass and composition in relation to lower extremity performance in men and women aged 70-79: the health, aging and body composition study. J Am Geriatr Soc. 2002;50:897-904.
8. Schwartz RS. Sarcopenia and physical performance in old age: introduction. Muscle Nerve Suppl. 1997;5:S10-S12.
9. Bohannon RW, Corrigan D. A broad range of forces is encompassed by the maximum manual muscle test grade of five. Percept Mot Skills. 2000;90:747-750.
10. Xue QL, Bandeen-Roche K, Varadhan R, et al. Initial manifestations of frailty criteria and the development of frailty phenotype in the women's health and aging study II. J Gerontol A Biol Sci Med Sci. 2008;63:984-990.
11. U.S. Department of Health and Human Services. Centers for Medicare & Medicaid Services, Medicare benefit policy manual; Home Health Services; 2011; ch 7; pp 61-64. http://www.cms.gov/Regulations-and-Guidance/Guidance/Manuals/downloads/bp102c07.pdf
12. Chang M, Cohen-Mansfield J, Ferrucci L, et al. Incidence of loss of ability to walk 400 meters in a functionally limited older population. J Am Geriatr Soc. 2004;52:2094-2098.
13. Shumway-Cook A, Patla AE, Stewart A, et al. Environmental demands associated with community mobility in older adults with and without mobility disabilities. Phys Ther. 2002;82:670-681.
14. Perry J, Garrett M, Gronley JK, et al. Classification of walking handicap in the stroke population. Stroke. 1995; 26:982-989
15. Maffiuletti NA. Assessment of hip and knee muscle function in orthopaedic practice and research. J Bone Joint Surg Am. 2010;92:220-229.
16. Balague F, Nordin M, Sheikhzadeh A, et al. Recovery of impaired muscle function in severe sciatica. Eur Spine J. 2001;10:242-249.
17. Cyriax JH. Textbook of orthopaedic medicine: diagnosis of soft tissue lesions, vol. 1. 8th ed. London: Bailliere Tindall; 1982:14-21.
18. Rikli R, Jones J. Development and validation of a functional fitness test for community-residing older adults. J Aging Phys Activity. 1999;7:129-161.
19. Rikli R, Jones J. Functional fitness normative scores for community-residing older adults, ages 60-94. J Aging Phys Activity. 1999;7:162-181.
20. Knepler C, Bohannon RW. Subjectivity of forces associated with manual muscle test scores of 3+, 4-, and 4. Percept Motor Skills. 1998;87:1123-1128.
21. Bohannon RW. Objective measures. Phys Ther. 1989;69: 590-593.
22. Florence JM, Pandya S, King WM, et al. Intrarater reliability of manual muscle test (medical research council scale) grades in Duchenne's muscular dystrophy. Phys Ther. 1992;72:115-122; discussion 122-126.
23. Wadsworth CT, Krishnan R, Sear M, et al. Intrarater reliability of manual muscle testing and hand-held dynametric muscle testing. Phys Ther. 1987;67:1342-1347.
24. Frese F, Brown M, Norton BJ. Clinical reliability of manual muscle testing: middle trapezius and gluteus medius muscles. Phys Ther. 1987;67:1072-1076.
25. Beasley WC. Quantitative muscle testing: Principles and application to research and clinical services. Arch Phys Med Rehabil. 1961;42:398-425.
26. Wintz M. Variations in current manual muscle testing. Phys Ther Rev. 1959;39:466-475.
27. Cuthbert SCJ, Goodheart GJ. On the reliability and validity of manual muscle testing: a literature review. Chiropr Osteopat. 2007;15:4.
28. Bohannon RW. Manual muscle testing: does it meet the standards of an adequate screening test? Clin Rehabil. 2005;19:662-667.
29. Lamb R. Manual muscle testing. In: Rothstein JM, ed. Measurement in physical therapy. New York: Churchill-Livingstone; 1985; pp 47-55.
30. Palmer ML, Epler ME. Fundamentals of musculoskeletal assessment techniques. 2nd ed. Philadelphia: Lippincott Williams & Wilkins; 1998.
31. Mulroy SJ, Lassen KD, Chambers SH, et al. The ability of male and female clinicians to effectively test knee extension strength using manual muscle testing. J Orthop Sports Phys Ther. 1997;26:192-199.
32. Edwards RHT, McDonnell M. Hand-held dynamometer for evaluating voluntary muscle function. Lancet. 1971;9: 757-758.
33. Marino M, Nicholas JA, Gleim GW, et al. The efficacy of manual assessment of muscle strength using a new device. Am J Sports Med. 1982;10:360-364.
34. Bohannon RW. Hand-held dynamometry: factors influencing reliability and validity. Clin Rehabil. 1998;11: 263-264.
35. Wikholm JB, Bohannon RW. Hand-held dynamometry measurements: tester strength makes a difference. J Ortho Sports Phys Ther. 1991;12:191-198.

Other Readings

Cameron D, Bohannon RW. Criterion validity of lower extremity Motricity Index scores. Clin Rehabil. 2000;14: 208-211.

Ciesla N, Dinglas V, Fan E, et al. Manual muscle testing: a method of measuring extremity muscle strength applied to critically ill patients. J Vis Exp. 2011;50:26-32.

Robles PG, Mathur S, Janaudis-Fereira T, et al. Measurement of peripheral muscle strength in individuals with chronic obstructive pulmonary disease: a systematic review. J Cardiopulm Rehabil Prev. 2011;31:11-24.

3

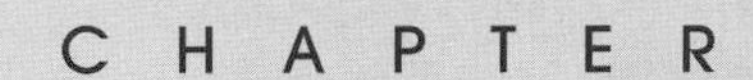

Testing the Muscles of the Neck

- Capital Extension
- Cervical Extension
- Combined Neck Extension
- Capital Flexion
- Cervical Flexion
- Combined Cervical Flexion
- Combined Flexion to Isolate a Single Sternocleidomastoid
- Cervical Rotation

Note: This section of the book on testing the neck muscles is divided into tests for capital and cervical extension and flexion and their combination. This distinction was first described by Perry and Nickel as a necessary and effective way of managing nuchal weakness or paralysis.[1] All muscles acting on the head are inserted on the skull. Those muscles that lie behind the coronal midline are termed capital extensors. Motion is centered at the atlanto-occipital and atlantoaxial joints.[2,3]

CAPITAL EXTENSION

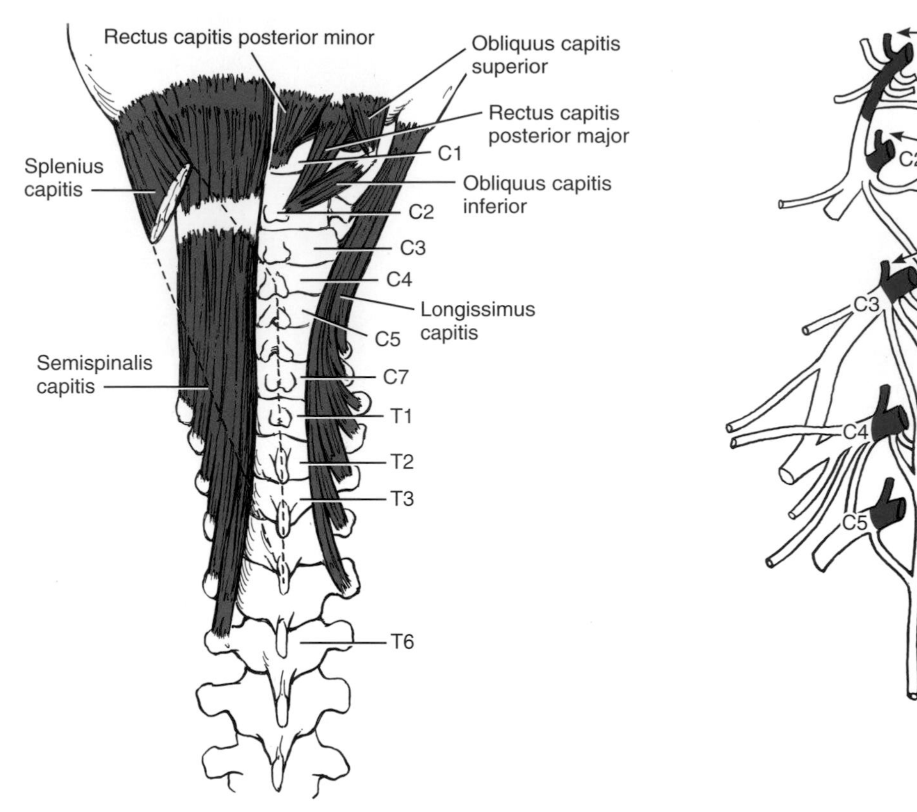

FIGURE 3-1

FIGURE 3-2

Range of Motion
0° to 25°

Table 3-1 CAPITAL EXTENSION

I.D.	Muscle	Origin	Insertion
56	Rectus capitis posterior major	Axis (spinous process)	Occiput (inferior nuchal line laterally)
57	Rectus capitis posterior minor	Atlas (tubercle of posterior arch)	Occiput (inferior nuchal line medially)
60	Longissimus capitis	T1-T5 vertebrae (transverse processes) C4-C7 vertebrae (articular processes)	Temporal bone (mastoid process, posterior surface)
58	Obliquus capitis superior	Atlas (transverse process)	Occiput (between superior and inferior nuchal lines)
59	Obliquus capitis inferior	Axis (lamina and spinous process)	Atlas (transverse process, inferior-posterior surface)
61	Splenius capitis	Ligamentum nuchae C7-T4 vertebrae (spinous processes)	Temporal bone (mastoid process) Occiput (below superior nuchal line)
62	Semispinalis capitis (distinct medial part often named Spinalis capitis)	C7-T6 vertebrae (transverse processes) C4-C6 vertebrae (articular processes)	Occiput (between superior and inferior nuchal lines)
124	Trapezius (upper)	Occiput (external protuberance and superior nuchal line, middle 1/3) C7 (spinous process) Ligamentum nuchae	Clavicle (posterior border of lateral 1/3)
63	Spinalis capitis	Medial part of Semispinalis capitis, usually blended inseparably	Occiput (between superior and inferior nuchal lines)
Other			
83	Sternocleidomastoid (posterior)		

Grade 5 (Normal) and Grade 4 (Good)

Position of Patient: Prone with head off end of table. Arms at sides.

Position of Therapist: Standing at side of patient next to the head. One hand provides resistance over the occiput (Figure 3-3). The other hand is placed beneath the overhanging head, prepared to support the head should it give way with resistance, which is applied directly opposite to the movement of the head.

Test: Patient extends head by tilting chin upward in a nodding motion. (Cervical spine is not extended.)

Instructions to Patient: "Look at the wall. Hold it. Don't let me tilt your head down."

Grading

Grade 5 (Normal): Patient completes available range of motion without substituting cervical extension. Tolerates maximum resistance. (This is a strong muscle group.)

Grade 4 (Good): Patient completes available range of motion without substituting cervical extension. Tolerates strong to moderate resistance.

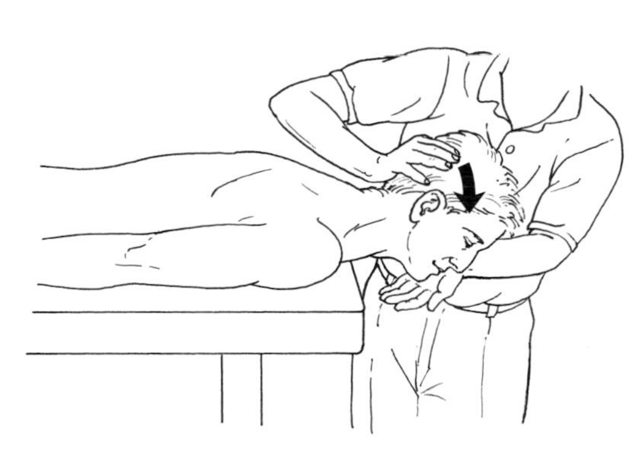

FIGURE 3-3

Grade 3 (Fair)

Position of Patient: Prone with head off end of table and supported by therapist. Arms at sides.

Position of Therapist: Standing at side of patient's head. One hand should remain under the head to catch it should the muscles fail to hold position (Figure 3-4).

Instructions to Patient: "Look at the wall."

Test: Patient completes available range of motion with no resistance.

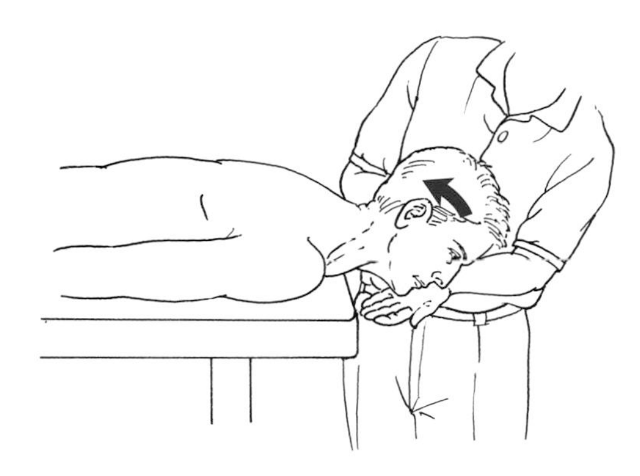

FIGURE 3-4

Grade 2 (Poor), Grade 1 (Trace), and Grade 0 (Zero)

Position of Patient: Supine with head on table. Arms at sides. Note: The gravity minimized position (side-lying) is not recommended for any of the tests of the neck for grades 2 (Poor) and below because test artifacts are created by the therapist in attempting to support the head without providing assistance to the motion.

Position of Therapist: Standing at end of table facing patient. Head is supported with two hands under the occiput. Fingers should be placed just at the base of the occiput lateral to the vertebral column to attempt to palpate the capital extensors (Figure 3-5). Head may be slightly lifted off table to reduce friction.

Test: Patient attempts to look back toward therapist without lifting the head from the table.

Instructions to Patient: "Tilt your chin up," OR "Look back at me. Don't lift your head."

Grading

Grade 2 (Poor): Patient completes limited range of motion.

Grade 1 (Trace) and Grade 0 (Zero): Palpation of the capital extensors at the base of the occiput just lateral to the spine may be difficult; the splenius capitis lies most lateral and the recti lie just next to the spinous process.

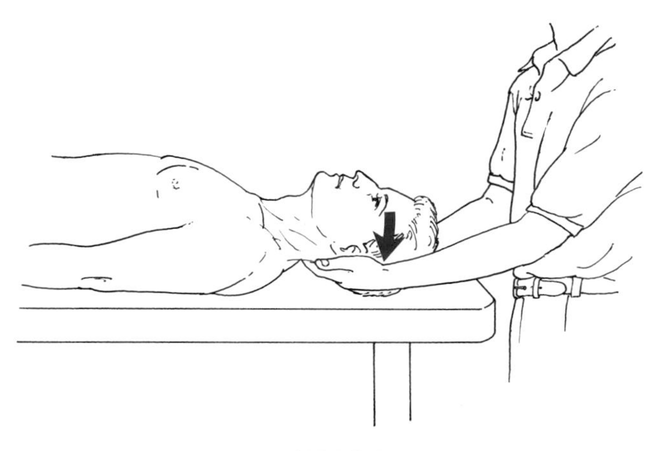

FIGURE 3-5

Helpful Hints

- Clinicians are reminded that the head is a very heavy object suspended on thin support. Whenever testing with the patient's head off the table, extreme caution should be used for the patient's safety, especially in the presence of suspected or known neck or trunk weakness. Always place a hand under the head to catch it should the muscles give way.
- Significant weakness of the capital extensor muscles combined with laryngeal and pharyngeal weakness can result in a nonpatent airway. There also may be inability to swallow. Both of these problems occur because the loss of capital extensors leaves the capital flexors unopposed, and the resultant head position favors the chin tucked on the chest, especially in the supine position.[1] This problem is not limited to patients with severe polio paralysis; it is also evident in patients with severe rheumatoid arthritis. Patients with chronic forward head posture also commonly have weak cervical extensors.

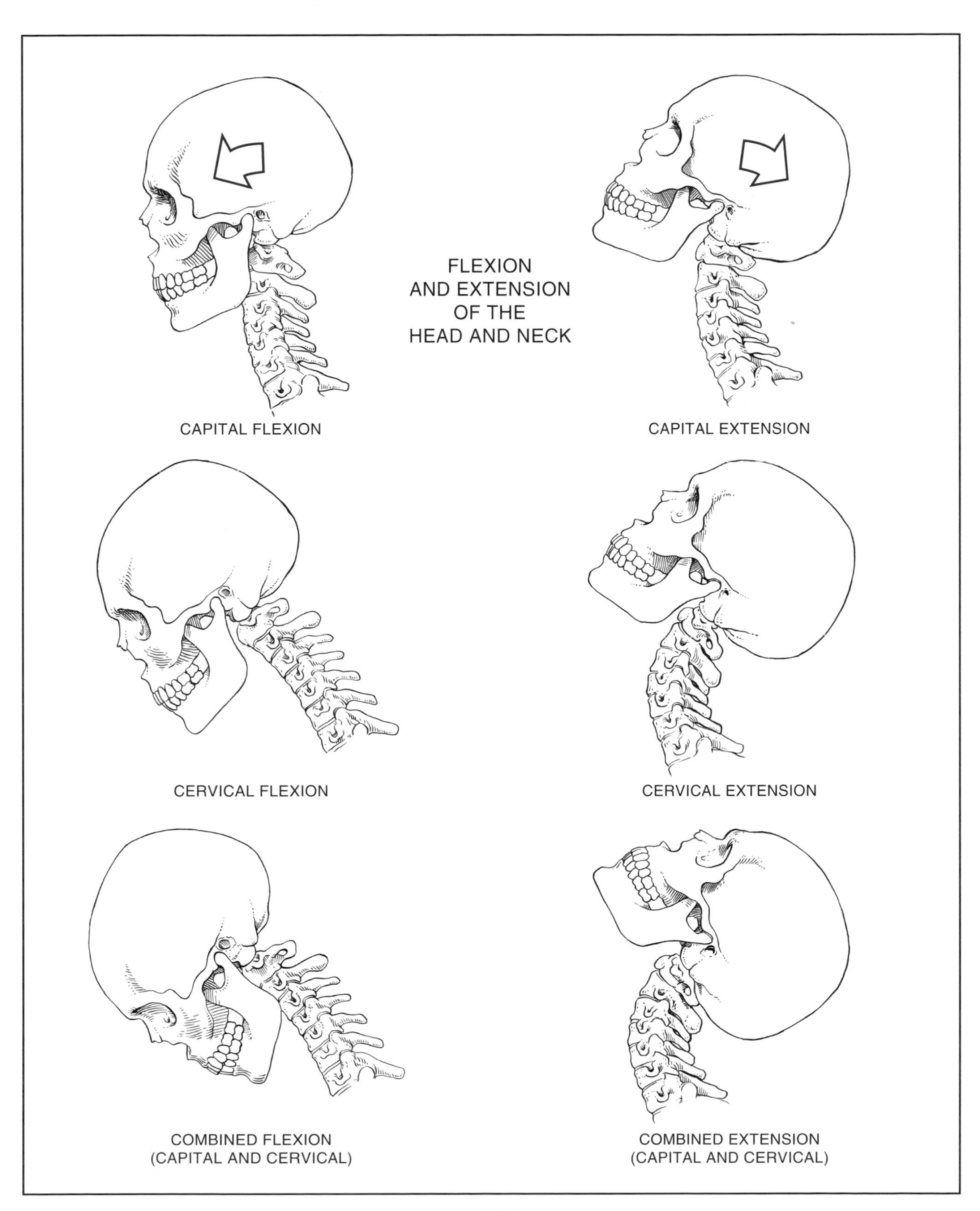
FLEXION
AND EXTENSION
OF THE
HEAD AND NECK
CAPITAL FLEXION
CAPITAL EXTENSION
CERVICAL FLEXION
CERVICAL EXTENSION
COMBINED FLEXION
(CAPITAL AND CERVICAL)
COMBINED EXTENSION
(CAPITAL AND CERVICAL)

PLATE 1

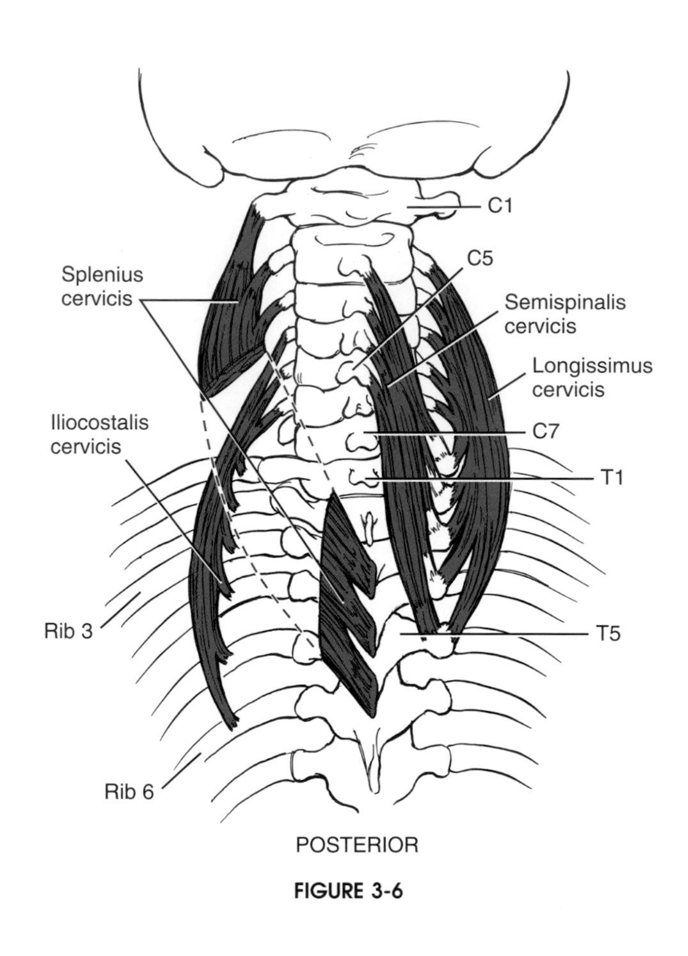

FIGURE 3-6

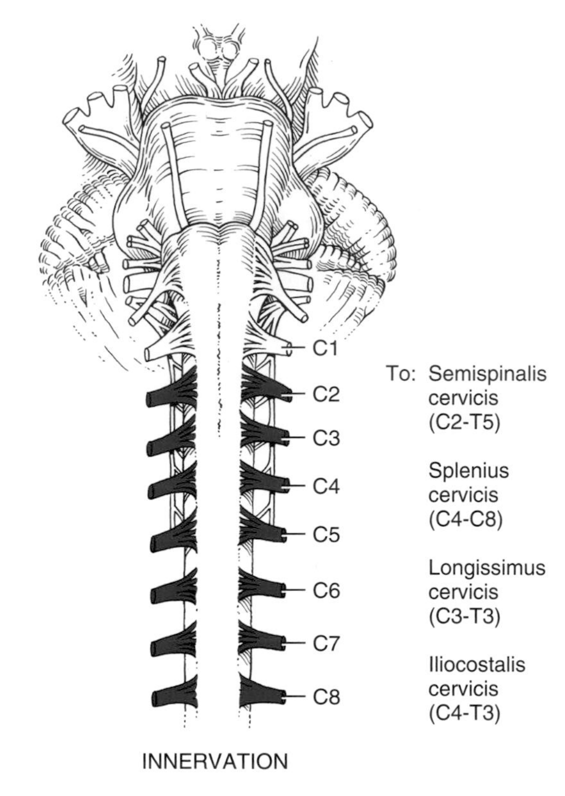

FIGURE 3-7

Range of Motion

0° to less than 30°

Table 3-2 CERVICAL EXTENSION

I.D.	Muscle	Origin	Insertion
64	Longissimus cervicis	T1-T5 vertebrae (transverse processes) variable	C2-C6 vertebrae (transverse processes)
65	Semispinalis cervicis	T1-T5 vertebrae (transverse processes)	Axis (C2)-C5 vertebrae (spinous processes)
66	Iliocostalis cervicis	Ribs 3-6 (angles)	C4-C6 vertebrae (transverse processes, posterior tubercles)
67	Splenius cervicis (may be absent or variable)	T3-T6 vertebrae (spinous processes)	C1-C3 vertebrae (transverse processes)
124	Trapezius (upper)	Occiput (protuberance and superior nuchal line, middle 1/3) C7 (spinous process) Ligamentum nuchae T1-T12 vertebrae occasionally	Clavicle (posterior border of lateral 1/3)
68	Spinalis cervicis (often absent)	C7 and often C6 vertebrae (spinous processes) Ligamentum nuchae T1-T2 vertebrae occasionally	Axis (spinous process) C2-C3 vertebrae (spinous processes)
Others			
69	Interspinales cervicis		
70	Intertransversarii cervicis		
71	Rotatores cervicis		
94	Multifidi		
127	Levator scapulae		

The cervical extensor muscles are limited to those that act only on the cervical spine with motion centered in the lower cervical spine.[2,3]

Grade 5 (Normal) and Grade 4 (Good)

Position of Patient: Prone with head off end of table. Arms at sides.

Position of Therapist: Standing next to patient's head. One hand is placed over the parieto-occipital area for resistance (Figure 3-8). The other hand is placed below the chin, ready to catch the head if it gives way suddenly during resistance.

Test: Patient extends neck without tilting chin.

Instructions to Patient: "Push up on my hand but keep looking at the floor. Hold it. Don't let me push it down."

Grading

Grade 5 (Normal): Patient completes full range of motion and holds against maximum resistance. Therapist must use clinical caution because these muscles are not strong, and their maximum effort will not tolerate much resistance.

Grade 4 (Good): Patient completes full range of motion against moderate resistance.

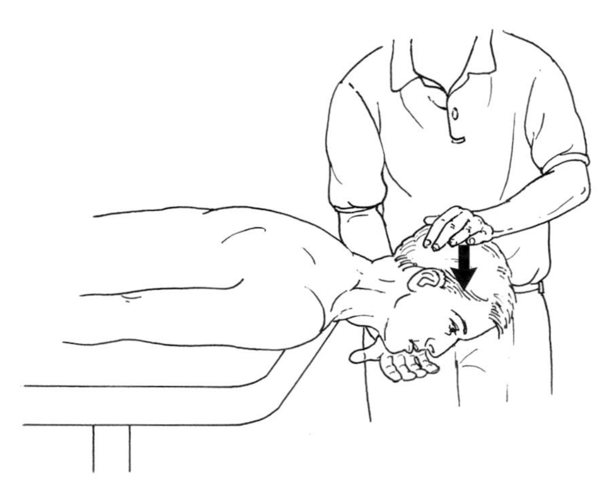

FIGURE 3-8

Grade 3 (Fair)

Position of Patient: Prone with head off end of table. Arms at sides.

Position of Therapist: Standing next to patient's head with one hand supporting (or ready to support) the forehead (Figure 3-9).

Test: Patient extends neck without looking up or tilting chin.

Instructions to Patient: "Lift your forehead from my hand and keep looking at the floor."

Grading

Grade 3 (Fair): Patient completes range of motion but takes no resistance.

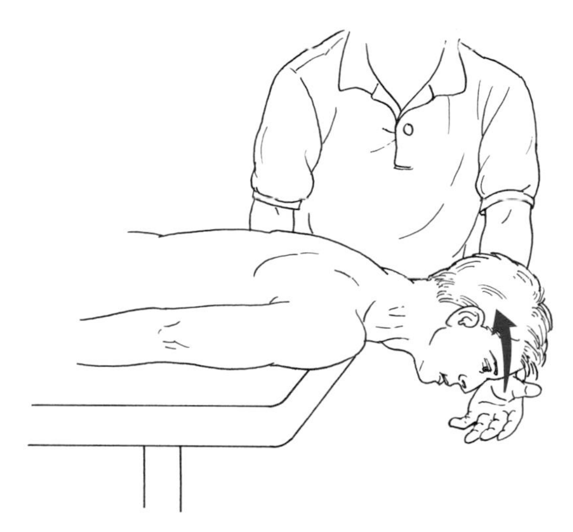

FIGURE 3-9

Alternate Test for Grade 3: This test should be used if there is known or suspected trunk extensor weakness. The therapist should always have an assistant participate to provide protective guarding under the patient's forehead. This test is identical to the preceding Grade 3 test except that stabilization is provided by the therapist if needed to accommodate trunk weakness. Stabilization is provided to the upper back by the forearm placed over the upper back with the hand cupped over the shoulder (Figure 3-10).

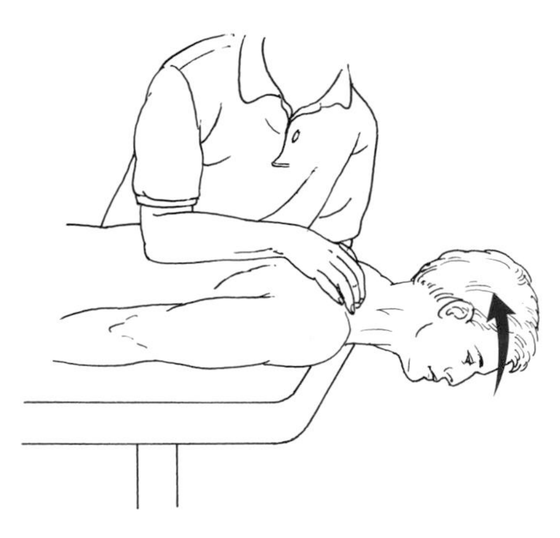

FIGURE 3-10

Grade 2 (Poor), Grade 1 (Trace), and Grade 0 (Zero)

Position of Patient: Supine with head fully supported by table. Arms at sides.

Position of Therapist: Standing at head end of table facing the patient. Both hands are placed under the head. Fingers are distal to the occiput at the level of the cervical vertebrae for palpation (Figure 3-11).

Test: Patient attempts to extend neck into table.

Instructions to Patient: "Try to push your head down into my hands."

Grading

Grade 2 (Poor): Patient moves through small range of neck extension by pushing into therapist's hands.

Grade 1 (Trace): Contractile activity palpated in cervical extensors.

Grade 0 (Zero): No palpable muscle activity.

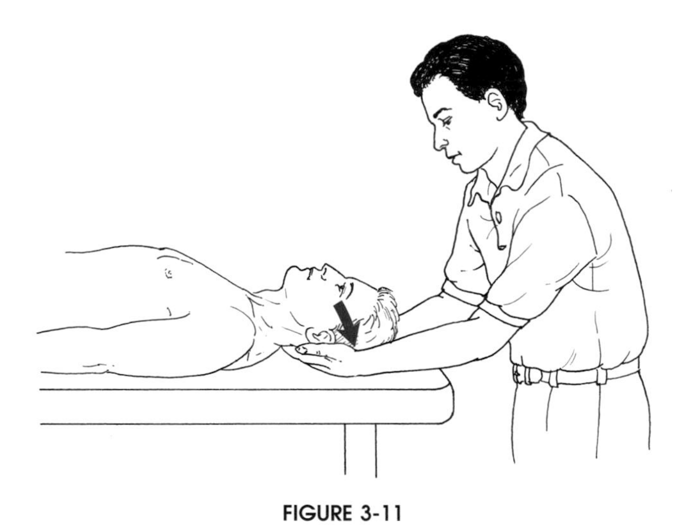

FIGURE 3-11

(Capital plus Cervical)

Range of Motion
0° to 45°

Grade 5 (Normal) and Grade 4 (Good)

Position of Patient: Prone with head off end of table. Arms at sides.

Position of Therapist: Standing next to patient's head. One hand is placed over the parieto-occipital area to give resistance, which is directed both down and forward (Figure 3-12). The other hand is below the chin ready to catch the head if muscles give way during resistance.

Test: Patient extends head and neck through available range of motion by lifting head and looking up.

Instructions to Patient: "Lift your head and look at the ceiling. Hold it. Don't let me push your head down."

Grading

Grade 5 (Normal): Patient completes available range of motion against maximum resistance.

Grade 4 (Good): Patient completes available range of motion against moderate resistance.

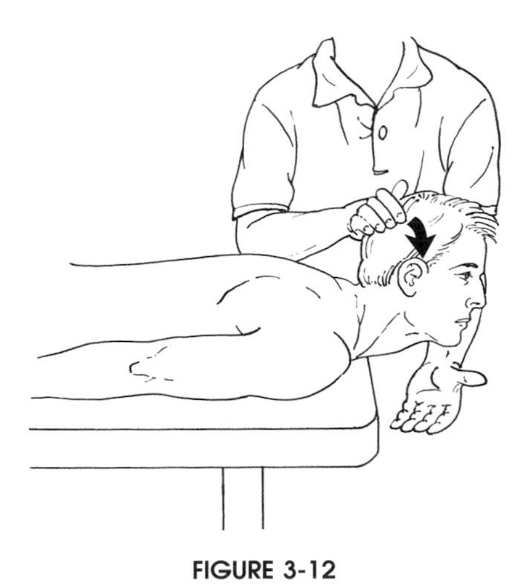

FIGURE 3-12

Grade 3 (Fair)

Position of Patient: Patient prone with head off end of table. Arms at sides.

Position of Therapist: Standing next to patient's head.

Test: Patient extends head and neck by raising head and looking up (Figure 3-13).

Instructions to Patient: "Raise your head from my hand and look up to the ceiling."

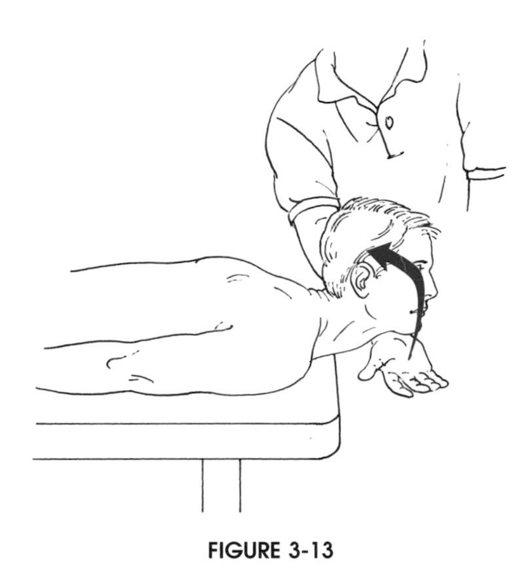

FIGURE 3-13

COMBINED NECK EXTENSION

(Capital plus Cervical)

Grading

Grade 3 (Fair): Patient completes available range of motion without resistance except that of gravity.

Alternate Test for Grade 3: This test is used when the patient has trunk or hip extensor weakness. The test is identical to the previous test except that stabilization of the upper back is provided by the therapist (Figure 3-14).

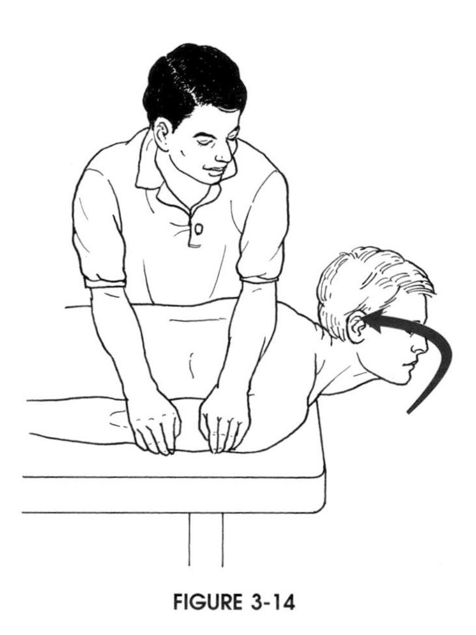

FIGURE 3-14

Helpful Hint

Extensor muscles on the right (or left) may be tested by having the patient rotate the head to the right (or left) and extend the head and neck.

Grade 2 (Poor), Grade 1 (Trace), and Grade 0 (Zero)

Position of Patient: Patient prone with head fully supported on table. Arms at sides.

Position of Therapist: Standing next to patient's upper trunk. Both hands on cervical region and base of occiput for palpation.

Test: Patient attempts to raise head and look up.

Instructions to Patient: "Try to raise your head off the table and look at the ceiling."

Grading

Grade 2 (Poor): Patient moves through partial range of motion.

Grade 1 (Trace): Palpable contractile activity in both capital and cervical extensor muscles, but no movement.

Grade 0 (Zero): No palpable activity in muscles.

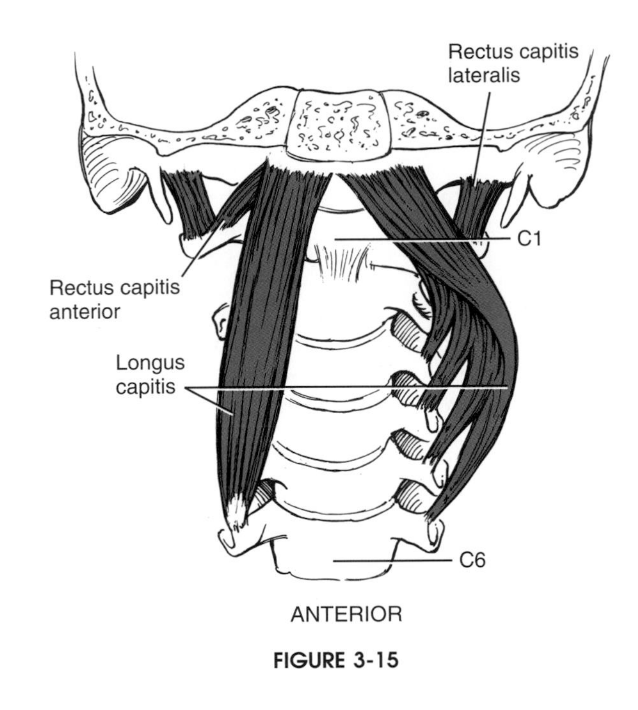

FIGURE 3-15

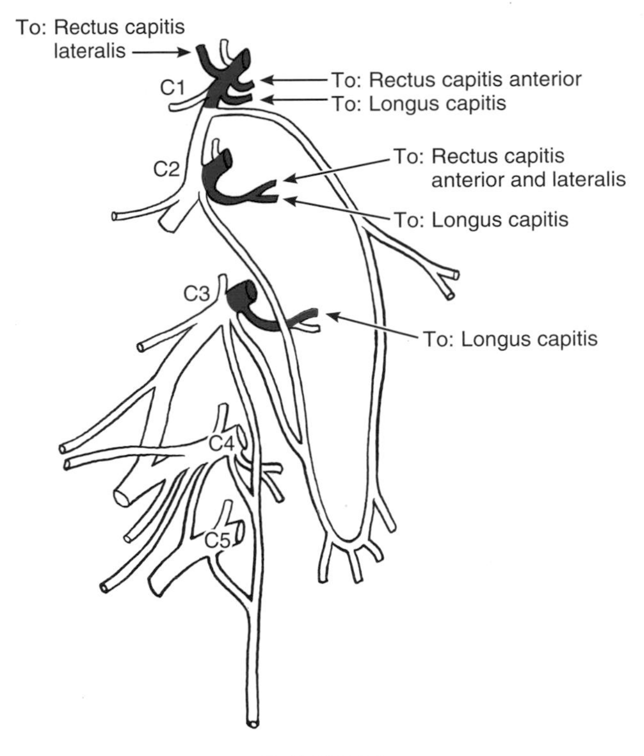

FIGURE 3-16

Range of Motion
0° to 10°-15°

Table 3-3 CAPITAL FLEXION

I.D.	Muscle	Origin	Insertion
72	Rectus capitis anterior	Atlas (C1) transverse process and lateral mass	Occiput (basilar part, inferior surface)
73	Rectus capitis lateralis	Atlas (transverse process)	Occiput (jugular process)
74	Longus capitis	C3-C6 vertebrae (transverse processes, anterior tubercles)	Occiput (basilar part, inferior surface)
Others			
Suprahyoids			
75	Mylohyoid		
76	Stylohyoid		
77	Geniohyoid		
78	Digastric		

All muscles that act on the head are inserted on the skull. Those that are anterior to the coronal midline are termed capital flexors. Their center of motion is in the atlanto-occipital or atlantoaxial joints.[2,3]

Starting Position of Patient: In all capital, cervical, and combined flexion tests, patient is supine with head supported on table and arms at sides (Figure 3-17). See Position of Patient and Helpful Hints (page 22).

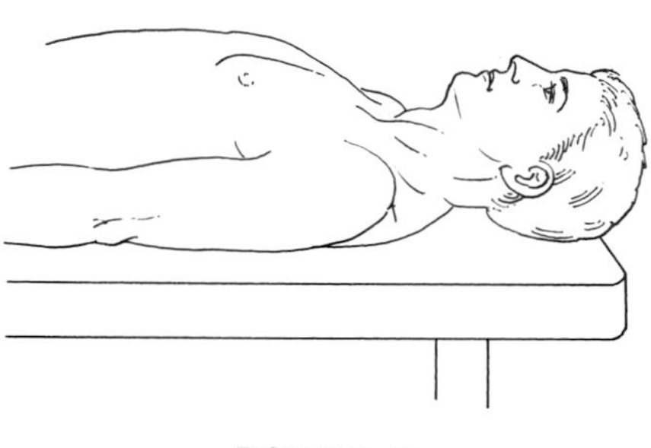

FIGURE 3-17

Grade 5 (Normal) and Grade 4 (Good)

Position of Patient: Supine with head on table. Arms at sides.

Position of Therapist: Standing at head of table facing patient. Both hands are cupped under the mandible to give resistance in an upward and backward direction (Figure 3-18).

Test: Patient tucks chin into neck without raising head from table. No motion should occur at the cervical spine. This is the downward motion of nodding.

Instructions to Patient: "Tuck your chin. Don't lift your head from the table. Hold it. Don't let me lift up your chin."

Grading

Grade 5 (Normal): Patient completes available range of motion against maximum resistance. These are very strong muscles.

Grade 4 (Good): Patient completes available range of motion against moderate resistance.

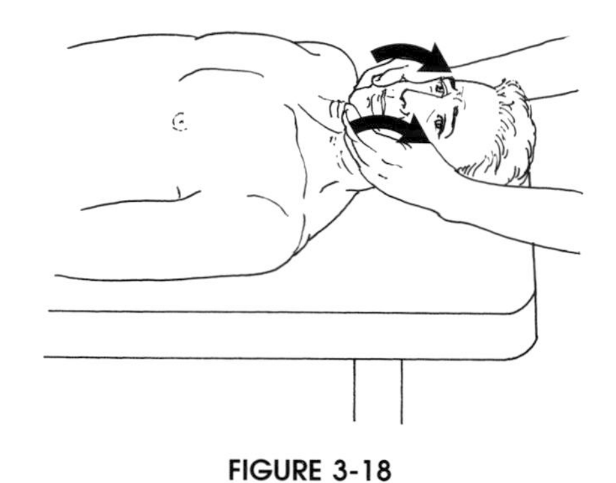

FIGURE 3-18

Grade 3 (Fair)

Position of Patient: Supine with head supported on table. Arms at sides.

Position of Therapist: Standing at head of table facing patient.

Test: Patient tucks chin without lifting head from table (Figure 3-19).

Instructions to Patient: "Tuck your chin into your neck. Do not raise your head from the table."

Grading

Grade 3 (Fair): Patient completes available range of motion with no resistance.

Grade 2 (Poor), Grade 1 (Trace), and Grade 0 (Zero)

Position of Patient: Supine with head supported on table. Arms at sides.

Position of Therapist: Standing at head of table facing patient.

Test: Patient attempts to tuck chin (Figure 3-20).

Instructions to Patient: "Try to tuck your chin into your neck."

Grading

Grade 2 (Poor): Patient completes partial range of motion.

Grade 1 (Trace): Contractile activity may be palpated in capital flexor muscles but it is difficult and only minimal pressure should be used.

Grade 0 (Zero): No contractile activity.

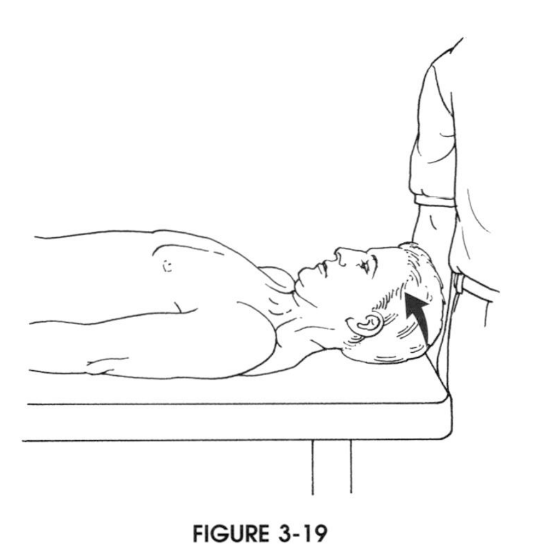

FIGURE 3-19

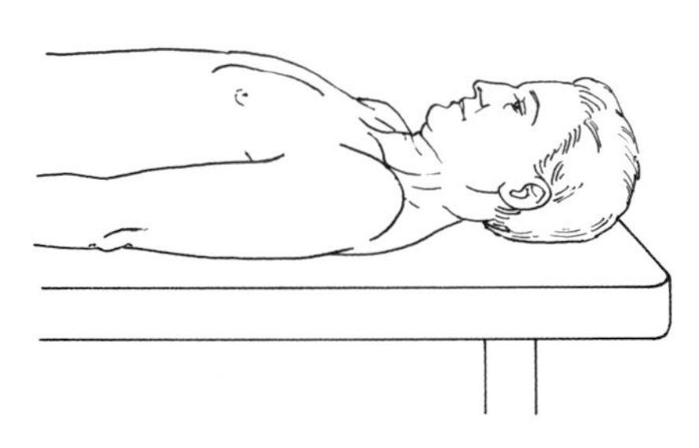

FIGURE 3-20

Helpful Hints

- Palpation of the small and deep muscles of capital flexion may be a difficult task unless the patient has severe atrophy. It is NOT recommended that much pressure be put on the neck in such attempts. Remember that the ascending arterial supply (carotids) to the brain runs quite superficially in this region.
- In patients with lower motor neuron lesions that do not affect the cranial nerves, capital flexion is seldom lost. This can possibly be attributed to the suprahyoid muscles, which are innervated by cranial nerves. Activity of the suprahyoid muscles can be identified by control of the floor of the mouth and the tongue as well as by the absence of impairment of swallowing or speech.[1]
- When capital flexion is impaired or absent, there usually is serious impairment of the cranial nerves, and other central nervous system (CNS) signs are present that may require further evaluation by the physical therapist.

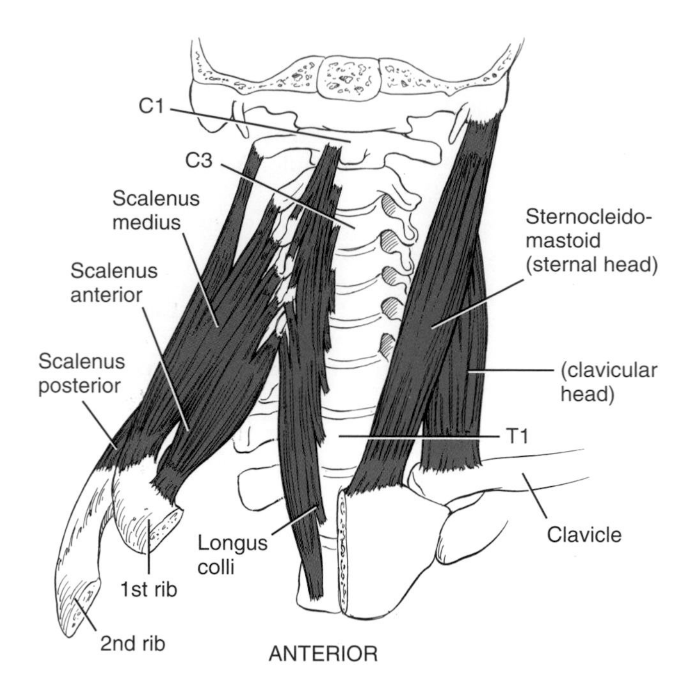

FIGURE 3-21

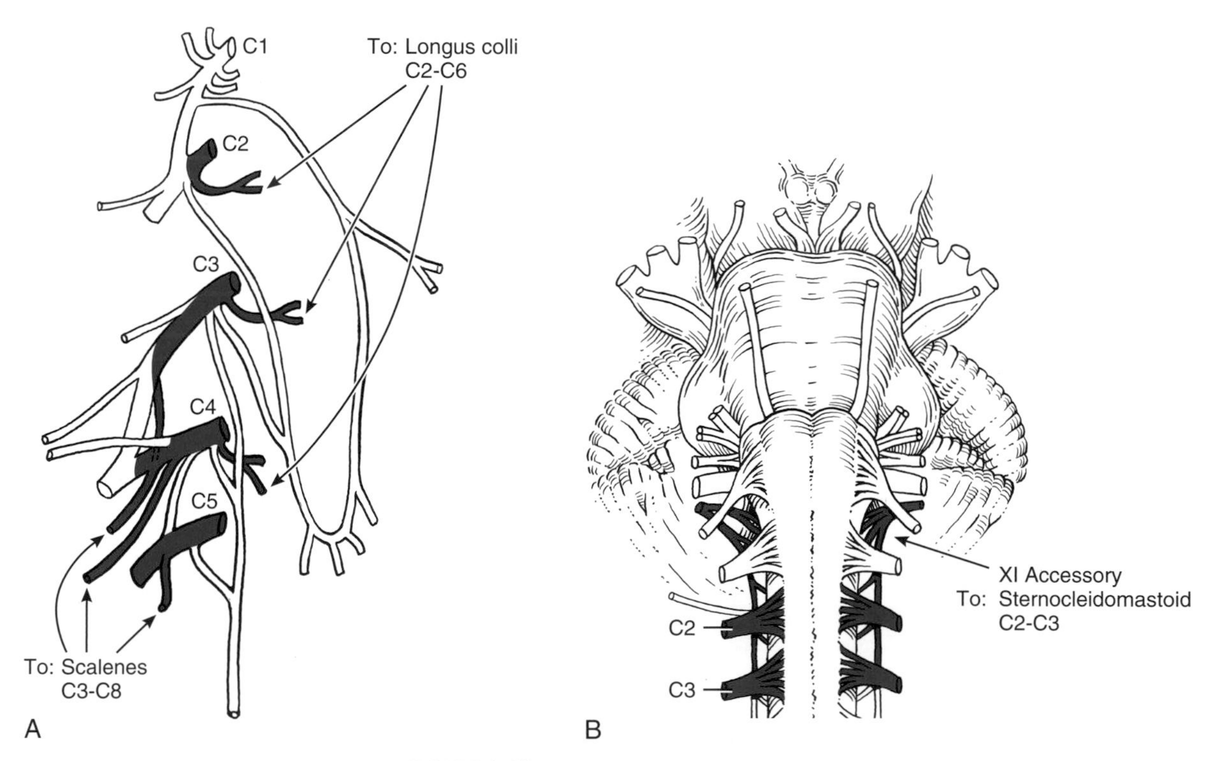

FIGURE 3-22

Range of Motion
0° to 35°-45° Note: Women have greater cervical lordosis than men, so it is likely that they will have a greater arc of motion.

Table 3-4 CERVICAL FLEXION

I.D.	Muscle	Origin	Insertion
83	Sternocleidomastoid		
	Sternal head	Sternum (Manubrium, upper anterior aspect)	Two heads blend in middle of neck; occiput (lateral half of superior nuchal line)
	Clavicular head	Clavicle (medial 1/3 superior and anterior surfaces)	Temporal bone (mastoid process)
79	Longus colli		
	Superior oblique head	C3-C5 vertebrae (transverse processes)	Atlas (anterior arch, tubercle)
	Vertical intermediate head	T1-T3 and C5-C7 vertebrae (anterolateral bodies)	C2-C4 vertebrae (anterior bodies)
	Inferior oblique head	T1-T3 vertebrae (anterior bodies)	C5-C6 vertebrae (transverse processes, anterior tubercles)
80	Scalenus anterior	C3-C6 vertebrae (transverse processes, anterior tubercles)	First rib (scalene tubercle)
Others			
81	Scalenus medius		
82	Scalenus posterior		
Infrahyoids			
84	Sternothyroid		
85	Thyrohyoid		
86	Sternohyoid		
87	Omohyoid		

The muscles of cervical flexion act only on the cervical spine with the center of motion in the lower cervical spine.[2,3]

Grade 5 (Normal) and Grade 4 (Good)

Position of Patient: Refer to starting position for all flexion tests. Supine with arms at side. Head supported on table.

Position of Therapist: Standing next to patient's head. Hand for resistance is placed on patient's forehead. Use two fingers only (Figure 3-23). Other hand may be placed on chest, but stabilization is needed only when the trunk is weak.

Test: Patient flexes neck by lifting head straight up from the table without tucking the chin. This is a weak muscle group.

Instructions to Patient: "Lift your head from the table; keep looking at the ceiling. Do not lift your shoulders off the table. Hold it. Don't let me push your head down."

Grading

Grade 5 (Normal): Patient completes available range of motion against moderate two-finger resistance.

Grade 4 (Good): Patient completes available range of motion against mild two-finger resistance.

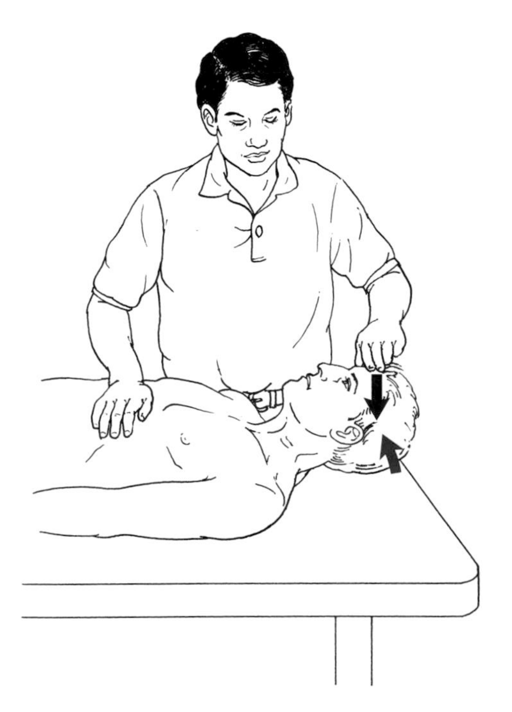

FIGURE 3-23

Grade 3 (Fair)

Positions of Patient and Therapist: Same as for previous test. No resistance is used on the forehead.

Test: Patient flexes neck, keeping eyes on the ceiling (Figure 3-24).

Instructions to Patient: "Bring your head off the table, keeping your eyes on the ceiling. Keep your shoulders completely on the table."

Grading

Grade 3 (Fair): Patient completes available range of motion.

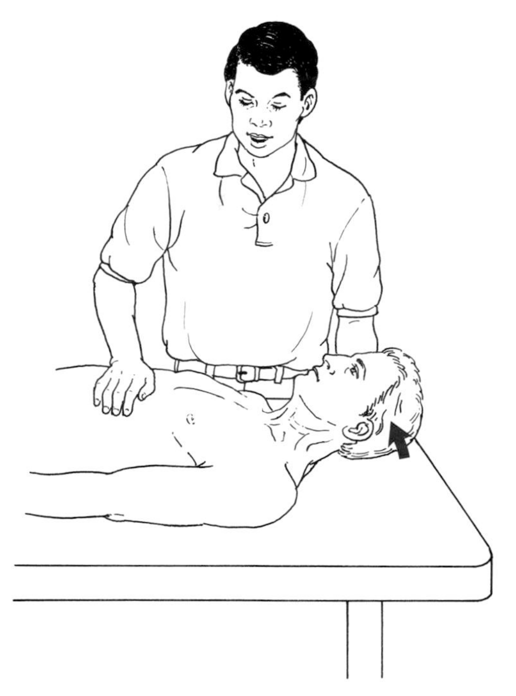

FIGURE 3-24

Grade 2 (Poor), Grade 1 (Trace), and Grade 0 (Zero)

Position of Patient: Supine with head supported on table. Arms at sides.

Position of Therapist: Standing at head of table facing patient. Fingers of both hands (or just the index finger) are placed over the sternocleidomastoid muscles to palpate them during test (Figure 3-25).

Test: Patient rolls head from side to side, keeping head supported on table.

Instructions to Patient: "Roll your head to the left and then to the right."

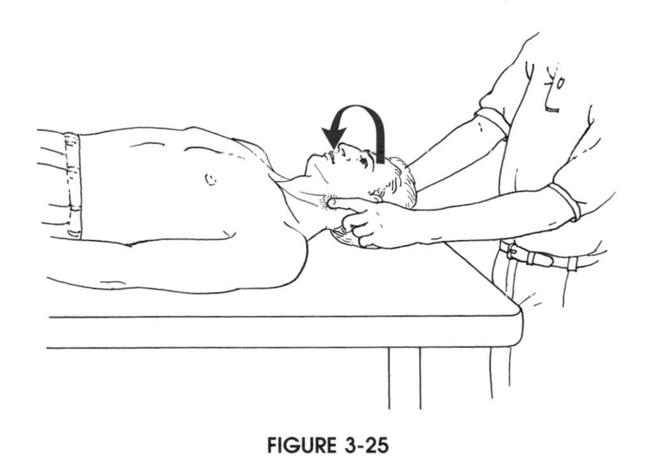

FIGURE 3-25

Grading

Grade 2 (Poor): Patient completes partial range of motion. The right sternocleidomastoid produces the roll to the left side and vice versa.

Grade 1 (Trace): No motion occurs, but contractile activity in one or both muscles can be detected.

Grade 0 (Zero): No motion and no contractile activity detected.

Substitution

The platysma may attempt to substitute for weak or absent sternocleidomastoid muscles during cervical or combined flexion. When this occurs, the corners of the mouth pull down; a grimacing expression or "What do I do now?" expression is seen. Superficial muscle activity will be apparent over the anterior surface of the neck, with skin wrinkling.

COMBINED CERVICAL FLEXION

(Capital plus Cervical)

Grade 5 (Normal) and Grade 4 (Good)

Position of Patient: Supine with head supported on table. Arms at sides.

Position of Therapist: Standing at side of table at level of shoulder. Hand placed on forehead of patient to give resistance (Figure 3-26). One arm may be used to provide stabilization of the thorax if there is trunk weakness. In such cases, the forearm is placed across the chest at the distal margin of the ribs. Although this arm does not offer resistance, considerable force may be required to maintain the trunk in a stable position. In a large patient, both arms may be required to provide such stabilization, the lower arm anchoring the pelvis. Therapist must use caution and not place too much weight or force over vulnerable nonbony areas like the abdomen.

Test: Patient flexes head and neck, bringing chin to chest.

Instructions to Patient: "Bring your head up until your chin is on your chest, and don't raise your shoulders. Hold it. Don't let me push it down."

Grading

Grade 5 (Normal): Patient completes available range of motion and tolerates strong resistance. (This combined flexion test is stronger than the capital or cervical component alone.)

Grade 4 (Good): Patient completes available range of motion and tolerates moderate resistance.

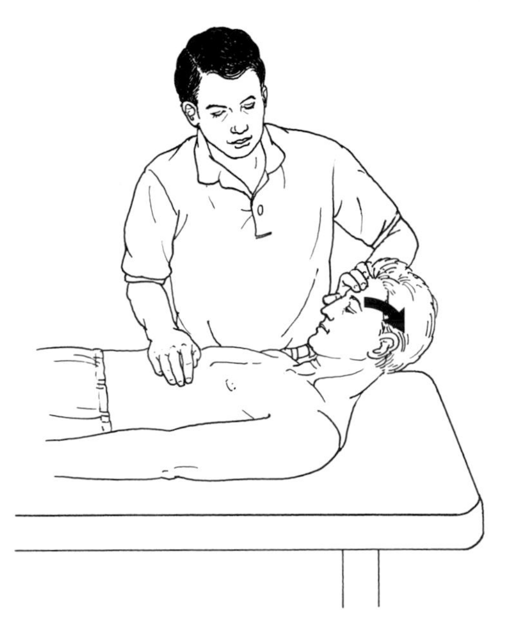

FIGURE 3-26

Grade 3 (Fair)

Position of Patient: Supine with head supported on table. Arms at sides.

Position of Therapist: Standing at side of table at about chest level. No resistance is given to the head motion. In the presence of trunk weakness, the thorax is stabilized.

Test: Patient flexes neck with chin tucked until the available range is completed (Figure 3-27).

Instructions to Patient: "Bring your chin up on your chest. Don't raise your shoulders."

Grading

Grade 3 (Fair): Patient completes available range of motion without resistance.

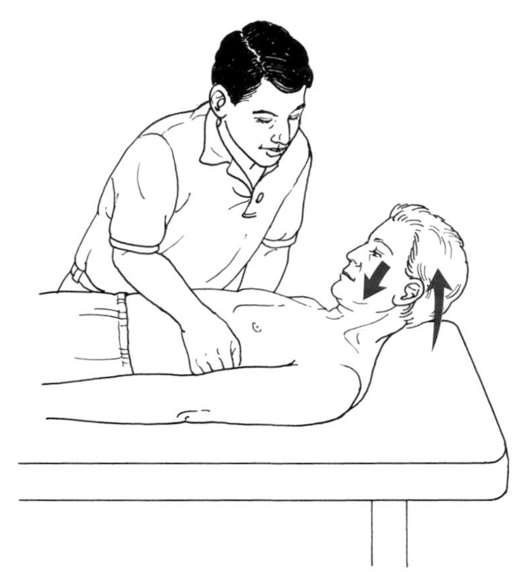

FIGURE 3-27

Grade 2 (Poor), Grade 1 (Trace), and Grade 0 (Zero)

Position of Patient: Supine with head fully supported on table. Arms at sides.

Position of Therapist: Standing at head of table facing the patient. Fingers of both hands or preferably just the index finger should be used to palpate the sternocleidomastoid muscles bilaterally.

Test: Patient attempts to roll the head from side to side. The sternocleidomastoid on one side rotates the head to the opposite side. Most of the capital flexors rotate the head to the same side.

Instructions to Patient: "Try to roll your head to the right and then back and all the way to the left."

Grading

Grade 2 (Poor): Patient completes partial range of motion.

Grade 1 (Trace): Muscle contractile activity palpated, but no motion occurs. Use considerable caution when palpating anterior neck.

Grade 0 (Zero): No palpable contractile activity.

Helpful Hints

If the capital flexor muscles are weak and the sternocleidomastoid is relatively strong, the latter muscle action will increase the extension of the cervical spine because its posterior insertion on the mastoid process makes it a weak extensor. This is true only if the capital flexors are not active enough to pre-fix the head in flexion. When the capital flexors are normal, they fix the spine in flexion, and the sternocleidomastoid functions in its flexor mode. If the capital flexors are weak, the head can be raised off the table, but it will be in a position of capital extension with the chin leading.

COMBINED FLEXION TO ISOLATE A SINGLE STERNOCLEIDOMASTOID

Range of Motion
0° to 45°-55°

This test should be performed when there is suspected or known asymmetry of strength in these neck flexor muscles.

Grade 5 (Normal), Grade 4 (Good), and Grade 3 (Fair)

Position of Patient: Supine with head supported on table and turned to the left (to test right sternocleidomastoid).

Position of Therapist: Standing at head of table facing patient. One hand is placed on the temporal area above the ear for resistance (Figure 3-28).

Test: Patient raises head from table.

Instructions to Patient: "Lift up your head, keeping your head turned."

Grading

Grade 5 (Normal): Patient completes available range of motion and takes strong resistance. This is usually a very strong muscle group.

Grade 4 (Good): Patient completes available range of motion and takes moderate resistance.

Grade 3 (Fair): Patient completes available range of motion with no resistance (Figure 3-29).

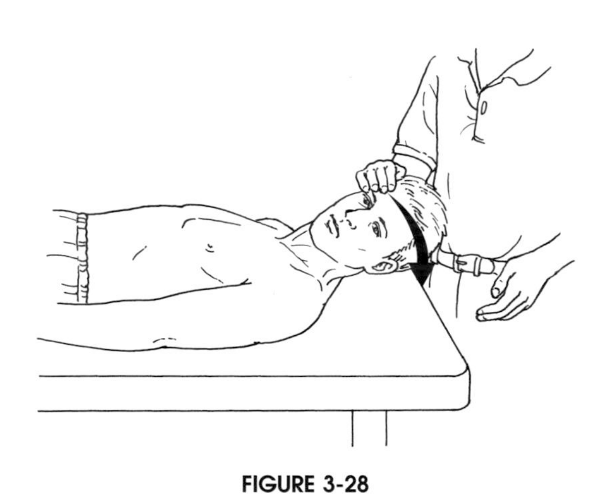

FIGURE 3-28

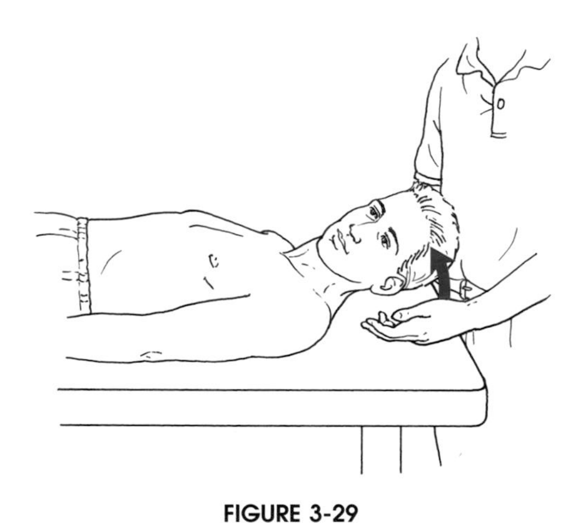

FIGURE 3-29

Grade 2 (Poor), Grade 1 (Trace), and Grade 0 (Zero)

Position of Patient: Supine with head supported on table.

Position of Therapist: Standing at head of table facing patient. Fingers are placed along the side of the head and neck so that they (or just the index finger) can palpate the sternocleidomastoid (see Figure 3-25).

Test: Patient attempts to roll head from side to side.

Instructions to Patient: "Roll your head to the right and then to the left."

Grading

Grade 2 (Poor): Patient completes partial range of motion.

Grade 1 (Trace): Palpable contractile activity in the sternocleidomastoid, but no movement.

Grade 0 (Zero): No palpable contractile activity.

Grade 5 (Normal), Grade 4 (Good), and Grade 3 (Fair)

Position of Patient: Supine with cervical spine in neutral (flexion and extension). Head supported on table with face turned as far to one side as possible. Sitting is an alternative position for all tests.

Position of Therapist: Standing at head of table facing patient. Hand for resistance is placed over the side of head above ear (Grades 5 and 4 only).

Test: Patient rotates head to neutral against maximum resistance. This is a strong muscle group. Repeat for rotators on the opposite side. Alternatively, have patient rotate from left side of face on table to right side of face on table.

Instructions to Patient: "Turn your head and face the ceiling. Hold it. Do not let me turn your head back."

Grading

Grade 5 (Normal): Patient rotates head through full available range of motion to both right and left against maximum resistance.

Grade 4 (Good): Patient rotates head through full available range of motion to both right and left against moderate resistance.

Grade 3 (Fair): Patient rotates head through full available range of motion to both right and left without resistance.

Grade 2 (Poor), Grade 1 (Trace), and Grade 0 (Zero)

Position of Patient: Sitting. Trunk and head may be supported against a high-back chair. Head posture neutral.

Position of Therapist: Standing directly in front of patient.

Test: Patient tries to rotate head from side to side, keeping the neck in neutral (chin neither down nor up).

Instructions to Patient: "Turn your head as far to the left as you can. Keep your chin level." Repeat for turn to right.

Grading

Grade 2 (Poor): Patient completes partial range of motion.

Grade 1 (Trace): Contractile activity in sternocleidomastoid or posterior muscles visible or evident by palpation. No movement.

Grade 0 (Zero): No palpable contractile activity.

Participating Muscles in Cervical Rotation (with reference numbers)

56. Rectus capitis posterior major
59. Obliquus capitis inferior
60. Longissimus capitis
61. Splenius capitis
62. Semispinalis capitis
65. Semispinalis cervicis
67. Splenius cervicis
71. Rotatores cervicis
74. Longus capitis
79. Longus colli (Inferior oblique)
80. Scalenus anterior
81. Scalenus medius
82. Scalenus posterior
83. Sternocleidomastoid
124. Trapezius
127. Levator scapulae

REFERENCES

Cited References

1. Perry J, Nickel VL. Total cervical spine fusion for neck paralysis. J Bone Joint Surg Am. 1959;41:37-60.
2. Fielding JW. Cineroentgenography of the normal cervical spine. J Bone Joint Surg Am. 1957;39:1280-1288.
3. Ferlic D. The range of motion of the "normal" cervical spine. Johns Hopkins Hosp Bull. 1962;110:59.

Other Readings

Bible JE, Biswas D, Miller CP, et al. Normal functional range of motion of the cervical spine during 15 activities of daily living. J Spinal Disord Tech. 2010;23:15-21.

Buford JA, Yoder SM, Heiss DG, et al. Actions of the scalene muscles for rotation of the cervical spine in macaque and human. J Orthop Sports Phys Ther. 2002;32:488-496.

Chan WC, Sze KL, Samartzis D, et al. Structure and biology of the intervertebral disk in health and disease. Orthop Clin North Am. 2011;42:447-464, vii. Review.

Cattrysse E, Provyn S, Kool P, et al. Morphology and kinematics of the atlanto-axial joints and their interaction during manual cervical rotation mobilization. Man Ther. 2011;16(5):481-486.

Dugailly PM, Sobczak S, Moiseev F, et al. Musculoskeletal modeling of the suboccipital spine: kinematics analysis, muscle lengths, and muscle moment arms during axial rotation and flexion extension. Spine. 2011;36:E413-E422.

Eriksson PO, Zafar H, Nordh E. Concomitant mandibular and head-neck movements during jaw opening-closing in man. J Oral Rehabil. 1998;25:859-870.

Falla D, Jull G, Dall'Alba P, et al. An electromyographic analysis of the deep cervical flexor muscles in performance of craniocervical flexion. Phys Ther. 2003;83:899-906.

Morishita Y, Falakassa J, Naito M, et al. The kinematic relationships of the upper cervical spine. Spine. 2009;34:2642-2645.

Okada E, Matsumoto M, Ichihara D, et al. Aging of the cervical spine in healthy volunteers: a 10-year longitudinal magnetic resonance imaging study. Spine. 2009;34:706-712.

Okada E, Matsumoto M, Ichihara D, et al. Cross-sectional area of posterior extensor muscles of the cervical spine in asymptomatic subjects: a 10-year longitudinal magnetic resonance imaging study. Eur Spine J. 2011;20:1567-1573.

Raybaud C. Anatomy and development of the craniovertebral junction. Neurol Sci. 2011;32 Suppl 3:S267-S270. Review.

Reynolds J, Marsh D, Koller H, et al. Cervical range of movement in relation to neck dimension. Eur Spine J. 2009;18:863-868.

Stemper BD, Pintar FA, Rao RD. The influence of morphology on cervical injury characteristics. Spine. 2011;36(25 Suppl):S180-S186. Review.

Takebe K, Vitti M, Basmajian JV. The functions of semispinalis capitis and splenius capitis muscles: an electromyographic study. Anat Rec. 1974;179:477-480.

Zafar H, Nordh E, Eriksson PO. Temporal coordination between mandibular and head-neck movements during jaw opening-closing tasks in man. Arch Oral Biol. 2000;45:675-682.

Wilke HJ, Zanker D, Wolfram U. Internal morphology of human facet joints: comparing cervical and lumbar spine with regard to age, gender and the vertebral core. J Anat. 2012;220:233-241.

CHAPTER 4

Testing the Muscles of the Trunk and Pelvic Floor

TRUNK EXTENSION

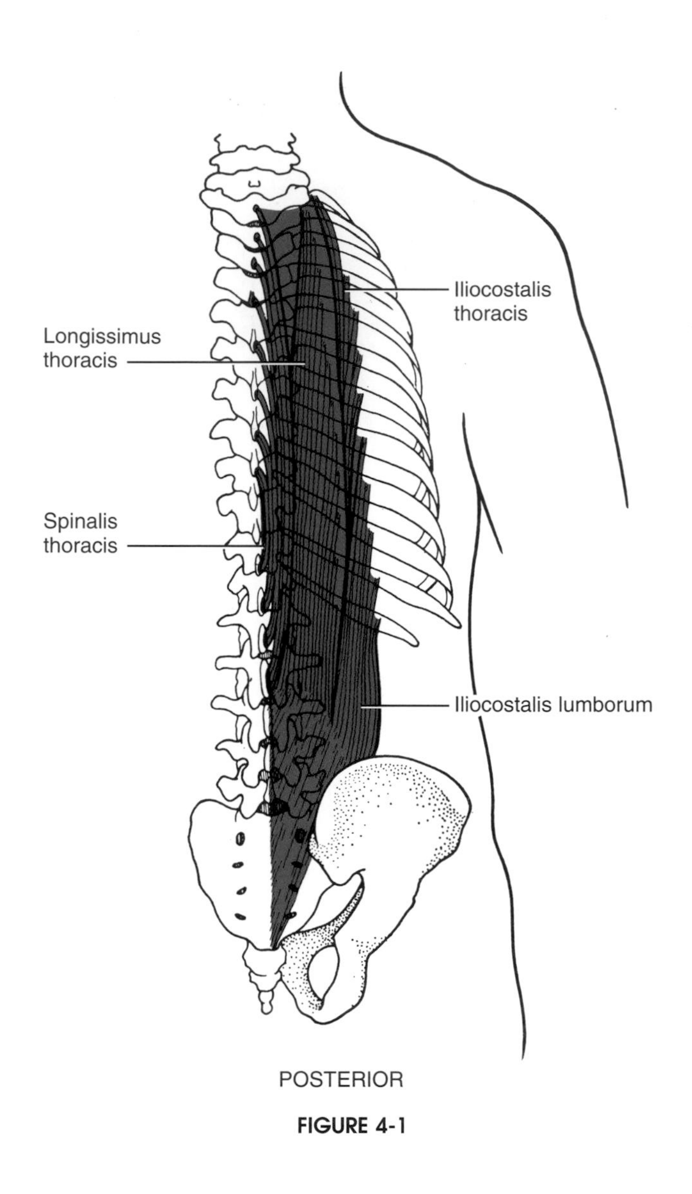

FIGURE 4-1

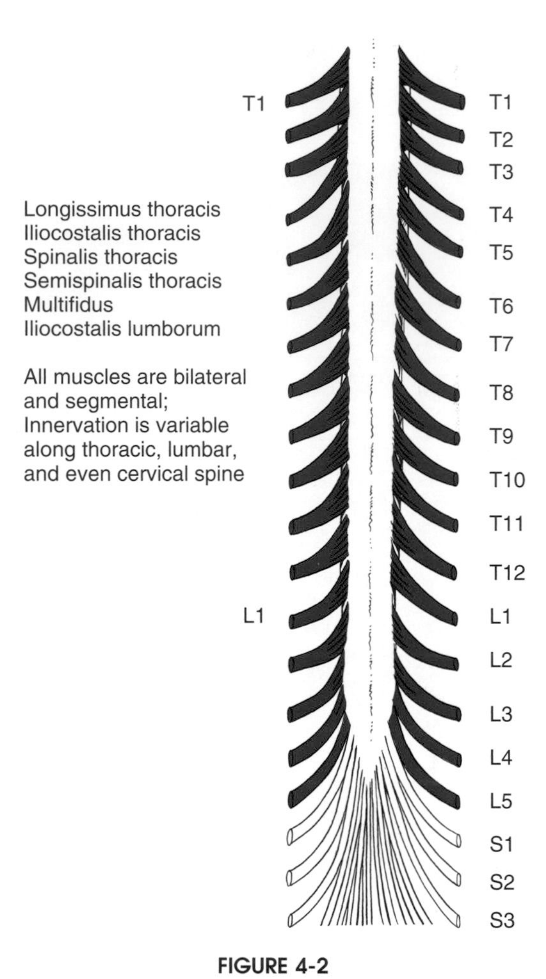

FIGURE 4-2

Range of Motion
Thoracic spine: 0° to 10° Lumbar spine: 0° to 25°

Table 4-1 TRUNK EXTENSION

I.D.	Muscle	Origin	Insertion
89	Iliocostalis thoracis	Ribs 12 up to 7 (angles)	Ribs 6 up to 1 (angles) C7 vertebra (transverse processes)
90	Iliocostalis lumborum	Tendon of erector spinae (anterior surface) Thoracolumbar fascia Sacrum (posterior surface)	Ribs 6-12 (angles)
91	Longissimus thoracis	Tendon of erector spinae Thoracolumbar fascia L1-L5 vertebrae (transverse processes)	T1-T12 vertebrae (transverse processes) Ribs 2-12 (between angles and tubercles)
92	Spinalis thoracis (often indistinct)	Common tendon of erector spinae T11-L2 vertebrae (spinous processes)	T1-T4 vertebrae (or to T8, spinous processes) Blends with semispinalis thoracis
93	Semispinalis thoracis	T6-T10 vertebrae (transverse processes)	C6-T4 vertebrae (spinous processes)
94	Multifidi	Sacrum (posterior) Erector spinae (aponeurosis) Ilium (PSIS) and crest Sacroiliac ligaments L1-L5 vertebrae (mamillary processes) T1-T12 vertebrae (transverse processes) C4-C7 vertebrae (articular processes)	Spinous processes of higher vertebra (may span 2-4 vertebrae before inserting)
95, 96	Rotatores thoracis and lumborum (11 pairs)	Thoracic and lumbar vertebrae (transverse processes; variable in lumbar area)	Next highest vertebra (lower border of lamina)
97, 98	Interspinales thoracis and lumborum	Thoracis: (3 pairs) between spinous processes of contiguous vertebrae (T1-T2; T2-T3; T11-T12) Lumborum: (4 pairs) lie between the 5 lumbar vertebrae; run between spinous processes	See origin
99	Intertransversarii thoracis and lumborum	Thoracis: (3 pairs) between transverse processes of contiguous vertebrae T10-T12 and L1 Lumborum: medial muscles; accessory process of superior vertebra to mamillary process of vertebra below Lateral muscles: fill space between transverse processes of adjacent vertebrae	See origin
100	Quadratus lumborum	Ilium (crest and inner lip) Iliolumbar ligament	12th rib (lower border) L1-L4 vertebrae (transverse processes) T12 vertebra (body)
Other			
182	Gluteus maximus (provides stable base for trunk extension by stabilizing pelvis)		

LUMBAR SPINE

Grade 5 (Normal) and Grade 4 (Good)

Note: The Grades 5 and 4 tests for spine extension are different for the lumbar and thoracic spines. Beginning at Grade 3, the tests for both spinal levels are combined.

Position of Patient: Prone with hands clasped behind head.

Position of Therapist: Standing so as to stabilize the lower extremities just above the ankles if the patient has Grade 5 hip extensor strength (Figure 4-3).

Alternate Position: Therapist stabilizes the lower extremities using body weight and both arms placed across the pelvis if the patient has hip extension weakness. It is very difficult to stabilize the pelvis adequately in the presence of significant hip weakness (Figure 4-4).

Test: Patient extends the lumbar spine until the entire trunk is raised from the table (clears umbilicus).

Instructions to Patient: "Raise your head, shoulders, and chest off the table. Come up as high as you can."

Grading

Grade 5 (Normal) and Grade 4 (Good): The therapist distinguishes between Grade 5 and Grade 4 muscles by the nature of the response (see Figures 4-3 and 4-4). The Grade 5 muscle holds like a lock; the Grade 4 muscle yields slightly because of an elastic quality at the end point. The patient with Grade 5 back extensor muscles can quickly come to the end position and hold that position without evidence of significant effort. The patient with Grade 4 back extensors can come to the end position but may waver or display some signs of effort.

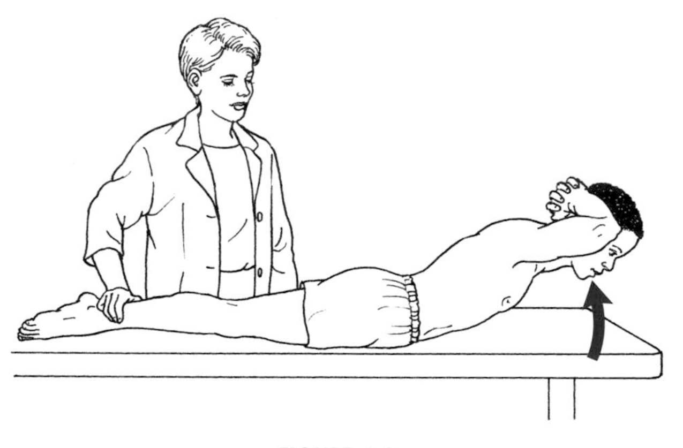

FIGURE 4-3

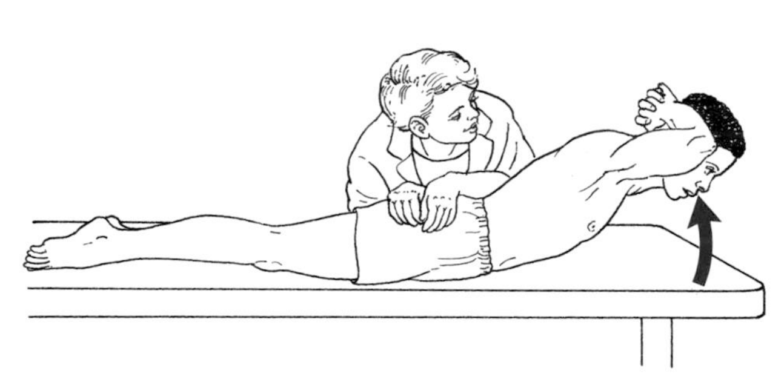

FIGURE 4-4

Alternative Grade 5 Sorensen Lumbar Spine Extension Test

The Biering-Sorensen test or Sorensen test is a global measure of back extension endurance capacity.[1]

Position of Patient: Prone with the trunk flexed off the end of the table at a level between the anterior superior iliac spine (ASIS) and umbilicus. The arms are folded across the chest. The pelvis, hips, and legs are stabilized on the table (Figure 4-5).

Position of Therapist: Kneeling above patient so as to stabilize the lower limbs and pelvis at the ankles.

Test: Patient lifts the trunk to the horizontal and maintains the position as long as possible. The therapist uses a stopwatch to time the effort, activating it at the "begin" command and stopping it when the patient shows obvious signs of fatigue and begins to falter.[1]

Instructions to Patient: "When I say 'begin,' raise your head, chest, and trunk from the table and hold the position as long as you can. I will be timing you. Let me know if you have any back pain."

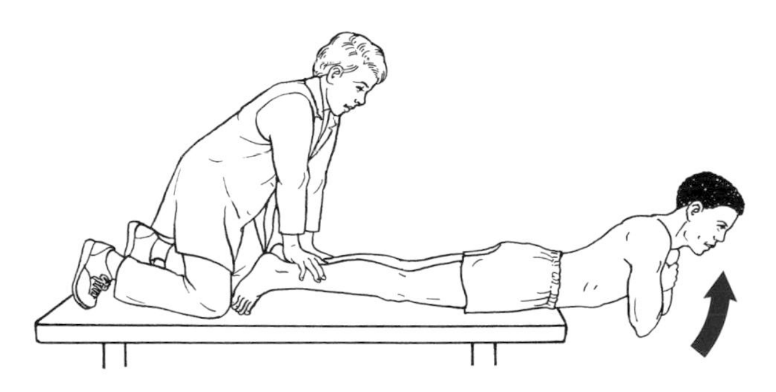

FIGURE 4-5

Helpful Hints

- Low levels of endurance of back muscles are reported as cause and effect of low back pain.[2]
- The Sorensen test has been validated as a differential diagnostic test for low back pain.[3,4] Individuals with low back pain have significantly lower hold times than those without low back pain. In subjects with low back pain, the mean endurance time ranges from 39.55 to 54.5 seconds in mixed-gender groups (compared with 80 to 194 seconds for men and 146 to 227 seconds for women without pain).[2]
- The mean endurance time for all subjects (with and without low back pain) in one study was 113 ± 46 seconds.[2] Men had higher mean endurance than women.
- Because average endurance times have not been established for older individuals, caution should be exercised when testing individuals aged 60 years and older.
- A significant difference was found in the endurance time across the age groups,[2] indicating that a decrease in endurance time should be expected with increasing age. Some age-based norms are listed in Table 4-2.
- More recent data suggest that normative values vary by specific populations and by specific anthropomorphic characteristics such as body mass index and torso length.[2,5]
- The multifidus demonstrates more electromyogram (EMG) activity and faster fatigue rates than the iliocostalis lumborum.[6]

Table 4-2 AGE-BASED NORMS FOR SORENSEN TEST

Age	Mean Hold Time in Seconds (SD)* Males	Mean Hold Time in Seconds (SD) Females
19-29	140[5]	130[5]
30-39	140[5]	120
35-39	97 (43)[2]	93 (55)[2]
40-44	101 (57)[2]	80 (55)[2]
40-49	110[5]	90[5]
45-49	99 (58)[2]	102 (64)[2]
50-54	89 (55)[2]	69 (60)[2]
50-59	90[5]	80[5]
60+	80[5]	90[5]

*Numbers in parentheses refer to standard deviation (SD). The standard deviation is only available for some age groups.
[2]Data from 508 subjects with and without back pain that comprised equal groups of blue and white collar male and female subjects. Modified Sorensen test performed (arms at sides).
[5]Data from 561 healthy, nonsmoking subjects in Nigeria without low back pain, performing a modified Sorensen test (arms at sides).

THORACIC SPINE

Grade 5 (Normal) and Grade 4 (Good)

Position of Patient: Prone with head and upper trunk extending off the table from about the nipple line (Figure 4-6).

Position of Therapist: Standing so as to stabilize the lower limbs at the ankle.

Test: Patient extends thoracic spine to the horizontal.

Instructions to Patient: "Raise your head, shoulders, and chest to table level."

Grading

Grade 5 (Normal): Patient is able to raise the upper trunk quickly from its forward flexed position to the horizontal (or beyond) with ease and no sign of exertion (Figure 4-7).

Grade 4 (Good): Patient is able to raise the trunk to the horizontal level but does it somewhat laboriously.

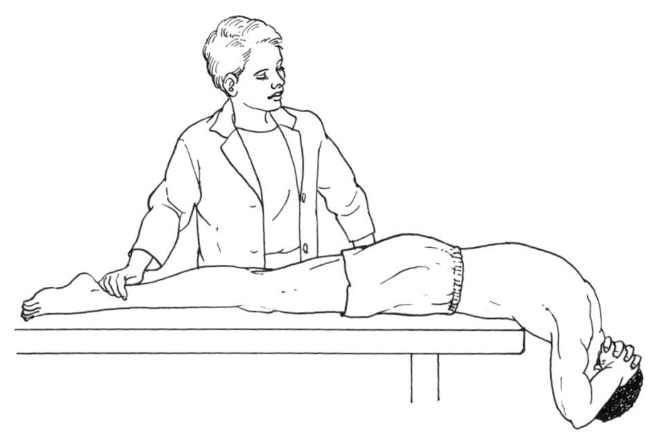

FIGURE 4-6

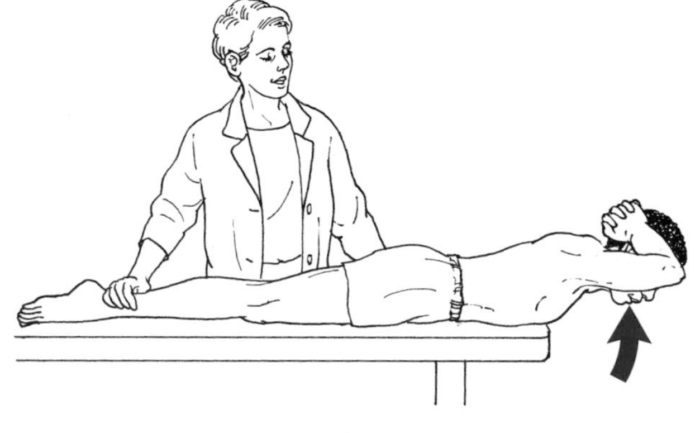

FIGURE 4-7

LUMBAR AND THORACIC SPINE

Grade 3 (Fair)

Position of Patient: Prone with arms at sides.

Position of Therapist: Standing at side of table. Lower extremities are stabilized just above the ankles.

Test: Patient extends spine, raising body from the table so that the umbilicus clears the table (Figure 4-8).

Instructions to Patient: "Raise your head, arms, and chest from the table as high as you can."

Grading

Grade 3 (Fair): Patient completes the range of motion.

Grade 2 (Poor), Grade 1 (Trace), and Grade 0 (Zero)

These tests are identical to the Grade 3 test except that the therapist must palpate the lumbar and thoracic spine extensor muscle masses adjacent to both sides of the spine. The individual muscles cannot be isolated (Figures 4-9 and 4-10).

Grading

Grade 2 (Poor): Patient completes partial range of motion.

Grade 1 (Trace): Contractile activity is detectable but no movement.

Grade 0 (Zero): No contractile activity.

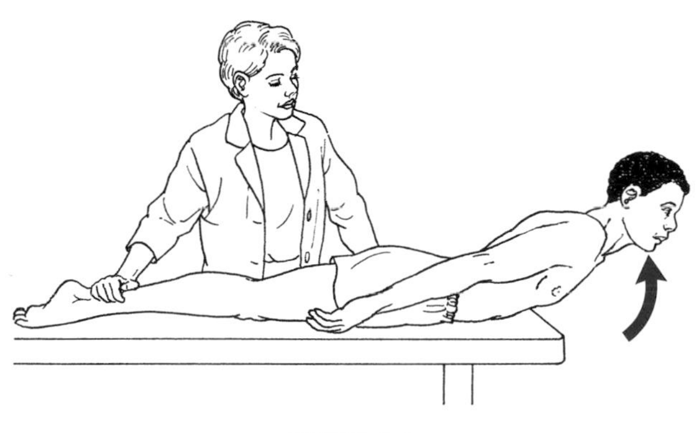

FIGURE 4-8

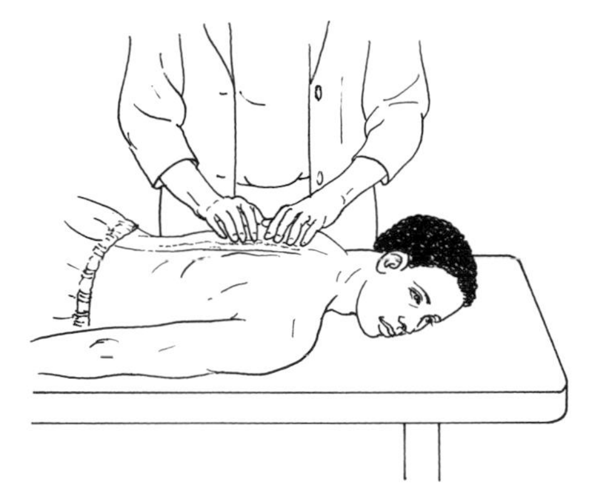

FIGURE 4-10

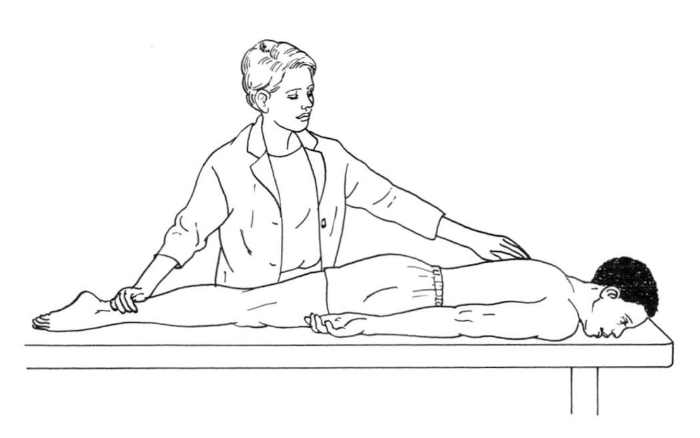

FIGURE 4-9

Helpful Hints

- Tests for hip extension and neck extension should precede tests for trunk extension.
- When the spine extensors are weak and the hip extensors are strong, the patient will be unable to raise the upper trunk from the table. Instead, the pelvis will tilt posteriorly while the lumbar spine moves into flexion (low back flattens).
- If the hip extensor muscles are Grade 4 or better, it may be helpful to use belts to anchor hips to the table, especially if the patient is much larger or stronger than the testing therapist.
- When the back extensors are strong and the hip extensors are weak, the patient can hyperextend the low back (increased lordosis) but will be unable to raise the trunk without very strong stabilization of the pelvis by the therapist.
- If the neck extensors are weak, the therapist may need to support the head as the patient raises the trunk.
- The position of the arms in external rotation and fingertips lightly touching the side of the head provides added resistance for Grades 5 and 4; the weight of the head and arms essentially substitutes for manual resistance by the therapist.
- If the patient is unable to provide stabilization through the weight of the legs and pelvis (such as in paraplegia or amputee), the test should be done on a mat table. Position the subject with both legs and pelvis off the mat. This allows the pelvis and limbs to contribute to stabilization, and the therapist holding the lower trunk has a chance to provide the necessary support. (If a mat table is not available, an assistant will be required, and the lower body may rest on a chair.)
- The Modified Sorensen test is the Sorensen test but performed with arms at the patient's sides.

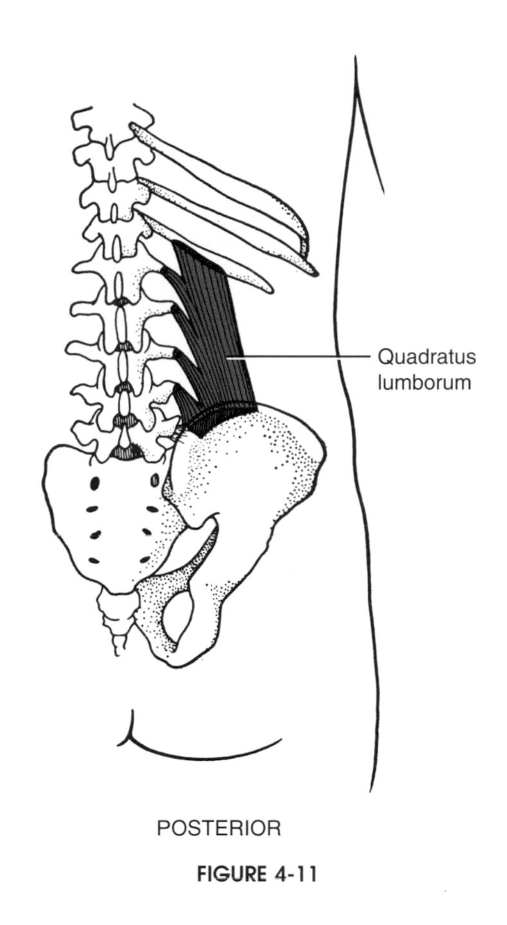

FIGURE 4-11

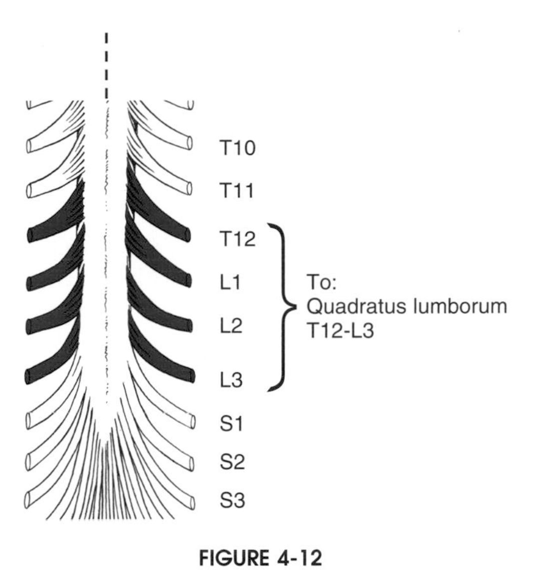

FIGURE 4-12

Range of Motion

Approximates pelvis to lower ribs; range not precise

Table 4-3 ELEVATION OF THE PELVIS

I.D.	Muscle	Origin	Insertion
100	Quadratus lumborum	Ilium (crest and inner lip) Iliolumbar ligament	Rib 12 (lower border) L1-L4 vertebrae (transverse processes, apex) T12 vertebra (body; occasionally)
110	Obliquus externus abdominis	Ribs 5-12 (interdigitating on external and inferior surfaces)	Iliac crest (outer border) Aponeurosis from 9th costal cartilage to ASIS; both sides meet at midline to form linea alba Pubic symphysis (upper border)
111	Obliquus internus abdominis	Iliac crest (anterior 2/3 of intermediate line) Thoracolumbar fascia Inguinal ligament (lateral 2/3 of upper aspect)	Ribs 9-12 (inferior border and cartilages by digitations that appear continuous with internal intercostals) Ribs 7-9 (cartilages) Aponeurosis to linea alba
Others			
130	Latissimus dorsi (arms fixed)		
90	Iliocostalis lumborum		

Grade 5 (Normal) and Grade 4 (Good)

Position of Patient: Supine or prone with hip and lumbar spine in extension. The patient grasps edges of the table to provide stabilization during resistance (not illustrated).

Position of Therapist: Standing at foot of table facing patient. Therapist grasps test limb with both hands just above the ankle and pulls caudally with a smooth, even pull (Figure 4-13). Resistance is given as in traction.

Test: Patient hikes the pelvis on one side, thereby approximating the pelvic rim to the inferior margin of the rib cage.

Instructions to Patient: "Hike your pelvis to bring it up to your ribs. Hold it. Don't let me pull your leg down."

Grading

Grade 5 (Normal): This motion, certainly not attributed solely to the quadratus lumborum, is one that tolerates a huge amount of resistance that is not readily broken when the muscles involved are Grade 5.

Grade 4 (Good): Patient tolerates very strong resistance. Testing this movement requires more than a bit of clinical judgment.

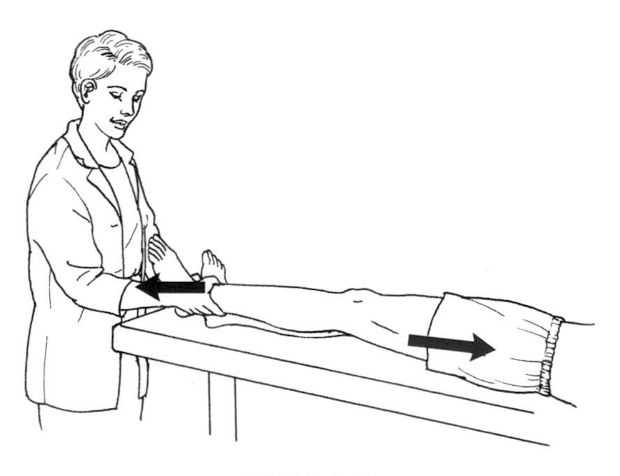

FIGURE 4-13

Grade 3 (Fair) and Grade 2 (Poor)

Position of Patient: Supine or prone. Hip in extension; lumbar spine neutral or extended.

Position of Therapist: Standing at foot of table facing patient. One hand supports the leg just above the ankle; the other is under the knee so the limb is slightly off the table to decrease friction (Figure 4-14).

Test: Patient hikes the pelvis unilaterally to bring the rim of the pelvis closer to the inferior ribs.

Instructions to Patient: "Bring your pelvis up to your ribs."

Grading

Grade 3 (Fair): Patient completes available range of motion.

Grade 2 (Poor): Patient completes partial range of motion.

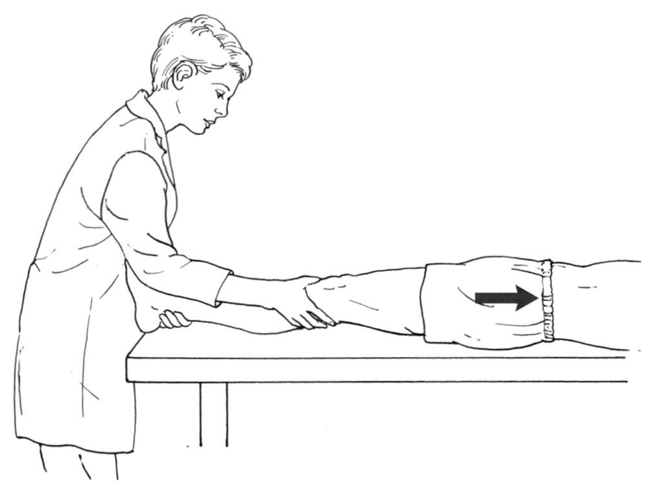

FIGURE 4-14

Grade 1 (Trace) and Grade 0 (Zero)

These grades should be avoided to ensure clinical accuracy. The principal muscle involved in pelvic elevation, the quadratus lumborum, lies deep to the paraspinal muscle mass and can rarely be palpated. In people who have extensive truncal atrophy, paraspinal muscle activity may be palpated, and possibly, but not necessarily convincingly, the quadratus lumborum can be palpated.

Substitution

The patient may attempt to substitute with trunk lateral flexion, primarily using the abdominal muscles. The spinal extensors may be used without the quadratus lumborum. In neither case can manual testing detect an inactive quadratus lumborum.

Helpful Hints

- The quadratus lumborum hikes the ipsilateral hip when the spine is fixed.
- It should be noted that the quadratus lumborum may have functions other than hip hiking, such as maintaining upright posture, though these functions have been less well studied. Quadratus lumborum strength has also been linked to low back pain and thus may deserve closer analysis.[6]

Side Bridge Endurance Test

Quadratus lumborum oblique and transverse muscles are elicited without generating large compression forces on the lumbar spine.[7,8]

Position of Patient: Side-lying with legs extended, resting on the lower forearm with the elbow flexed to 90°. Upper arm is crossed over chest.

Position of Therapist: Standing or sitting in front of patient holding a stopwatch. Patient is given feedback regarding posture; the hips and trunk should be level throughout the test (Figure 4-15).

Test: Patient lifts hip off the table, holding the elevated position in a straight line with the body on a flexed elbow. This position is maintained until the patient loses posture form, fatigues, or complains of pain. The therapist times the effort.

Instructions to the Patient: "When I say 'go!' lift your hip off the table, keeping it in a straight line with your body for as long as you can. I will be timing you."

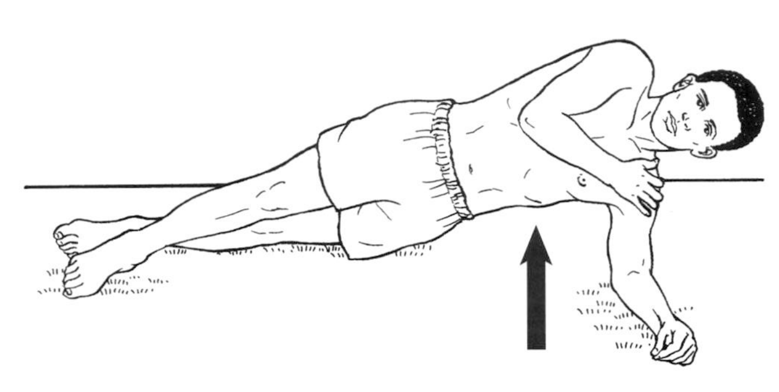

FIGURE 4-15

Helpful Hint

Despite the high reliability of the side bridge test, significant changes in hold times must be observed to confidently assess a true change in strength. Therefore, the patient's rating of perceived exertion (RPE) would help inform clinical decision making.[9] Mean hold times range from 20 to 203 seconds (mean 104.8 seconds) for the right side bridge test and from 19 to 251 seconds (mean of 103.0 seconds) for the left side bridge test.[9] Males demonstrated longer endurance times than females.

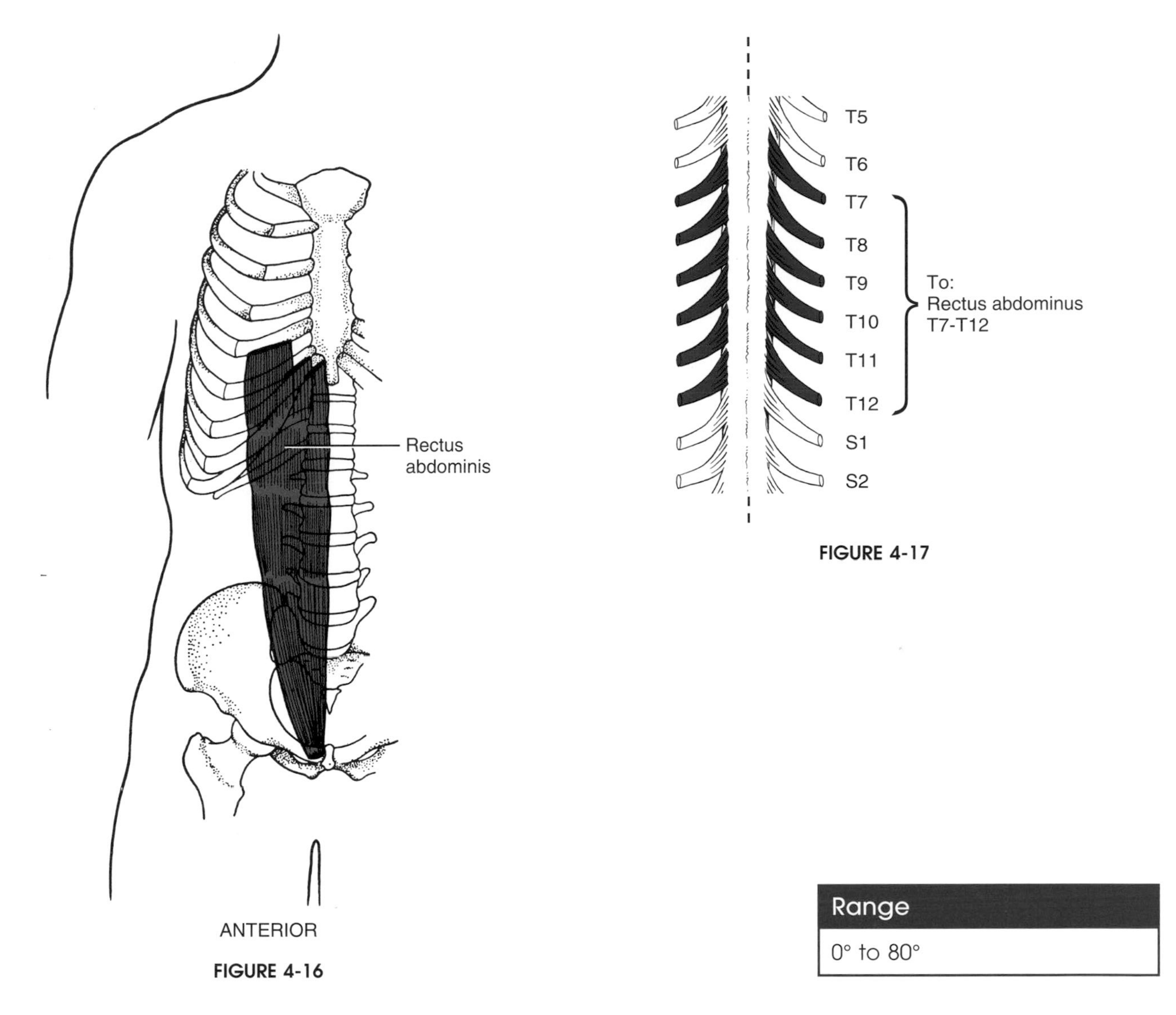

FIGURE 4-16

FIGURE 4-17

Range
0° to 80°

Table 4-4 TRUNK FLEXION

I.D.	Muscle	Origin	Insertion
113	Rectus abdominis (paired muscle)	Pubis Lateral fibers (tubercle on crest and pecten pubis) Medial fibers (ligamentous covering of symphysis attaches to contralateral muscle)	Ribs 5-7 (costal cartilages) Sternum (xiphoid ligaments)
110	Obliquus externus abdominis	Ribs 5-12 (interdigitating on external and inferior surfaces)	Iliac crest (outer border) Aponeurosis from 9th costal cartilage to ASIS; both sides meet at midline to form linea alba
111	Obliquus internus abdominis	Iliac crest (anterior 2/3 of intermediate line) Thoracolumbar fascia Inguinal ligament (lateral 2/3 of upper aspect)	Ribs 9-12 (inferior border and cartilages by digitations that appear continuous with internal intercostals) Ribs 7-9 (cartilages) Aponeurosis to linea alba
Others			
174	Psoas major		
175	Psoas minor		

Trunk flexion has multiple elements that include cervical, thoracic, and lumbar motion. Measurement is difficult at best and may be done in a variety of ways with considerable variability in results.

The neck flexors should be eliminated as much as possible by asking the patient to maintain a neutral neck position with the chin pointed to the ceiling to avoid neck flexion.

Grade 5 (Normal)

Position of Patient: Supine with fingertips lightly touching the back of the head (Figure 4-18).

Position of Therapist: Standing at side of table at level of patient's chest to be able to ascertain whether scapulae clear table during test (see Figure 4-18). For a patient with no other muscle weakness, the therapist does not need to touch the patient. If, however, the patient has weak hip flexors (refer to page 206), the therapist should stabilize the pelvis by leaning across the patient on the forearms (Figure 4-19).

Test: Patient flexes trunk through range of motion, lifting the trunk until scapulae clear table. The neck should not flex.

Instructions to Patient: "Keep your chin pointed toward the ceiling and lift your head, shoulders, and back off the table."

Grading

Grade 5 (Normal): Patient completes range of motion until inferior angles of scapulae are off the table. (Weight of the arms serves as resistance.)

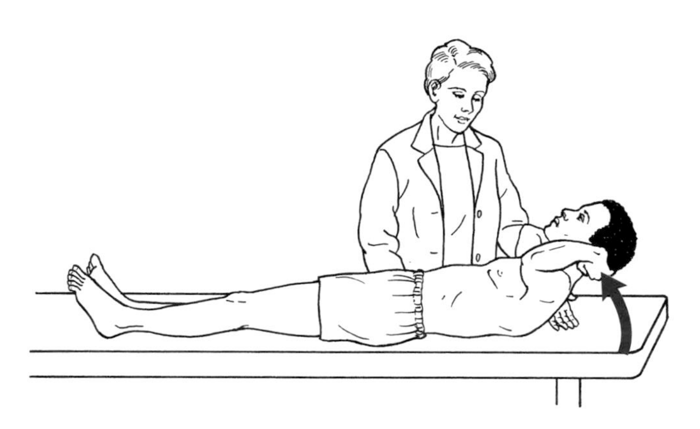

FIGURE 4-18

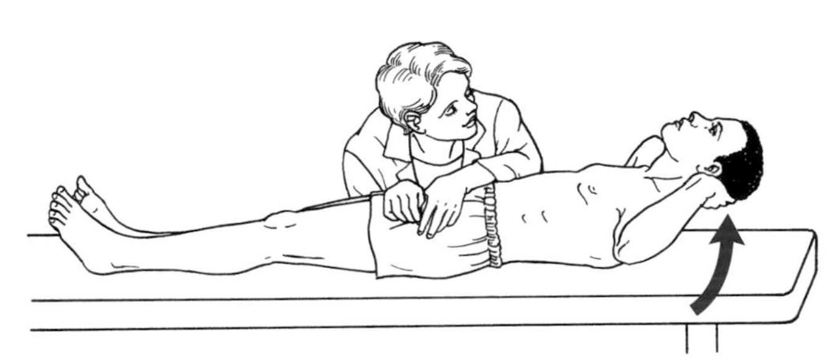

FIGURE 4-19

Grade 4 (Good)

Position of Patient: Supine with arms crossed over chest (Figure 4-20).

Test: Other than patient's position, all other aspects of the test are the same as for Grade 5.

Grading

Grade 4 (Good): Patient completes range of motion and raises trunk until scapulae are off the table. Resistance of arms is reduced in the cross-chest position.

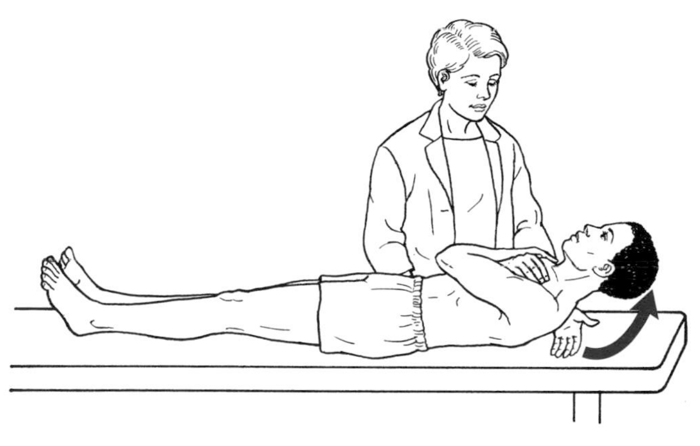

FIGURE 4-20

Grade 3 (Fair)

Position of Patient: Supine with arms outstretched in full extension above plane of body (Figure 4-21).

Test: Except for the patient's position, all other aspects of the test are the same as for Grade 5. Patient lifts trunk until inferior angles of scapulae are off the table. Position of the outstretched arms "neutralizes" resistance by bringing the weight of the arms closer to the center of gravity.

Instructions to Patient: "Keep your chin pointed to the ceiling as you raise your head, shoulders, and arms off the table."

Grading

Grade 3 (Fair): Patient completes range of motion and lifts trunk until inferior angles of scapulae are off the table.

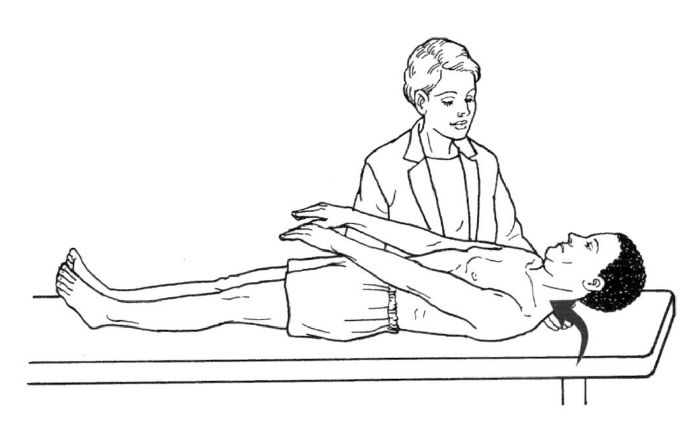

FIGURE 4-21

Grade 2 (Poor), Grade 1 (Trace), and Grade 0 (Zero)

Testing trunk flexion is rather clear-cut for Grades 5, 4, and 3. When testing Grade 2 and below, the results may be ambiguous, but observation and palpation are critical for defendable results. To determine Grades 2 to 0, the patient will be asked, in sequence, to raise the head, do an assisted forward lean, and cough.

Position of Patient: Supine with arms at sides. Knees flexed.

Position of Therapist: Standing at side of table. The hand used for palpation is placed at the midline of the thorax over the linea alba, and the four fingers of both hands are used to palpate the rectus abdominis (Figure 4-22).

Test and Instructions to Patient: The therapist tests for Grades 2, 1, and 0 in a variety of ways to make certain that muscle contractile activity that may be present is not missed.

Grading

Sequence 1: Head raise (Figure 4-23): Ask the patient to lift the head from the table. If the scapulae do not clear the table, the Grade is 2 (Poor). If the patient cannot lift the head, proceed to Sequence 2.

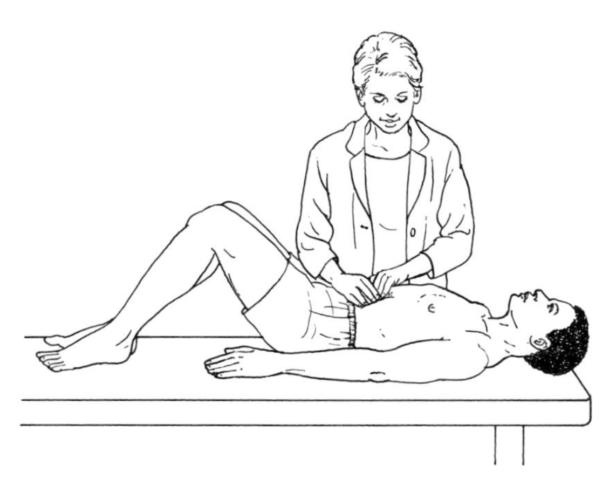

FIGURE 4-22

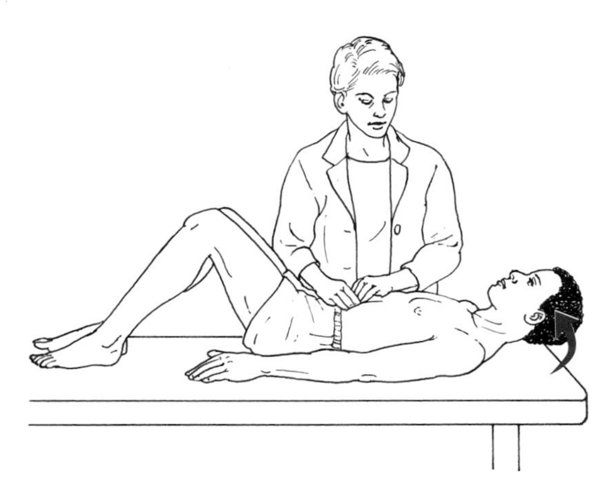

FIGURE 4-23

Sequence 2: Assisted forward lean (Figure 4-24): The therapist cradles the upper trunk and head off the table and asks the patient to lean forward. If there is depression of the rib cage, the Grade is 2 (Poor). If there is no depression of the rib cage but visible or palpable contraction occurs, the Grade assigned should be 1 (Trace). If there is no activity, the Grade is 0; proceed to Sequence 3.

Sequence 3: Cough (Figure 4-25): Ask the patient to cough. If the patient can cough to any degree and depression of the rib cage occurs, the Grade is 2 (Poor). (If the patient coughs, regardless of its effectiveness, the abdominal muscles are automatically brought into play.) If the patient cannot cough but there is palpable rectus abdominis activity, the Grade is 1 (Trace). Lack of any demonstrable activity is Grade 0 (Zero).

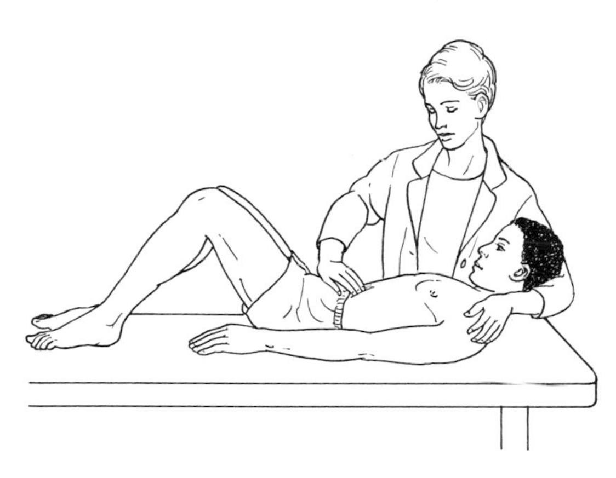

FIGURE 4-24

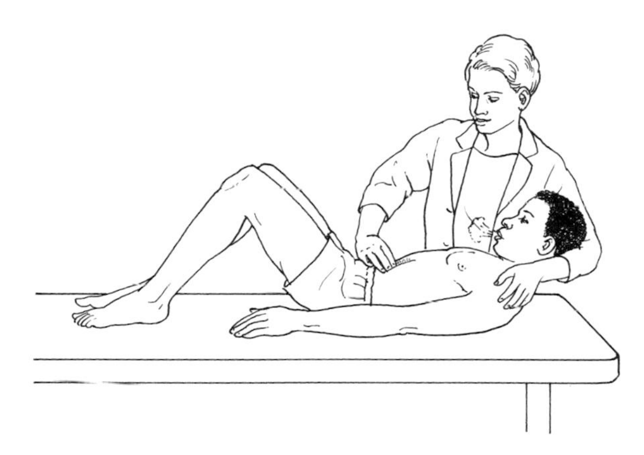

FIGURE 4-25

Helpful Hints

- If the abdominal muscles are weak, reverse action of the hip flexors may cause lumbar lordosis. When this occurs, the patient should be positioned with the hips extended to disallow the hip flexors to contribute to the test motion.[10]
- In all tests observe any deviations of the umbilicus. (This is not to be confused with the response to light stroking, which elicits superficial reflex activity.) In response to muscle testing, if there is a difference in the segments of the rectus abdominis, the umbilicus will deviate toward the stronger part (i.e., cranially if the upper parts are stronger, caudally if the lower parts are stronger, and laterally if one or more segment of *one* rectus is paralyzed).
- If the extensor muscles of the lumbar spine are weak, contraction of the abdominal muscles can cause posterior tilt of the pelvis. If this situation exists, tension of the hip flexor muscles would be useful to stabilize the pelvis; therefore, the therapist should position the patient in hip and knee flexion.
- The thoracic flexion muscle test should be done absolutely correctly—that is, with the neck in neutral to avoid undue strain on the neck and in the presence of known or suspected osteoporosis. Trunk flexion is contraindicated in the presence of osteoporosis secondary to the risk of vertebral fracture. To avoid thoracic flexion, instruct the patient to keep the chin pointed to the ceiling and the elbows flat.
- To avoid cervical strain, have the patient avoid clasping the head with the hands. The hands should not carry any of the head's weight.
- The abdominal muscles are activated the most when slight spine flexion occurs without active hip flexion.[7]
- Leg support during a pelvic tilt and fixed feet during spine and hip flexion exercises may decrease the intensity of rectus abdominus activity. Having the feet on the floor or fixed activates the hip flexors.[10]
- Spine flexion with knees and hips bent with feet in the air neutralizes the pelvic lordosis, reduces tension on the psoas muscle, decreases involvement of the hip flexors and decreases the compressive load of the spinal segments.[10]
- In summary, to ensure the patient's spine safety, remember these important guidelines:[10]

  a. Avoid active hip flexion or fixed feet.
  b. Do not allow the patient to pull the head up with the hands behind the head.
  c. Knees and hips should be flexed during upper body exercises.

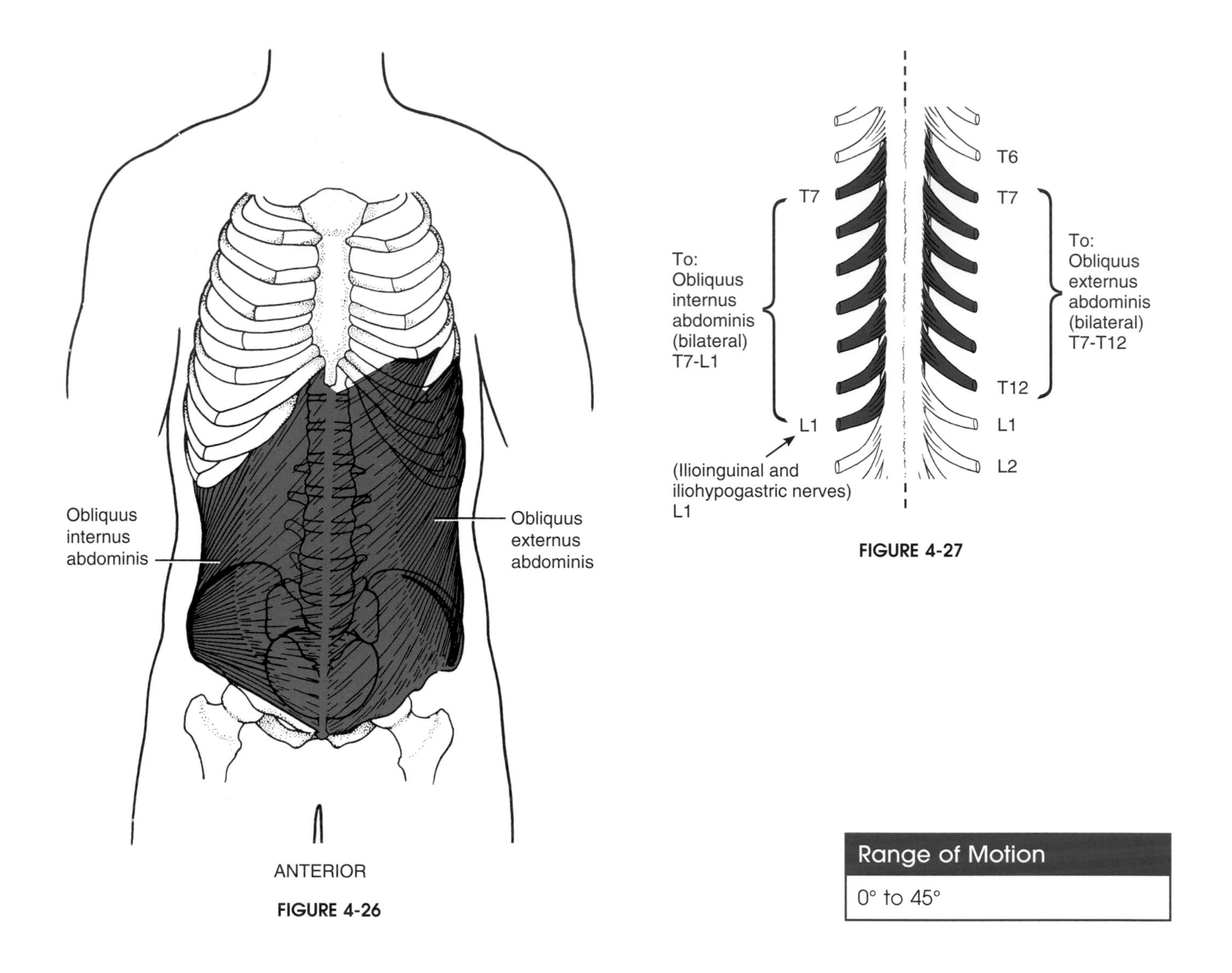

FIGURE 4-26

FIGURE 4-27

Range of Motion
0° to 45°

Table 4-5 TRUNK ROTATION

I.D.	Muscle	Origin	Insertion
110	Obliquus externus abdominis	Ribs 5-12 (interdigitating on external and inferior surfaces)	Iliac crest (outer border) Aponeurosis from 9th costal cartilage to ASIS; both sides meet at midline to form linea alba Pubic symphysis (upper border)
111	Obliquus internus abdominis	Iliac crest (anterior 2/3 of intermediate line) Thoracolumbar fascia Inguinal ligament (lateral 2/3 of upper aspect)	Ribs 9-12 (inferior border and cartilages by digitations that appear continuous with internal intercostals) Ribs 7-9 (cartilages) Aponeurosis to linea alba
Other			
	Deep back muscles (1 side)		

CAUTION: Trunk rotation must be used with caution in patients with known or suspected osteoporosis.

Grade 5 (Normal)

Position of Patient: Supine with fingertips to the side of the head.

Position of Therapist: Standing at patient's waist level.

Test: With chin pointed to the ceiling, patient flexes trunk and rotates to one side. This movement is then repeated on the opposite side so that the muscles on both sides can be examined.

Right elbow to left knee tests the right external obliques and the left internal obliques. Left elbow to right knee tests the left external obliques and the right internal obliques (Figure 4-28). When the patient rotates to one side, the internal oblique muscle is palpated on the side toward the turn; the external oblique muscle is palpated on the side away from the direction of turning (Figure 4-29).

Substitution

If the pectoralis major is active (inappropriately) in this test of trunk rotation at any grade, the shoulder will shrug or be raised from the table, and there is limited rotation of the trunk.

Instructions to Patient: "With your chin pointed to the ceiling, lift your head and shoulders from the table, taking your right elbow toward your left knee. Then, with your chin pointed to the ceiling, lift your head and shoulders from the table, taking your left elbow toward your right knee."

Grading

Grade 5 (Normal): The scapula corresponding to the side of the external oblique function must clear the table for a Grade 5.

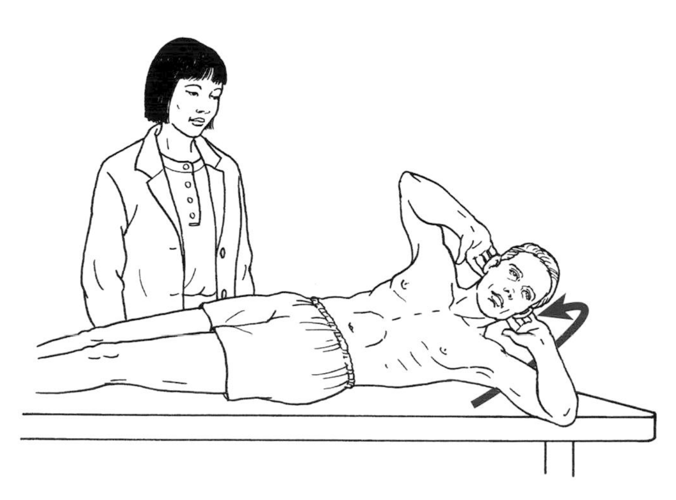

FIGURE 4-28

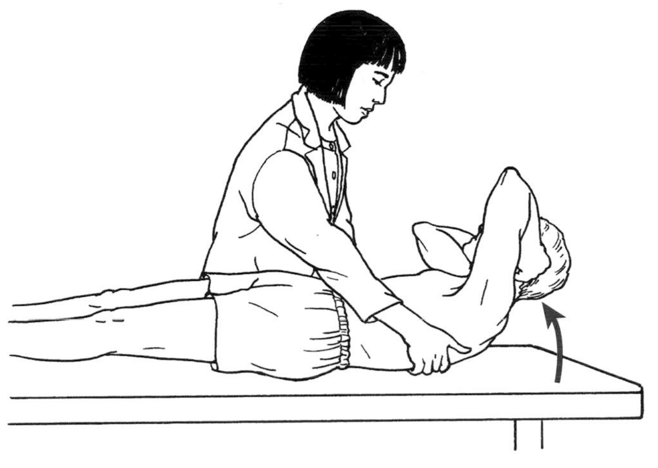

FIGURE 4-29

Grade 4 (Good)

Position of Patient: Supine with arms crossed over chest.

Test: Other than patient's position, all other aspects of the test are the same as for Grade 5. The test is done first to one side (Figure 4-30) and then to the other.

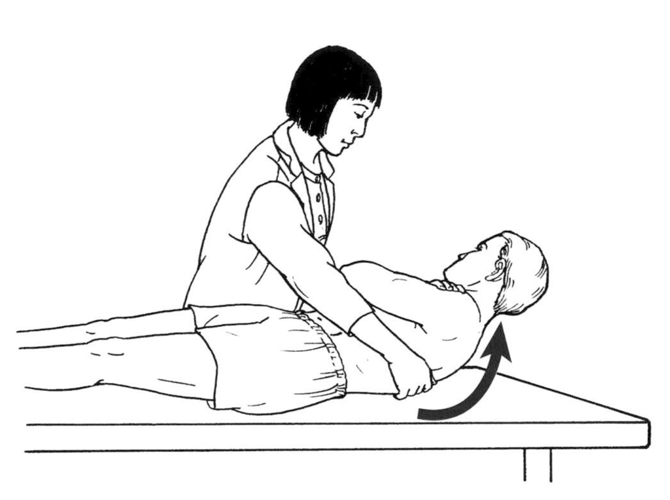

FIGURE 4-30

Grade 3 (Fair)

Position of Patient: Supine with arms outstretched above plane of body.

Test: Position of therapist and instructions are the same as for Grade 5. The test is done first to the left (Figure 4-31) and then to the right (Figure 4-32).

Grading

Grade 3 (Fair): Patient is able to raise the scapula off the table. The therapist may use one hand to check for scapular clearance (see Figure 4-32).

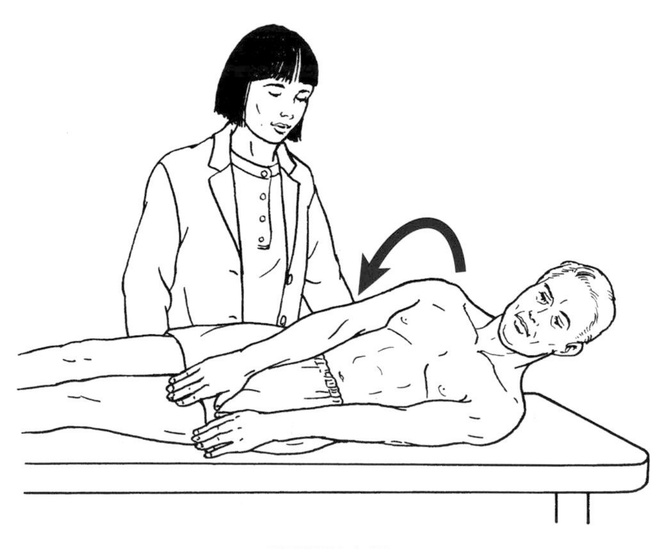

FIGURE 4-31

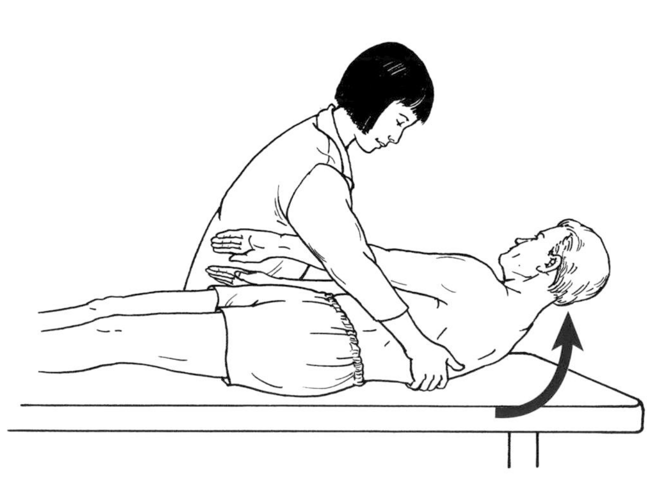

FIGURE 4-32

Grade 2 (Poor)

Position of Patient: Supine with arms outstretched above plane of body.

Position of Therapist: Standing at level of patient's waist. Therapist palpates the external oblique first on one side and then on the other, with one hand placed on the lateral part of the anterior abdominal wall distal to the rib cage (Figure 4-33). Continue to palpate the muscle distally in the direction of its fibers until reaching the ASIS.

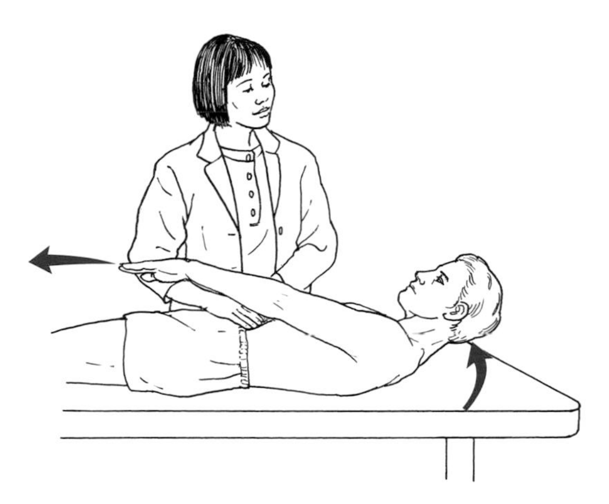

FIGURE 4-33

At the same time, the internal oblique muscle on the opposite side of the trunk is palpated. The internal oblique muscle lies under the external oblique, and its fibers run in the opposite diagonal direction.

Therapists may remember this palpation procedure better if they think of positioning their two hands as if both hands were to be in the pants pockets or grasping the abdomen in pain. (The external obliques run from out to in; the internal obliques run from in to out.)

Instructions to Patient: "Keeping your chin pointed to the ceiling, lift your head and reach toward your right knee." (Repeat to left side for the opposite muscle.)

Test: Patient attempts to raise body and turn toward the right. Repeat toward left side.

Grading

Grade 2 (Poor): Patient is unable to clear the inferior angle of the scapula from the table on the side of the external oblique being tested. The therapist must, however, be able to observe depression of the rib cage during the test activity.

Grade 1 (Trace) and Grade 0 (Zero)

Position of Patient: Supine with arms at sides. Hips flexed with feet flat on table.

Position of Therapist: Head is supported as patient attempts to turn to one side (Figure 4-34). (Turn to the other side in a subsequent test.) Under normal conditions, the abdominal muscles stabilize the trunk when the head is lifted. In patients with abdominal weakness, the supported head permits the patient to recruit abdominal muscle activity without having to overcome the entire weight of the head.

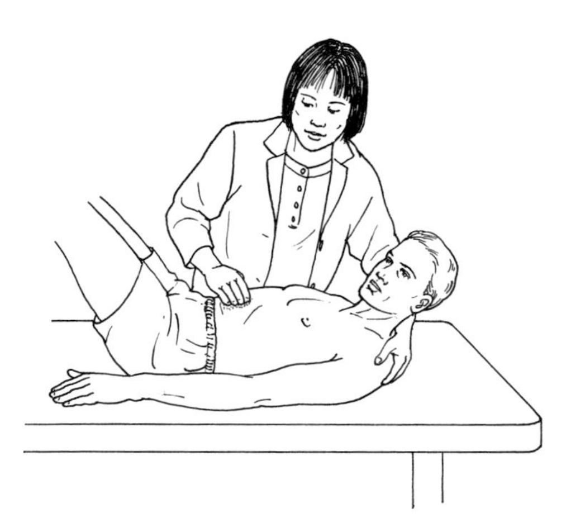

FIGURE 4-34

One hand palpates the internal obliques on the side toward which the patient turns (not illustrated) and the external obliques on the side away from the direction of turning (see Figure 4-34). The therapist assists the patient to raise the head and shoulders slightly and turn to one side. This procedure is used when abdominal muscle weakness is profound.

Instructions to Patient: "Try to lift up and turn to your right." (Repeat for turn to the left.)
Test: Patient attempts to flex trunk and turn to either side.

Grading

Grade 1 (Trace): The therapist can see or palpate muscular contraction.

Grade 0 (Zero): No response from the obliquus internus or externus muscles.

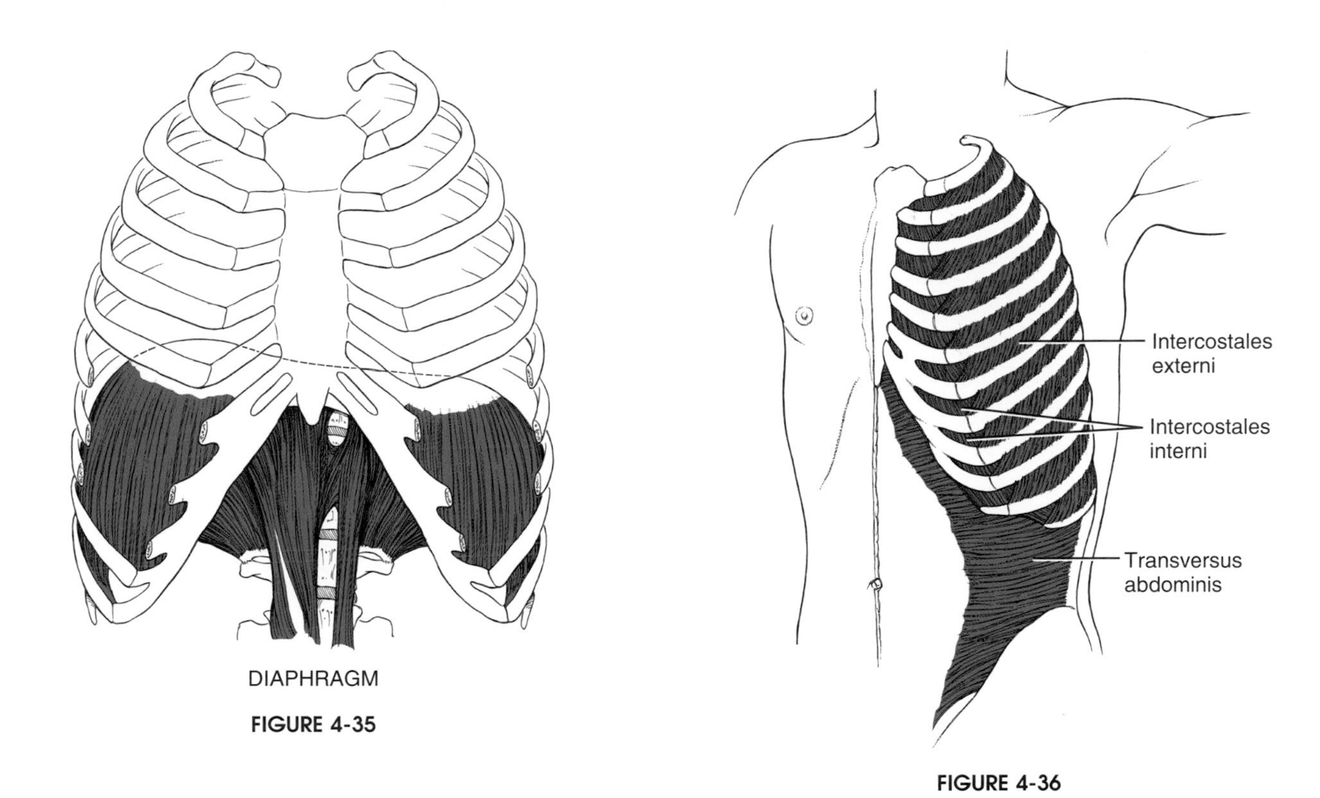

FIGURE 4-35

FIGURE 4-36

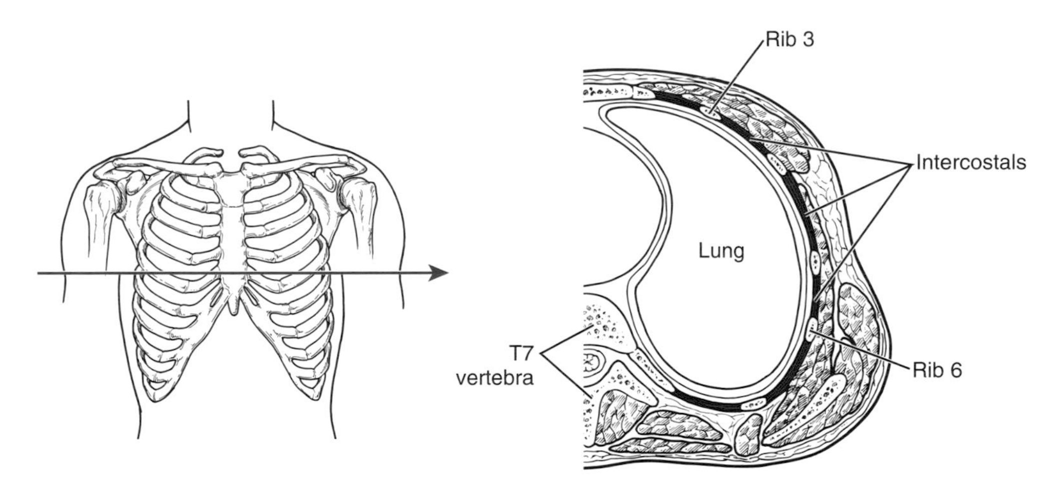

FIGURE 4-37 Arrow indicates level of cross section.

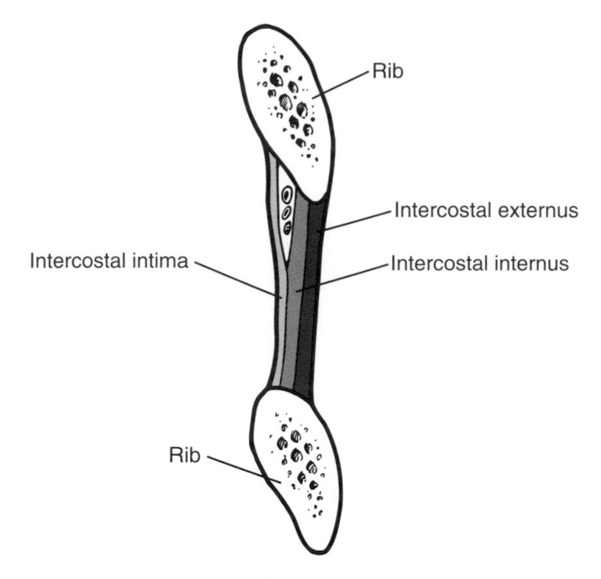

FIGURE 4-38

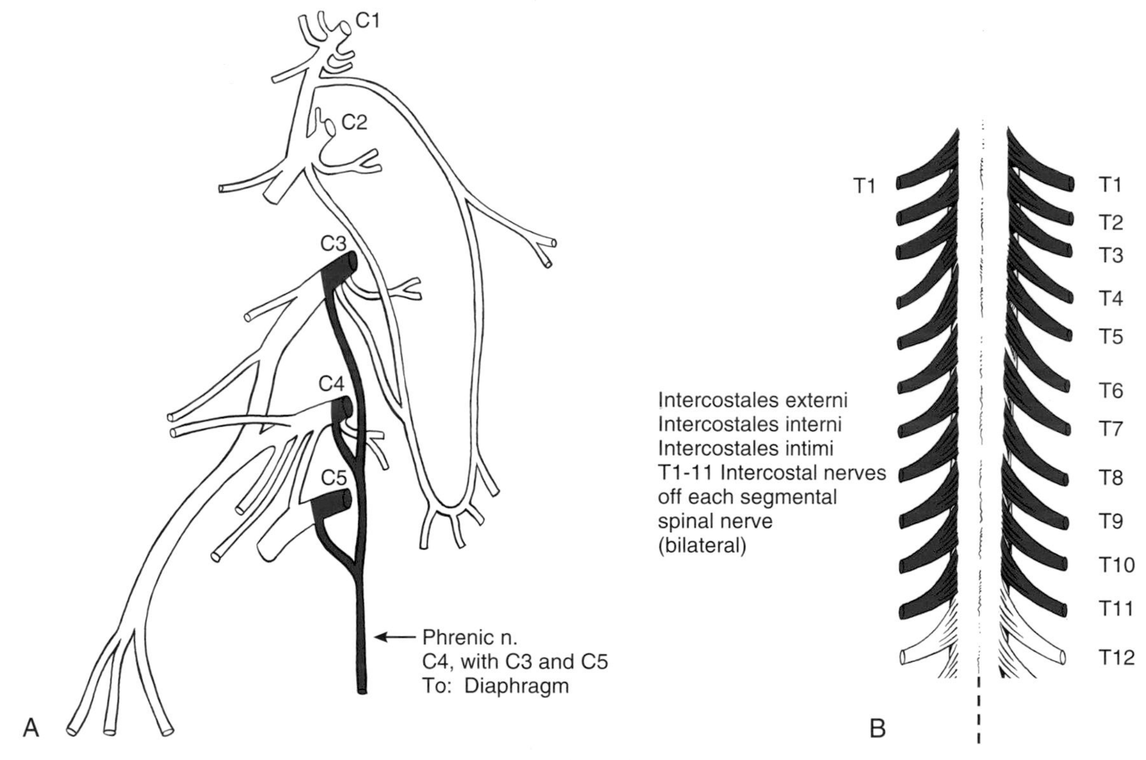

FIGURE 4-39

Range of Motion

Normal range of motion of the chest wall during quiet inspiration is about 0.75 inch, with gender variations. Normal chest expansion in forced inspiration varies from 2.0 to 2.5 inches at the level of the xiphoid.[11]

Table 4-6 MUSCLES OF QUIET INSPIRATION

I.D.	Muscle	Origin	Insertion
101	Diaphragm (formed of 3 parts from the circumference of the thoracic outlet)		Fibers all converge on central tendon of diaphragm; middle of central tendon is below and partially blended with pericardium
	Sternal	Xiphoid process (posterior)	
	Costal	Ribs 7-12 (internal surfaces of costal cartilages and ribs on each side) Interdigitates with transversus abdominis	
	Lumbar	Medial and lateral arcuate ligaments (aponeurotic arches) L1-L2 (left crus, bodies) L1-L3 (right crus, bodies)	
102	Intercostales externi (11 pairs)	Ribs 1-11 (lower borders and tubercles; costal cartilages)	Ribs 2-12 (upper margins of rib below; last 2 end in free ends of the costal cartilages) External intercostal membrane
103	Intercostales interni (11 pairs)	Sternum (anterior) Ribs 1-11 (ridge on inner surface) Costal cartilages of same rib Internal intercostal membrane	Upper border of rib below Fibers run obliquely to the external intercostals
104	Intercostales intimi (innermost intercostals) Often absent	Ribs 1-11 (costal groove)	Rib below (upper margin) Fibers run in same pattern as internal intercostals
107	Levatores costarum (12 pairs)	C7-T11 vertebrae (transverse processes, tip)	Rib below vertebra of origin (external surface)
80	Scalenus anterior	C3-C6 vertebrae (transverse processes, anterior tubercles)	1st rib (scalene tubercle)
81	Scalenus medius	C2 (axis)-C7 vertebrae (transverse processes, posterior tubercles) C1 (atlas) sometimes	1st rib (superior surface)
82	Scalenus posterior	C4-C6 vertebrae (transverse processes posterior tubercle, variable)	2nd rib (outer surface)
Others			
100	Quadratus lumborum		
131	Pectoralis major (arms fixed)		

THE DIAPHRAGM

The diaphragm performs 70 to 80% of the effort of quiet inspiration. The remainder is performed by the intercostals, scalenes, and sternocleidomastoid muscles.[12]

Preliminary Examination

Uncover the patient's chest and abdominal area so that the motions of the chest and abdominal walls can be observed. Watch the normal respiration pattern and observe differences in the motion of the chest wall and epigastric area and note any contraction of the neck muscles and the abdominal muscles.

Epigastric rise and flaring of the lower margin of the rib cage during inspiration indicate that the diaphragm is active. The rise on both sides of the linea alba should be symmetrical. During quiet inspiration, epigastric rise reflects the movement of the diaphragm descending over one intercostal space.[13,14] In deeper inspiratory efforts, the diaphragm may move across three or more intercostal spaces.

An elevation and lateral expansion of the rib cage are indicative of intercostal activity during inspiration. Exertional chest expansion measured at the level of the xiphoid process is 2.0 to 2.5 inches (the expansion may exceed 3.0 inches in more active young people and athletes).[12]

All Grades (5 to 0)

Position of Patient: Supine.

Position of Therapist: Standing next to patient at approximately waist level. One hand is placed lightly on the abdomen in the epigastric area just below the xiphoid process (Figure 4-40). Resistance is given (by same hand) in a downward direction.

Test: Patient inhales with maximal effort and holds maximal inspiration.

Instructions to Patient: "Take a deep breath ... as much as you can ... hold it. Push against my hand. Don't let me push you down."

Grading

Grade 5 (Normal): Patient completes full inspiratory (epigastric) excursion and holds against maximal resistance. A Grade 5 diaphragm takes high resistance in the range of 100 pounds.[15]

Grade 4 (Good): Completes maximal inspiratory excursion but yields against heavy resistance.

Grade 3 (Fair): Completes maximal inspiratory expansion but cannot tolerate manual resistance.

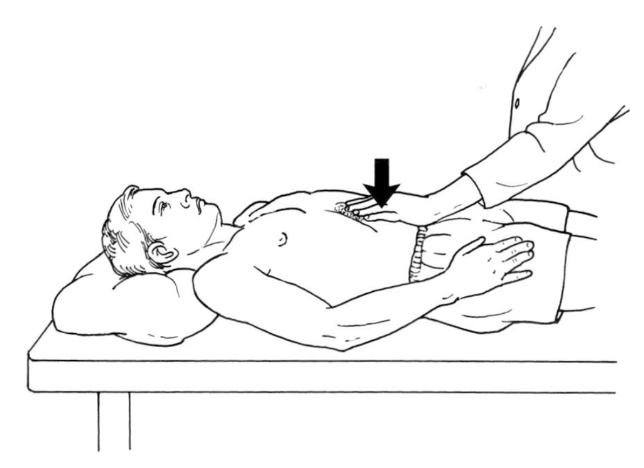

FIGURE 4-40

Grade 2 (Poor): Observable epigastric rise without completion of full inspiratory expansion.

Grade 1 (Trace): Palpable contraction is detected under the inner surface of the lower ribs, provided that the abdominal muscles are relaxed (Figure 4-41). Another way to detect minimal epigastric motion is by instructing the patient to "sniff" with the mouth closed.

Grade 0 (Zero): No epigastric rise and no palpable contraction of the diaphragm occur.

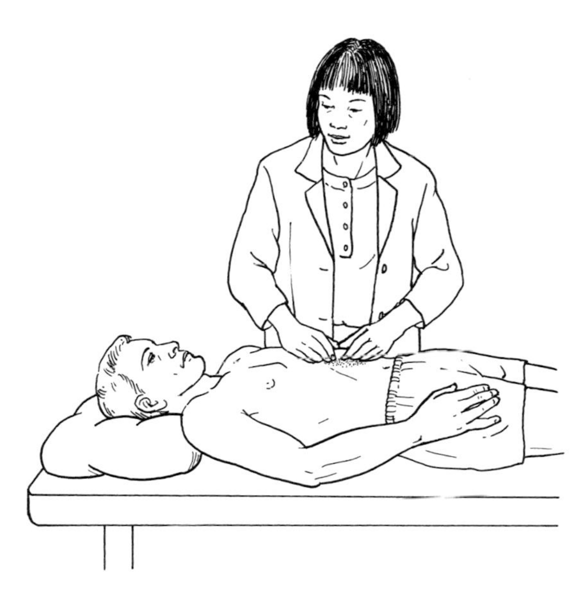

FIGURE 4-41

Substitution

Patient may attempt to substitute for an inadequate diaphragm by hyperextending the lumbar spine in an effort to increase the response to the therapist's manual resistance.[15] The abdominal muscles also may contract, but both motions are improper attempts to follow the instruction to push up against the therapist's hand.

THE INTERCOSTALS

There is no method of direct assessment of the strength of the intercostal muscles. An indirect method measures the difference in magnitude of chest excursion between maximal inspiration and the girth of the chest at the end of full expiration.

Position of Patient: Supine on a firm surface. Arms at sides.

Position of Therapist: Standing at side of table. Tape measure placed lightly around thorax at level of xiphoid.

Test: Patient holds maximal inspiration for measurement and then holds maximal expiration for a second measurement. (A pneumograph may be used for the same purpose if one is available.) The difference between the two measurements is recorded as chest expansion.

Instructions to Patient: "Take a big breath in and hold it. Now blow it all out and hold it."

Grading

There are no classic 5 to 0 grades given for the intercostal muscles. Instead, a flexible metal or new cloth tape is used to measure chest expansion.

Helpful Hint

The scalene muscles, as assessed via needle EMG examination, are active with every inspiratory effort and should be considered a primary muscle of inspiration.[16]

FORCED EXPIRATION

Coughing often is used as the clinical test for forced expiration. An effective cough requires the use of all muscles of active expiration in contrast to quiet expiration, which is the passive relaxation of the muscles of inspiration. It must be recognized, however, that a patient may not have an effective cough because of inadequate laryngeal control or low vital capacity.

Grading

The usual muscle test grades do not apply here; thus, the following scale to assess the cough is used:

Functional: Normal or only slight impairment:
- Crisp or explosive expulsion of air
- Volume is sharp and clearly audible
- Able to clear airway of secretions

Weak Functional: Moderate impairment that affects the degree of active motion or endurance:
- Decreased volume and diminished air movement
- Appears labored
- May take several attempts to clear airway

Nonfunctional: Severe impairment:
- No clearance of airway
- No expulsion of air
- Cough attempt may be nothing more than an effort to clear the throat

Zero: Cough is absent.

Table 4-7 MUSCLES OF FORCED EXPIRATION

I.D.	Muscle	Origin	Insertion
110	Obliquus externus abdominis	Ribs 5-12 (interdigitating on external and inferior surfaces)	Iliac crest (outer border) Aponeurosis from 9th costal cartilage to ASIS; both sides meet at midline to form linea alba Pubic symphysis (upper border)
111	Obliquus internus	Iliac crest (anterior 2/3 of intermediate line) Thoracolumbar fascia Inguinal ligament (lateral 2/3 of upper aspect)	Ribs 9-12 (inferior border and abdominis cartilages by digitations that appear continuous with internal intercostals) Ribs 7-9 (cartilages) Aponeurosis to linea alba Pubic crest and pecten pubis
112	Transverse abdominis	Inguinal ligament (lateral 1/3) Iliac crest (anterior 2/3, inner lip) Thoracolumbar fascia Ribs 7-12 (costal cartilages interdigitate with diaphragm)	Linea alba (blends with broad aponeurosis) Pubic crest and pecten pubis (to form falx inguinalis)
113	Rectus abdominis	Arises via 2 tendons: Lateral: pubic crest (tubercle) and pecten pubis Medial: symphysis pubis (ligamentous covering)	Ribs 5-7 (costal cartilages) Costoxiphoid ligaments
103	Intercostales interni	Ribs 1-11 (inner surface) Sternum (anterior) Internal intercostal membrane	Ribs 2-12 (upper border of rib below rib of origin)
130	Latissimus dorsi	T6-T12 and all lumbar and sacral vertebrae (spinous processes via supraspinous ligaments) Iliac crest (posterior) Thoracolumbar fascia Ribs 9-12 (interdigitates with external abdominal oblique)	Humerus (floor of intertubercular sulcus) Deep fascia of arm
Other			
106	Transversus thoracis		

Alternative Measurement of Inspiration and Expiration Muscle Strength

Measurements of maximal inspiratory pressure (MIP) and maximal expiratory pressure (MEP) may serve as a means of measuring ventilatory muscle strength, although not the strength of any single muscle. The MIP reflects the strength of the diaphragm and other inspiratory muscles, whereas the MEP reflects the strength of the abdominal muscles and other expiratory muscles.

Equipment: Either a manual pressure gauge (Figure 4-42) or an electronic pressure gauge (Figure 4-43) is used. The device should contain a small hole (1 mm diameter and 20 to 30 mm in length), which allows air to escape. This prevents the patient from generating pressure by using the cheek muscles. Place a new cardboard mouthpiece or a clean rubber mouthpiece with flanges on the device for each patient use.

Maximal Inspiratory Pressure

Position of Patient: Seated in a chair, with a nose clip applied to the nose (Figure 4-44).

Position of Therapist: Standing or sitting in front of seated patient so as to read the gauge (see Figure 4-44).

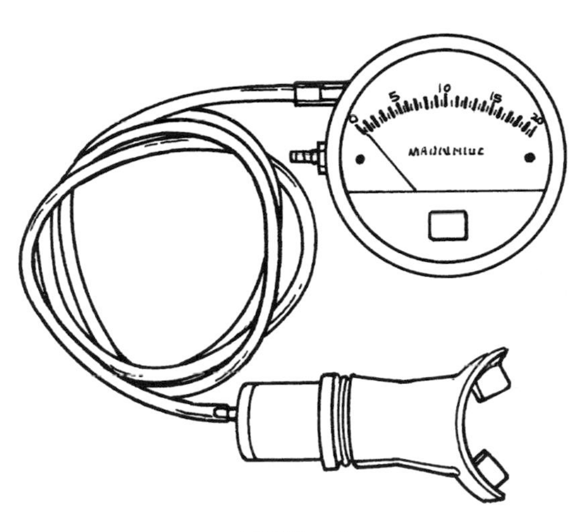

FIGURE 4-42

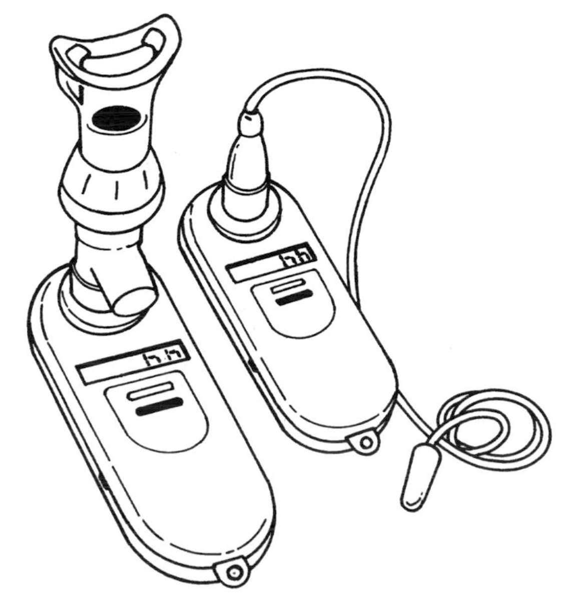

FIGURE 4-43

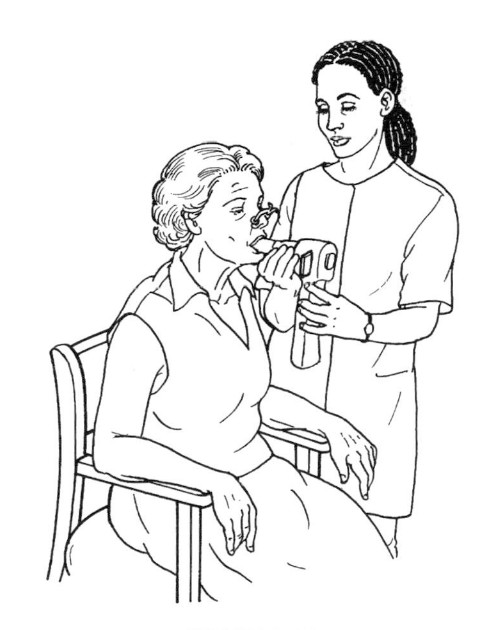

FIGURE 4-44

Test: Demonstrate the maneuver and then have the patient repeat it. Patient first exhales completely, then sucks in as hard as possible. The patient should maintain inspiratory pressure for at least 1.5 seconds; the largest negative pressure sustained for at least 1 second should be recorded. Allow the patient to rest for about one minute and then repeat the maneuver five times. Provide verbal or visual feedback after each maneuver, but do not allow trunk flexion or extension during the test. The goal is for the variability among measurements to be less than 10 cmH_2O. Measurements should be rounded to the nearest 5 cmH_2O. Table 4-8 lists maximum inspiration pressure values.

Instructions to Patient: "Seal your lips firmly around the mouthpiece, exhale slowly and completely, and then pull in hard, like you are trying to suck up a thick milkshake."

Maximal Expiratory Pressure

Position of Patient: Seated in a chair, with a nose clip applied to the nose.

Position of Therapist: Standing or sitting in front of seated patient so as to read the gauge.

Test: Demonstrate the maneuver and have the patient repeat it. Patient first inhales completely, then blows out as hard as possible. The patient should maintain expiratory pressure for at least 1.5 seconds. The largest positive pressure sustained for at least 1 second should be recorded. Allow the patient to rest for about one minute and then repeat the maneuver five times. Provide verbal or visual feedback after each maneuver but do not allow trunk flexion or extension during the test. The goal is for the variability among measurements to be less than 10 cmH_2O. Measurements should be rounded to the nearest 5 cmH_2O (see Table 4-8).

Instructions to Patient: "I want you to inhale completely as you push the mouthpiece firmly against your lips and teeth, and then push (or blow) as hard as possible, like you are trying to fill a very stiff balloon."

Helpful Hint

Some patients with orofacial muscle weakness may not be able to obtain a good seal with the lips. It is permissible to allow such patients to use their hand to press their lips against the mouthpiece during each maneuver. Alternatively, the therapist can press the patient's lips against the mouthpiece as necessary to obtain a good seal or a face mask interface can be substituted.

Table 4-8 MAXIMUM INSPIRATION PRESSURE (MIP) AND MAXIMUM EXPIRATION PRESSURE (MEP) GRADING*

Age Group	MIP Values†		MEP Values‡
Adolescents (ages 13-17)[17]	Male:	114-121	131-161
	Female:	65-85	92-95
Adults (ages 18-65)[18]	Male:	92-121	140
	Female:	68-79	95
Older adults (ages 65-85)[19]	Male:	65-90	140-190
	Female:	45-60	90-130

*Reference ranges derived from population-based studies with good reference equations.
†Mean values in cmH_2O.
‡These mean MEP are under estimates because the mouthpiece was used between the teeth instead of against the lips and teeth.[20]

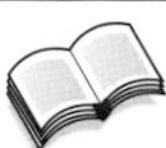

The Functional Anatomy of Coughing

Cough is an essential procedure to maintain airway patency and to clear the pharynx and bronchial tree when secretions accumulate. A cough may be a reflex or voluntary response to irritation anywhere along the airway downstream from the nose.

The cough reflex occurs as a result of stimulation of the mucous membranes of the pharynx, larynx, trachea, or bronchial tree. These tissues are so sensitive to light touch that any foreign matter or other irritation initiates the cough reflex. The sensory (afferent) limb of the reflex carries the impulses set up by the irritation via the glossopharyngeal and vagus cranial nerves to the fasciculus solitarius in the medulla, from which the motor impulses (efferent) then move out to the muscles of the pharynx, palate, tongue, and larynx and to the muscles of the abdominal wall and chest and the diaphragm. The reflex response is a deep inspiration (about 2.5 liters of air) followed quickly by a forced expiration, during which the glottis closes momentarily, trapping air in the lungs.[21] The diaphragm contracts spasmodically, as do the abdominal muscles and intercostal muscles. This raises the intrathoracic pressure (to above 200 mm Hg) until the vocal cords are forced open, and the explosive outrush of air expels mucus and foreign matter. The expiratory airflow at this time may reach a velocity of 500 mph or higher.[22] Important to the reflex action is that the bronchial tree and laryngeal walls collapse because of the strong compression of the lungs, causing an invagination so that the high linear velocity of the airflow moving past and through these tissues dislodges mucus or foreign particles, thus producing an effective cough.

The three phases of cough—inspiration, compression, and forced expiration—are mediated by the muscles of the thorax and abdomen as well as those of the pharynx, larynx, and tongue. The deep inspiratory effort is supported by the diaphragm, intercostals, and arytenoid abductor muscles (the posterior cricoarytenoids), permitting inhalation of more than 1.5 liters of air.[23] The palatoglossus and styloglossus elevate the tongue and close off the oropharynx from the nasopharynx. The compression phase requires the lateral cricoarytenoid muscles to adduct and close the glottis.

The strong expiratory movement is augmented by strong contractions of the thorax muscles, particularly the latissimus dorsi and the oblique and transverse abdominal muscles. The abdominal muscles raise intra-abdominal pressure, forcing the relaxing diaphragm up and drawing the lower ribs down and medially. Elevation of the diaphragm raises the intrathoracic pressure to about 200 mm Hg, and the explosive expulsion phase begins with forced abduction of the glottis.

Functional Assessment of Coughing

It is generally accepted that if an individual's forced vital capacity (FVC) is ≥60% of the predicted value, the inspired volume is sufficient to generate a functional, effective cough.[24] FVC can be measured with a simple spirometer (Figure 4-45). A forced expiratory volume ≥60% of the individual's measured FVC should be adequate for sufficiently forceful expulsion.[25] A peak cough flow rate of 160 L/min is highly predictive of successful secretion clearance and subsequent extubation and decannulation in patients with neuromuscular disease.[26]

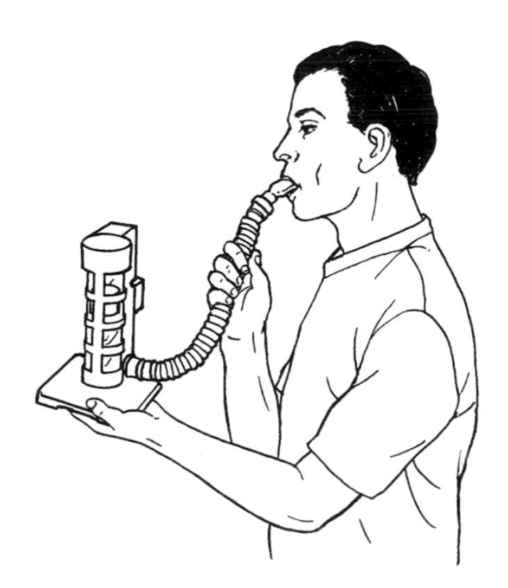

FIGURE 4-45

PELVIC FLOOR

The pelvic floor muscles form the "floor" of the pelvis and perform four important functions:

Supportive: by counteracting passive gravitational pull and dynamic intraabdominal pressures impacting the pelvic viscera in conjunction with the inner core muscles forming the canister theory of core stabilization.[27]

Sphincteric: by shortening in an anterosuperior direction, these muscles squeeze off the urethra, vagina, and anorectal junction to maintain urinary and fecal continence.[28]

Sexual: by rhythmically contracting during orgasm to enhance sexual satisfaction.

Postural stabilizer: by working with the transverse abdominus, multifidi, and pulmonary diaphragm, the pelvic floor creates the bottom of the inner core "canister" (Figure 4-46).

Poor pelvic floor strength is associated with pelvic organ prolapse and urinary or fecal incontinence. Ninety-seven percent of women will experience some level of supportive dysfunction in their lifetime, leading to "falling" of the bladder, rectum, uterus, or small intestine.[29] Urinary or fecal incontinence is experienced by as many as 72% of women of all ages.[30] Fecal incontinence is thought to be grossly underreported because of the associated social stigma. However, urinary incontinence is amenable to treatment, with reports of an 84% success rate using the Kegel exercise (controlled voluntary contractions used to strengthen the pelvic floor).[31]

Sexual dysfunction may be related to weak pelvic floor musculature and urinary incontinence.[32,33] Thirty-one percent of men and 43% of women between the ages of 18 and 59 years report concerns during physical intimacy, some of which are related to urinary incontinence and a weak pelvic floor.[34] Up to 80% of aging women have similar concerns.[35]

The pelvic floor muscles can become weakened from childbirth,[36] poor patterns of muscle recruitment, medical comorbidities such as diabetes, abdominopelvic surgical procedures, constipation, chronic cough, hormonal changes, and loss of muscle mass with aging. Because of the frequency of pelvic floor weakness, pelvic floor muscle strength should be routinely assessed to rule out muscle weakness, spasm, or dyscoordination in the presence of lumbopelvic, urologic, gynecologic, sexual, or gastrointestinal dysfunction.

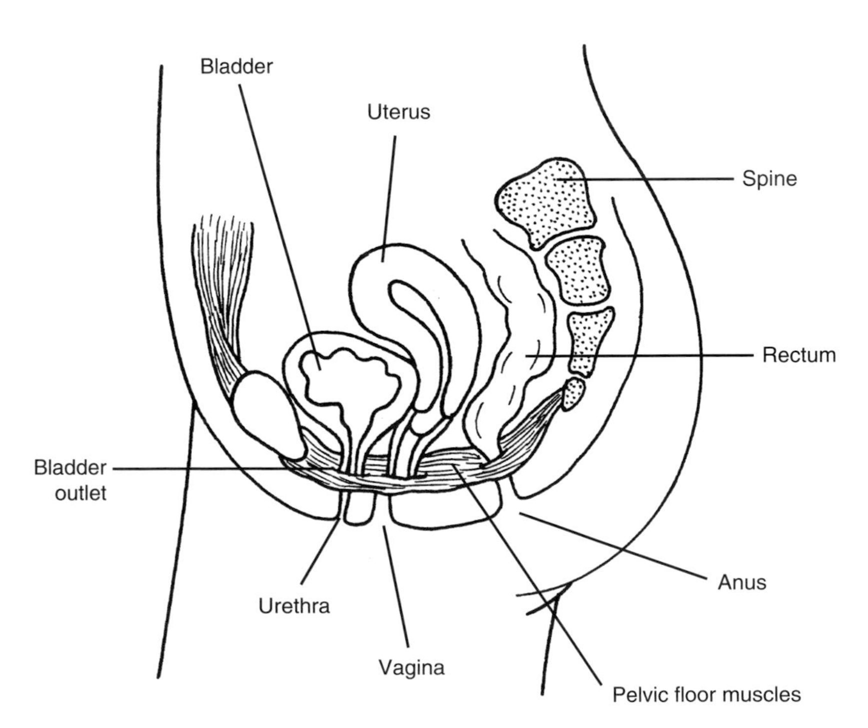

FIGURE 4-46 Pelvic floor muscles serve as a sling for the female organs.

Methods used to assess the strength and function of the pelvic floor muscles include the following:

- Presence of pelvic floor muscle activation: clinical observation, external perineal palpation, vaginal or rectal digital palpation, EMG, and pressure gauges.
- Quantification of pelvic floor muscle strength: manual muscle testing with rectal or vaginal palpation, vaginal cones,[37] and vaginal squeeze pressure.[38]
- Additional visualization of the pelvic floor musculature may be done with abdominal or pelvic two-dimensional ultrasound,[39] ultrasound, and magnetic resonance imaging.[40]

Anatomy of the Pelvic Floor

Muscles of the pelvic floor are difficult to visualize, particularly because most students do not have the opportunity to dissect this region in anatomy class. In both males and females, there are five muscles of the urogenital region that differ in size and disposition in relation to the male and female external genitalia. These five muscles are grouped into superficial and deep layers. Superficial muscles include three portions of the levator ani (puborectalis, pubococcygeus, iliococcygeus) and the ischiococcygeus. Connective tissue and the deep transverse perinei comprise the deep layer (Figure 4-47).

The superficial layer is the outermost layer; it resembles a sling and is shaped like a figure eight. Although the superficial layer is relatively thin in terms of mass, it is highly sensitive. This area is responsible for controlling the anal and urethral sphincters, so these muscles play an important role in continence. In order to work effectively the sphincters need the support of the rest of the pelvic floor, particularly the connective tissue elements. Additionally, because the abdominals share the same connective tissue attachments as the pelvic floor musculature, in many women they too need to be strengthened, along with the pelvic floor musculature.

The deep layer of the pelvic floor is the real workhorse of the pelvic floor. The deep pelvic floor muscles have the highest resting muscle tone in the body and play a vital role in movement, posture, and breathing. These muscles must continuously support the weight of the pelvic and abdominal organs when the person is upright (see Figure 4-46). The deep pelvic floor is sometimes called the pelvic diaphragm. Like its companion, "the roof" or the pulmonary diaphragm, it has minimal sensory innervation and its movement is not felt directly. When it works well, the pelvic floor functions like a well-balanced trampoline and has amazing tensile strength and elasticity. It plays a crucial role in ensuring spinal stability and free locomotion. Deep abdominal muscles in front, the multifidi around the spine, and the pulmonary diaphragm all must work together synergistically with the pelvic diaphragm. Thus "there is no core without the floor" (Table 4-9).

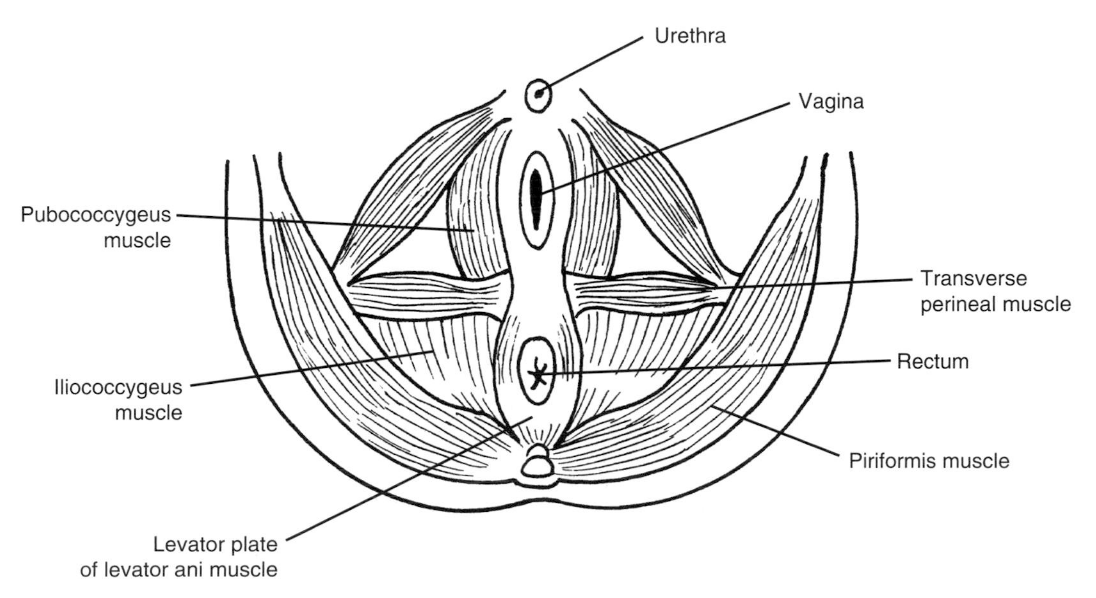

FIGURE 4-47

Table 4-9 MUSCLES OF THE PELVIC FLOOR (PERINEUM)

I.D.	Muscle	Origin	Insertion
120	Bulbocavernosus	Surrounds the orifice of the vagina	Blends with sphincter ani externus
121	Ischiococcygeus	Inner surface of the ischial tuberosity	Tendinous aponeurosis attached to the sides and under surface of the crus clitoridus.
118	Transversus perinei superficialis (indistinct, often missing)	Medial/anterior ischial tuberosity	Perineal body
119	Transversus perinei profundus	Inner surface ramus of the ischium	Blends into perineal body and vaginal wall
122	Sphincter urethrae	Superior: encircle lower end of the urethra Inferior: transverse perineal ligament	Interlace with fibers from the opposite side
Others			
115	Puborectalis		
115	Levator ani: Puborectalis Iliococcygeus Pubococcygeus		

Testing the Muscles of the Pelvic Floor

Test Description and Procedure

In a separate treatment room the patient is asked to sit and chat with the therapist who explains the pelvic exam in total detail. It is not uncommon for therapists to have patients sign a consent form prior to beginning the exam. The patient should be advised that she can stop the exam at any time for any reason. Once the patient thoroughly understands the exam, the therapist instructs her to disrobe from the waist down, cover herself with a sheet provided by the therapist, and lie supine on a plinth. The therapist leaves the room while the patient is preparing for the test. Once the therapist returns, the patient is asked to roll her legs into external rotation and abduction (hook lying). After the patient is relaxed, the therapist dons sterile gloves that contain no allergens or other potentially irritating material. The therapist may apply a nonallergenic lubricant to the gloves. While standing slightly to the side of the patient, the therapist pushes the sheet drape aside to locate needed landmarks, replaces the drape, and then slowly inserts the middle finger, index and middle finger, or middle and ring finger, into the vagina. If a patient has complaints of pelvic pain usually only one finger is used. Once fingers are in place the patient is asked to "pull my fingers up and in" a total of three to four times. Contractions are maintained for 1 to 2 seconds (Figure 4-48).

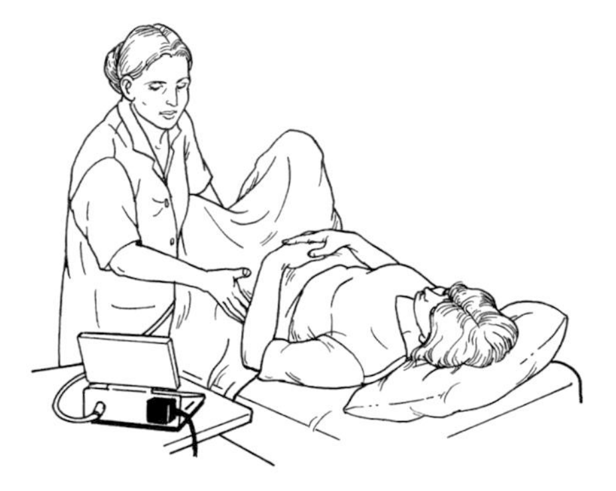

FIGURE 4-48

Grading

There are several grading scales, but the scale used most commonly is the Modified Oxford Scale.[41] The Modified Oxford Scale is a 6-point scale where half numbers of + and – can be added when a contraction is considered to fall between two full grades so that the scale expands to a 15-point scale (when both + and – are used):

0 = No contraction detected
1 = Flicker
2 = Weak (the patient is able to contract the pelvic floor muscles well enough to partially encircle the therapist's fingers)

3 = Moderate (the patient is able to fully encircle the therapist's fingers)
4 = Good (the patient is able to fully encircle the therapist's fingers and partially pull the fingers further into the vaginal cavity)
5 = Strong (the patient is able to fully encircle the therapist's fingers with a *strong* contraction *and* pull the fingers fully up and into the vaginal canal)

The Modified Oxford Scale has fair reliability among experienced therapists.[42] Test accuracy may be enhanced with visual examination during the actual manual muscle test. Visual observation can confirm perineal tightening and whether the fingers are drawn up and in, but most therapists do not observe the movement out of respect for the patient.

The Perineometer

The perineometer was developed to specifically determine the amount of contractile force a woman can generate with the pelvic floor musculature (Figure 4-49). The portion of the perineometer that is inserted into the vagina is typically ~28 mm in diameter with an active measurement length of ~55 mm. Different types of perineometers are available and each works on the same principle as a blood pressure monitor.

Test Procedure. The perineometer is first covered with a sterile sheath and then inserted into the vagina. A sterile hypoallergenic gel may be used on the sheath. The patient is then asked to perform a Kegel exercise, exerting as much force against the probe as possible (squeezing it). The therapist must make sure the patient is *not* holding her breath while performing the pelvic contraction. The patient performs three contractions with a 10-second rest between each contraction; the therapist records the highest force output or the average of the three. One advantage of the perineometer over MMT is that duration of contraction hold can be determined. The reliability of the perineometer is comparable to that of manual muscle testing. Inter- and intra-rater reliability have been established.[43]

Risk Management Considerations

Vaginal, rectal, and instrumented testing of the pelvic floor is typically taught at the post-entry level. Given the sensitivity of this examination, there should be a compelling reason to perform it based on the patient's subjective complaint or previous test findings. An appropriate level of patient education to ensure informed consent should also be provided. Before engaging in this new area of practice, therapists should review their state's practice laws to ensure that pelvic floor examination is included within the physical therapist's scope of practice. Additionally, each therapist must be able to demonstrate competence through evidence of training specific to pelvic floor rehabilitation, including internal assessment and treatment, before entering this new area of practice.

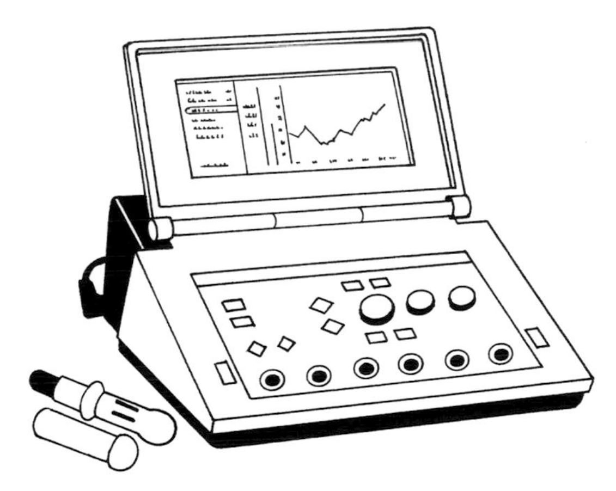

FIGURE 4-49

REFERENCES

Cited References

1. Moreau CE, Green BN, Johnson CD, et al. Isometric back extension endurance tests: a review of the literature. J Manip Physiol Ther. 2001;24:110-122.
2. Alaranta H, Hurri H, Heliovaara M, et al. Non-dynamometric trunk performance tests: reliability and normative data. Scand J Rehabil Med. 1994;26:211-215.
3. Biering-Sorensen F. Physical measurements as risk indicators for low-back trouble over a one-year period. Spine. 1984;9:106-119.
4. Luoto S, Heliovaara M, Hurri H, et al. Static back endurance and the risk of low-back pain. Clin Biomech. 1995;10:323-324.
5. Adedoyin RA, Mbada CE, Farotimi AO, et al. Endurance of low back musculature: normative data for adults. J Back Musculoskelet Rehabil. 2011;24:101-109.
6. Ng JFK, Richardson C, Jull GA. Electromyographic amplitude and frequency changes in the iliocostalis lumborum and multifidus muscles during a trunk holding test. Phys Ther. 1997;77:954-961.
7. Kavcic N, Grenier S, McGill SM. Determining the stabilizing role of individual torso muscles during rehabilitation exercises. Spine. 2004;29:1254-1265.
8. Juker D, McGill S, Kropf P, et al. Quantitative intramuscular myoelectric activity of lumbar portions of psoas and the abdominal wall during a wide variety of tasks. Med Sci Sports Exerc. 1998;30:301-310.
9. Evans K, Refshauge KM, Adams R. Trunk muscle endurance tests: reliability, and gender differences in athletes. J Sci Med Sport. 2007;10:447-455.
10. Monfort-Pañego M, Vera-García FJ, Sànchez-Zuriaga D, et al. Electromyographic studies in abdominal exercises. A literature synthesis. J Manipulative Physiol Ther. 2009;32: 232-244.
11. Carlson B. Normal chest excursion. Phys Ther. 1973;53: 10-14.
12. Reid WD, Dechman G. Considerations when testing and training the respiratory muscles. Phys Ther. 1995;75: 971-982.
13. Wade OL. Movements of the thoracic cage and diaphragm in respiration. J Physiol (Lond). 1954;124:193-212.
14. Stone DJ, Keltz H. Effect of respiratory muscle dysfunction on pulmonary function. Am Rev Respir Dis. 1964:88: 621-629.
15. Dail CW. Muscle breathing patterns. Med Art Sci. 1956; 10:2-8.
16. DeTroyer A, Estenne M. Coordination between rib cage muscles and diaphragm during quiet breathing in humans. J Appl Physiol. 1984;57:899-906.
17. Leech JA, Ghezzo H, Stevens D, et al. Respiratory pressures and function in young adults. Am Rev Respir Dis. 1983;128:17.
18. Harik-Khan RI, Wise RA, Fozard JL. Determinants of maximal inspiratory pressure: the Baltimore Longitudinal Study of Aging. Am J Respir Crit Care Med. 1998;158(5 Pt 1):1459-1564.
19. Enright PL, Kronmal RA, Manolino TA, et al. Respiratory muscle strength in the elderly. Correlates and reference values. Am J Respir Crit Care Med. 1994;149:430.
20. Bruschi C, Cerveri I, Zoia MC, et al. Reference values of maximal respiratory mouth pressures: a population-based study. Am Rev Respir Dis. 1992;146:790-793.
21. Guyton AC, Hall JE. Textbook of Medical Physiology. 10th ed. Philadelphia: W.B. Saunders; 2000.
22. Comroe JH Jr. Special acts involving breathing. In: Physiology of Respiration: An Introductory Text. 2nd ed. Chicago: Year Book Medical Publishers; 1974:230.
23. Starr JA. Manual techniques of chest physical therapy and airway clearance techniques. In: Zadai CC, ed. Pulmonary Management in Physical Therapy. New York: Churchill-Livingstone; 1992:142-148.
24. Frownfelter D, Massery M. Facilitating airway clearance with coughing techniques. In: Frownfelter D, Dean E, eds. Cardiovascular and Pulmonary Physical Therapy: Evidence and Practice. 4th ed. St. Louis, MO: Mosby Elsevier; 2006:363-376.
25. Evans JA, Whitelaw WA. The assessment of maximal respiratory mouth pressures in adults. Respir Care. 2009; 54: 1348.
26. Bach JR, Saporito LR. Criteria for extubation and tracheostomy tube removal for patients with ventilatory failure: a different approach to weaning. Chest. 1996;110: 1566-1571.
27. Neumann P, Grimmer-Somers KA, Gill V, et al. Rater reliability of pelvic floor muscle strength. Aust N Z Continence J. 2007;13:9-14.
28. Retzky SS, Rogers RM. Urinary incontinence in women. Ciba Clin Symp. 1995;47(3):2-32.
29. Swift SE. The distribution of pelvic organ support in a population of female subjects seen for routine gynecologic health care. Am J Obstet Gynecol. 2000;183:277-285.
30. Hunskaar S, Burgio K, Diokno A, et al. Epidemiology and natural history of urinary incontinence (UI). In: Abrams P, Cardozo L, Khoury S, Wein A, eds. Incontinence. Plymouth, UK: Plymbridge Distributors Ltd; 2002:165-201.
31. Kegel AH. Progressive resistance exercise in the functional restoration of the perineal muscles. Am J Obstet Gynecol. 1948;56:238-249.
32. Lewis RW, Fugl-Meyer KS, Corona G, et al. Definitions/epidemiology/risk factors for sexual dysfunction. J Sex Med. 2010;7(4 Pt 2):1598-1607.
33. Knoepp LR, Shippey SH, Chen CC, et al. Sexual complaints, pelvic floor symptoms, and sexual distress in women over forty. J Sex Med. 2010;7:3675-3682.
34. Laumann EO, Paik A, Rosen RC. Sexual dysfunction in the United States: prevalence and predictors. JAMA. 1999;281:537-544. Erratum in JAMA 1999;281(13): 1174.
35. Dennerstein L, Randolph J, Taffe J, et al. Hormones, mood, sexuality, and the menopausal transition. Fertil Steril. 2002;77(suppl 4):S42-S48.
36. Dietz HP, Schierlitz L. Pelvic floor trauma in childbirth—myth or reality? Aust N Z J Obstet Gynaecol. 2005;45: 3-11.
37. Plevnik S. A new method for testing and strengthening of pelvic floor muscles [abstract]. In: Proceeding of the 15th Annual Meeting of the International Continence Society. London, UK, September 1985.
38. Bø K, Sherburn M. Evaluation of female pelvic-floor muscle function and strength. Phys Ther. 2005;85: 269-282.
39. Dietz H, Jarvis S, Vancaillie T. The assessment of levator muscle strength: a validation of three ultrasound techniques. Int Urogynecol J Pelvic Floor Dysfunct. 2002;13: 156-159.
40. Bø K, Lilleås F, Talseth T, et al. Dynamic MRI of pelvic floor muscles in an upright sitting position. Neurourol Urodyn. 2001;20:167-174.

41. Laycock J. Clinical evaluation of the pelvic floor. In: Schussler B, Laycock J, Norton P, et al, eds. Pelvic Floor Re-education. London, UK: Springer-Verlag; 1994: 42-48.
42. Ferreira CH, Barbosa PB, de Oliveira Souza F, et al. Inter-rater reliability study of the modified Oxford Grading Scale and the Peritron manometer. Physiotherapy. 2011;97(2): 132-138.
43. Hundley AF, Wu JM, Visco AG. A comparison of perineometer to brink score for assessment of pelvic floor muscle strength. Am J Obstet Gynecol. 2005;192:1583-1591.

Other Readings

Sartore A, Pregazzi R, Bortoli P, et al. The urine stream interruption test and pelvic muscle function in the puerperium. Inter J Gynec Obstet. 2002;78:235-239.

Sampselle CM, DeLancey JO. The urine stream interruption test and pelvic muscle function. Nurs Res. 1992;41:73-77.

Lewis RW, Fugl-Meyer KS, Corona G, et al. Definitions/epidemiology/risk factors for sexual dysfunction. J Sex Med. 2010;7(4 Pt 2):1598-1607.

Knoepp LR, Shippey SH, Chen CC, et al. Sexual complaints, pelvic floor symptoms, and sexual distress in women over forty. J Sex Med. 2010;7:3675-3682.

Travell JG, Simons DG. Myofascial Pain and Dysfunction: The Trigger Point Manual, vol 2. Baltimore, MD: Williams and Wilkins; 1992.

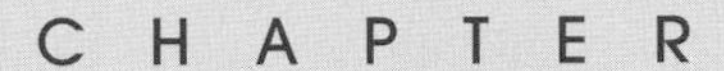

CHAPTER 5

Testing the Muscles of the Upper Extremity

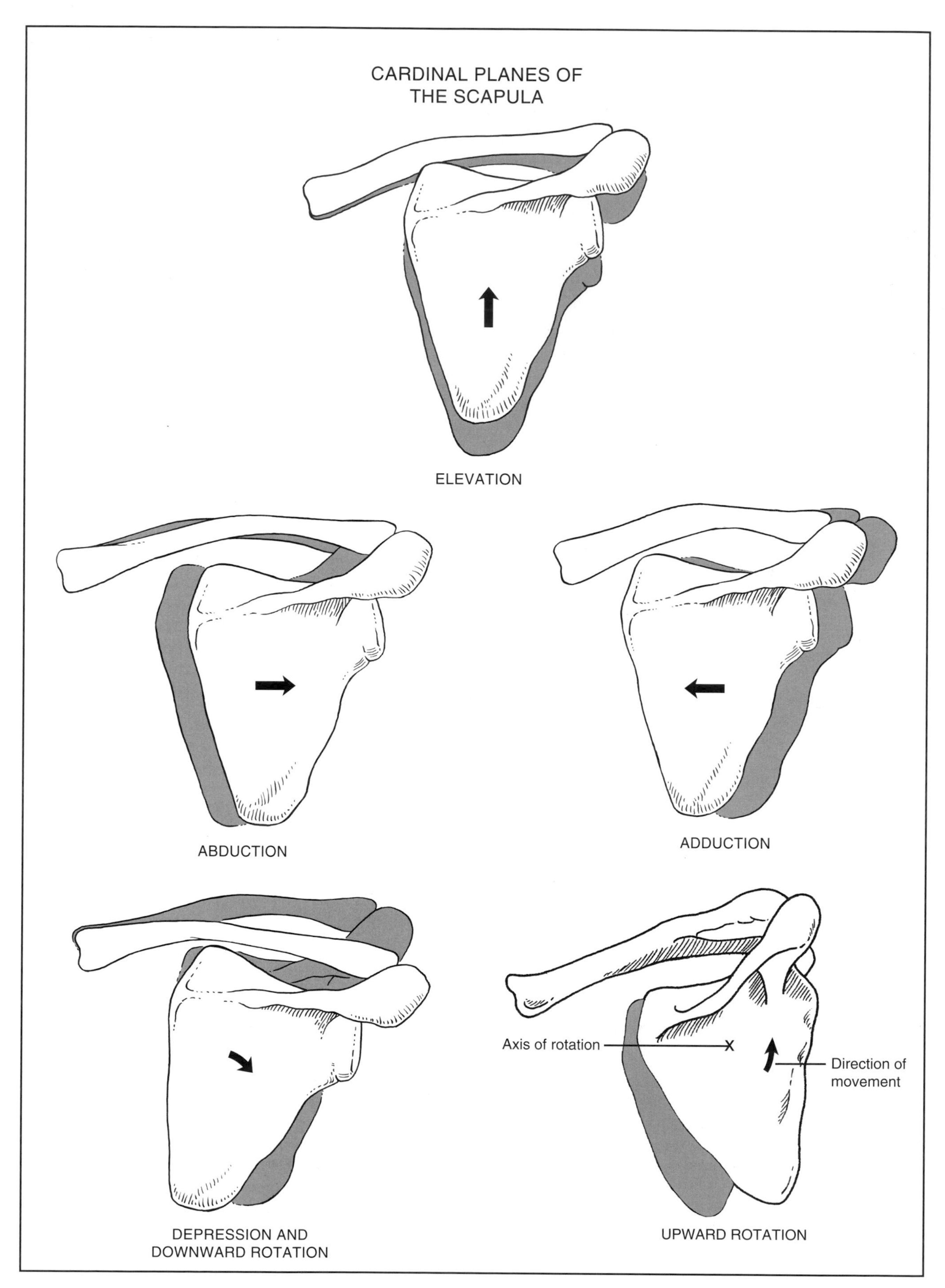
CARDINAL PLANES OF
THE SCAPULA
ELEVATION
ABDUCTION
ADDUCTION
DEPRESSION AND
DOWNWARD ROTATION
Axis of rotation
Direction of
movement
UPWARD ROTATION

PLATE 2

(Serratus anterior)

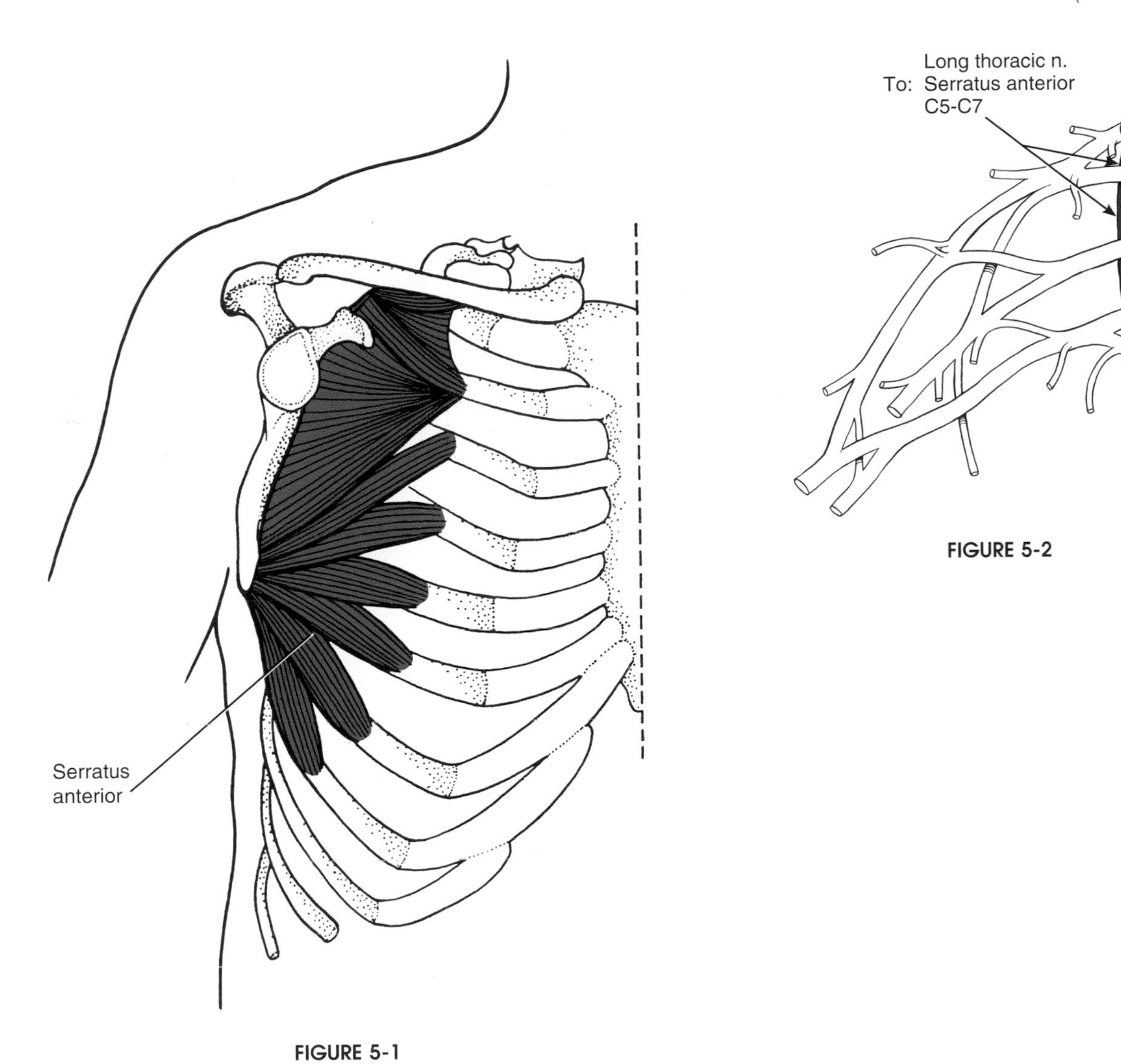

FIGURE 5-1

FIGURE 5-2

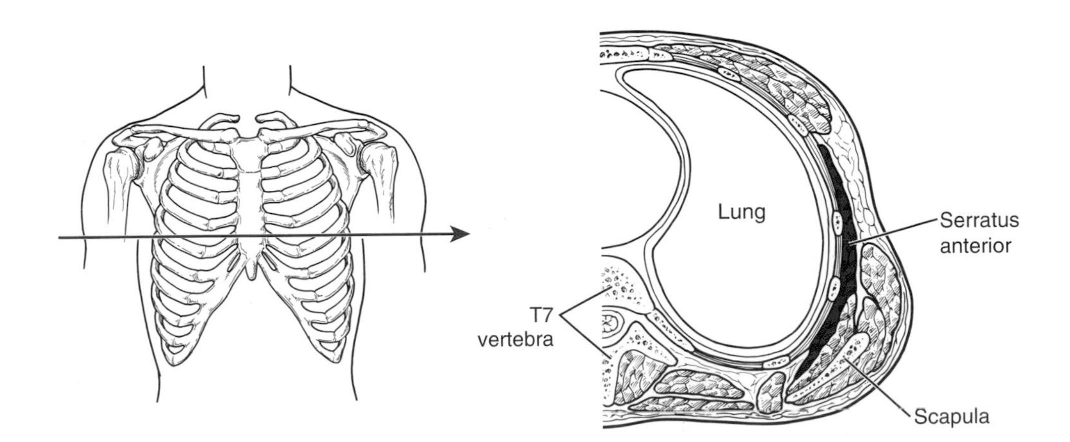

FIGURE 5-3 Arrow indicates level of cross section.

SCAPULAR ABDUCTION AND UPWARD ROTATION

(Serratus anterior)

Range of Motion
Reliable values not available

Table 5-1 SCAPULAR ABDUCTION AND UPWARD ROTATION

I.D.	Muscle	Origin	Insertion
128	Serratus anterior	Ribs 1-8 and often 9 and 10 (by digitations along a curved line) Intercostal fascia Aponeurosis of intercostals	Scapula (ventral surface of vertebral border) 1st digitation (superior angle) 2nd to 4th digitations (costal surface of entire vertebral border) Lower 4th or 5th digitations (costal surface of inferior angle)

INTRODUCTION TO SCAPULAR-THORACIC MUSCLE TESTING

A primary role of the thoracic-scapular muscles is to provide stabilization of the scapula so that the scapular-humeral muscles may work efficiently to produce movement at the glenohumeral joint. Stabilization of upward rotation of the scapula is a primary consideration when evaluating function of the shoulder girdle. In the absence of strong scapular-thoracic muscles, dyskinesia may occur at the glenohumeral joint such that the scapula may rotate downward rather than the humerus moving upward. This in turn decreases the sub-acromial space contributing to impingement syndromes at the glenohumeral joint. External resistance to the upper extremity that often occurs with lifting activities may exacerbate this problem. Also, the more elevation of the upper extremity that is required for the task, the higher the risk for impingement.

The serratus often is graded incorrectly, perhaps because the muscle arrangement and the bony movement are unlike those of axial structures. The test procedure is in keeping with known kinesiologic and pathokinesiologic principles. The scapular muscles, however, do need further dynamic testing with electromyography, magnetic resonance imaging, and other modern technology before completely reliable functional diagnoses can be made.

The supine position, although best for isolating the serratus anterior, is not recommended at any grade level. The supine position allows too much substitution that may not be noticeable. Lying supine on the table gives added stabilization to the scapula so that it does not "wing" and protraction of the arm may be performed by the clavicular portion of the pectoralis minor.

Preliminary Examination

Observation of the scapulae, both at rest and during active and passive shoulder flexion, is a routine part of the test. Examine the patient in the sitting position with hands in the lap.

Palpate the vertebral borders of both scapulae with the thumbs; place the web of the thumb below the inferior angle; the fingers extend around the axillary borders (Figure 5-4).

Specific Elements

Position and symmetry of scapulae: Determine the position of the scapulae at rest and whether the two sides are symmetrical, although minor asymmetry is normal.

The normal scapula lies close to the rib cage with the vertebral border nearly parallel to and from 1 to 3 inches lateral to the spinous processes. The inferior angle is on the chest wall. The most prominent abnormal posture of the scapula is "winging," in which the vertebral border tilts away from the rib cage, a sign indicative of serratus

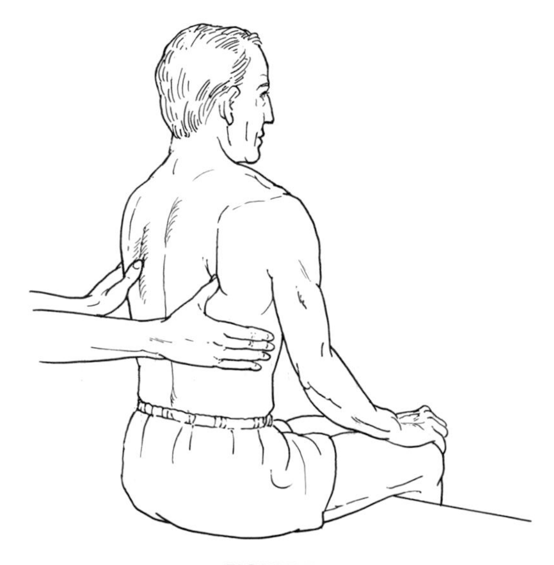

FIGURE 5-4

Preliminary Examination Continued

anterior weakness (Figure 5-5). Other abnormal postures are abduction and downward rotation of the scapula. If the inferior angle of the scapula is tilted away from the rib cage, check for tightness of the pectoralis minor, weakness of the trapezius, and spinal deformity.

Scapulohumeral rhythm improves the shoulder's range of motion and consists of integrated movements of the glenohumeral, scapulothoracic, acromioclavicular, and sternoclavicular joints. It occurs in sequential fashion to allow full functional motion of the shoulder complex. To complete 180° of shoulder abduction, the overall ratio of glenohumeral to scapulothoracic motion is 2:1.

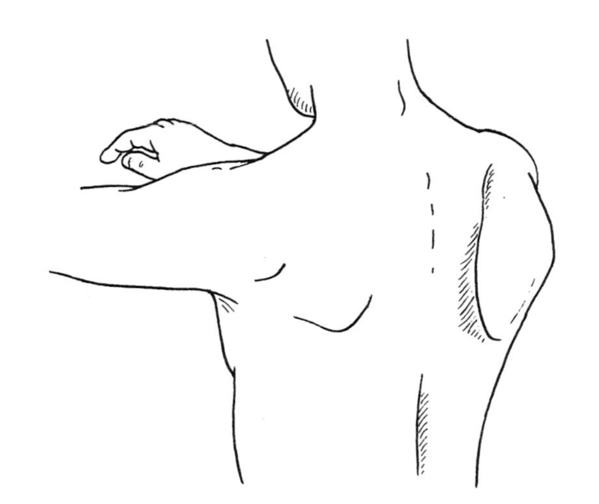

FIGURE 5-5

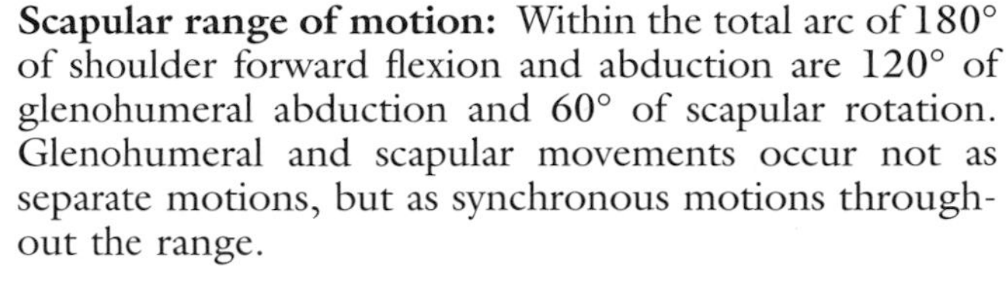

Scapular range of motion: Within the total arc of 180° of shoulder forward flexion and abduction are 120° of glenohumeral abduction and 60° of scapular rotation. Glenohumeral and scapular movements occur not as separate motions, but as synchronous motions throughout the range.

a. The scapula sits against the thorax (T) during the first phase of shoulder abduction and flexion to provide initial stability as the humerus (H) abducts and flexes to 30°.
b. From 30° to 90° of flexion and abduction, the glenohumeral (G-H) joint contributes another 30° of motion, whereas the scapula upwardly rotates 30°. The upward rotation is accompanied by clavicular elevation through the sternoclavicular and acromioclavicular joints (Figure 5-6, *A*).
c. The second phase (90° to 180°) is made up of 60° of glenohumeral abduction and flexion and an additional 30° of scapular upward rotation. The scapular rotation is associated with 5° of elevation at the sternoclavicular joint and 25° of rotation at the acromioclavicular joint (Figure 5-6, *B*).

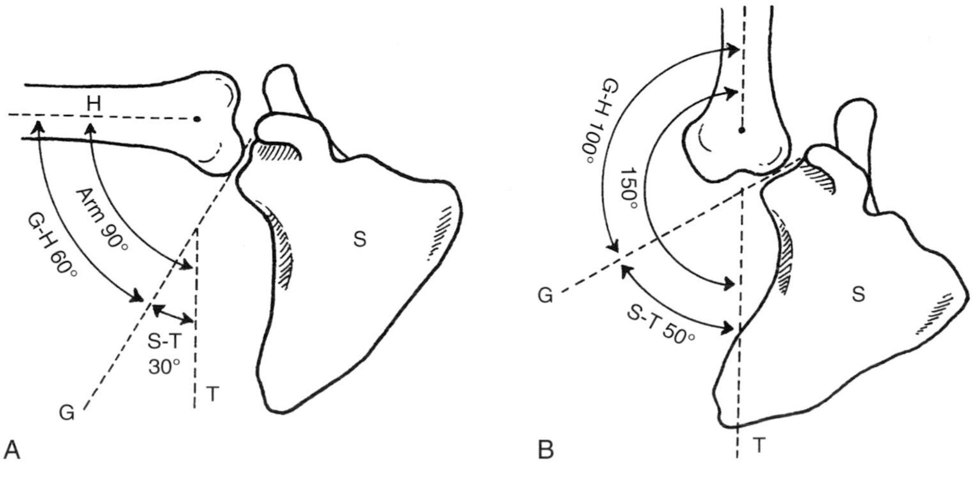

FIGURE 5-6

Preliminary Examination Continued

Passively raise the test arm completely above the head in forward flexion to determine scapular mobility. The scapula should start to rotate at about 30°, although there is considerable individual variation. Scapular rotation continues until about –20° to –30° from full flexion.

Check that the scapula basically remains in its rest position at ranges of shoulder flexion less than 30° of forward flexion (the position is variable among subjects). If the scapula moves a lot as the glenohumeral joint moves through from 0 to 60°—that is, if in this range they move as a unit—there is limited glenohumeral motion. Above 30° and to about 150° or 160° in both active and passive motion, the scapula moves in concert with the humerus.

The serratus should always be tested in shoulder flexion to minimize the synergy with the trapezius.

If the scapular position at rest is normal, ask the patient to raise the test arm above the head in the sagittal plane. If the arm can be raised well above 90° (glenohumeral muscles must be at least Grade 3 to do this), observe the direction and amount of scapular motion that occur. Normally, the scapula rotates forward in a motion that is controlled by the serratus, and if erratic or "uncoordinated" motion occurs, the serratus is most likely weak. The normal amount of motion of the vertebral border from the start position is about the breadth of two fingers (Figure 5-7). If the patient is able to raise the arm with simultaneous rhythmical scapular upward rotation, proceed with the test sequence for Grades 5 and 4.

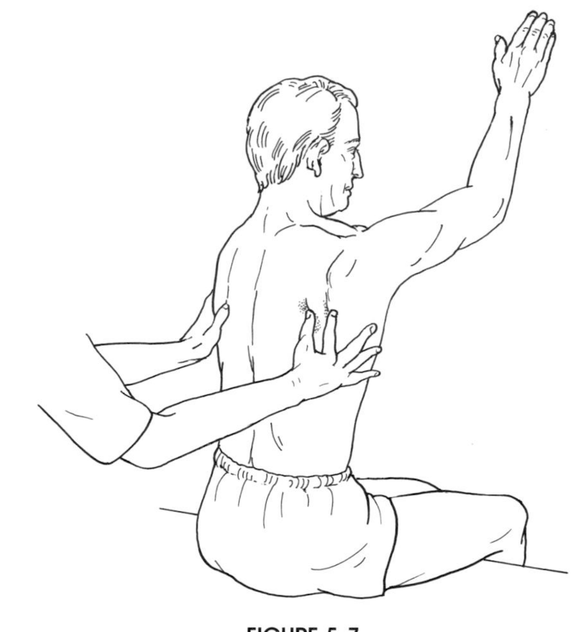

FIGURE 5-7

Scapula abnormal position at rest: If the scapula is positioned abnormally at rest (i.e., downwardly rotated, abducted, or winging), the patient will not be able to flex the arm above 90°. Proceed to tests described for Grades 2, 1, and 0.

The serratus anterior never can be graded higher than the grade given to shoulder flexion. If the patient has a weak deltoid, the lever for testing is gone, and the arm cannot be used to apply resistance.

Helpful Hint

Thoracic spine extension is necessary to achieve full shoulder flexion. If a person is kyphotic, arm elevation will be sacrificed and a 10° to 20° deficit of shoulder flexion will be noted.

Grade 5 (Normal) and Grade 4 (Good)

Position of Patient (All Grades): Short sitting over end or side of table. Hands on lap.

Position of Therapist: Standing at test side of patient. Hand giving resistance is on the arm proximal to the elbow (Figure 5-8). The other hand uses the web space along with the thumb and index finger to palpate the edges of the scapula at the inferior angle and along the vertebral and axillary borders.

Test: Patient raises arm to approximately 130° of flexion with the elbow extended. (Examiner is reminded that the arm can be elevated up to 60° without using the serratus.) The scapula should rotate (glenoid facing up) and abduct without winging.

Instructions to Patient: "Raise your arm forward over your head. Keep your elbow straight; hold it! Don't let me push your arm down."

Grading

Grade 5 (Normal): Scapula maintains its abducted and rotated position against maximal resistance given on the arm just above the elbow in a downward direction.

Grade 4 (Good): Scapular muscles "give" or "yield" against maximal resistance given on the arm. The glenohumeral joint is held rigidly in the presence of a strong deltoid, but the serratus yields, and the scapula moves in the direction of adduction and downward rotation.

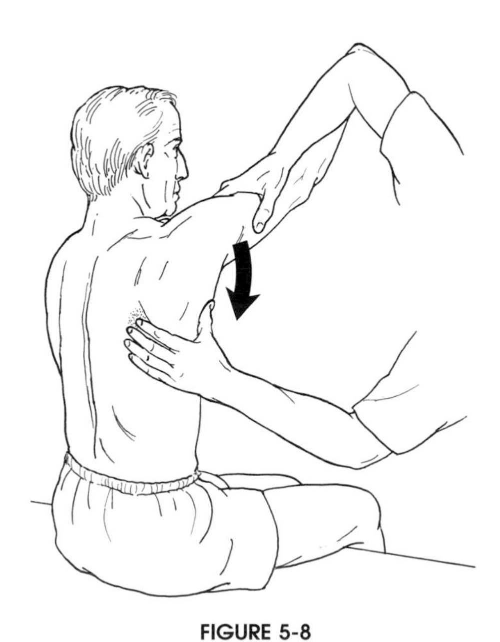

FIGURE 5-8

Grade 3 (Fair)

Positions of Patient and Therapist: Same as for Grade 5 test.

Test: Patient raises the arm to approximately 130° of flexion with the elbow extended (Figure 5-9).

Instructions to Patient: "Raise your arm forward above your head."

Grading

Grade 3 (Fair): Scapula moves through full range of motion without winging but can tolerate no resistance other than the weight of the arm.

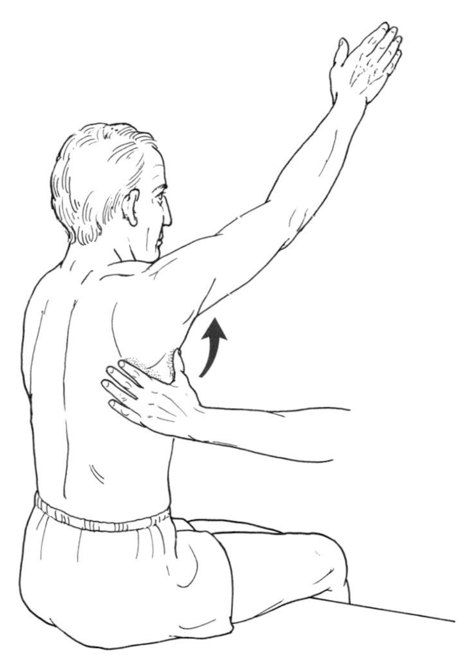

FIGURE 5-9

SCAPULAR ABDUCTION AND UPWARD ROTATION

(Serratus anterior)

Alternate Test (Grades 5, 4, and 3)

Position of Patient: Short sitting with arm forward flexed to about 130° and then protracted in that plane as far as it can move.

Position of Therapist: Standing at test side of patient. Hand used for resistance grasps the forearm just above the wrist and gives resistance in a downward and backward direction. The other hand stabilizes the trunk just below the scapula on the same side; this prevents trunk rotation.

The examiner should select a spot on the wall or ceiling that can serve as a target for the patient to reach toward in line with about 130° of flexion.

Test: Patient abducts and upwardly rotates the scapula by protracting and elevating the arm to about 130° of flexion. The patient then holds against maximal resistance.

Instructions to Patient: "Bring your arm up, and reach for the target on the wall."

Grading

Same as for primary test.

Grade 2 (Poor)

Position of Patient: Short sitting with arm flexed above 90° and supported by examiner.

Position of Therapist: Standing at test side of patient. One hand supports the patient's arm at the elbow, maintaining it above the horizontal (Figure 5-10). The other hand is placed at the inferior angle of the scapula with the thumb positioned along the axillary border and the fingers along the vertebral border (see Figure 5-10).

Test: Therapist monitors scapular motion by using a light grasp on the scapula at the inferior angle. Therapist must be sure not to restrict or resist motion. The scapula is observed to detect winging.

Instructions to Patient: "Hold your arm in this position" (i.e., above 90°). "Let it relax. Now hold your arm up again. Let it relax."

Grading

Grade 2 (Poor): If the scapula abducts and rotates upward as the patient attempts to hold the arm in the elevated position, the weakness is in the glenohumeral muscles. The serratus is awarded a grade of 2. The serratus is graded 2– (Poor–) if the scapula does not smoothly abduct and upwardly rotate without the weight of the arm or if the scapula moves toward the vertebral spine.

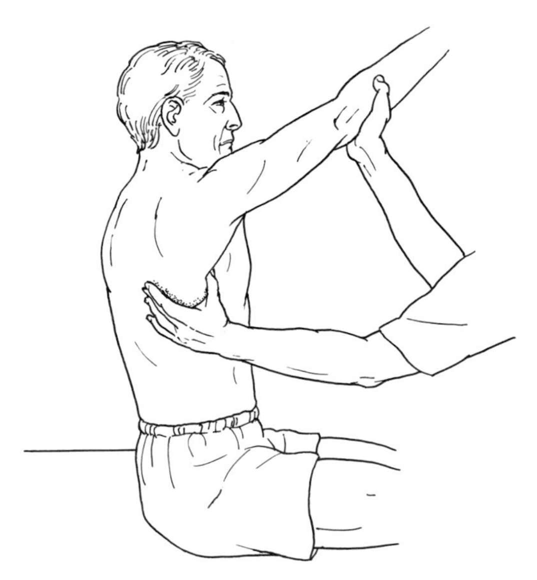

FIGURE 5-10

Grade 1 (Trace) and Grade 0 (Zero)

Position of Patient: Short sitting with arm forward flexed to above 90° (supported by therapist).

Position of Therapist: Standing in front of and slightly to one side of patient. Support the patient's arm at the elbow, maintaining it above 90° (Figure 5-11). Use the other hand to palpate the serratus with the tips of the fingers just in front of the inferior angle along the axillary border (see Figure 5-11).

Test: Patient attempts to hold the arm in the test position.

Instructions to Patient: "Try to hold your arm in this position."

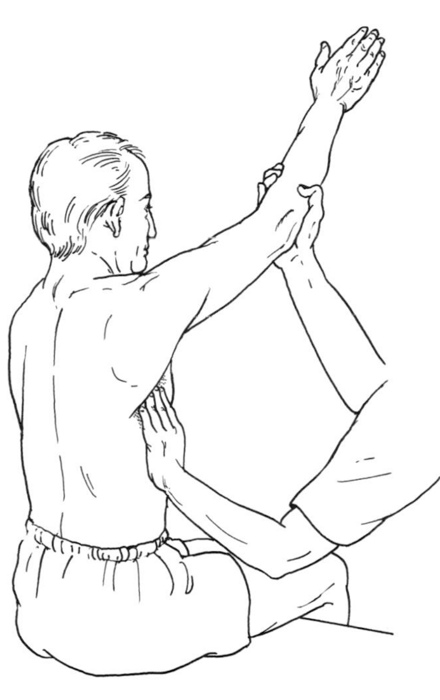

FIGURE 5-11

Alternate Test for Grade 1

Position of Patient: Lying on table with arm forward flexed to 90° (supported by therapist).

Position of Therapist: Standing to the same side as arm being tested. Support the patient's arm at the elbow, maintaining the arm above 90° (Figure 5-12). Use the other hand to palpate the serratus with tips of fingers just in front of the inferior angle along the axillary border.

Test: Patient attempts to hold the arm in the test position.

Instructions to Patient: "Try to hold your arm in this position."

Grading

Grade 1 (Trace): Muscle contraction is palpable.

Grade 0 (Zero): No contractile activity.

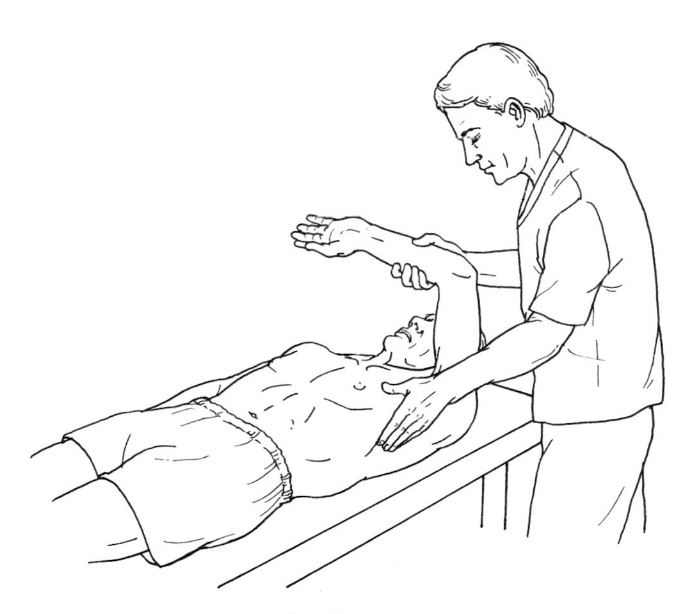

FIGURE 5-12

SCAPULAR ELEVATION

(Trapezius, upper fibers)

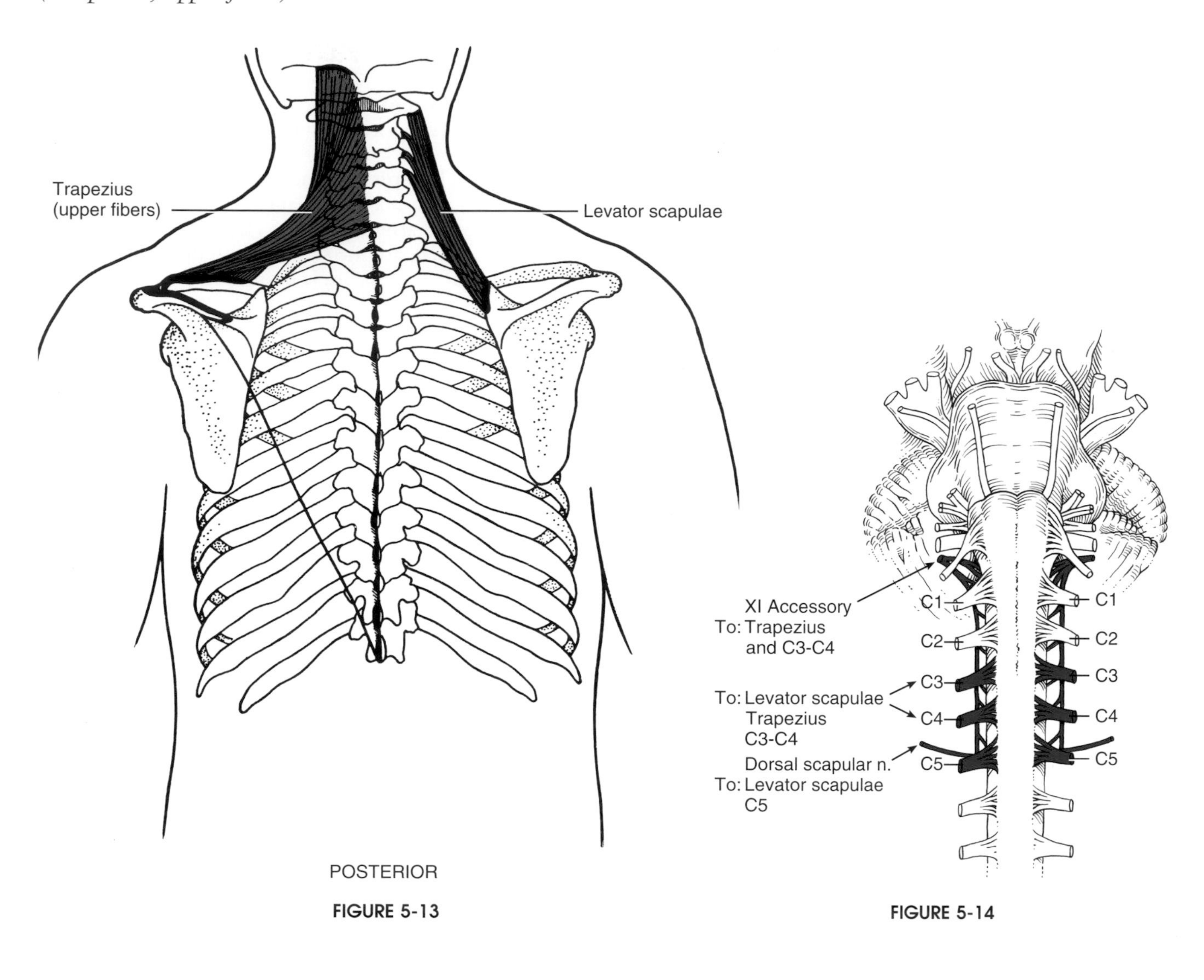

FIGURE 5-13

FIGURE 5-14

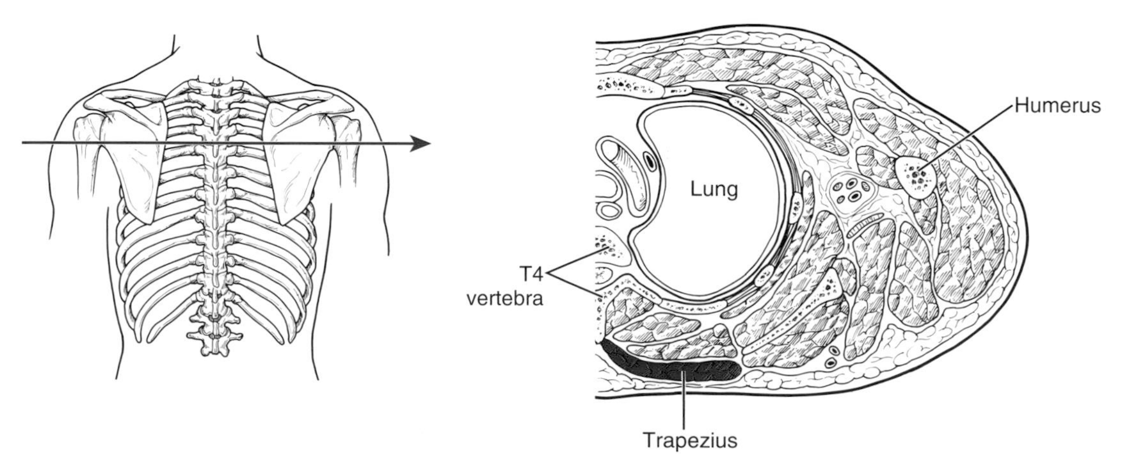

FIGURE 5-15 Arrow indicates level of cross section.

(Trapezius, upper fibers)

Range of Motion
Reliable data not available

Table 5-2 SCAPULAR ELEVATION

I.D.	Muscle	Origin	Insertion
124	Trapezius (upper fibers)	Occiput (external protuberance and superior nuchal line, medial 1/3) Ligamentum nuchae C7 vertebra (spinous process)	Clavicle (posterior border of lateral 1/3)
127	Levator scapulae	C1-C4 vertebrae (transverse processes)	Scapula (vertebral border between superior angle and root of scapular spine)
Others			
125	Rhomboid major	See Table 5-3	See Plate 3
126	Rhomboid minor	See Table 5-5	

Grade 5 (Normal) and Grade 4 (Good)

Position of Patient: Short sitting over end or side of table. Hands relaxed in lap.

Position of Therapist: Standing behind patient. Hands contoured over top of both shoulders to give resistance in a downward direction. The therapist's arms should be nearly straight, transferring the therapist's body weight through the arms to provide enough resistance to this typically strong muscle.

Test: It is important to examine the patient's shoulders and scapula from a posterior view and to note any asymmetry of shoulder height, muscular bulk, or scapular winging. This kind of asymmetry is common and can be caused by carrying purses or briefcases habitually on one side (Figure 5-16).

Patient elevates ("shrugs") shoulders. In the sitting position, the test is almost always performed on both sides simultaneously.

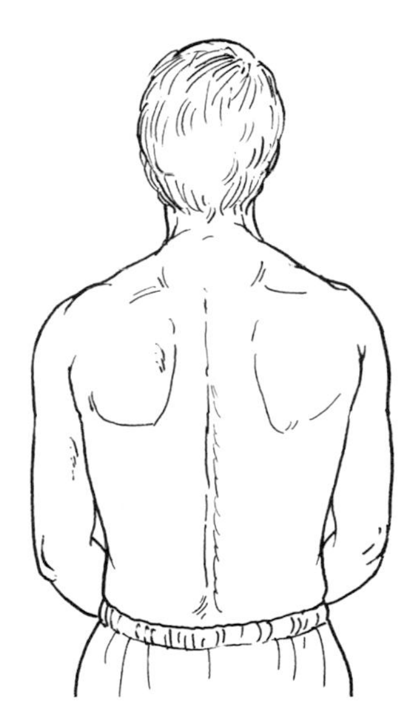

FIGURE 5-16

SCAPULAR ELEVATION

(Trapezius, upper fibers)

Grade 5 (Normal) and Grade 4 (Good) Continued

Instructions to Patient: "Shrug your shoulders." OR "Raise your shoulders toward your ears. Hold it. Don't let me push them down."

Grading

Grade 5 (Normal): Patient shrugs shoulders through available range of motion and holds against maximal resistance (Figure 5-17).

Grade 4 (Good): Patient shrugs shoulders against strong to moderate resistance. The shoulder muscles may "give" at the end point.

Grade 3 (Fair)

Position of Patient and Therapist: Same as those used for Grade 5 test except that no resistance is given (Figure 5-18).

Test: Patient elevates shoulders through range of motion.

Instructions to Patient: "Raise your shoulders toward your ears." OR "Shrug your shoulders."

Grading

Grade 3 (Fair): Elevates shoulders through range but takes no resistance.

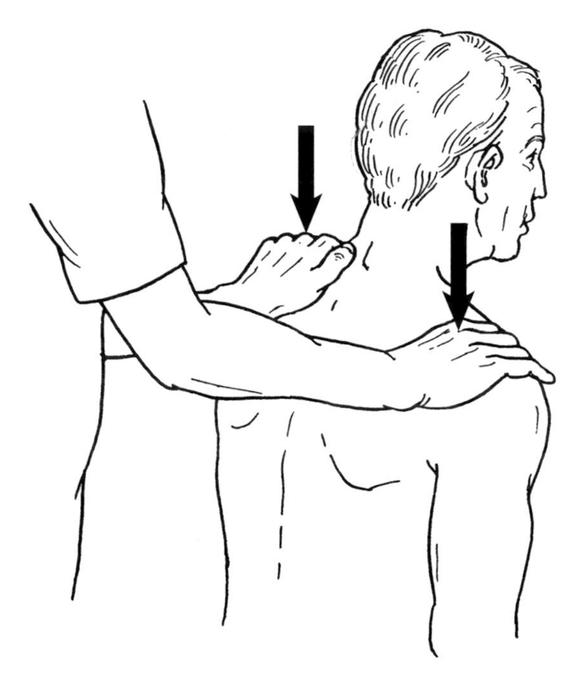

FIGURE 5-17

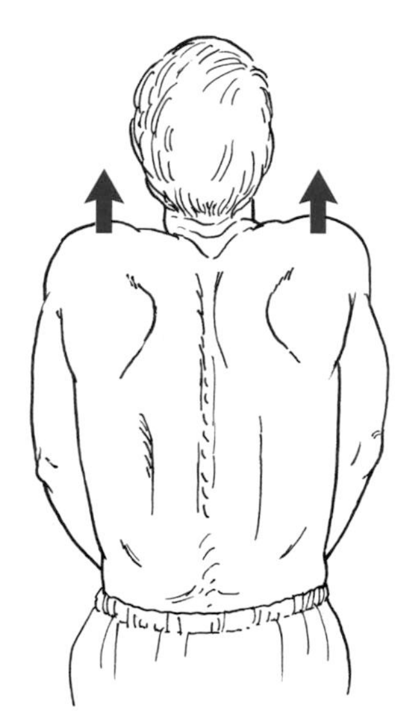

FIGURE 5-18

Grade 2 (Poor), Grade 1 (Trace), and Grade 0 (Zero)

Position of Patient: Prone or supine, fully supported on table. If prone, head is turned to one side for patient comfort (Figure 5-19). If supine, head is in neutral position.

Position of Therapist: Standing at test side of patient. Support test shoulder in palm of one hand. The other hand palpates the upper trapezius near its insertion above the clavicle. A second site for palpation is the upper trapezius just adjacent to the cervical vertebrae.

Test: With the therapist supporting the shoulder, the patient elevates the shoulder (usually done unilaterally) toward the ear.

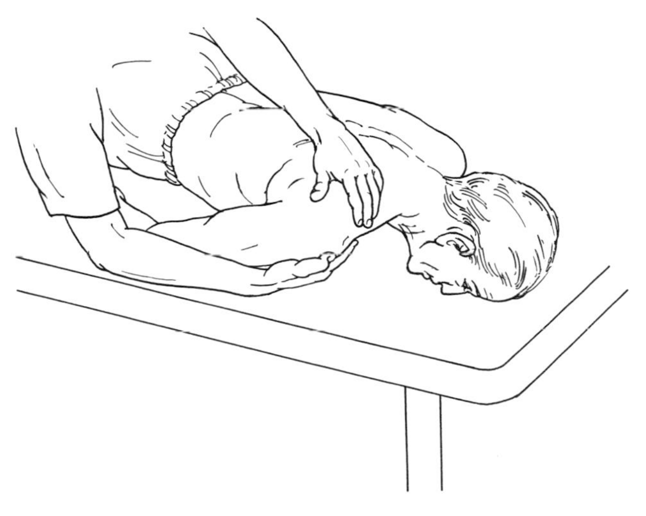

FIGURE 5-19

Instructions to Patient: "Raise your shoulder toward your ear."

Grading

Grade 2 (Poor): Patient completes full range of motion in gravity-eliminated position.

Grade 1 (Trace): Upper trapezius fibers can be palpated at clavicle or neck. The levator muscle lies deep and is more difficult to palpate in the neck (between the sternocleidomastoid and the trapezius). It can be felt at its insertion on the vertebral border of the scapula superior to the scapular spine.

Helpful Hints

- If the patient cannot assume the sitting position for testing for any reason, the tests for Grade 5 and Grade 4 in the supine position will be quite inaccurate. If the Grade 3 test is done in the supine position, it will require manual resistance because gravity is neutralized.
- If the prone position is not comfortable, the tests for Grades 2, 1, and 0 may be performed with the patient supine, but palpation in such cases will be less than optimal.
- In the prone position, the turned head offers a disadvantage. When the face is turned to either side, there is more trapezius activity and less levator activity on that side.
- Use the same lever (hand placement for resistance) in all subsequent scapular testing.

SCAPULAR ADDUCTION

(Trapezius, middle fibers)

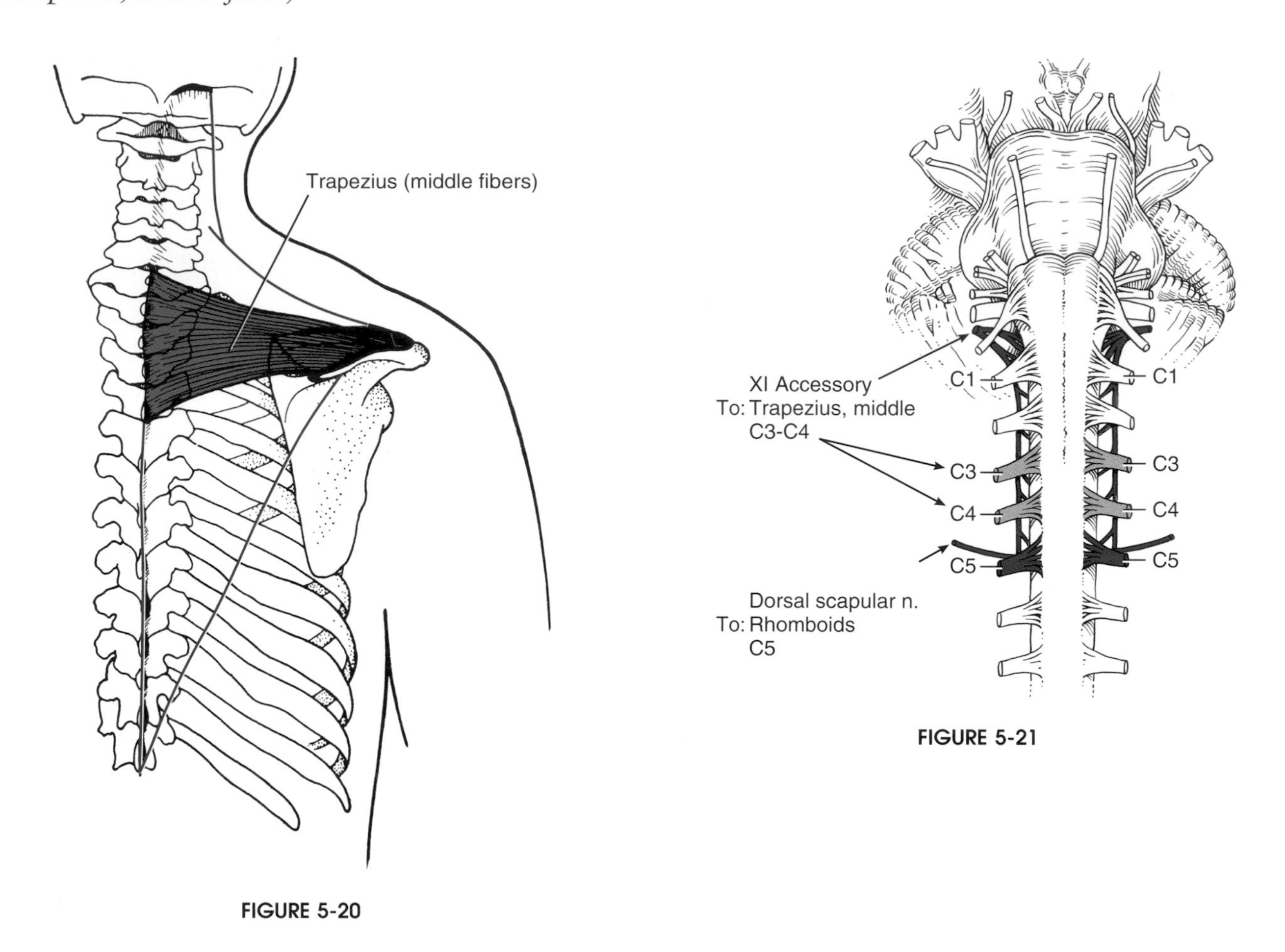

FIGURE 5-20

FIGURE 5-21

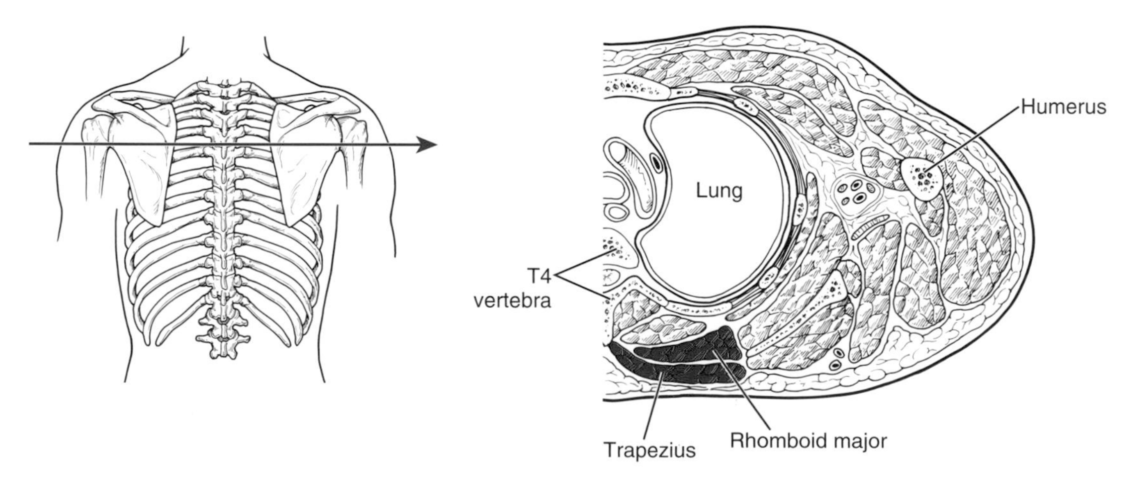

FIGURE 5-22 Arrow indicates level of cross section.

(Trapezius, middle fibers)

Range of Motion
Reliable data not available

Table 5-3 SCAPULAR ADDUCTION (RETRACTION)

I.D.	Muscle	Origin	Insertion
124	Trapezius (middle fibers)	T1-T5 vertebrae (spinous processes) Supraspinous ligaments	Scapula (medial acromial margin and superior lip of crest on scapular spine)
125	Rhomboid major	T2-T5 vertebrae (spinous processes) Supraspinous ligaments	Scapula (vertebral border between root of spine and inferior angle)
Others			
126	Rhomboid minor	See Table 5-5	
124	Trapezius (upper and lower)	See Tables 5-3, 5-4	
127	Levator scapulae	See Table 5-2	See Plate 3

Grade 5 (Normal), Grade 4 (Good), and Grade 3 (Fair)

Position of Patient: Prone with shoulder at edge of table. Shoulder is abducted to 90°. Elbow is flexed to a right angle (Figure 5-23). Head may be turned to either side for comfort.

Position of Therapist: Standing at test side close to patient's arm. Stabilize the contralateral scapular area to prevent trunk rotation. There are two ways to give resistance; one does not require as much strength as the other.

1. When the posterior deltoid is Grade 3 or better: The hand for resistance is placed over the distal end of the humerus, and resistance is directed downward toward the floor (see Figure 5-23). The wrist also may be used for a longer lever, but the lever selected should be maintained consistently throughout the test.
2. When the posterior deltoid is Grade 2 or less: Resistance is given in a downward direction (toward floor) with the hand contoured over the shoulder joint (Figure 5-24). This placement of resistance requires less adductor muscle strength by the patient than is needed in the test described in the preceding paragraph.

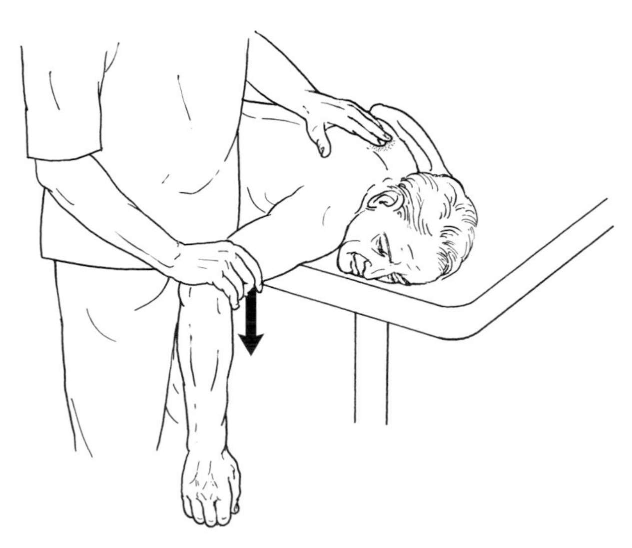

FIGURE 5-23

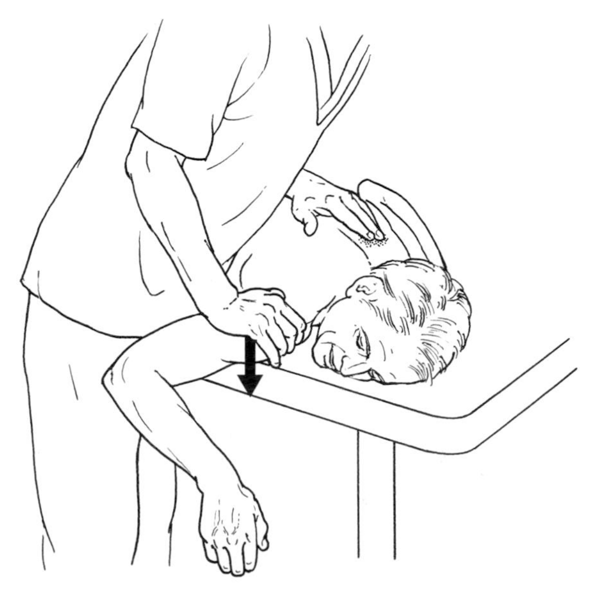

FIGURE 5-24

SCAPULAR ADDUCTION

(Trapezius, middle fibers)

Grade 5 (Normal), Grade 4 (Good), and Grade 3 (Fair) Continued

The fingers of the other hand can palpate the middle fibers of the trapezius at the spine of the scapula from the acromion to the vertebral column if necessary (Figure 5-25).

Test: Patient horizontally abducts arm and adducts scapula.

Instructions to Patient: "Lift your elbow toward the ceiling. Hold it. Don't let me push it down."

Grading

Grade 5 (Normal): Completes available scapular adduction range and holds end position against maximal resistance.

Grade 4 (Good): Tolerates strong to moderate resistance.

Grade 3 (Fair): Completes available range but without manual resistance (see Figure 5-25).

Grade 2 (Poor), Grade 1 (Trace), and Grade 0 (Zero)

Position of Patient and Therapist: Same as for normal test except that the therapist uses one hand to cradle the patient's shoulder and arm, thus supporting the arm's weight (Figure 5-26), and the other hand for palpation.

Test: Same as that for Grades 5 to 3.

Instruction to Patient: "Try to lift your elbow toward the ceiling."

Grading

Grade 2 (Poor): Completes full range of motion without the weight of the arm.

Grade 1 (Trace) and Grade 0 (Zero): A Grade 1 (Trace) muscle exhibits contractile activity or slight movement. There will be neither motion nor contractile activity in the Grade 0 (Zero) muscle.

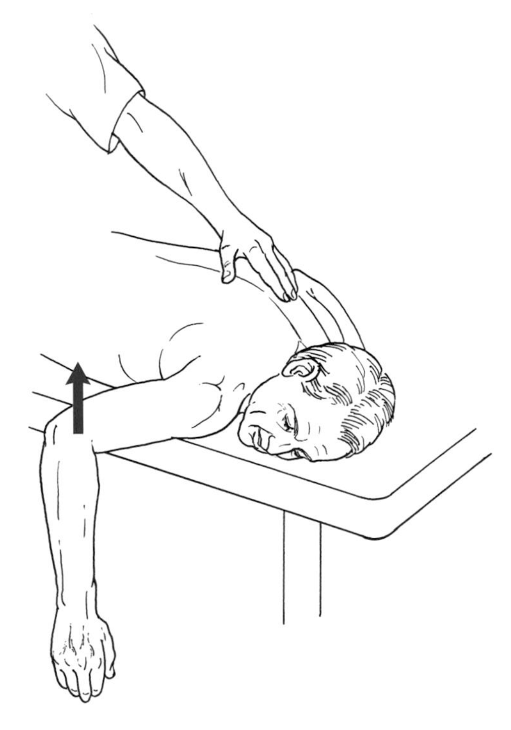

FIGURE 5-25

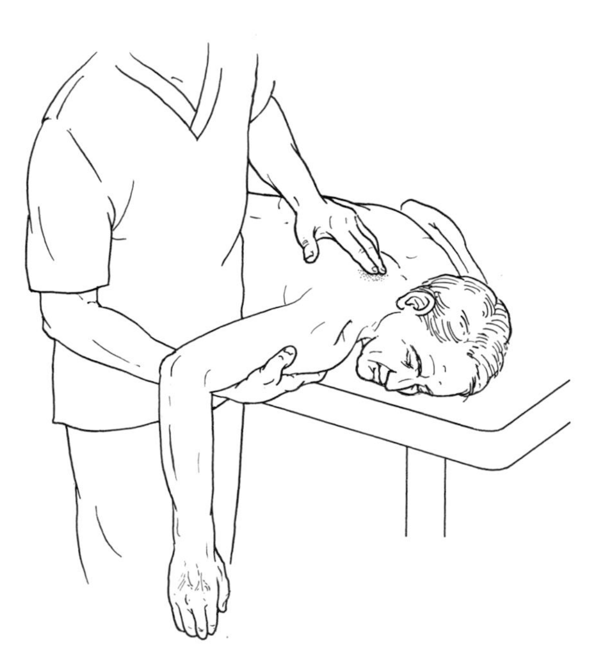

FIGURE 5-26

Alternate Test for Grades 5, 4, and 3

Position of Patient: Prone. Place scapula in full adduction. Arm is in horizontal abduction (90°) with shoulder externally rotated and elbow fully extended.

Position of Therapist: Standing near shoulder on test side. Stabilize the opposite scapular region to avoid trunk rotation. For Grades 5 and 4, give resistance toward the floor at the distal humerus or at the wrist, maintaining consistency of location of resistance.

Instructions to Patient: "Keep your shoulder blade close to the spine. Don't let me draw it away."

Test: Patient maintains scapular adduction.

Substitutions

- By the rhomboids: The rhomboids can substitute for the trapezius in adduction of the scapula. They cannot, however, substitute for the upward rotation component. When substitution by the rhomboids occurs, the scapula will adduct and rotate downward.
- By the posterior deltoid: If the scapular muscles are absent and the posterior deltoid acts alone, horizontal abduction occurs at the shoulder joint but there is no scapular adduction.

Helpful Hint

When the posterior deltoid muscle is weak, support the patient's shoulder with the palm of one hand and allow the patient's elbow to flex. Passively move the scapula into adduction via horizontal abduction of the arm. Have the patient hold the scapula in adduction as the examiner slowly releases the shoulder support. Observe whether the scapula maintains its adducted position. If it does, it is Grade 3 (Fair).

SCAPULAR DEPRESSION AND ADDUCTION

(Trapezius, lower fibers)

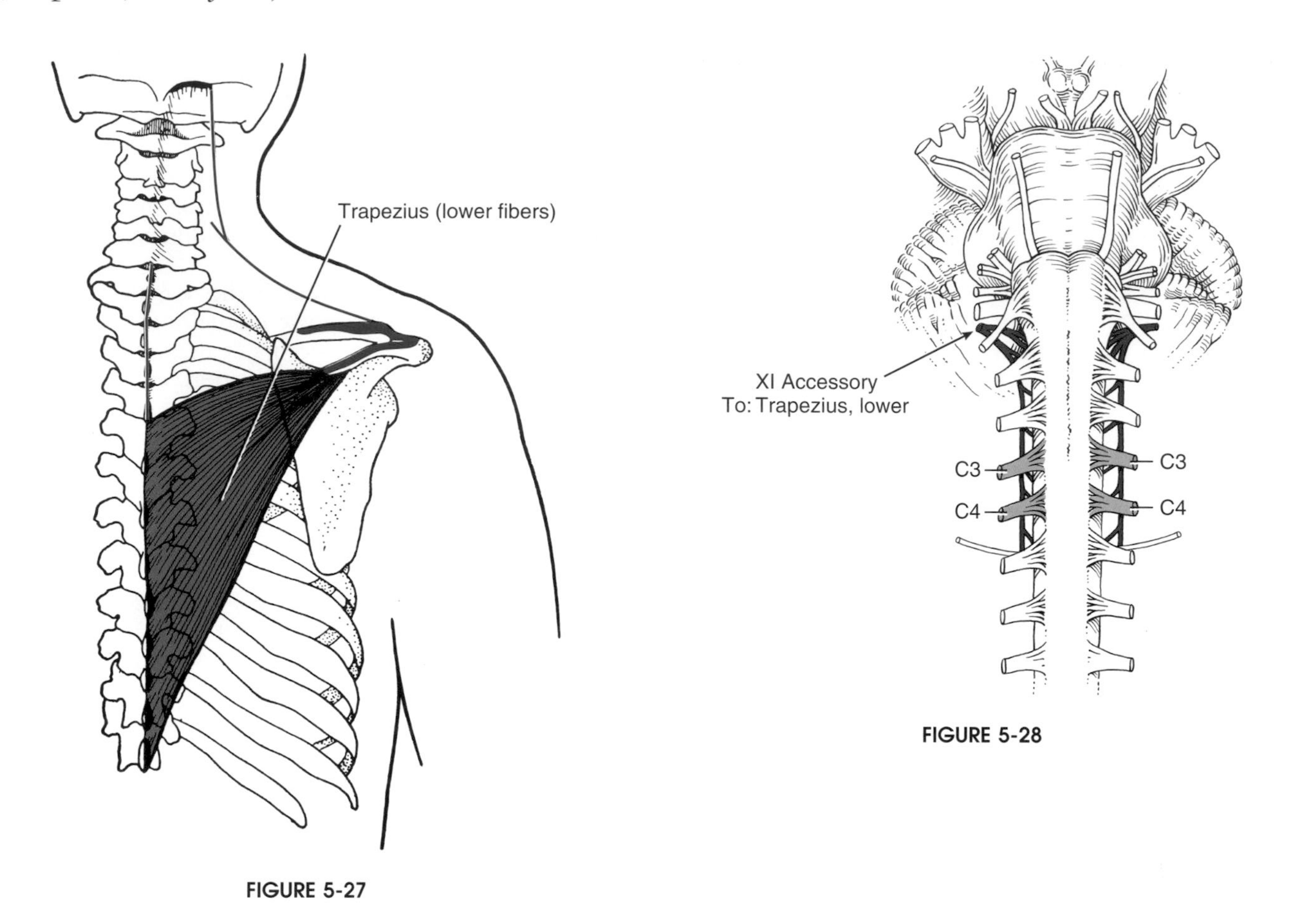

FIGURE 5-27

FIGURE 5-28

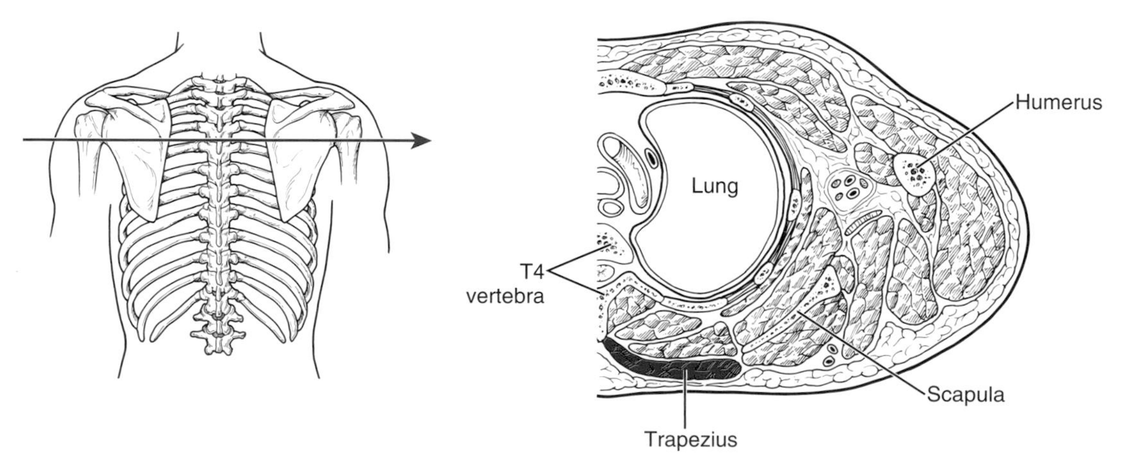

FIGURE 5-29 Arrow indicates level of cross section.

Range of Motion
Reliable data not available

(Trapezius, lower fibers)

Table 5-4 SCAPULAR DEPRESSION AND ADDUCTION

I.D.	Muscle	Origin	Insertion
124	Trapezius (middle and lower fibers)	T1-T5 vertebrae (spinous processes) Supraspinous ligaments T6-T12 vertebrae (spinous processes)	Scapula (spine, medial end, and tubercle at lateral apex via aponeurosis)
Others			
130	Latissimus dorsi	Spines of the 6 lower thoracic vertebrae, thoracolumbar fascia, crest of the ilium, lowest 4 ribs	Anterior humerus, lower margin of the intertubercular sulcus
131	Pectoralis major	Sternal half of clavicle, entire anterior surface of the sternum	Lateral lip of the intertubercular sulcus of anterior humerus
129	Pectoralis minor	Ribs 3-5, intercostal cartilage	Coracoid process

Grade 5 (Normal) Grade 4 (Good), and Grade 3 (Fair)

Position of Patient: Prone with test arm over head to about 145° of abduction (in line with the fibers of the lower trapezius). Forearm is in midposition with the thumb pointing toward the ceiling. Head may be turned to either side for comfort.

Position of Therapist: Standing at test side. Hand giving resistance is contoured over the distal humerus just proximal to the elbow (Figure 5-30). Resistance will be given straight downward (toward the floor). For a less rigorous test, resistance may be given over the axillary border of the scapula.

Fingertips of the opposite hand palpate (for Grade 3) below the spine of the scapula and across to the thoracic vertebrae, following the muscle as it curves down to the lower thoracic vertebrae.

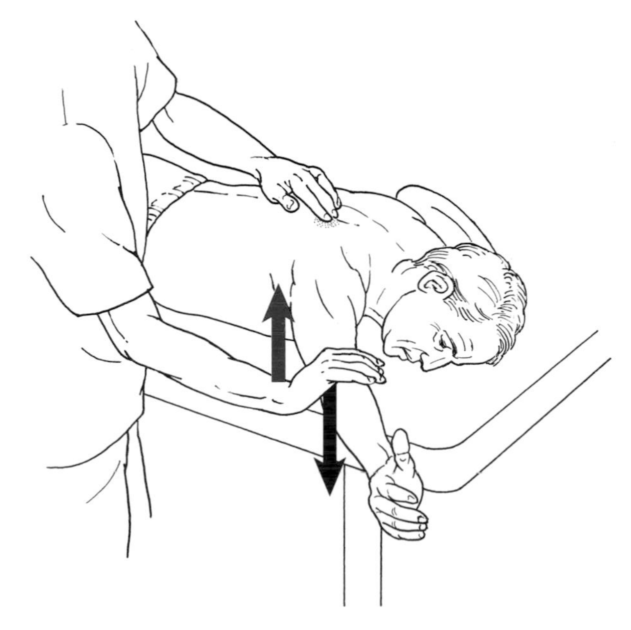

FIGURE 5-30

Test: Patient raises arm from the table to at least ear level and holds it strongly against resistance. Alternatively, preposition the arm in elevation diagonally over the head and ask the patient to hold it strongly against resistance.

Instructions to Patient: "Raise your arm from the table as high as possible. Hold it. Don't let me push it down."

Grading

Grade 5 (Normal): Completes available range and holds it against maximal resistance. This is a strong muscle.

Grade 4 (Good): Takes strong to moderate resistance.

Grade 3 (Fair): Same procedure is used, but patient tolerates no manual resistance (Figure 5-31).

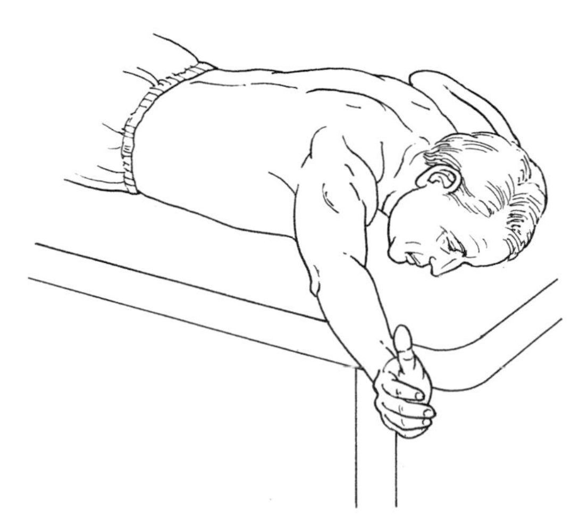

FIGURE 5-31

SCAPULAR DEPRESSION AND ADDUCTION

(Trapezius, lower fibers)

Grade 2 (Poor), Grade 1 (Trace), and Grade 0 (Zero)

Position of Patient: Same as for Grade 5.

Position of Therapist: Standing at test side. Support patient's arm under the elbow (Figure 5-32).

Test: Patient attempts to lift the arm from the table. If the patient is unable to lift the arm because of a weak posterior and middle deltoid, the examiner should lift and support the weight of the arm.

Instructions to Patient: "Try to lift your arm from the table past your ear."

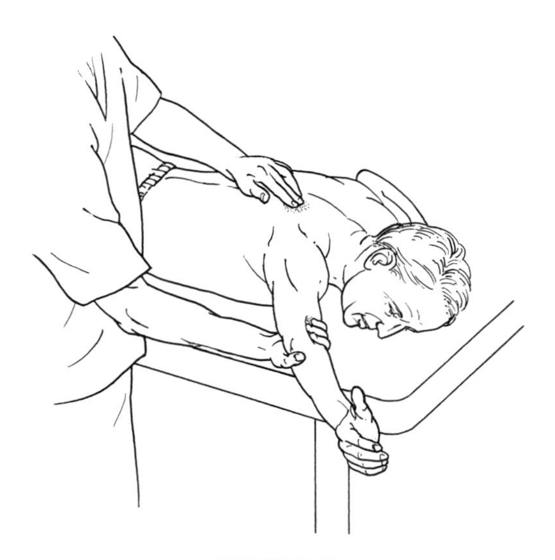

FIGURE 5-32

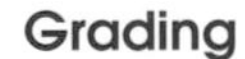

Grading

Grade 2 (Poor): Completes full scapular range of motion without the weight of the arm.

Grade 1 (Trace): Contractile activity can be palpated in the triangular area between the root of the spine of the scapula and the lower thoracic vertebra (T7-T12), that is, the course of the fibers of the lower trapezius.

Grade 0 (Zero): No palpable contractile activity.

Helpful Hints

- If shoulder range of motion is limited in flexion and abduction, the patient's arm should be positioned over the side of the table and supported by the examiner at its maximal range of elevation as the start position.
- Examiners are reminded of the test principle that the same lever arm must be used in sequential testing (over time) for valid comparison of results.
- If the patient cannot isolate this test or substitutes away from test position, the grade is 0 (zero).

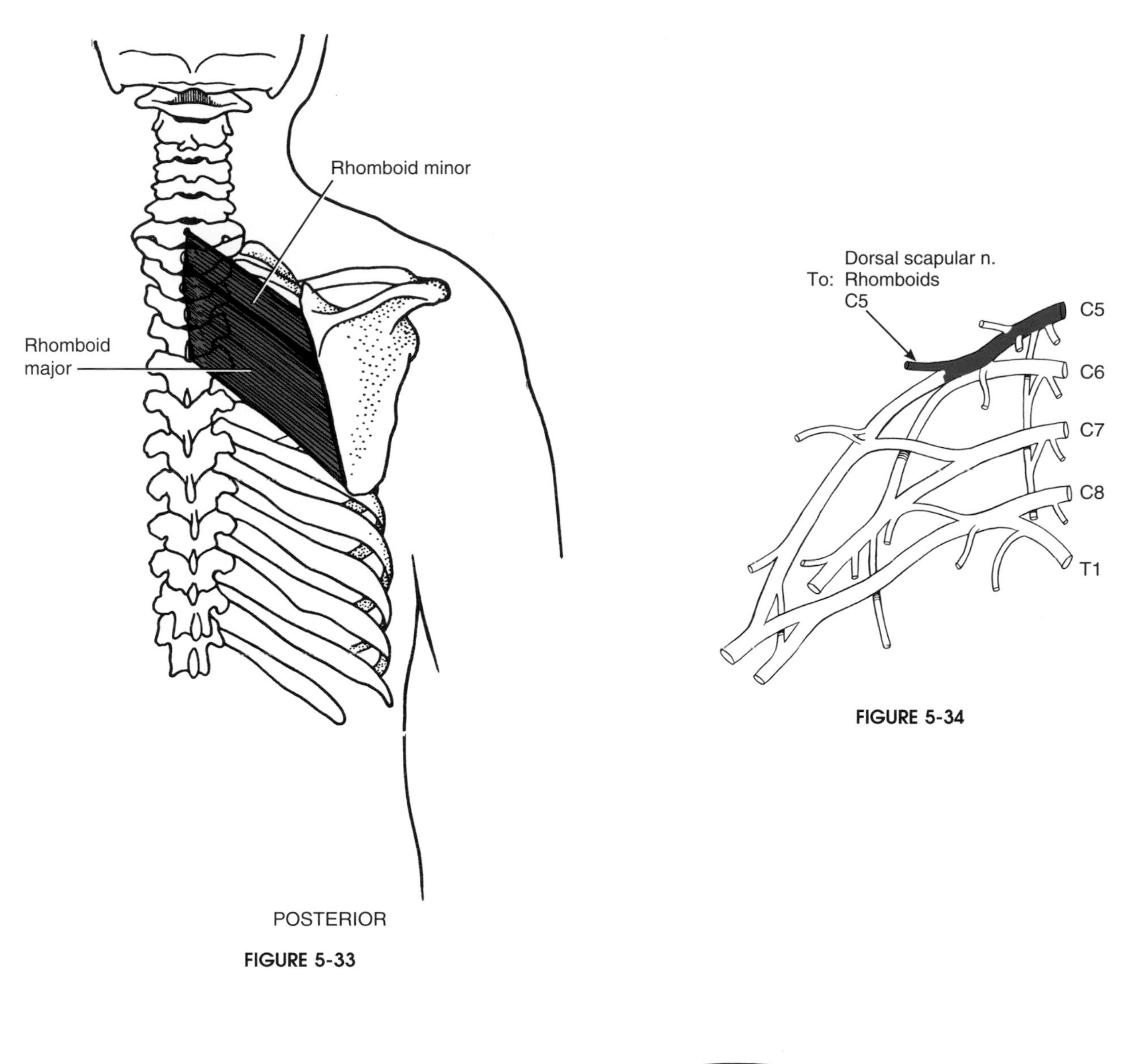

FIGURE 5-33

FIGURE 5-34

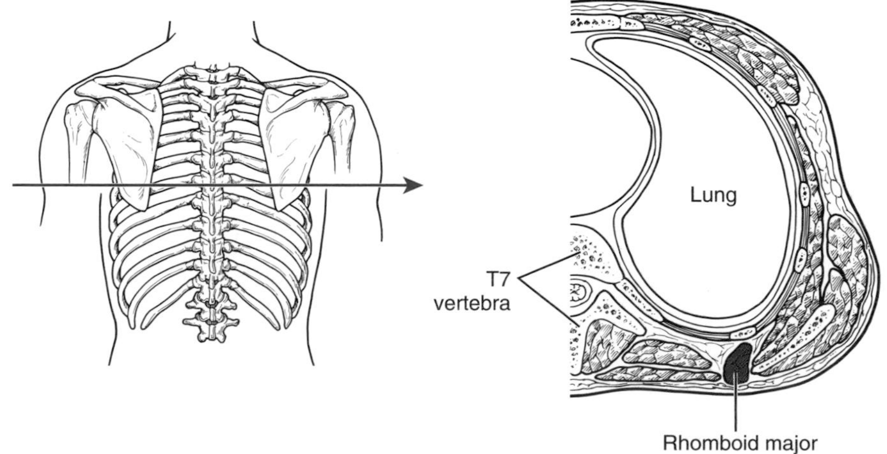

FIGURE 5-35 Arrow indicates level of cross section.

SCAPULAR ADDUCTION AND DOWNWARD ROTATION

(Rhomboids)

Range of Motion
Reliable data not available

Table 5-5 SCAPULAR ADDUCTION AND DOWNWARD ROTATION

I.D.	Muscle	Origin	Insertion
125	Rhomboid major	T2-T5 vertebrae (spinous processes) Supraspinous ligaments	Scapula (vertebral border between root of spine and inferior angle)
126	Rhomboid minor	C7-T1 vertebrae (spinous processes) Ligamentum nuchae (lower)	Scapula (vertebral margin at root of spine)
Other			
127	Levator scapulae	See Table 5-2	See Plate 3

The test for the rhomboid muscles has become the focus of some clinical debate. Kendall and co-workers claim, with good evidence, that these muscles frequently are underrated; that is, they are too often graded at a level less than their performance.[1] At issue also is the confusion that can occur in separating the function of the rhomboids from those of other scapular or shoulder muscles, particularly the trapezius and the pectoralis minor. Because the rhomboids are innervated only by C5, a test for the rhomboids, correctly conducted, can confirm or rule out a nerve root lesion at this level. With these issues in mind, the authors present first their method and then, with the generous permission of Mrs. Kendall, her rhomboid test as another method of assessment.

Grade 5 (Normal), Grade 4 (Good), and Grade 3 (Fair)

Position of Patient: Prone. Head may be turned to either side for comfort. Shoulder is internally rotated and the arm is adducted across the back with the elbow flexed and hand resting on the back (Figure 5-36).

Position of Therapist: Standing at test side. When the shoulder extensor muscles are Grade 3 or higher, the hand used for resistance is placed on the humerus just above the elbow, and resistance is given in a downward and outward direction (Figure 5-37).

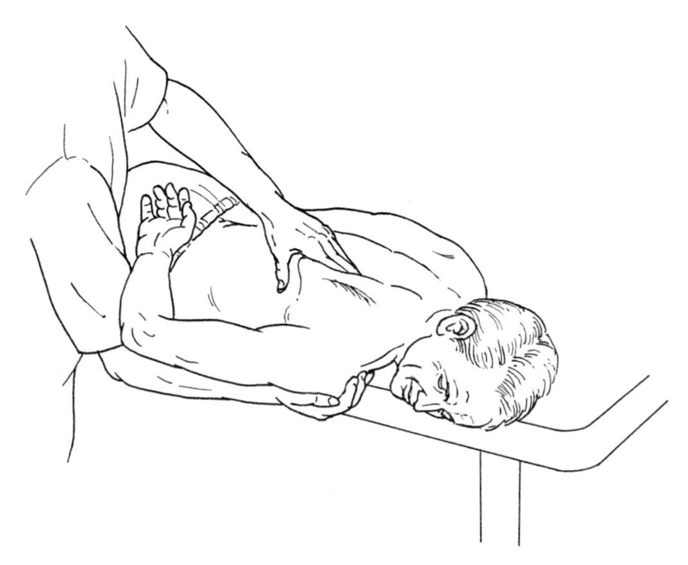

FIGURE 5-36

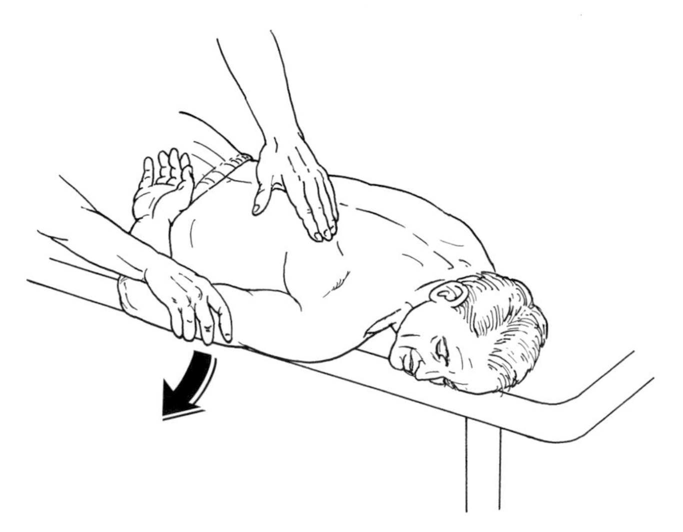

FIGURE 5-37

Grade 5 (Normal), Grade 4 (Good), and Grade 3 (Fair) Continued

When the shoulder extensors are weak, place the hand for resistance along the axillary border of the scapula (Figure 5-38). Resistance is applied in a downward and outward direction.

The fingers of the hand used for palpation are placed deep under the vertebral border of the scapula.

Test: Patient lifts the hand off the back, maintaining the arm position across the back at the same time the examiner is applying resistance above the elbow. With strong muscle activity, the therapist's fingers will "pop" out from under the edge of the scapular vertebral border (see Figure 5-36.)

Instructions to Patient: "Lift your hand. Hold it. Don't let me push it down."

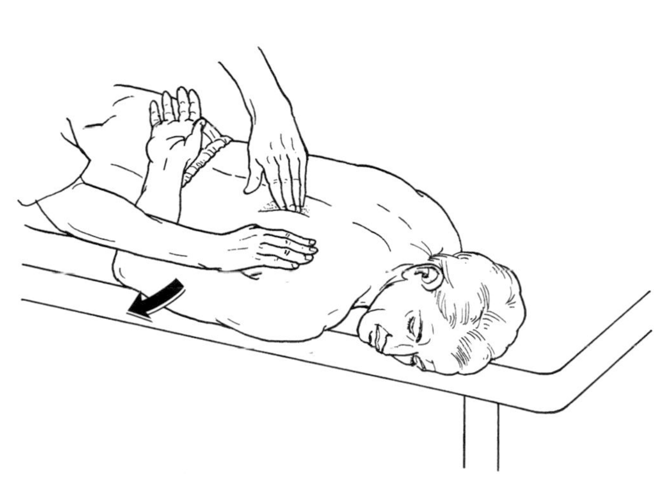

FIGURE 5-38

Grading

Grade 5 (Normal): Completes available range and holds against maximal resistance (Figure 5-39). The fingers will "pop out" from under the scapula when strong rhomboids contract.

Grade 4 (Good): Completes range and holds against strong to moderate resistance. Fingers usually will "pop out."

Grade 3 (Fair): Completes range but tolerates no manual resistance (Figure 5-40).

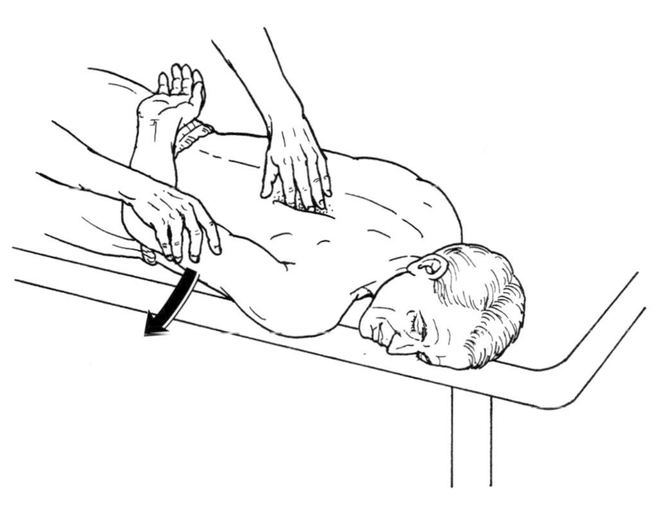

FIGURE 5-39

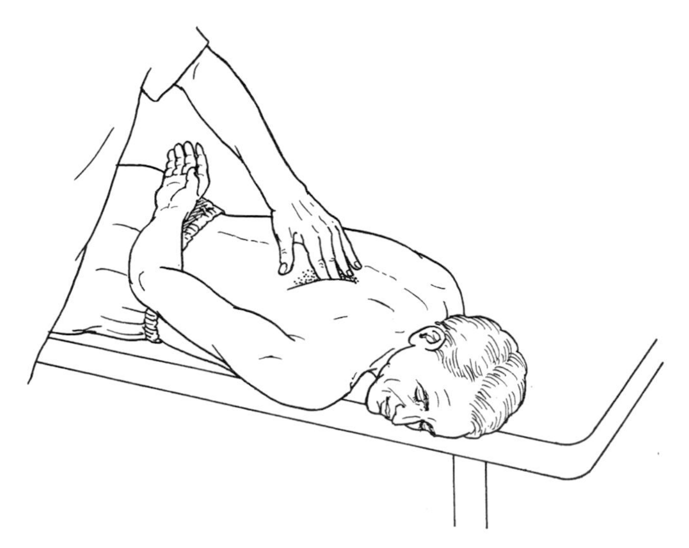

FIGURE 5-40

(Rhomboids)

Grade 2 (Poor), Grade 1 (Trace), and Grade 0 (Zero)

Position of Patient: Short sitting with shoulder internally rotated and arm extended and adducted behind back (Figure 5-41).

Position of Therapist: Standing at test side; support arm by grasping the wrist. The fingertips of one hand palpate the muscle under the vertebral border of the scapula.

Test: Patient attempts to move hand away from back.

Instructions to Patient: "Try to move your hand away from your back."

Grading

Grade 2 (Poor): Completes range of scapular motion.

Grades 1 (Trace) and 0 (Zero): A Grade 1 muscle has palpable contractile activity. A Grade 0 muscle shows no response.

Alternate Test for Grades 2, 1, and 0

Position of Patient: Prone with shoulder in about 45° of abduction and elbow at about 90° of flexion with the hand on the back.

Position of Therapist: Standing at test side; support arm by cradling it under the shoulder (Figure 5-42). Fingers used for palpation are placed firmly under the vertebral border of the scapula.

Test: Patient attempts to lift hand from back.

Instructions to Patient: "Try to lift your hand away from your back." OR "Lift your hand toward the ceiling."

Grading

Grade 2 (Poor): Completes partial range of scapular motion.

Grades 1 (Trace) and 0 (Zero): A Grade 1 (Trace) muscle has some palpable contractile activity. A Grade 0 muscle shows no contractile response.

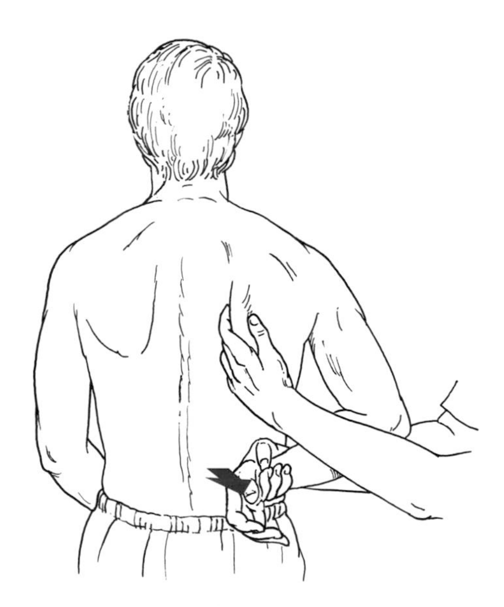

FIGURE 5-41

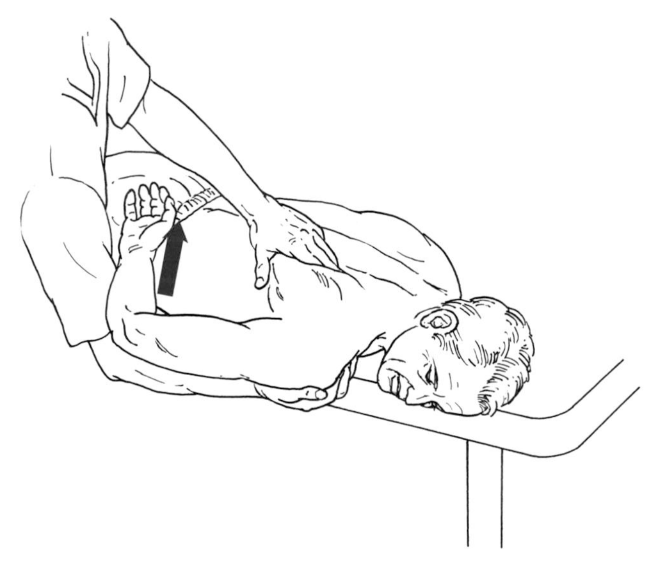

FIGURE 5-42

Alternate Rhomboid Test After Kendall[1]

As a preliminary to this rhomboid test, the shoulder adductors should be tested and found sufficiently strong to allow the arm to be used as a lever.

Position of Patient: Prone with head turned to side of test. Non-test arm is abducted with elbow flexed.

Test arm is near the edge of the table. Arm (humerus) is fully adducted and held firm to the side of the trunk in external rotation and some extension with elbow fully flexed. In this position the scapula is in adduction, elevation, and downward rotation (glenoid down).

Position of Therapist: Stand at test side. One hand used for resistance is cupped around the flexed elbow. The resistance applied by this hand will be in the direction of scapular abduction and upward rotation (out and up; Figure 5-43). The other hand is used to give resistance simultaneously. It is contoured over the shoulder joint and gives resistance caudally in the direction of shoulder depression.

Test: Examiner tests the ability of the patient to hold the scapula in its position of adduction, elevation, and downward rotation (glenoid down).

Instructions to Patient: "Hold your arm as I have placed it. Do not let me pull your arm forward." OR "Hold the position you are in; keep your shoulder blade against your spine as I try to pull it away."

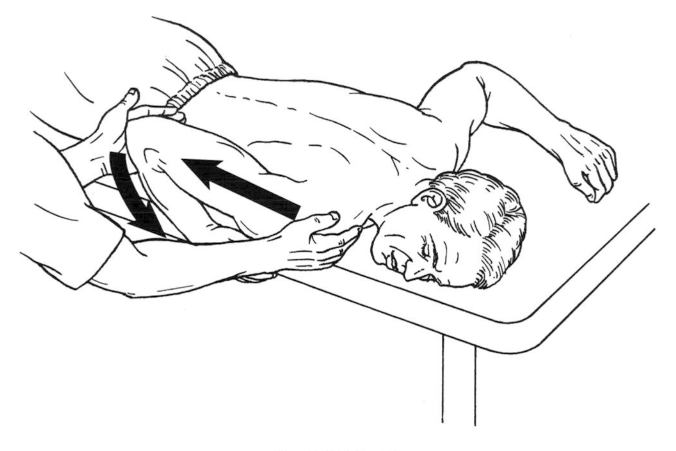

FIGURE 5-43

Helpful Hints

- Clinical weakness of the rhomboids is a strong diagnostic test for a subscapular nerve lesion or muscle tear.[2] Inability to lift the hand off the small of the back is diagnostic for a subscapular muscle tear.
- Using needle electromyography (EMG) on 11 male subjects, Smith and colleagues[3] found the posterior deltoid manual muscle test produced the greatest rhomboid EMG activity of eight manual muscle tests and 30% greater rhomboid activity than the muscle test shown in Figure 5-39. The manual muscle test described in Figure 5-39 produced greatest EMG activity in the latissimus dorsi and levator scapula muscles and equal activation in the middle trapezius, posterior deltoid, and rhomboids. The sitting position used in the posterior deltoid muscle test position described by Smith and colleagues requires the rhomboids to function as a scapular rotator and scapular retractor as opposed to the prone position, which only requires the rhomboids to act as a scapular retractor.[3,4]
- The Kendall test (see Figure 5-43) demonstrated greater EMG activity than the rhomboid test shown in Figure 5-39.[3]
- When the rhomboid test is performed with the hand behind the back, never allow the patient to lead the lifting motion with the elbow because this will activate the humeral extensors.

Substitution by Middle Trapezius

The middle fibers of the trapezius can substitute for the adduction component of the rhomboids. The middle trapezius cannot, however, substitute for the downward rotation component. When substitution occurs, the patient's scapula will adduct with no downward rotation (no glenoid down occurs). Only palpation can detect this substitution for sure.

SCAPULAR DEPRESSION

(Latissimus dorsi, Teres major, Posterior deltoid)

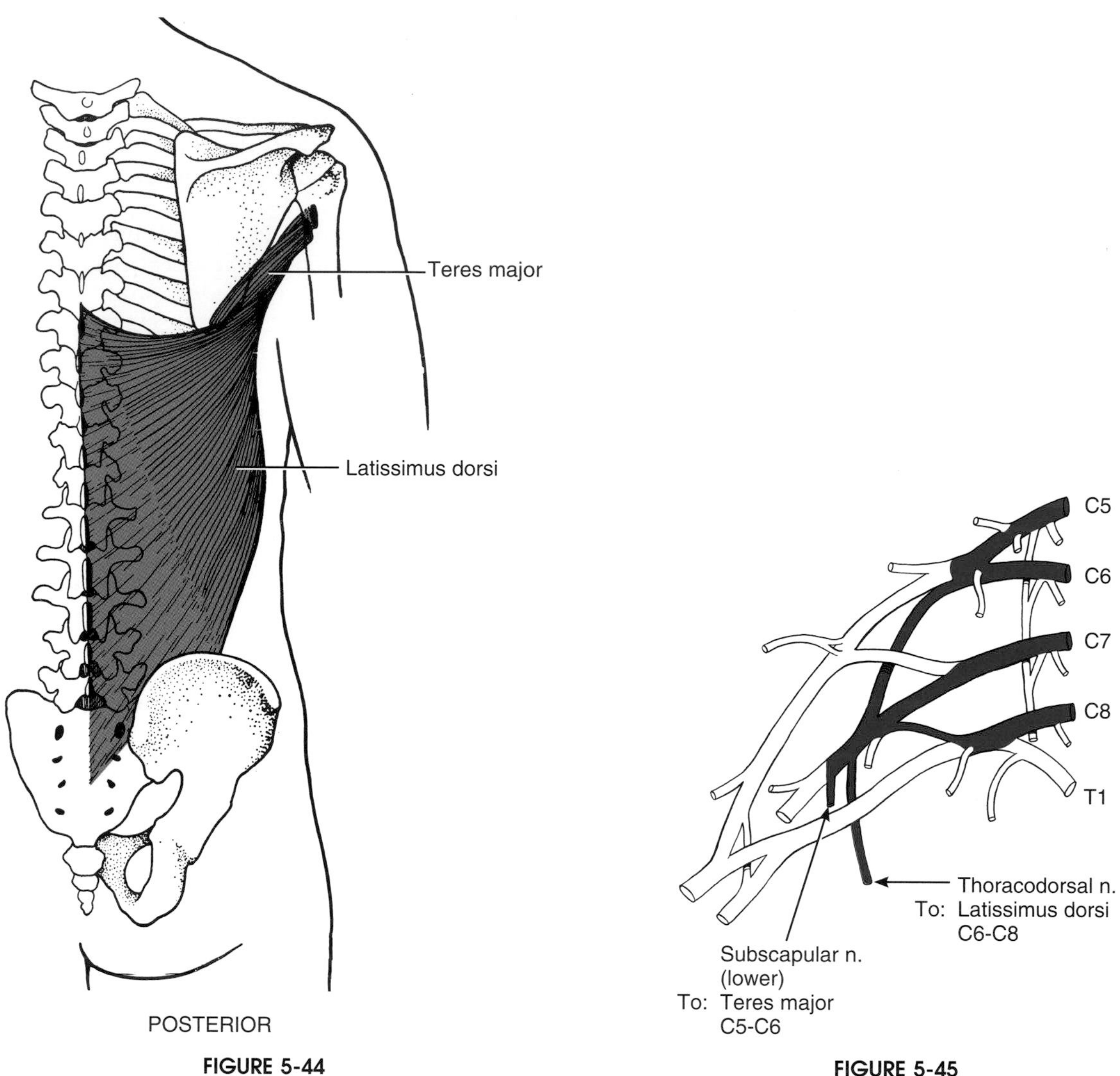

FIGURE 5-44

FIGURE 5-45

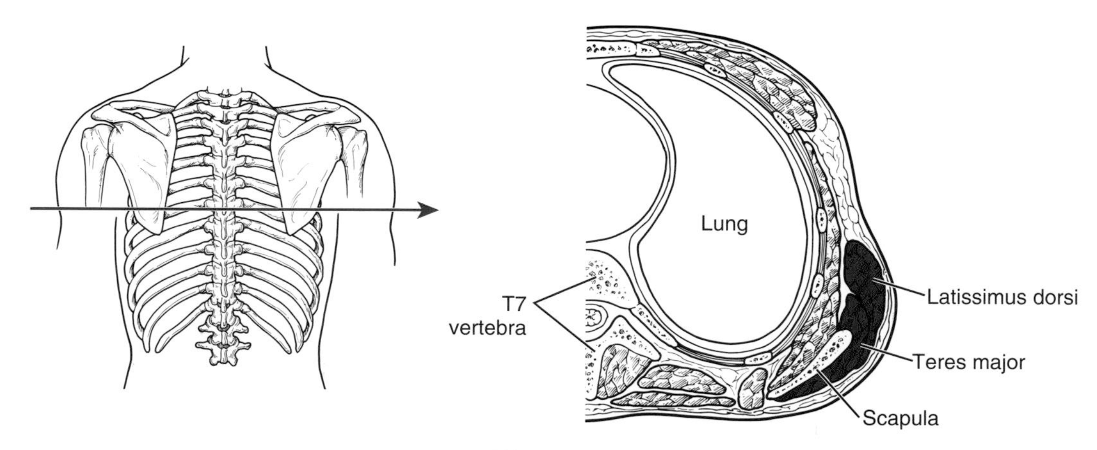

FIGURE 5-46

Before describing the test for scapular depression, a few words about the latissimus dorsi are warranted. This enormous muscle is anatomically complex and there are many movements at the humerus, scapula, and pelvis that require its participation. For example, when the humerus is fixed, the latissimus dorsi can lift the pelvis, which occurs during pressure relief in a wheelchair and during a sliding transfer. When the pelvis is fixed, the latissimus dorsi acts to depress the humerus and internally rotate, adduct, and extend the shoulder, particularly from a position of flexion. Importantly, the latissimus dorsi also depresses the scapula, which independently contributes to shoulder stability. The student will find the latissimus dorsi mentioned in other parts of this chapter as a participant in muscle actions in addition to scapular depression, further supporting the importance and complexity of this muscle.

The latissimus dorsi is a scapular depressor when the origin is fixed and a shoulder adductor and internal rotator when its insertion is fixed. The latissimus dorsi is included here because it is the prime mover of scapular depression with more fibers acting as depressors than as adductors or internal rotation.

Grade 5 (Normal) and Grade 4 (Good)

Test for Latissimus Dorsi

Position of Patient: Prone with head turned to test side; arms are at sides and shoulder is internally rotated (palm up). Test shoulder is "hiked" to the level of the chin.

Position of Therapist: Standing at test side. Grasp forearm above patient's wrist with both hands (Figure 5-47).

Test: Patient depresses arm caudally and in so doing approximates the rib cage to the pelvis.

Instructions to Patient: "Reach toward your feet. Hold it. Don't let me push your arm upward toward your head."

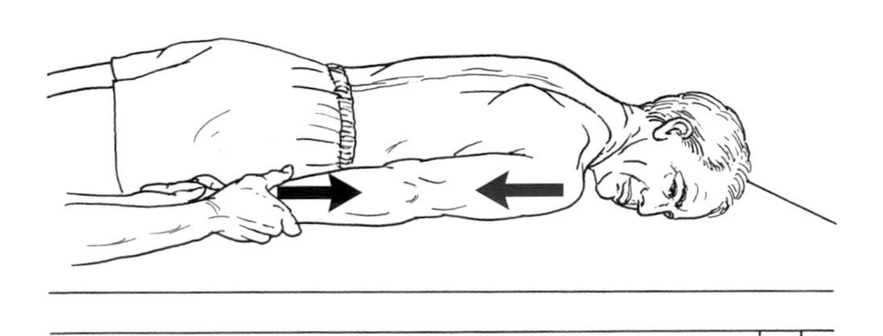

FIGURE 5-47

Grading

Grade 5: Patient completes available range against maximal resistance. If the therapist is unable to push the arm upward using both hands for resistance, test the patient in the sitting position as described in Test 3.

Grade 4: Patient completes available range of motion, but the shoulder yields at end point against strong resistance.

Alternate Test for Latissimus Dorsi

Position of Patient: Short sitting, with hands flat on table adjacent to hips (Figure 5-48).

If the patient's arms are too short to assume this position, provide a push-up block for each hand.

Position of Therapist: Standing behind patient. Fingers are used to palpate fibers of the latissimus dorsi on the lateral aspects of the thoracic wall (bilaterally) just above the waist (see Figure 5-48). (In this test the sternal head of the pectoralis major is equally active.)

Test: Patient pushes down on hands (or blocks) and lifts buttocks from table (see Figure 5-48).

Instructions to Patient: "Lift your bottom off the table."

Grading

Grade 5: Patient is able to lift buttocks clear of table.

Grade 4: There is no Grade 4 in this sequence because the prone test (Test 2) determines a grade of less than 5.

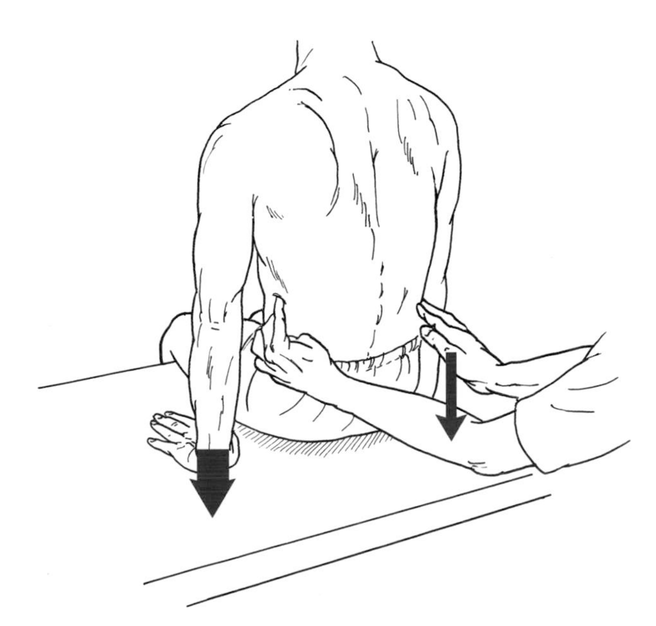

FIGURE 5-48

SCAPULAR DEPRESSION

(Latissimus dorsi, Teres major, Posterior deltoid)

Helpful Hints

- A person cannot complete a chin-up without tremendous participation of the latissimus dorsi. Thus, a chin-up (forearms supinated) or pull-up (forearms pronated) may be a more appropriate test for an active male and a flexed arm hang more appropriate for a female. The chin-up test is described in Chapter 8.
- It is impossible to isolate the latissimus dorsi muscle because its action changes when its origin or insertion is fixed. When its origin is fixed, the latissimus dorsi is a shoulder abductor, shoulder extender, and internal rotator as well as a scapular depressor. It also may assist in lateral flexion of the trunk. When its insertion is fixed, it assists in tilting the pelvis anteriorly and laterally. When acting bilaterally, it may assist in hyperextending the spine and anteriorly tilting the pelvis. It may also act as an accessory muscle of respiration.

INTRODUCTION TO SHOULDER MUSCLE TESTING

Movement at the shoulder girdle is complex in that it is composed of five distinct joints. The scapulothoracic joint, the glenohumeral joint, the subacromial joint, the acromioclavicular joint, and the sternoclavicular joint all contribute to producing normal movement at the shoulder girdle. Deficits in the function in any of the joints have to be compensated for by the remaining joints. As more dysfunction occurs in one or more joints, more compensation is likely to occur to achieve the end result of upper extremity function. Care needs to be taken when evaluating each of these joints to ascertain where movement is occurring and what muscle is responsible for producing the movement.

Scaption

Scaption is elevation of the shoulder girdle performed in the resting plane of the scapula. The plane is typically halfway between the plane of flexion and the plane of abduction. Although scaption is a very functional movement in that people rarely elevate their shoulder girdle in the cardinal planes of abduction and flexion, muscle testing is done in these cardinal planes. If strength testing in the cardinal planes of flexion and abduction are normal, the strength for the movement of scaption will also be normal.

Testing the Supraspinatus

Much controversy exists regarding the diagnosis of supraspinatus pathology. Two tests used to examine the supraspinatus muscle are the empty can test (also known as the Jobe test) and the full can test. In the full can test, the arm is externally rotated (thumb pointed up); in the empty can test the arm is internally rotated (thumb pointed down). In both tests the shoulder is in abduction but with 30° of flexion included. In a meta-analysis of physical examination tests of the shoulder,[5] the authors found the Jobe or empty can test had insufficient sensitivity and specificity to be clinically useful in diagnosing supraspinatus tendonitis or impingement but performed better in identifying a full-thickness or massive tear, especially in the presence of weakness in the Jobe test (sensitivity = 41%; specificity = 70%).[6] Furthermore, the empty can (thumb pointed down) and full can (thumb pointed up) positions were not statistically different in their performance of identifying pathology. Finally, in a study measuring the moment arm of three positions of the shoulder (neutral, Jobe, and abducted positions), the neutral position was found to be the most advantageous to isolate the supraspinatus, and therefore was recommended as the best position to test the supraspinatus.[7] In another study of six male volunteers, the empty and full can positions were equally effective in activating the supraspinatus muscle and statistically better than the horizontal abduction position.[8]

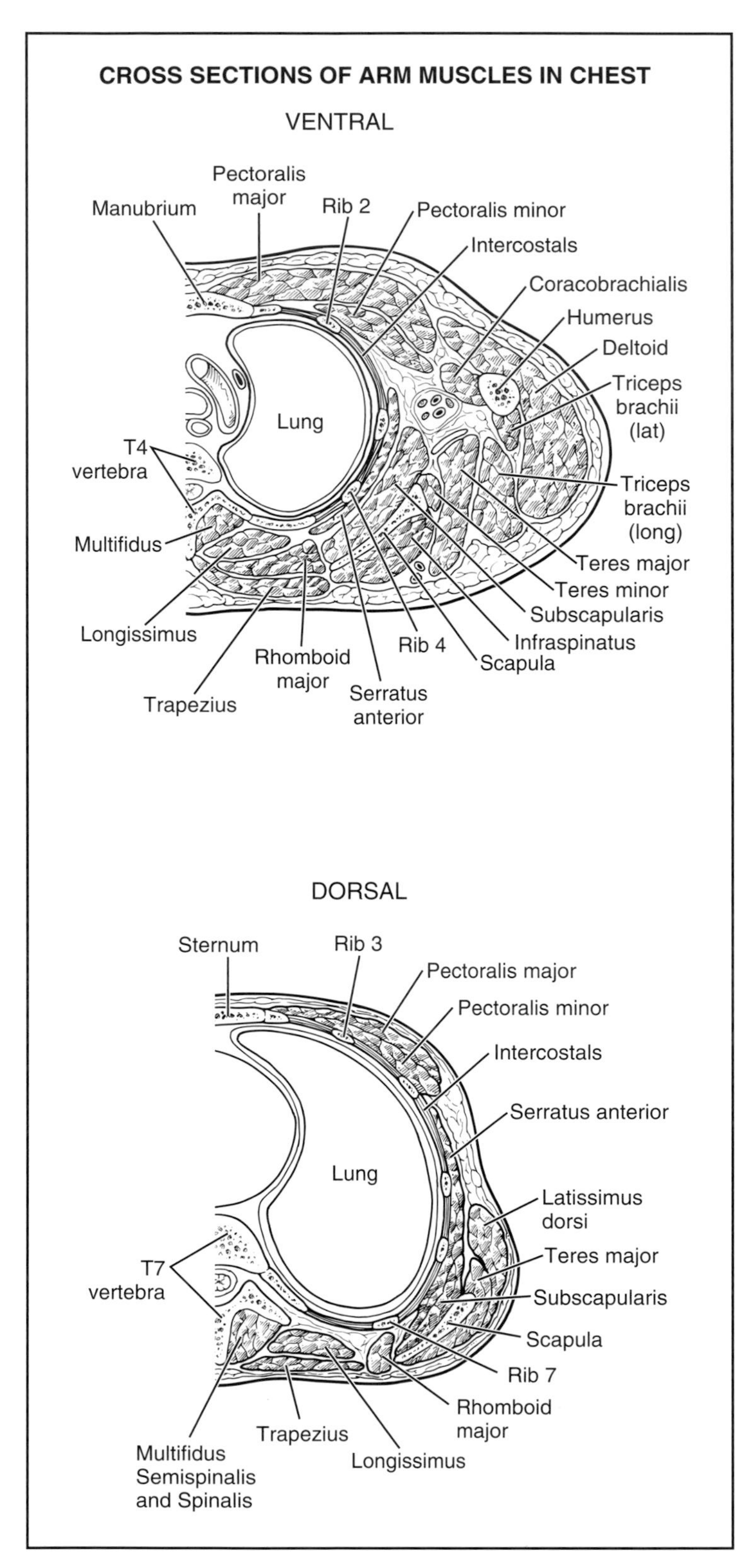
CROSS SECTIONS OF ARM MUSCLES IN CHEST
VENTRAL
Pectoralis major
Manubrium
Rib 2
Pectoralis minor
Intercostals
Coracobrachialis
Humerus
Deltoid
Triceps brachii (lat)
Lung
T4 vertebra
Triceps brachii (long)
Multifidus
Teres major
Teres minor
Subscapularis
Longissimus
Infraspinatus
Rib 4
Scapula
Rhomboid major
Trapezius
Serratus anterior
DORSAL
Sternum
Rib 3
Pectoralis major
Pectoralis minor
Intercostals
Serratus anterior
Lung
Latissimus dorsi
Teres major
T7 vertebra
Subscapularis
Scapula
Rib 7
Rhomboid major
Trapezius
Longissimus
Multifidus Semispinalis and Spinalis

PLATE 3

(Anterior deltoid, Supraspinatus, and Coracobrachialis)*

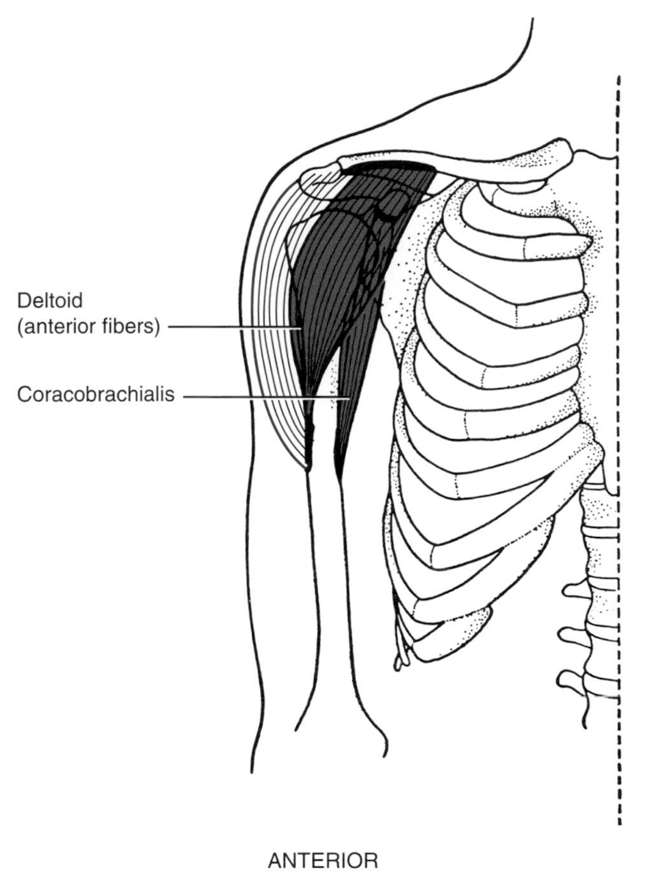

FIGURE 5-49

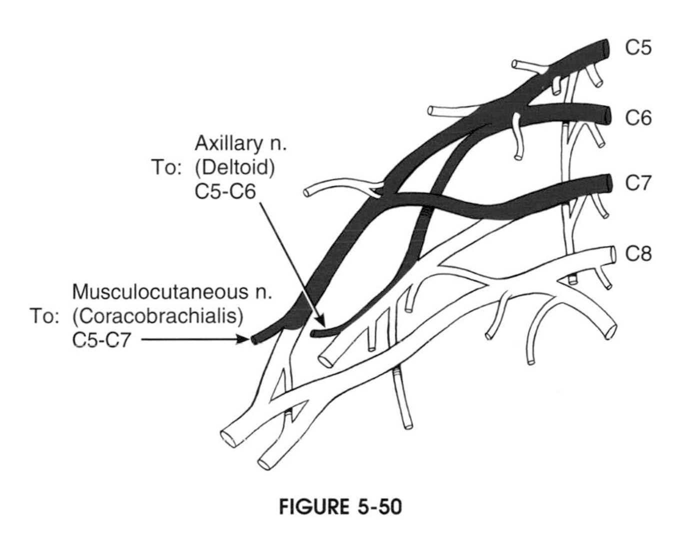

FIGURE 5-50

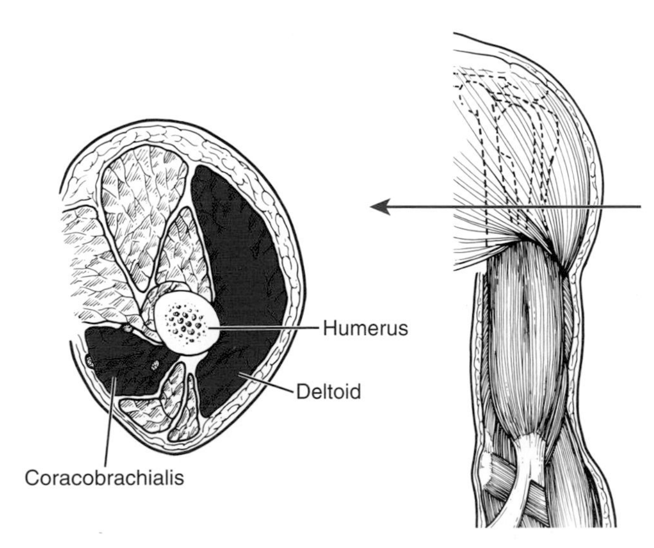

FIGURE 5-51

*The coracobrachialis muscle cannot be isolated, nor is it really palpable. It has no unique function. It is included here because classically it is considered a shoulder flexor and adductor.

SHOULDER FLEXION

(Anterior deltoid, Supraspinatus, and Coracobrachialis)

Range of Motion
0° to 80°

Table 5-6 SHOULDER FLEXION

I.D.	Muscle	Origin	Insertion
133	Deltoid (anterior)	Clavicle (anterior superior border of lateral 1/3 of shaft)	Humerus (deltoid tuberosity on shaft)
135	Supraspinatus	Scapula (supraspinous fossa) Supraspinatus fascia	Humerus (greater tubercle, highest facet) Articular capsule of glenohumeral joint
139	Coracobrachialis	Scapula (coracoid process at apex)	Humerus (shaft, medial surface at middle 1/3)
Others			
131	Pectoralis major (upper)	See Table 5-4	
133	Deltoid (middle)	Lateral margin and superior surface of the acromion	Deltoid tuberosity
128	Serratus anterior (via upwardly rotating scapula and preventing scapular adduction)	See Table 5-1	

Grade 5 (Normal) and Grade 4 (Good)

Position of Patient: Short sitting with arms at sides, elbow slightly flexed, forearm pronated.

Position of Therapist: Stand at test side. Hand giving resistance is contoured over the distal humerus just above the elbow. The other hand may stabilize the shoulder (Figure 5-52).

Test: Patient flexes shoulder to 90° without rotation or horizontal movement (see Figure 5-52). The scapula should be allowed to abduct and upwardly rotate.

Instructions to Patient: "Raise your arm forward to shoulder height. Hold it. Don't let me push it down."

Grading

Grade 5 (Normal): Holds end position (90°) against maximal resistance.

Grade 4 (Good): Holds end position against strong to moderate resistance.

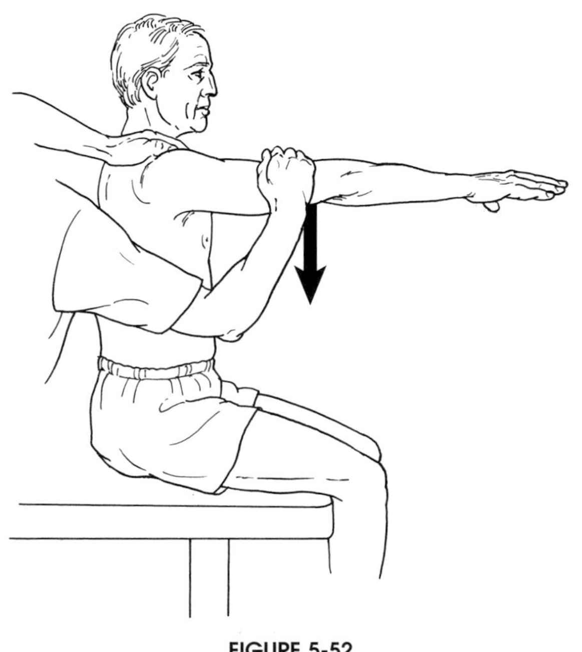

FIGURE 5-52

Grade 3 (Fair)

Position of Patient: Short sitting, arm at side with elbow slightly flexed and forearm pronated.

Position of Therapist: Stand at test side.

Test: Patient flexes shoulder to 90° (Figure 5-53).

Instructions to Patient: "Raise your arm forward to shoulder height."

Grading

Grade 3 (Fair): Completes test range (90°) but tolerates no resistance.

Grade 2 (Poor), Grade 1 (Trace), and Grade 0 (Zero)

Position of Patient: Short sitting with arm at side and elbow slightly flexed.

Position of Therapist: Stand at test side. Fingers used for palpation are placed over the superior and anterior surfaces of the deltoid over the shoulder joint (Figure 5-54).

Test: Patient attempts to flex shoulder to 90°.

Instructions to Patient: "Try to raise your arm."

Grading

Grade 2 (Poor): Completes partial range of motion since this is against gravity.

Grade 1 (Trace): Examiner feels or sees contractile activity in the anterior deltoid, but no motion occurs.

Grade 0 (Zero): No contractile activity.

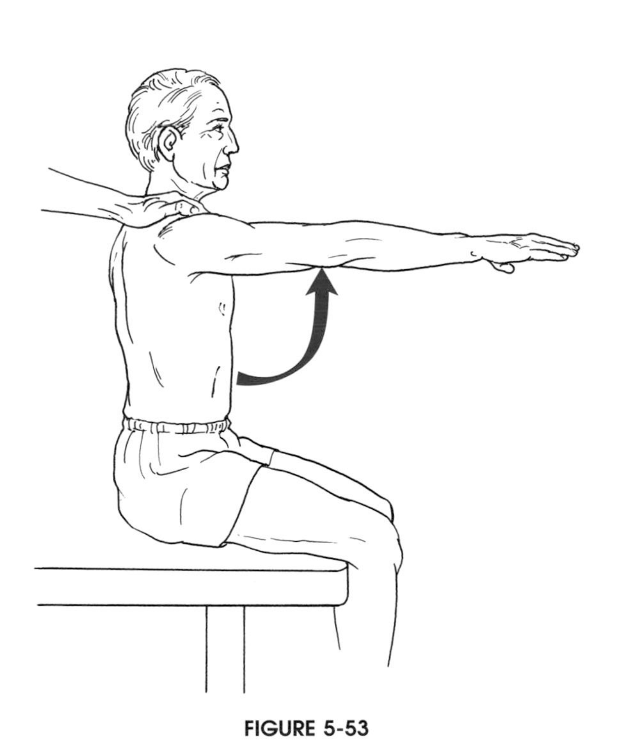

FIGURE 5-53

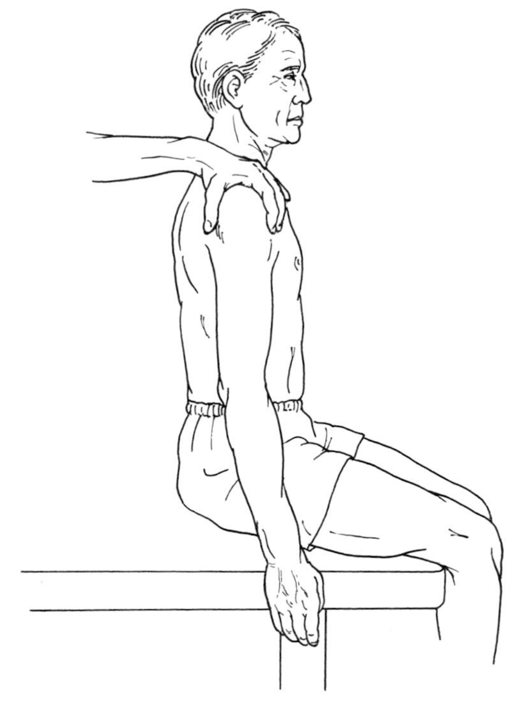

FIGURE 5-54

SHOULDER FLEXION

(Anterior deltoid, Supraspinatus, and Coracobrachialis)

Alternate Test for Grades 2, 1, and 0

If for any reason the patient is unable to sit, the test can be conducted in the side-lying position (test side up). In this posture, the examiner cradles the test arm at the elbow before asking the patient to flex the shoulder. For Grade 2 (Poor), the patient must complete full range of motion.

Substitutions

- In the absence of a deltoid, the patient may attempt to flex the shoulder with the biceps brachii by first externally rotating the shoulder (Figure 5-55). To avoid this, the arm should be kept in the midposition between internal and external rotation.
- Attempted substitution by the upper trapezius results in shoulder elevation.
- Attempted substitution by the pectoralis major results in horizontal adduction. It should be noted that substitution by the pectoralis major as a shoulder flexor can only occur up to about 70°.
- The patient may lean backward or try to elevate the shoulder girdle to assist in flexion.

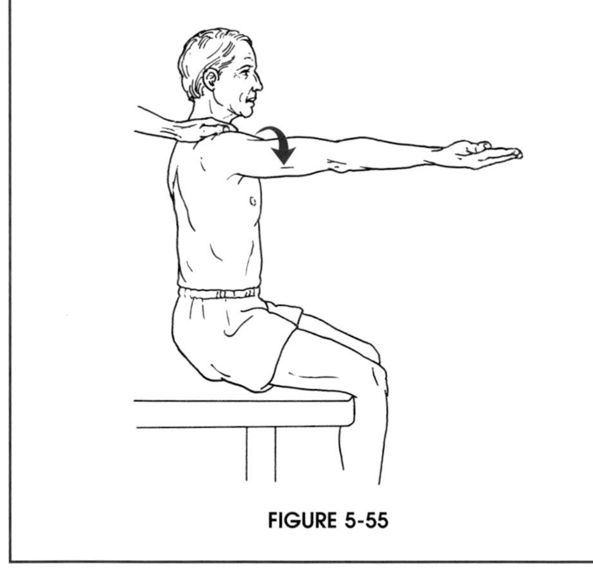

FIGURE 5-55

Helpful Hints

- Although the coracobrachialis is a minor contributor to shoulder flexion, it is deep-lying and may be difficult or impossible to palpate within a reasonable range of comfort for the patient.
- The supraspinatus initiates shoulder flexion with the anterior deltoid.[9,10] This action may help explain the difficulty patients with a massive tear of the rotator cuff have in initiating flexion.
- The supraspinatus has a role as a humeral head depressor during shoulder flexion.[10]

(Posterior deltoid)

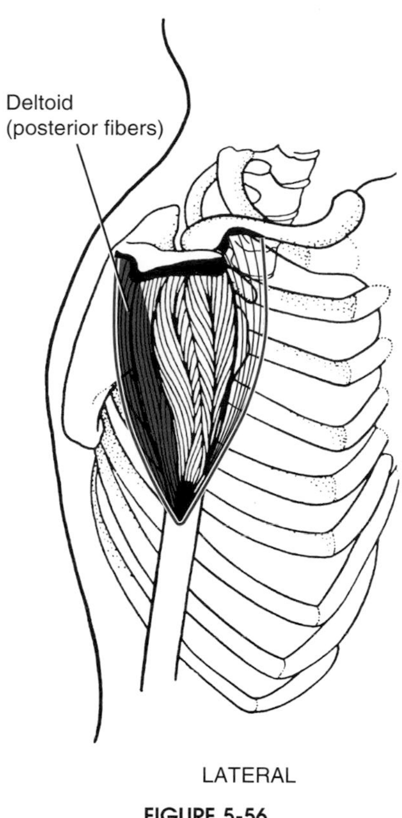

FIGURE 5-56

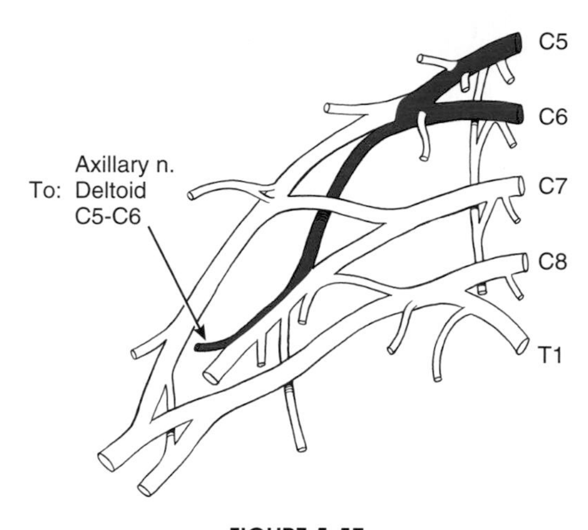

FIGURE 5-57

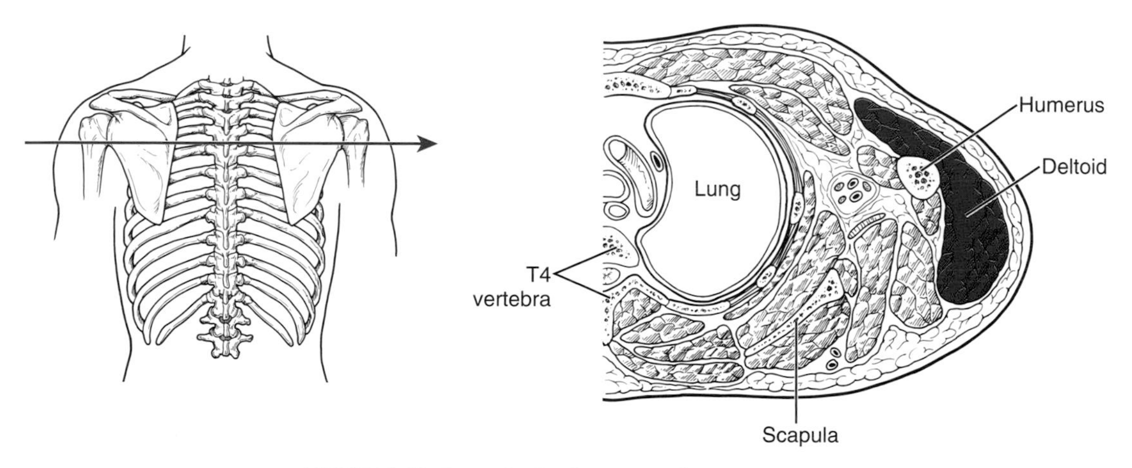

FIGURE 5-58 Arrow indicates level of cross section.

SHOULDER EXTENSION

(Posterior deltoid)

Range of Motion
0° to 45° (up to 60°)

Table 5-7 SHOULDER EXTENSION

I.D.	Muscle	Origin	Insertion
130	Latissimus dorsi	T6-T12, L1-L5, and sacral vertebrae (spinous processes) Supraspinous ligaments Ribs 9-12 (by slips interdigitating with obliquus abdominis externus) Ilium (crest, posterior) Thoracolumbar fascia	Humerus (intertubercular sulcus, floor) Deep fascia of arm
133	Deltoid (posterior)	Scapula (spine on lower lip of lateral and posterior borders)	Humerus (deltoid tuberosity on midshaft via humeral tendon)
138	Teres major	Scapula (dorsal surface of inferior angle)	Humerus (intertubercular sulcus, medial lip)
Other			
142	Triceps brachii (long head)		

Grade 5 (Normal) and Grade 4 (Good)

Position of Patient: Prone with arms at sides and shoulder internally rotated (palm up) (Figure 5-59).

Position of Therapist: Standing at test side. Hand used for resistance is contoured over the posterior arm just above the elbow.

Test: Patient raises arm off the table, keeping the elbow straight (Figure 5-60).

Instructions to Patient: "Lift your arm as high as you can. Hold it. Don't let me push it down."

Grading

Grade 5 (Normal): Completes available range and holds against maximal resistance.

Grade 4 (Good): Completes available range but yields against strong resistance.

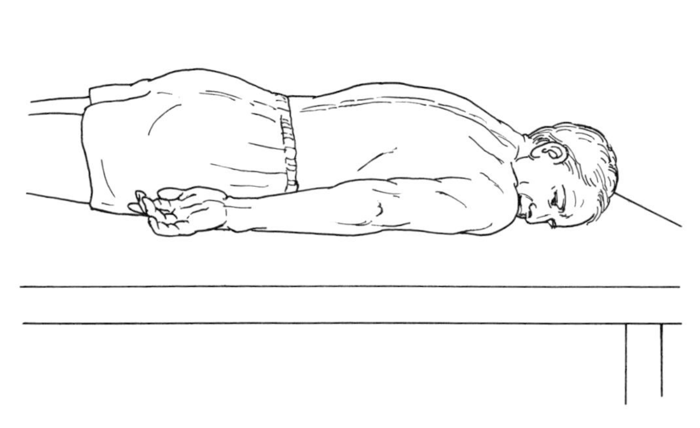

FIGURE 5-59

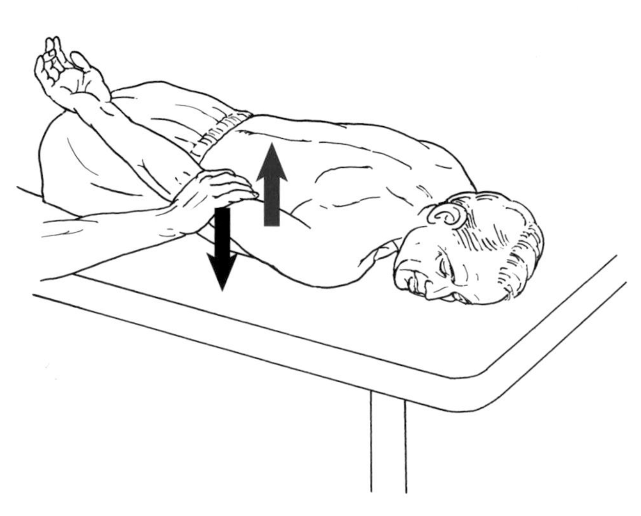

FIGURE 5-60

Shoulder Extension Grade 3 (Fair) and Grade 2 (Poor)

Position of Patient: Prone with head turned to one side. Arms at sides; test arm is internally rotated (palm up) (Figure 5-61).

Position of Therapist: Stand at test side.

Test: Patient raises arm off table (see Figure 5-61).

Instructions to Patient: "Lift your arm as high as you can."

Grading

Grade 3 (Fair): Completes available range of motion with no manual resistance.

Grade 2 (Poor): Completes partial range of motion.

Grade 1 (Trace) and Grade 0 (Zero)

Position of Patient: Prone with arms at sides and shoulder internally rotated (palm up).

Position of Therapist: Standing at test side. Fingers for palpation are placed on the posterior aspect of the upper arm (posterior deltoid) (Figure 5-62).

Palpate over the posterior shoulder just superior to the axilla for posterior deltoid fibers. Palpate the teres major on the lateral border of the scapula just below the axilla. The teres major is the lower of the two muscles that enter the axilla at this point; it forms the lower posterior rim of the axilla.

Test and Instructions to Patient: Patient attempts to lift arm from table on request.

Grading

Grade 1 (Trace): Palpable contractile activity in any of the participating muscles but no movement of the shoulder.

Grade 0 (Zero): No contractile response in participating muscles.

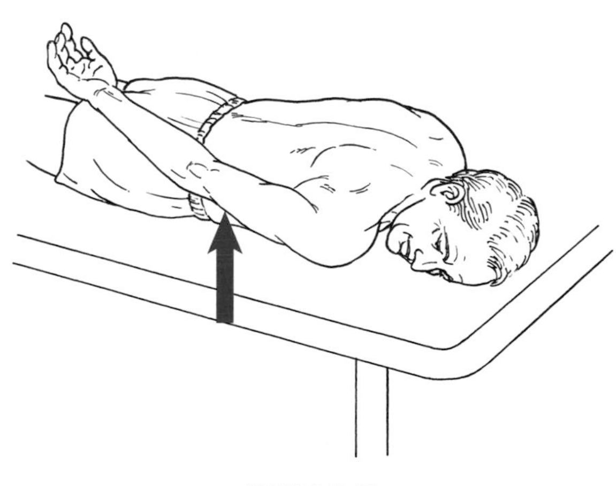

FIGURE 5-61

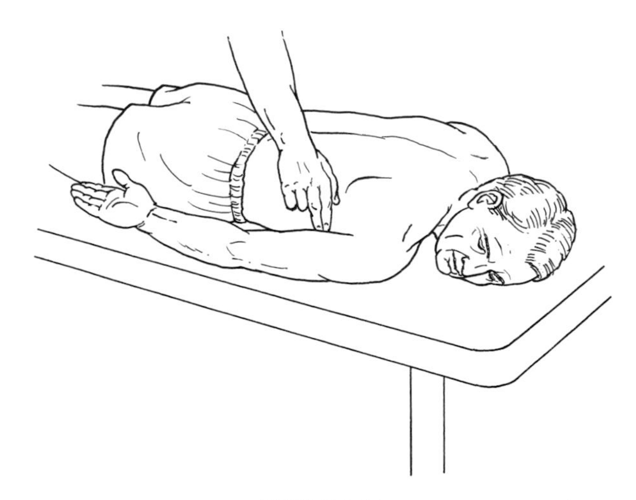

FIGURE 5-62

SHOULDER ABDUCTION

(Middle deltoid and Supraspinatus)

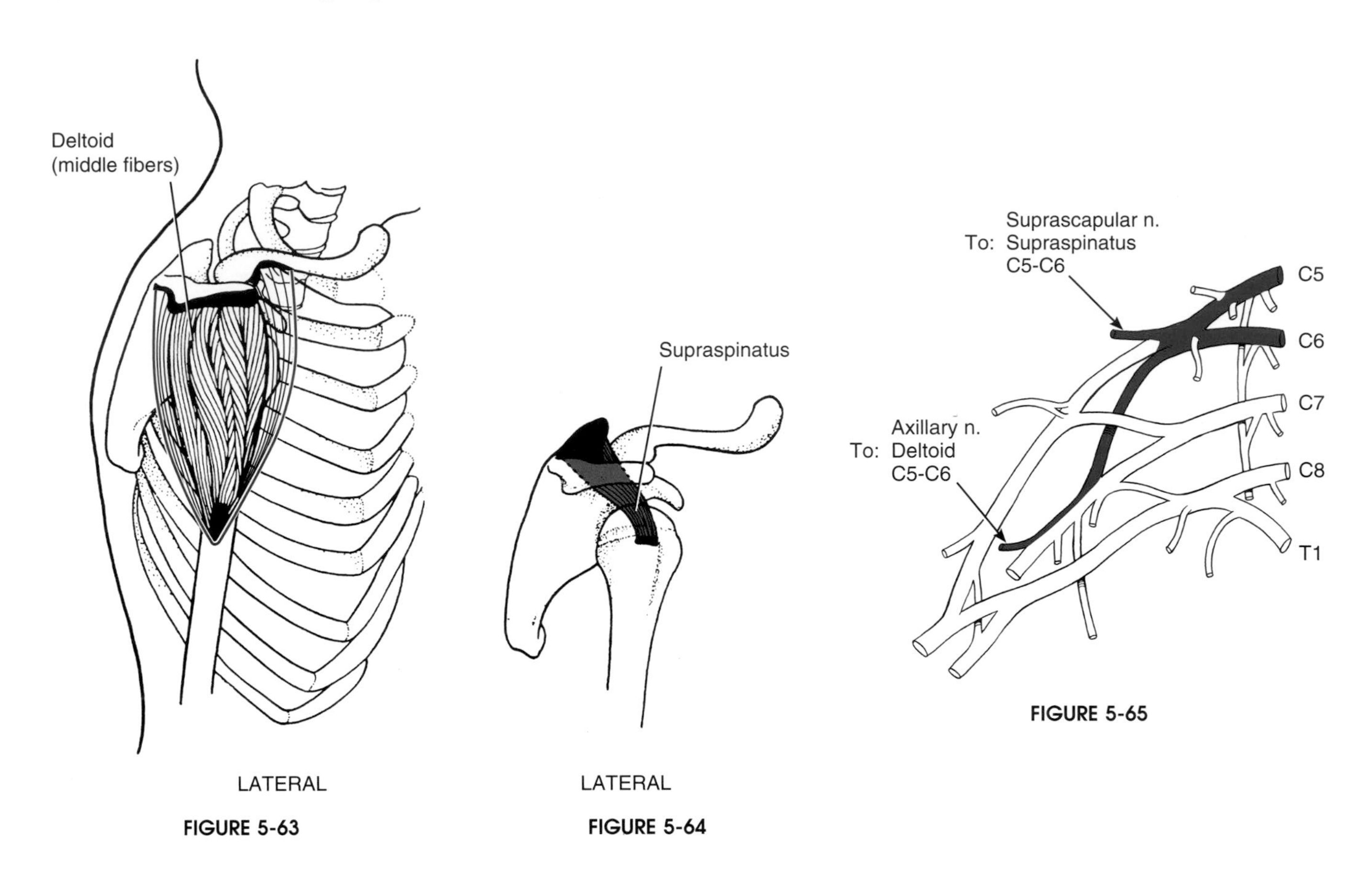

FIGURE 5-63

FIGURE 5-64

FIGURE 5-65

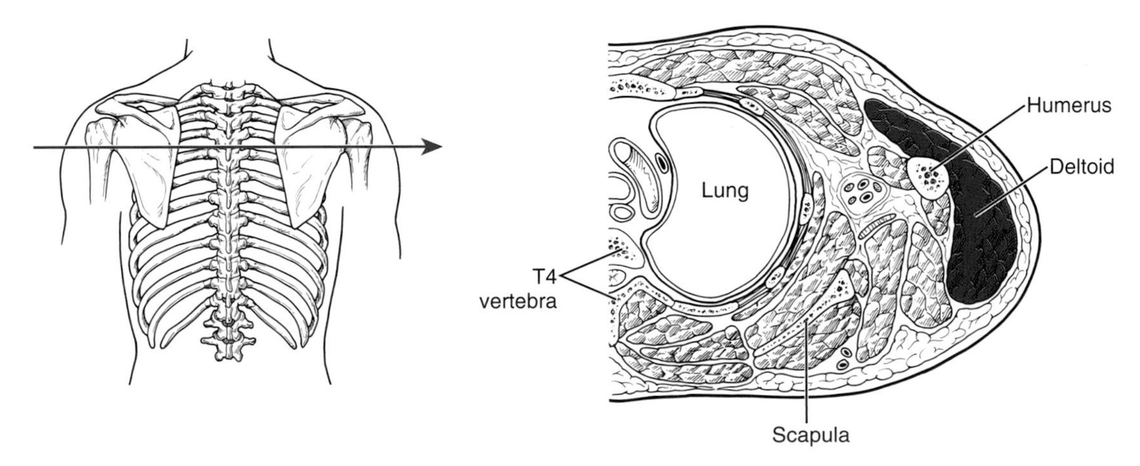

FIGURE 5-66 Arrow indicates level of cross section.

(Middle deltoid and Supraspinatus)

Range of Motion
0° to 180°

Table 5-8 SHOULDER ABDUCTION

I.D.	Muscle	Origin	Insertion
133	Deltoid (middle fibers)	Scapula (acromion, lateral margin, superior surface, and crest of spine)	Humerus (deltoid tuberosity on shaft via humeral tendon)
135	Supraspinatus	Scapula (supraspinous fossa, medial 2/3) Supraspinatus fascia	Humerus (greater tubercle, highest facet) Articular capsule of glenohumeral joint

Grade 5 (Normal), Grade 4 (Good), and Grade 3 (Fair)

Preliminary Evaluation: Examiner should check for full range of shoulder motion in all planes and should observe scapula for stability and smoothness of movement. (Refer to test for scapular abduction and upward rotation; see Figure 5-7).

Position of Patient: Short sitting with arm at side and elbow slightly flexed.

Position of Therapist: Standing behind patient. Hand giving resistance is contoured over arm just above elbow (Figure 5-67).

Test: Patient abducts arm to 90°.

Instructions to Patient: "Lift your arm out to the side to shoulder level. Hold it. Don't let me push it down."

Grading

Grade 5 (Normal): Holds end test position against maximal downward resistance.

Grade 4 (Good): Holds end test position against strong to moderate downward resistance.

Grade 3 (Fair): Completes range of motion to 90° with no manual resistance (Figure 5-68).

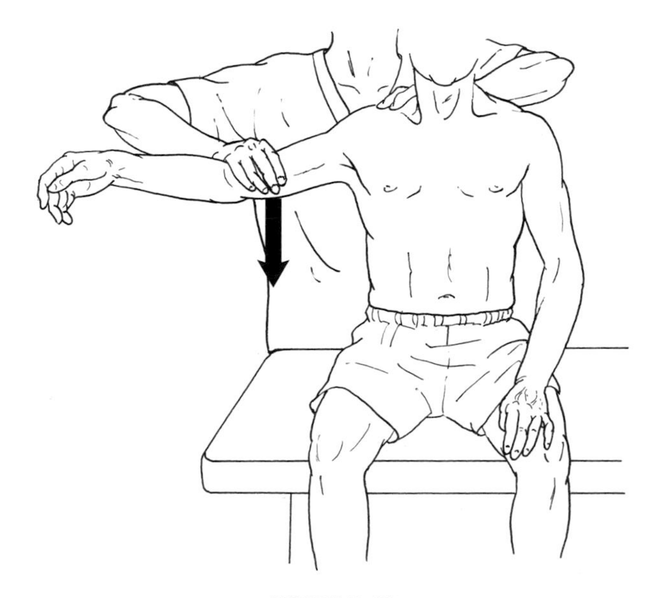

FIGURE 5-67

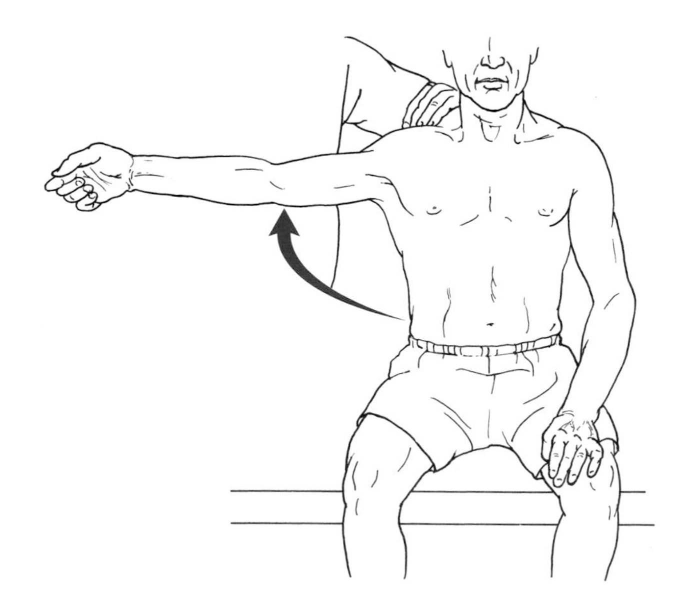

FIGURE 5-68

SHOULDER ABDUCTION

(Middle deltoid and Supraspinatus)

Grade 2 (Poor)

Position of Patient: Short sitting with arm at side and slight elbow flexion.

Position of Therapist: Standing behind patient to palpate muscles on test side. Palpate the deltoid (Figure 5-69) lateral to the acromial process on the superior aspect of the shoulder. The supraspinatus can be palpated by placing the fingers deep under the trapezius in the supraspinous fossa of the scapula.

Test: Patient attempts to abduct arm.

Instructions to Patient: "Try to lift your arm out to the side."

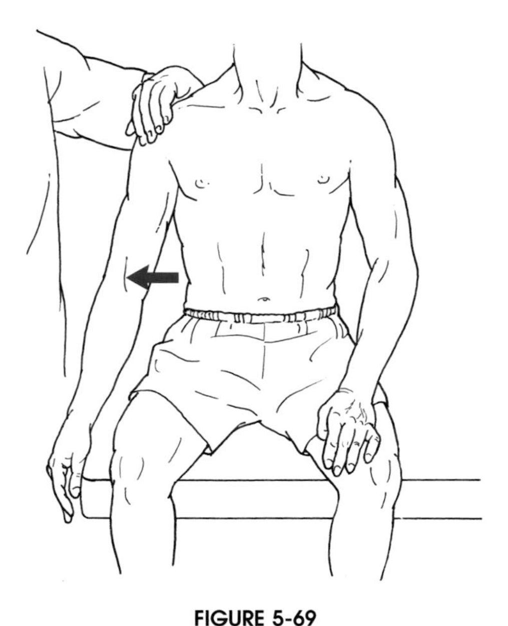

FIGURE 5-69

Alternate Test for Grade 2

Position of Patient: Supine. Arm at side supported on table (Figure 5-70).

Position of Therapist: Standing at test side of patient (therapist is shown on opposite side of test in figure to clearly illustrate test procedure). Hand used for palpation is positioned as described for Grade 2 test.

Test: Patient attempts to abduct shoulder by sliding arm on table without rotating it (see Figure 5-70).

Instructions to Patient: "Take your arm out to the side."

Grading

Grade 2 (Poor): Completes partial range of motion for sitting test and full range for supine test.

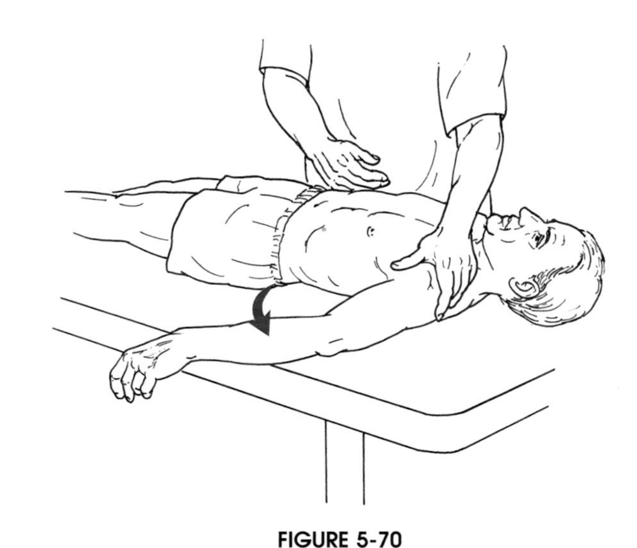

FIGURE 5-70

Grade 1 (Trace) and Grade 0 (Zero)

Position of Patient: Short sitting.

Position of Therapist: Standing behind and to the side of patient. Therapist cradles test arm with the shoulder in about 90° of abduction, providing limb support at the elbow (Figure 5-71).

Test: Patient tries to maintain the arm in abduction.

Instructions to Patient: "Try to hold your arm in this position."

Alternate Test for Grade 1 and Grade 0 (Supine)

Position of Patient: Supine with arm at side and elbow slightly flexed.

Position of Therapist: Standing at side of table at a place where the deltoid can be reached. Palpate the deltoid on the lateral surface of the upper one third of the arm (Figure 5-72).

Grading

Grade 1 (Trace): Palpable or visible contraction of deltoid with no movement.

Grade 0 (Zero): No contractile activity.

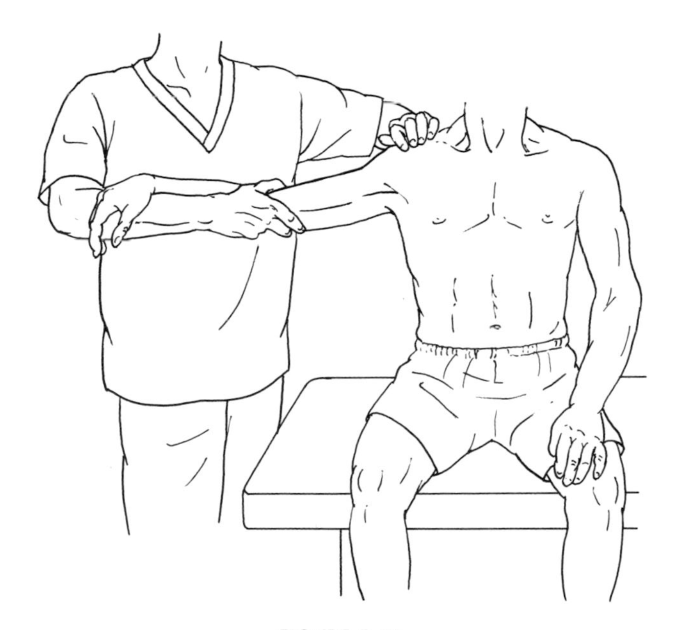

FIGURE 5-71

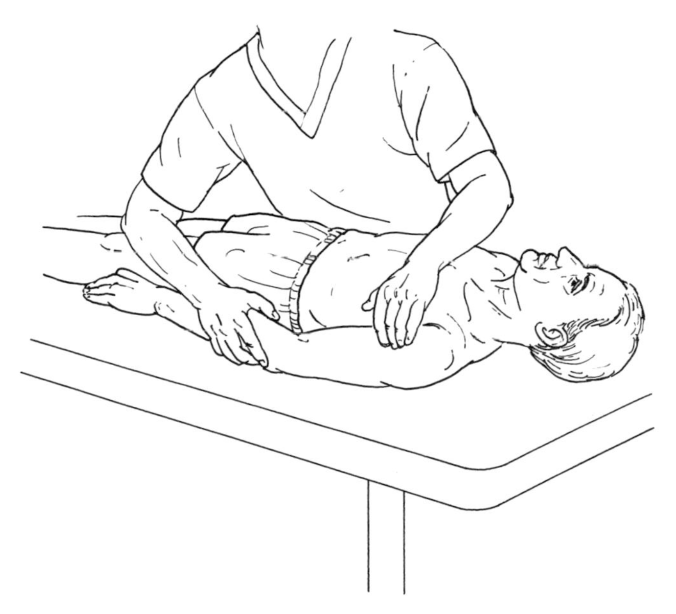

FIGURE 5-72

SHOULDER ABDUCTION

(Middle deltoid and Supraspinatus)

Substitution by Biceps Brachii

When a patient uses the biceps to substitute, the shoulder will externally rotate and the elbow will flex. The arm will be raised but not by the action of the abductor muscles. To avoid this substitution begin the test with the arm in a few degrees of elbow flexion, but do not allow active contraction of the biceps during the test.

Helpful Hints

- Turning the face to the opposite side and extending the neck will put the trapezius on slack and make the supraspinatus more accessible for palpation.
- The deltoid and supraspinatus work in tandem; when one is active in abduction, the other also will be active. Only when supraspinatus weakness is suspected is it necessary to palpate.
- Do not allow shoulder elevation or lateral flexion of the trunk to the opposite side because these movements can create an illusion of abduction.
- The tendon of the supraspinatus is most frequently injured of all the rotator cuff muscles because of its vulnerable position between the humeral head and acromion.[6]
- The supraspinatus is activated first when the patient abducts the arm from a neutral position of hanging at the side.[10] It functions to prevent the deltoid from superiorly translating the humeral head during abduction.[11]
- Peak activation of the supraspinatus is at 90°, which corresponds with the largest shoulder joint compressive loads when the forces of gravity are the greatest.[10]
- If the shoulder is painful in abduction, especially with lifting, then the resisted external rotation exercise is a good substitute exercise.[12,13]

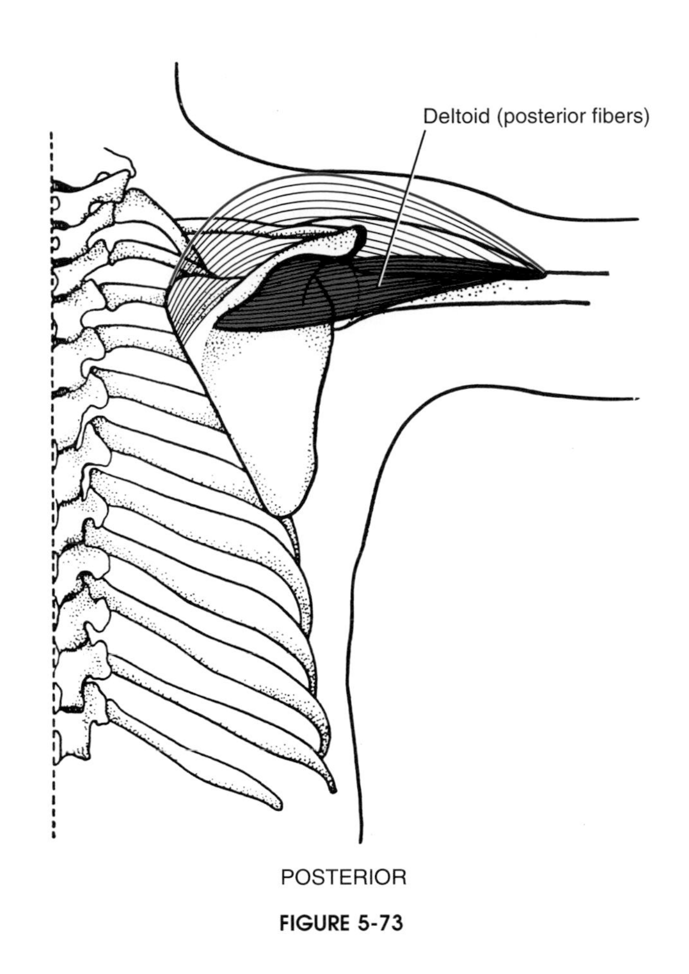

FIGURE 5-73

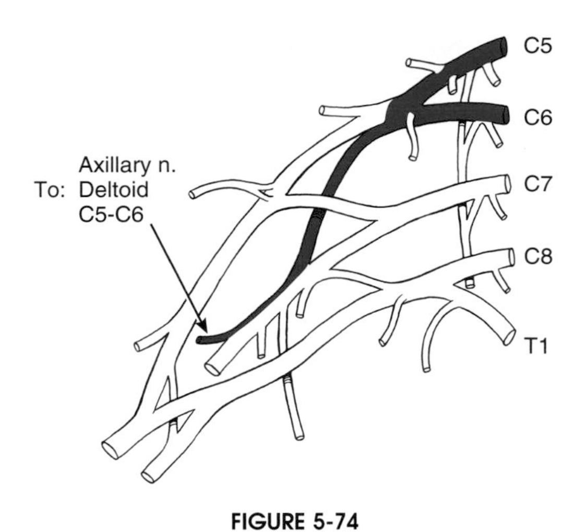

FIGURE 5-74

Range of Motion
When starting from a position of 90° of forward flexion: 0° to 90° (range, 90°)
When starting with the arm in full horizontal adduction: –40° to 90° (range, 130°)

Table 5-9 SHOULDER HORIZONTAL ABDUCTION

I.D.	Muscle	Origin	Insertion
133	Deltoid (posterior fibers)	Scapula (spine on lower lip of crest)	Humerus (deltoid tuberosity via humeral tendon)
Others			
136	Infraspinatus		
137	Teres minor		

SHOULDER HORIZONTAL ABDUCTION

(Posterior deltoid)

Grade 5 (Normal), Grade 4 (Good), and Grade 3 (Fair)

Position of Patient: Prone. Shoulder abducted to 90° and forearm off edge of table with elbow straight.

Position of Therapist: Standing at test side. Hand giving resistance is contoured over posterior arm just above the elbow (Figure 5-75).

Test: Patient horizontally abducts shoulder against maximal resistance.

Instructions to Patient: "Lift your elbow up toward the ceiling. Hold it. Don't let me push it down."

Grading

Grade 5 (Normal): Completes range and holds end position against maximal resistance.

Grade 4 (Good): Completes range and holds end position against strong to moderate resistance.

Grade 3 (Fair): Completes range of motion with no manual resistance (Figure 5-76). Note the elbow can be flexed for a Grade 3 (Fair).

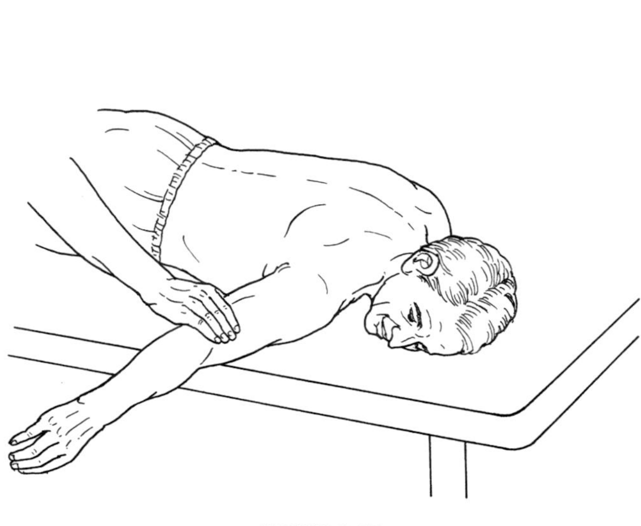

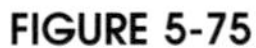

FIGURE 5-75

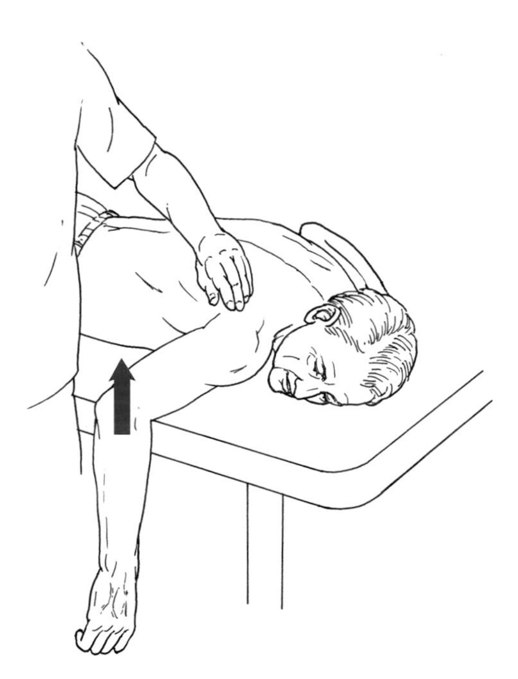

FIGURE 5-76

Grade 2 (Poor), Grade 1 (Trace), Grade 0 (Zero)

Position of Patient: Sitting over end or side of table.

Position of Therapist: Standing at test side. Support forearm under distal surface (Figure 5-77) and palpate over the posterior surface of the shoulder just superior to the axilla.

Test: Patient attempts to horizontally abduct the shoulder.

Instructions to Patient: "Try to move your arm backward."

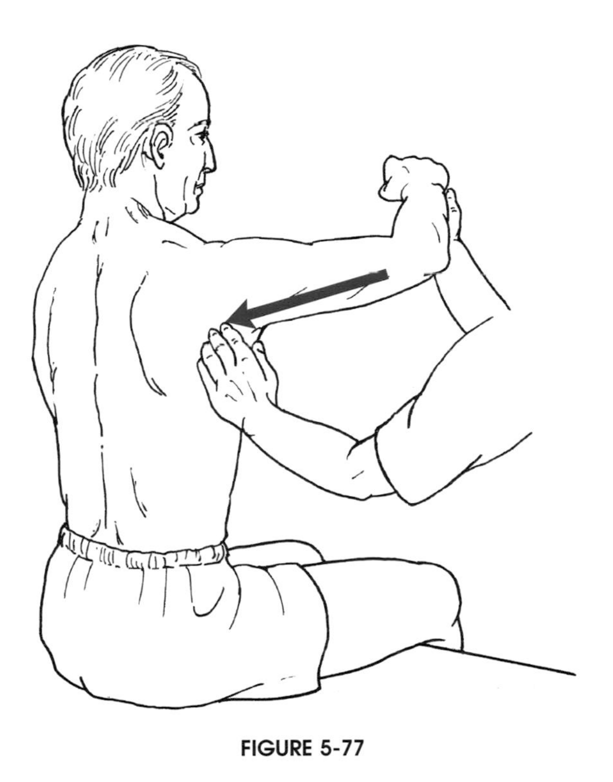

FIGURE 5-77

Alternate Test for Grades 2, 1, and 0

Position of Patient: Short sitting with arm supported on table (smooth surface) in 90° of abduction; elbow partially flexed.

Position of Therapist: Stand behind patient. Stabilize by contouring one hand over the superior aspect of the shoulder and the other over the scapula (Figure 5-78). Palpate the fibers of the posterior deltoid below and lateral to the spine of the scapula and on the posterior aspect of the proximal arm adjacent to the axilla.

Test: Patient slides (or tries to move) the arm across the table in horizontal abduction.

Instructions to Patient: "Slide your arm backward."

Grading

Grade 2 (Poor): Moves through full range of motion.

Grade 1 (Trace): Palpable contraction; no motion.

Grade 0 (Zero): No contractile activity.

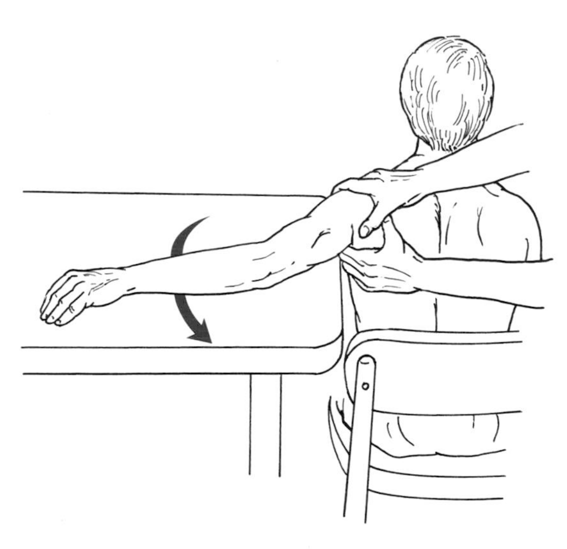

FIGURE 5-78

Helpful Hints

If the scapular muscles are weak, the examiner must manually stabilize the scapula to avoid scapular abduction.

Substitution by Triceps Brachii (Long Head)

Maintain the elbow in flexion to avoid substitution by the long head of the triceps.

SHOULDER HORIZONTAL ADDUCTION

(Pectoralis major)

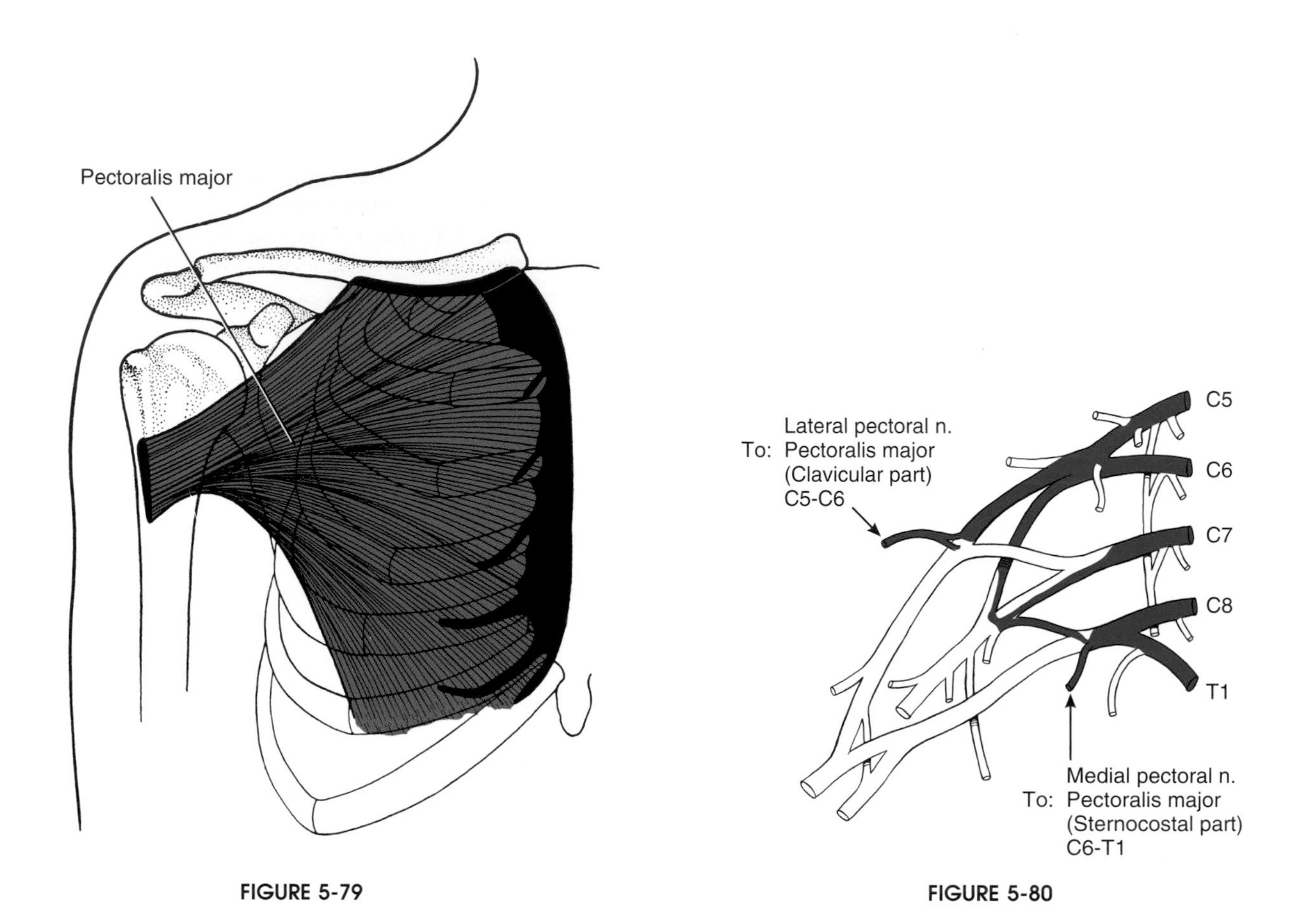

FIGURE 5-79

FIGURE 5-80

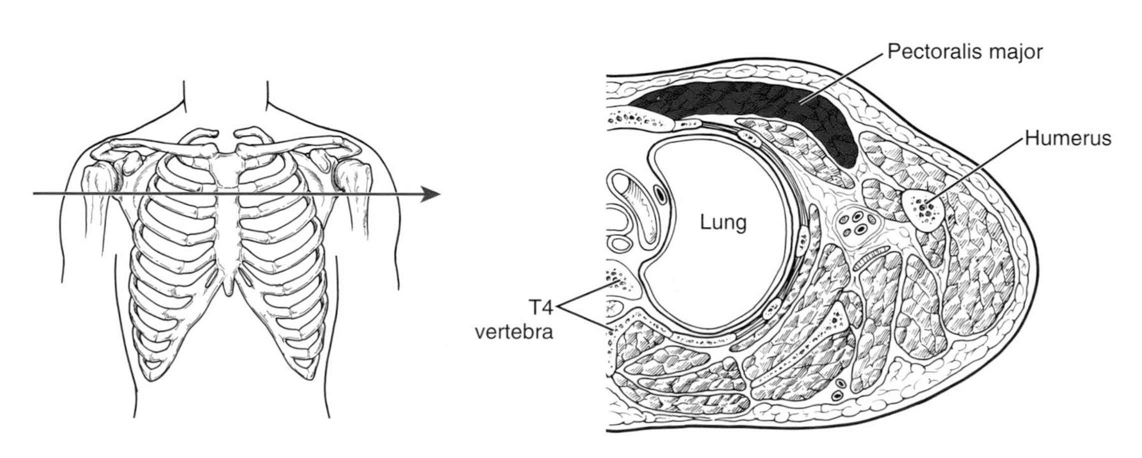

FIGURE 5-81 Arrow indicates level of cross section.

(Pectoralis major)

Range of Motion
0° to 130°
When starting from a position of 90° of forward flexion: 0° to –40° (range, 40°)
When starting with the arm in full horizontal abduction: 0° passing across the midline to –40° (range, 130°)

Table 5-10 SHOULDER HORIZONTAL ADDUCTION

I.D.	Muscle	Origin	Insertion
131	Pectoralis major	See Table 5-4	
	Clavicular part	Clavicle (sternal half of anterior surface)	Humerus (intertubercular sulcus, lateral lip)
	Sternal part	Sternum (anterior surface down to rib 6) Ribs 2-7 (costal cartilages) Aponeurosis of obliquus externus abdominis	Both parts converge on a bilaminar common tendon
Other			
133	Deltoid (anterior fibers)	See Table 5-6	

Preliminary Examination

The examiner begins with the patient supine and checks the range of motion and then tests both heads of the pectoralis major simultaneously. The patient is asked to move the arm in horizontal adduction, keeping it parallel to the floor without rotation.

If the arm moves across the body in a diagonal motion, test the sternal and clavicular heads of the muscle separately. Testing both heads of the pectoralis major separately should be routine in any patient with cervical spinal cord injury because of their different nerve root innervation.

Grade 5 (Normal) and Grade 4 (Good)

Position of Patient:

Whole Muscle: Supine. Shoulder abducted to 90°; elbow flexed to 90°.

Clavicular Head: Patient begins test with shoulder in 60° of abduction with elbow flexed. Patient then is asked to horizontally adduct the shoulder in a slightly upward diagonal direction.

Sternal Head: Patient begins test with shoulder in about 120° of abduction with elbow flexed. Patient is asked to horizontally adduct the shoulder in a slightly downward diagonal direction.

(Pectoralis major)

Grade 5 (Normal) and Grade 4 (Good) Continued

Position of Therapist: Standing at side of shoulder to be tested. Hand used for resistance is contoured around upper arm, just proximal to elbow. The other hand is used to check the activity of the pectoralis major on the upper aspect of the chest just medial to the shoulder joint (Figure 5-82). Palpation is not needed in a Grade 5 test, but it is prudent to assess activity if the muscle being tested is less than Grade 5.

Palpate the clavicular fibers of the pectoralis major up under the medial half of the clavicle (Figure 5-83). Palpate the sternal fibers on the chest wall at the lower anterior border of the axilla.

Test: When the *whole muscle* is tested, the patient horizontally adducts the shoulder through the available range of motion.

To test the *clavicular head,* the patient's motion begins at 60° of abduction and moves up and in across the body. The examiner applies resistance above the elbow in a downward direction (toward floor) and outward (i.e., opposite to the direction of the fibers of the clavicular head, which moves the arm diagonally up and inward) (Figure 5-84).

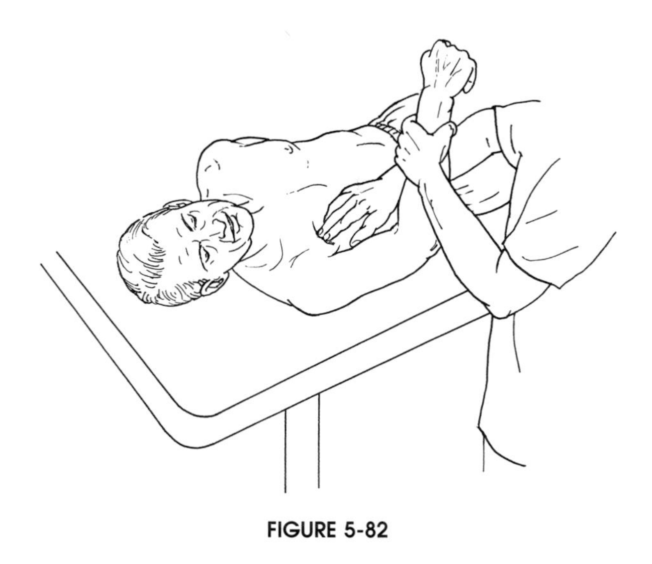

FIGURE 5-82

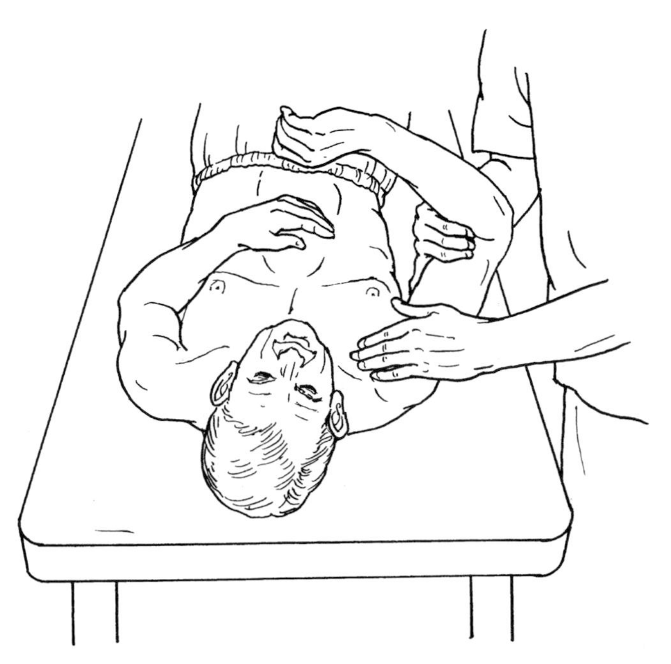

FIGURE 5-83

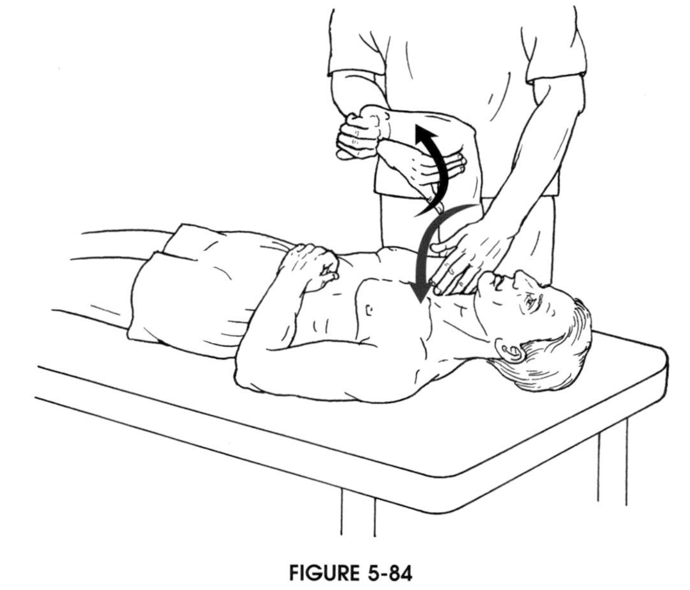

FIGURE 5-84

Grade 5 (Normal) and Grade 4 (Good) Continued

To test the *sternal head,* the motion begins at 120° of shoulder abduction and moves diagonally down and in toward the patient's opposite hip. Resistance is given above the elbow in an up and outward direction (Figure 5-85) (i.e., opposite to the motion of the sternal head, which is diagonally down and inward).

Instructions to Patient:

Both Heads: "Move your arm across your chest. Hold it. Don't let me pull it back."

Clavicular Head: "Move your arm up and in."

Sternal Head: "Move your arm down and in."

Grading

Grade 5 (Normal): Completes range of motion and takes maximal resistance.

Grade 4 (Good): Completes range of motion and takes strong to moderate resistance, but muscle exhibits some "give" at end of range.

Grade 3 (Fair)

Position of Patient: Supine. Shoulder at 90° of abduction and elbow at 90° of flexion.

Position of Therapist: Same as for Grade 5.

Test:

Both Heads: Patient horizontally adducts extremity across chest in a straight pattern with no diagonal motion (Figure 5-86).

Clavicular Head: Direction of motion by the patient is diagonally up and inward.

Sternal Head: Direction of motion is diagonally down and inward.

Instructions to Patient: Same as for the Grade 5 test, but no resistance is offered.

Grading

Grade 3 (Fair): Patient completes available range of motion in all three tests with no resistance other than the weight of the extremity.

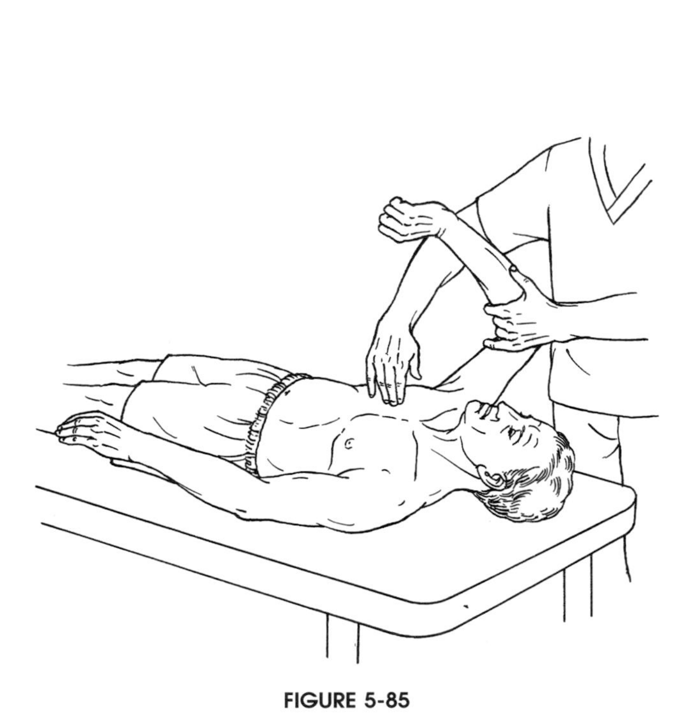

FIGURE 5-85

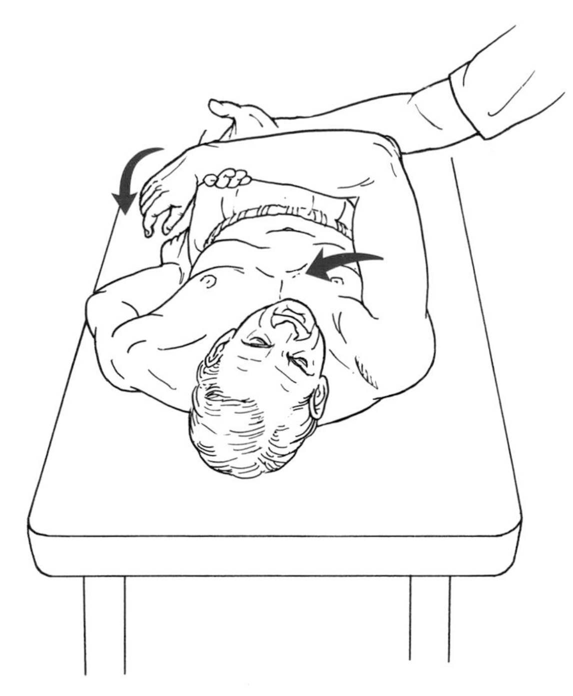

FIGURE 5-86

SHOULDER HORIZONTAL ADDUCTION

(Pectoralis major)

Grade 2 (Poor), Grade 1 (Trace), and Grade 0 (Zero)

Position of Patient: Supine. Arm is supported in 90° of abduction with elbow flexed to 90°.

Alternate Position: Patient is seated with test arm supported on table (at level of axilla) with arm in 90° of abduction midway between flexion and extension and elbow slightly flexed (Figure 5-87). Friction of the table surface should be minimized (as with a powder board).

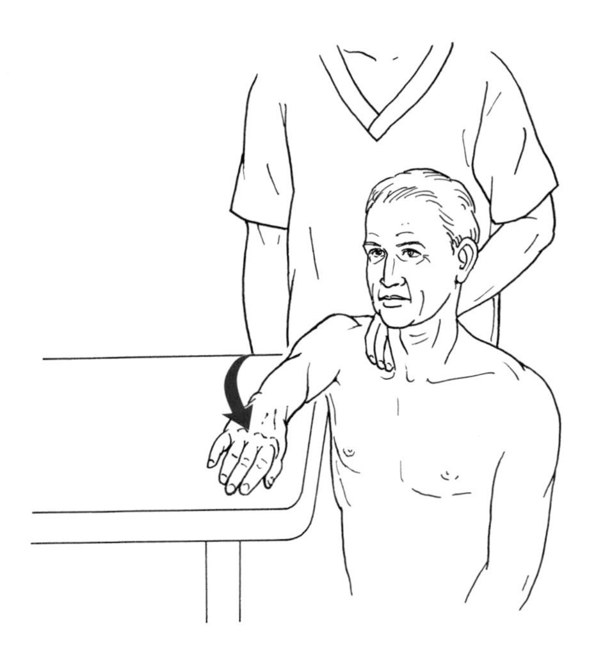

FIGURE 5-87

Position of Therapist: Standing at side of shoulder to be tested or behind the seated patient. When the patient is supine, support the full length of the forearm and hold the limb at the wrist (see Figure 5-84).

For both tests palpate the pectoralis major muscle on the anterior aspect of the chest medial to the shoulder joint (see Figure 5-82.)

Test: Patient attempts to horizontally adduct the shoulder. The use of the alternate test position, in which the arm moves across the table, precludes individual testing for the two heads.

Instructions to Patient: "Try to move your arm across your chest." In seated position: "Move your arm forward."

Grading

Grade 2 (Poor): Patient horizontally adducts shoulder through available range of motion with the weight of the arm supported by the examiner or the table.

Grade 1 (Trace): Palpable contractile activity.

Grade 0 (Zero): No contractile activity.

Helpful Hints

For grades 5 (normal) and 4 (good), This test requires resistance on the forearm, which in turn requires that the elbow flexors be strong. If they are weak, provide resistance on the arm just proximal to the elbow.

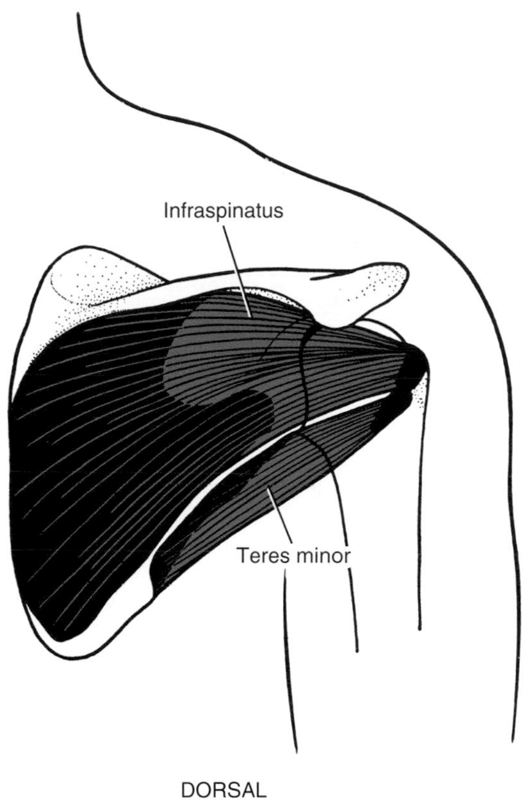

FIGURE 5-88

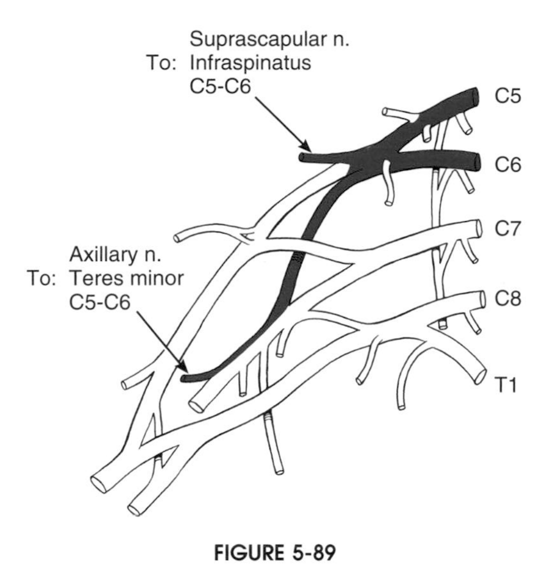

FIGURE 5-89

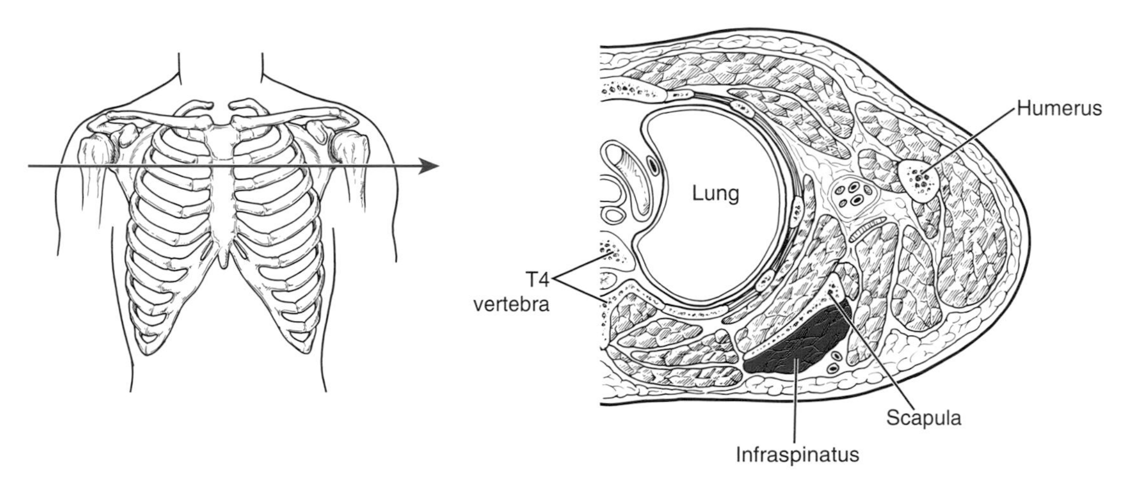

FIGURE 5-90 Arrow indicates level of cross section.

SHOULDER EXTERNAL ROTATION

(Infraspinatus and Teres minor)

Range of Motion
0° to 60°
(In the literature, range varies between 0° and 90°. Range also varies with elevation of arm.)

Table 5-11 SHOULDER EXTERNAL ROTATION

I.D.	Muscle	Origin	Insertion
136	Infraspinatus	Scapula (infraspinous fossa, medial 2/3) Infraspinous fascia	Humerus (greater tubercle, middle facet)
137	Teres minor	Scapula (lateral border, superior 2/3)	Humerus (greater tubercle, lowest facet) Humerus (shaft, distal to lowest facet) Capsule of glenohumeral joint
Other			
133	Deltoid (posterior)	Lower edge of the crest of the spine of the scapula	Deltoid tuberosity

Grade 5 (Normal), Grade 4 (Good), and Grade 3 (Fair)

Position of Patient: Prone with head turned toward test side. Shoulder abducted to 90° with arm fully supported on table; forearm hanging vertically over edge of table. Place a folded towel under the arm at the edge of the table if it has a sharp edge (Figure 5-91).

Position of Therapist: Standing at test side at level of patient's waist (see Figure 5-91). One hand is used to give resistance over the forearm, as near the wrist as possible, for Grades 5 and 4. The other hand supports the elbow to provide some counter-pressure at the end of the range.

Test: Patient moves forearm upward through the range of external rotation.

Instructions to Patient: "Raise your arm to the level of the table. Hold it. Don't let me push it down." Therapist may need to demonstrate the desired motion.

Grading

Grade 5 (Normal): Completes available range of motion and holds firmly against resistance.

Grade 4 (Good): Completes available range, but the muscle at end range yields or gives way.

Grade 3 (Fair): Completes available range of motion but is unable to take any manual resistance (Figure 5-92).

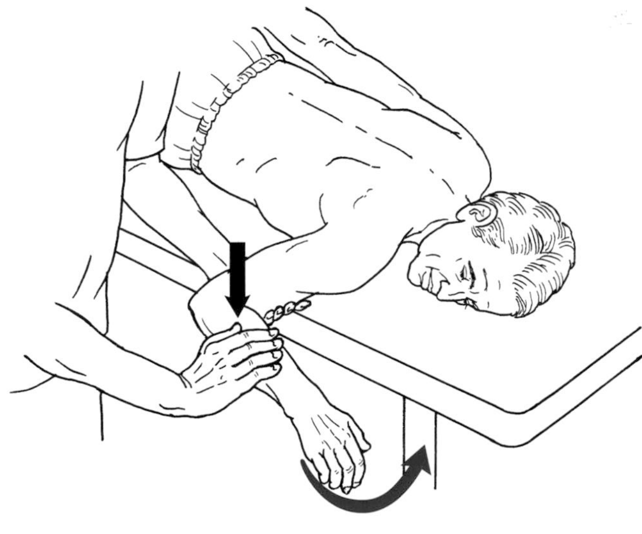

FIGURE 5-91

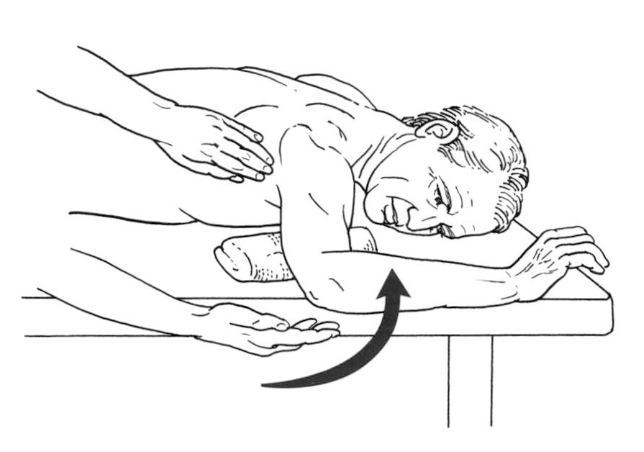

FIGURE 5-92

Alternate Position for Grade 3

Short sitting with elbow flexed to 90°. The therapist supports the patient's flexed elbow while the patient moves the forearm away from the body. Note the hand is eliminating friction (Figure 5-93).

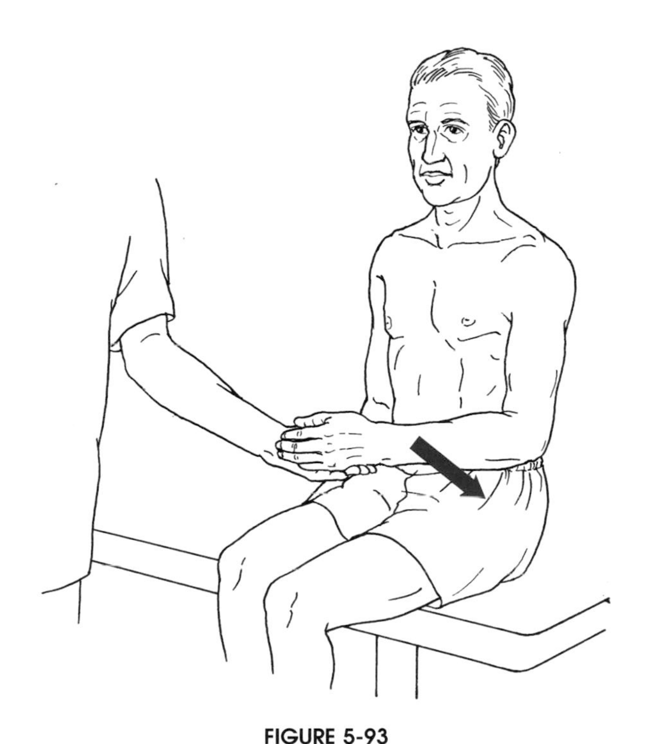

FIGURE 5-93

Alternate Position for Grades 4 and 5

Short sitting, with elbow flexed to 90°. The therapist stabilizes the elbow while the other hand provides resistance at the dorsal (extensor) surface of the forearm, just proximal to the wrist (Figure 5-94). The amount of resistance tolerated in this position may be much greater for Grades 5 and 4. Note: it is more difficult to isolate the external rotators in this position.

Test: Patient internally rotates arm, pushing forearm away from patient's abdomen.

Instructions to Patient: "Push your forearm away from your stomach."

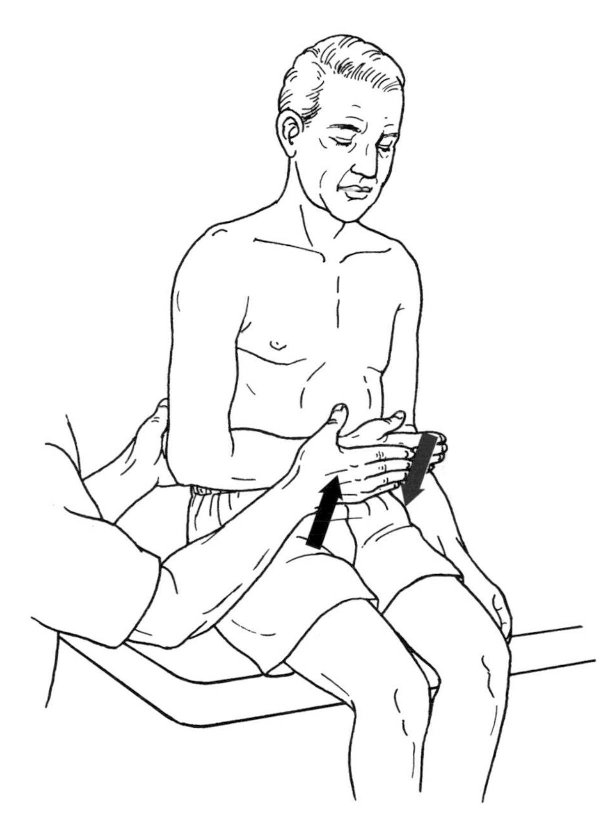

FIGURE 5-94

SHOULDER EXTERNAL ROTATION

(Infraspinatus and Teres minor)

Grade 2 (Poor), Grade 1 (Trace), and Grade 0 (Zero)

The test for Grade 2 and below is done in a short sitting position, with the shoulder in a neutral position and with gravity eliminated. Visualization is maximized in this position (Figure 5-95).

Position of Patient: Short sitting with elbow flexed to 90° and forearm in neutral rotation with hand facing forward.

Position of Therapist: Standing or sitting on a low stool at test side of patient at shoulder level. One hand stabilizes the outside of the flexed elbow while the other hand palpates for the tendon of the infraspinatus over the body of the scapula below the spine in the infraspinous fossa. Palpate the teres minor on the inferior margin of the axilla and along the axillary border of the scapula (Figure 5-96).

Test: Patient attempts to move forearm away from the stomach (see Figure 5-96).

Instructions to Patient: "Try to push your forearm away from your stomach."

Grading

Grade 2 (Poor): Completes available range in this gravity-eliminated position.

Grade 1 (Trace): Palpation of either or both muscles reveals contractile activity but no motion.

Grade 0 (Zero): No palpable or visible activity.

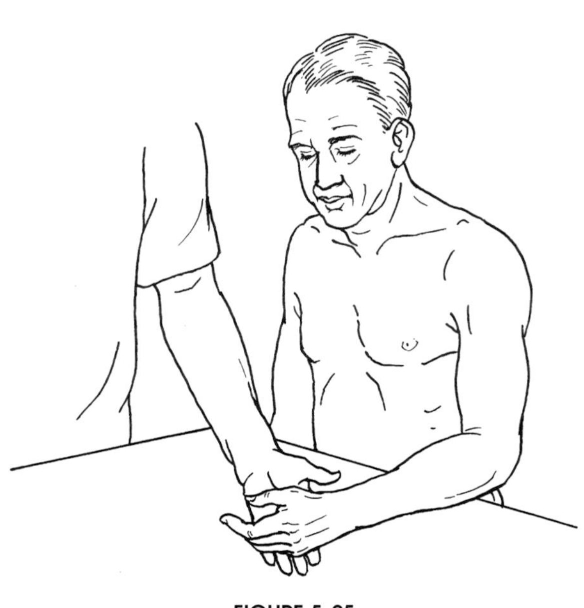

FIGURE 5-95

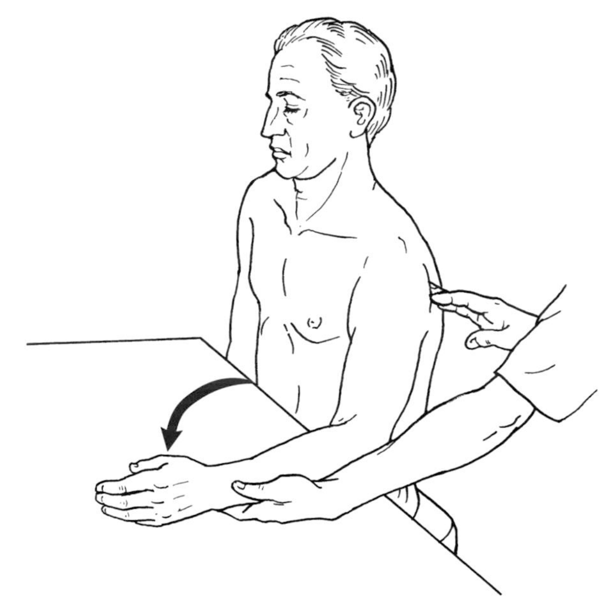

FIGURE 5-96

Helpful Hints

- Resistance in tests of shoulder rotation should be administered gradually and carefully because of the inherent instability of the shoulder and in the presence of pain, muscle tears, or instability.
- The therapist must be careful to discern whether supination occurs instead of the requested external rotation during the testing of Grade 2 and Grade 1 muscles because this motion can be mistaken for lateral rotation.
- Eliminating gravity for the Grade 2 test can be done by supporting the patient's forearm (see Figure 5-96) or by using a table to support the forearm. If using the table, the therapist should support the hand so as to eliminate friction (see Figure 5-95).
- Testing rotation in the supine position necessitates the greatest force at the beginning of the movement to overcome the largest gravitational moment arm at the beginning of the movement. Supine testing also provides a stabilizing effect on the scapula since the patient's body weight "pins" the scapula to the table.

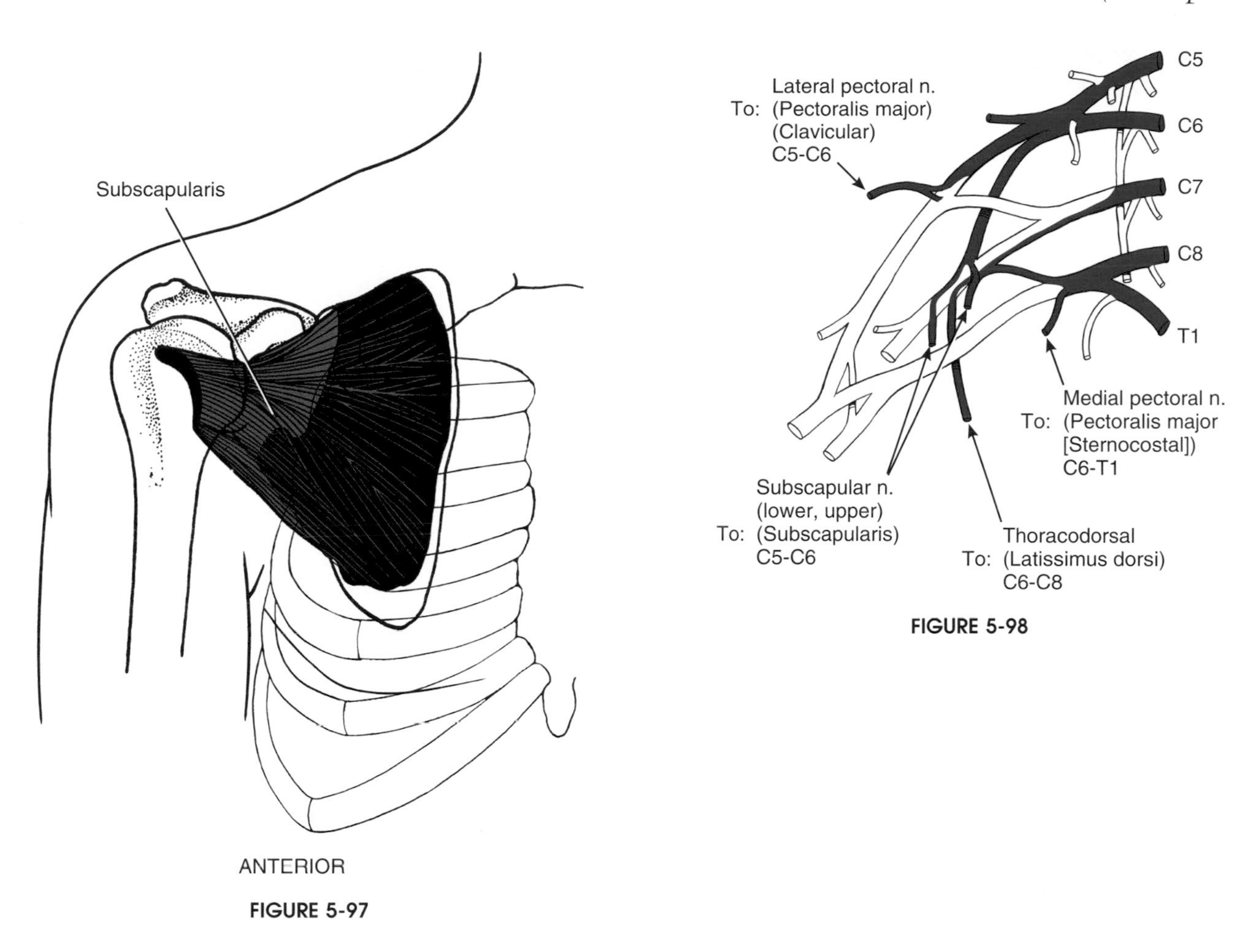

FIGURE 5-97

FIGURE 5-98

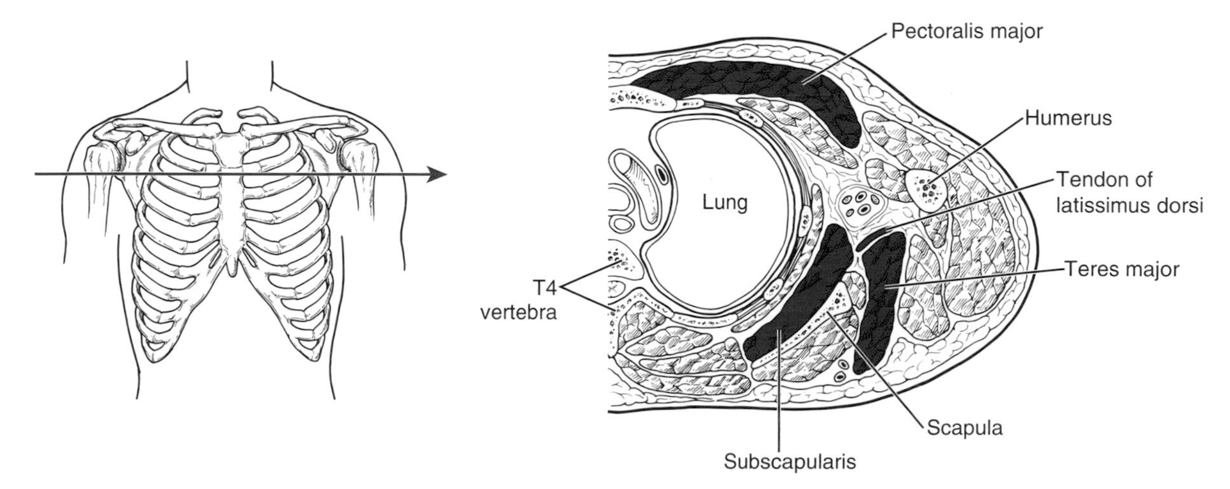

FIGURE 5-99 Arrow indicates level of cross section.

SHOULDER INTERNAL ROTATION

(Subscapularis)

Range of Motion
0° to 80°
(In the literature, range varies from 0° to 45° and to as high as 90°. Range also varies with elevation of arm.)

Table 5-12 SHOULDER INTERNAL ROTATION

I.D.	Muscle	Origin	Insertion
134	Subscapularis	Scapula (fills fossa on costal surface) Intermuscular septa Aponeurosis of subscapularis	Humerus (lesser tubercle) Capsule of glenohumeral joint (anterior)
131	Pectoralis major	Sternal half of clavicle, entire anterior surface of the sternum	Lateral lip of the intertubercular sulcus of anterior humerus
	Clavicular part	Clavicle (sternal half of anterior surface)	Humerus (intertubercular sulcus, lateral lip)
	Sternal part	Sternum (anterior surface down to rib 6) Ribs 2-7 (costal cartilages) Aponeurosis of obliquus externus abdominis	Both parts converge on a bilaminar common tendon
130	Latissimus dorsi	T6-T12, L1-L5, and sacral vertebrae (spinous processes) Supraspinous ligaments Ribs 9-12 (by slips which interdigitate with obliquus externus abdominus) Ilium (crest, posterior) Thoracolumbar fascia	Humerus (floor of intertubercular sulcus) Deep fascia of arm
138	Teres major	Scapula (dorsal surface of inferior angle)	Humerus (intertubercular sulcus, medial lip)
Other			
133	Deltoid (anterior)	See Table 5-6	

Grade 5 (Normal), Grade 4 (Good), and Grade 3 (Fair)

Position of Patient: Prone with head turned toward test side. Shoulder is abducted to 90° with folded towel placed under distal arm and forearm hanging vertically over edge of table.

Position of Therapist: Standing at test side. Hand giving resistance is placed on the volar side of the forearm just above the wrist. The other hand provides counterforce at the elbow (Figure 5-100). The resistance hand applies resistance in a downward and forward direction; the counterforce is applied backward and slightly upward. Stabilize the scapular region if muscles are weak or perform test in the supine position.

Test: Patient moves arm through available range of internal rotation (backward and upward).

Instructions to Patient: "Move your forearm up and back. Hold it. Don't let me push it down." Demonstrate the desired motion to the patient.

Grading

Grade 5 (Normal): Completes available range and holds firmly against strong resistance.

Grade 4 (Good): Completes available range, but there is a "spongy" feeling against strong resistance.

Grade 3 (Fair): Completes available range with no manual resistance (Figure 5-101).

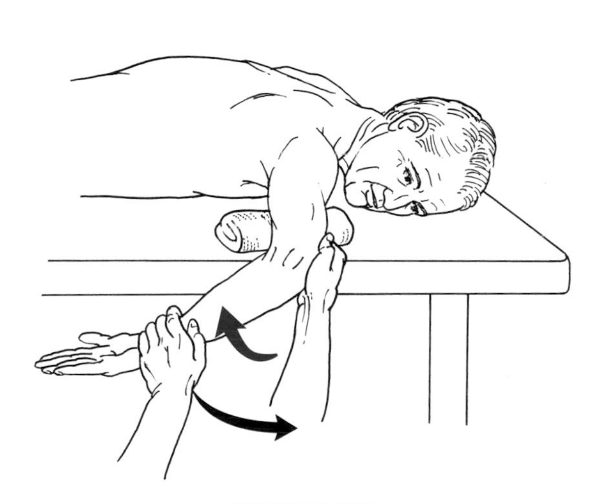

FIGURE 5-100

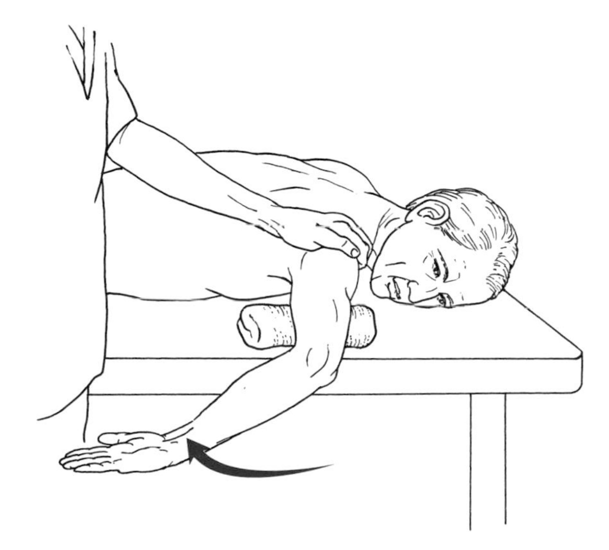

FIGURE 5-101

SHOULDER INTERNAL ROTATION

(Subscapularis)

Alternate Test for Grades 4 and 5

Sitting with elbow flexed to 90°. The therapist stabilizes the inside of the elbow while the other hand provides resistance at the volar (flexor) surface of the forearm, just proximal to the wrist (Figure 5-102). The amount of resistance tolerated in this position may be much greater for Grades 5 and 4.

Test: Patient internally rotates arm, pulling forearm toward abdomen.

Instructions to Patient: "Pull your forearm toward your stomach."

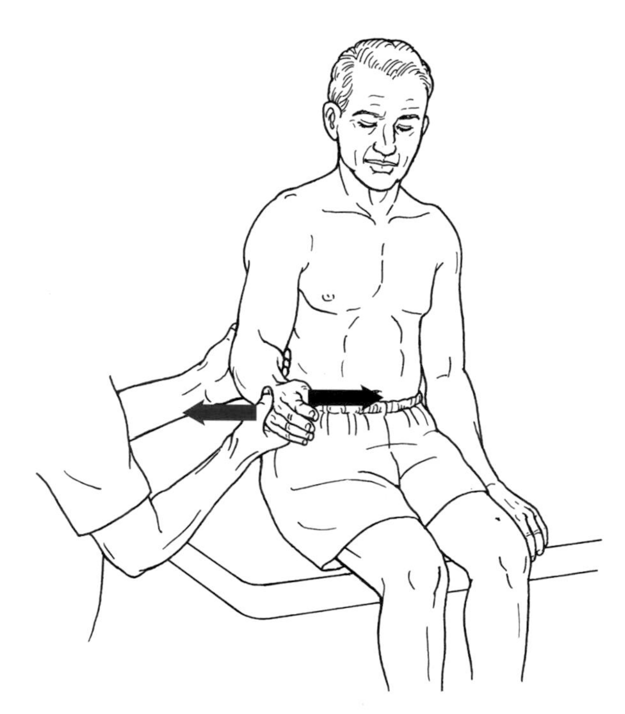

FIGURE 5-102

Grade 2 (Poor), Grade 1 (Trace), and Grade 0 (Zero)

The test for grade 2 and below is done in a sitting position, with the shoulder in a neutral position and with gravity eliminated. Visualization is maximized in this position.

Position of Patient: Short sitting with elbow flexed and forearm in neutral rotation.

Grade 2 (Poor), Grade 1 (Trace), and Grade 0 (Zero) Continued

Position of Therapist: Standing at test side or sitting on low stool. One hand stabilizes the forearm while the other hand palpates for the tendon of the subscapularis, deep in the axilla (Figure 5-103). Note: The hand of the examiner under the patient's hand will eliminate friction in the Grade 2 test if a flat surface is being used (Figure 5-104).

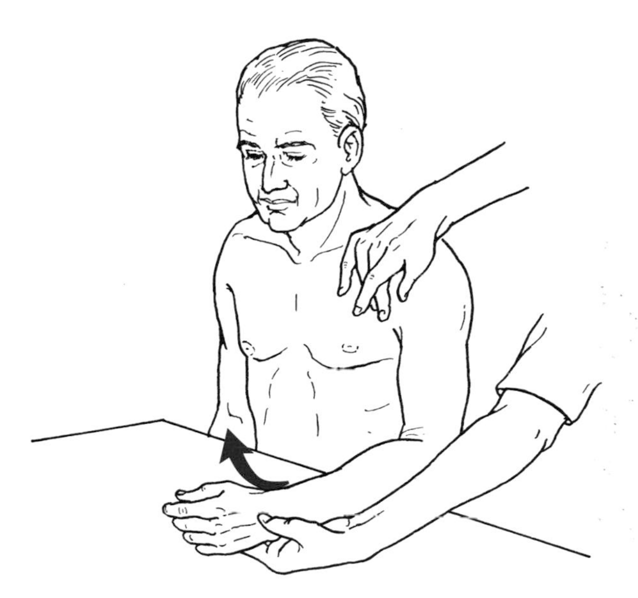

FIGURE 5-103

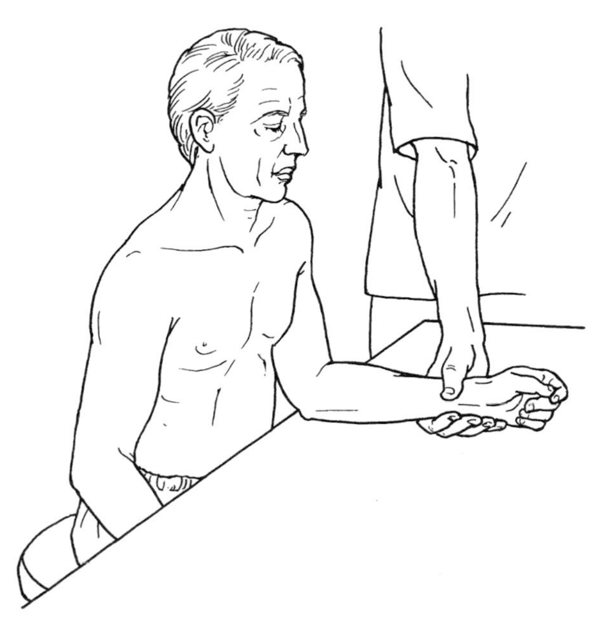

FIGURE 5-104

Test: Patient attempts to internally rotate arm, pulling forearm toward abdomen.

Instructions to Patient: "Try to pull your forearm toward your stomach."

Grading

Grade 2 (Poor): Completes available range.

Grade 1 (Trace): Palpable contraction occurs.

Grade 0 (Zero): No palpable contraction.

Helpful Hints

- Internal rotation is a stronger motion than external rotation. This is largely a factor of muscle mass.
- The subscapularis is important for anterior shoulder stability.[14]
- The muscle test for the subscapularis muscle is very similar to the clinical diagnostic test for subscapularis tears. Cleland describes the lift-off test with the patient sitting and the arm internally rotated behind the back. The test asks the patient to lift the arm off the back.[2]
- The Belly Press test[15] is an alternative test to the lift-off test, useful when pain or limited motion prevents the shoulder from getting into the position described by Cleland in the lift-off test.[16] It is performed in sitting or standing position with the palm of the hand placed against the belly, just below the level of the xiphoid process. The patient is instructed to maximally push the hand into the belly by internally rotating the shoulder. A positive test is indicated when the patient drops the elbow toward the torso (shoulder adduction and extension), indicating an inability to internally rotate the shoulder.
- Pain at the shoulder joint from a subscapularis tendonitis or partial subscapularis tendon tear may limit the ability to strongly resist internal rotation. Limited range may also prohibit the patient from assuming the position. In these cases, a sitting position is used.

ELBOW FLEXION

(Biceps, Brachialis, and Brachioradialis)

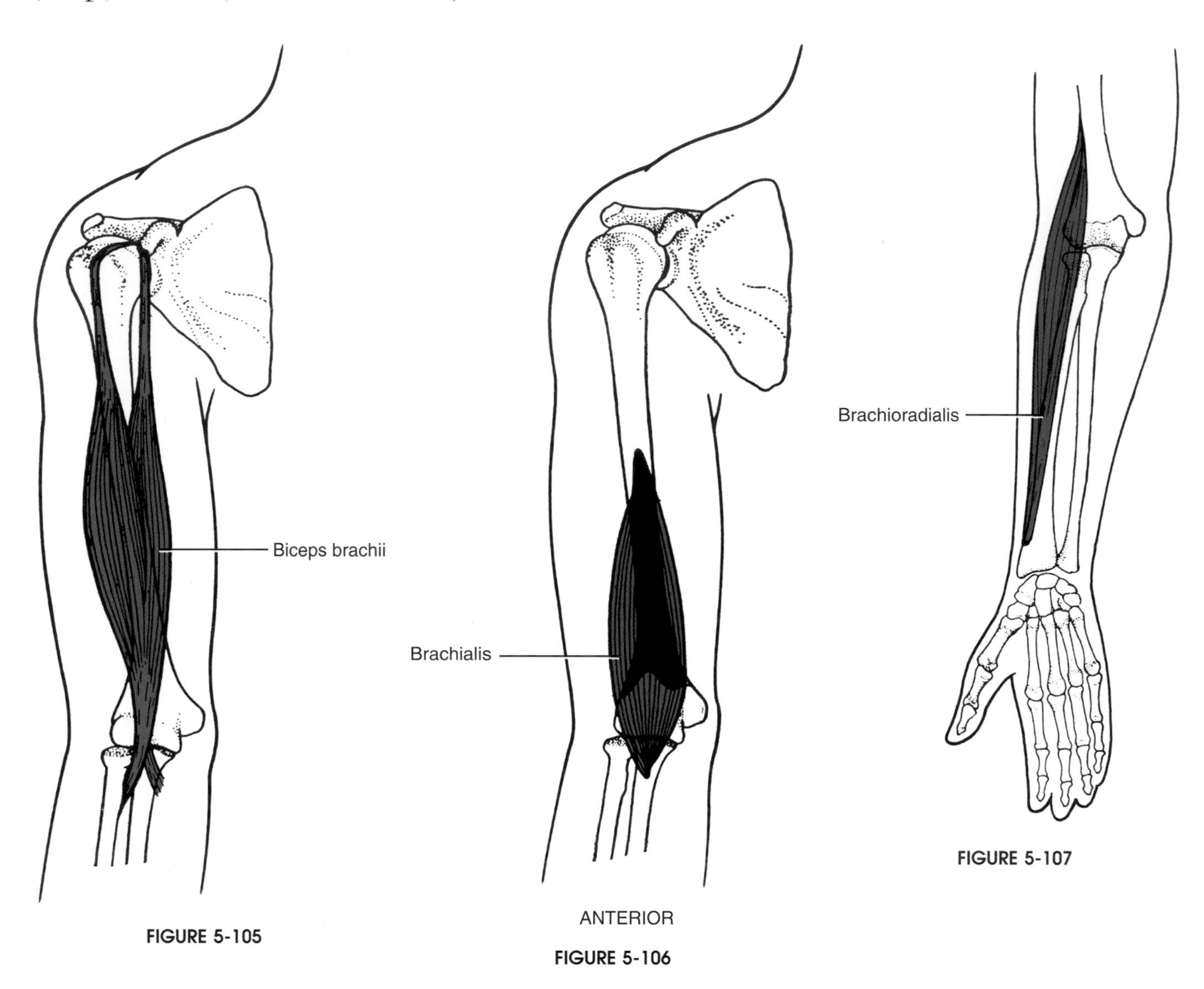

FIGURE 5-105

FIGURE 5-106

FIGURE 5-107

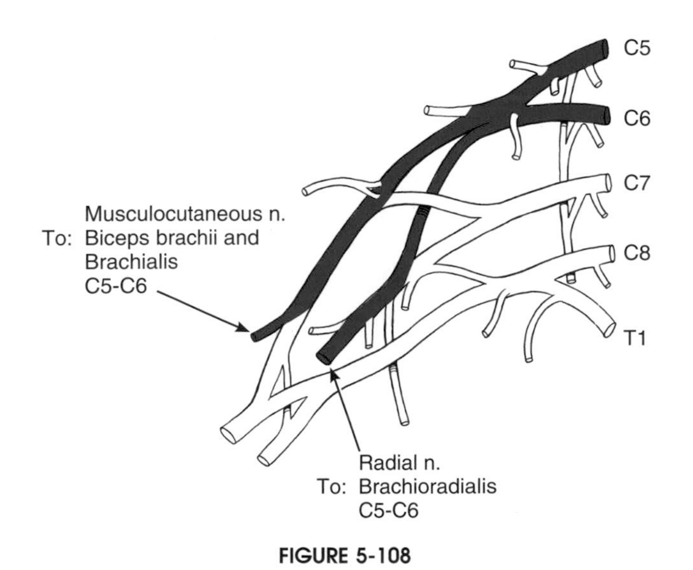

FIGURE 5-108

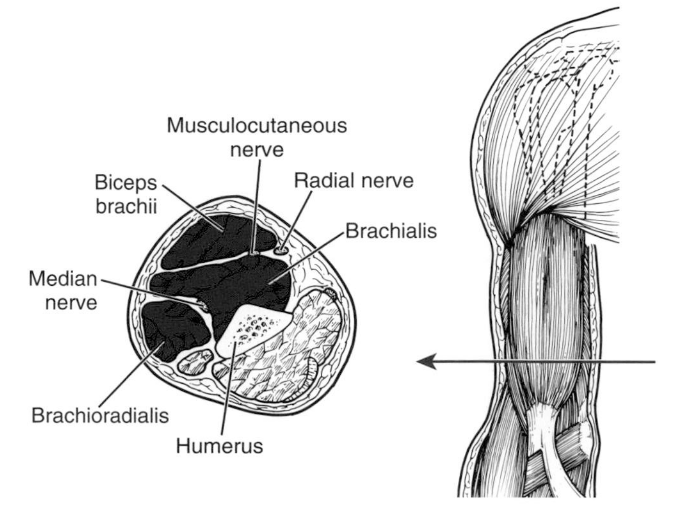

FIGURE 5-109 Arrow indicates level of cross section.

(Biceps, Brachialis, and Brachioradialis)

Range of Motion
0° to 150°

Table 5-13 ELBOW FLEXION

I.D.	Muscle	Origin	Insertion
140	Biceps brachii Short head Long head	Scapula (coracoid process, apex) Scapula (supraglenoid tubercle) Capsule of glenohumeral joint and glenoid labrum	Radius (radial tuberosity) Bicipital aponeurosis
141	Brachialis	Humerus (shaft anterior, distal 1/2) Intermuscular septa (medial)	Ulna (tuberosity and coronoid process)
143	Brachioradialis	Humerus (lateral supracondylar ridge, proximal 2/3) Lateral intermuscular septum	Radius (distal end just proximal to styloid process)
Others			
146	Pronator teres		
148	Extensor carpi radialis longus		
151	Flexor carpi radialis		
153	Flexor carpi ulnaris		See Plate 4

Grade 5 (Normal), Grade 4 (Good), and Grade 3 (Fair)

Position of Patient: Short sitting with arms at sides. The following are the positions of choice, but it is doubtful whether the individual muscles can be separated when strong effort is used. The brachialis in particular is independent of forearm position.

Biceps brachii: forearm in supination (Figure 5-110)

Brachialis: forearm in pronation (Figure 5-111)

Brachioradialis: forearm in midposition between pronation and supination (Figure 5-112)

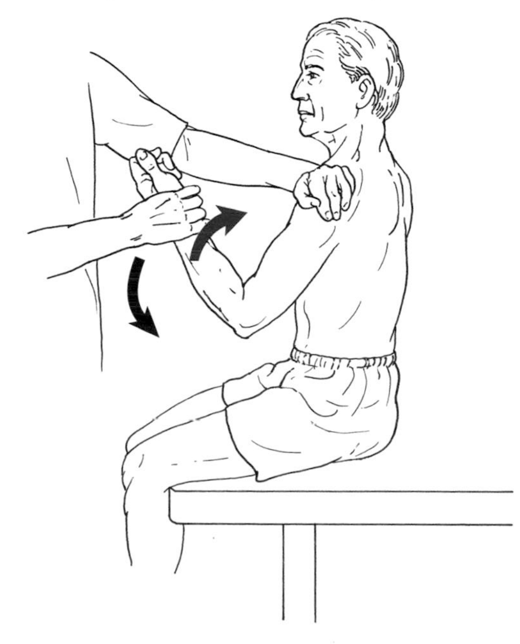

FIGURE 5-110

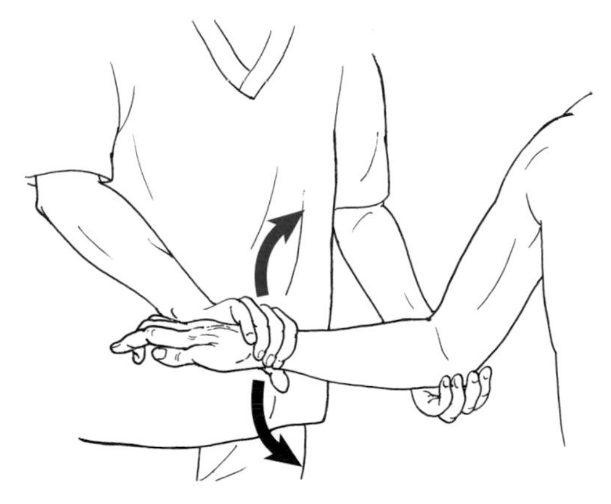

FIGURE 5-111

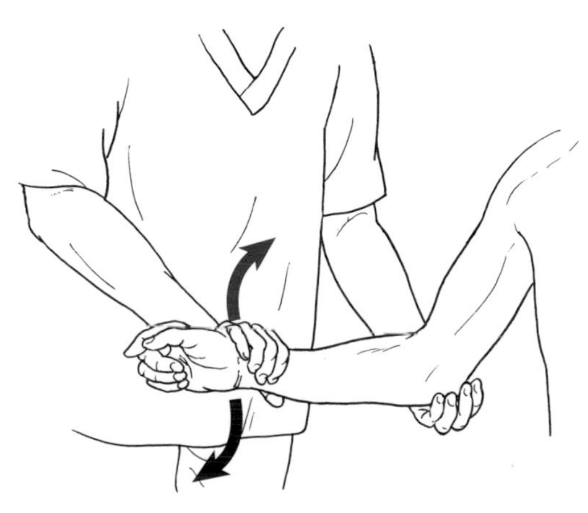

FIGURE 5-112

(Biceps, Brachialis, and Brachioradialis)

Grade 5 (Normal), Grade 4 (Good), and Grade 3 (Fair) Continued

Position of Therapist: Standing in front of patient toward the test side. Hand giving resistance is contoured over the volar (flexor) surface of the forearm proximal to the wrist (see Figure 5-110). The other forearm is placed over the anterior surface of the upper arm and applies counterforce by resisting any upper arm movement.

No resistance is given in a Grade 3 test, but the test elbow is cupped by the examiner's hand (Figure 5-113, biceps illustrated at end range).

Test (All Three Forearm Positions): Patient flexes elbow through range of motion.

Instructions to Patient (All Three Tests)
Grades 5 and 4: "Bend your elbow. Hold it. Don't let me pull it down."

Grade 3: "Bend your elbow."

Grading

Grade 5 (Normal): Completes available range and holds firmly against maximal resistance.

Grade 4 (Good): Completes available range against strong to moderate resistance, but the end point may not be firm.

Grade 3 (Fair): Completes available range with each forearm position with no manual resistance.

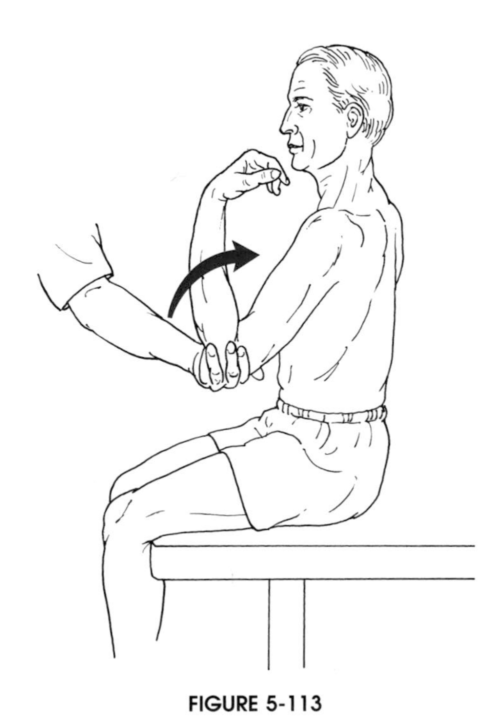

FIGURE 5-113

Grade 2 (Poor)

Position of Patient:
All Elbow Flexors: Short sitting with arm abducted to 90° and supported by examiner (Figure 5-114). Forearm is supinated (biceps), pronated (brachialis), and in mid-position (brachioradialis).

Alternate Position for Patients Unable to Sit: Supine. Elbow is flexed to about 45° with forearm supinated (for biceps; see Figure 5-114), pronated (for brachialis), and in midposition (for brachioradialis; Figure 5-115, biceps illustrated).

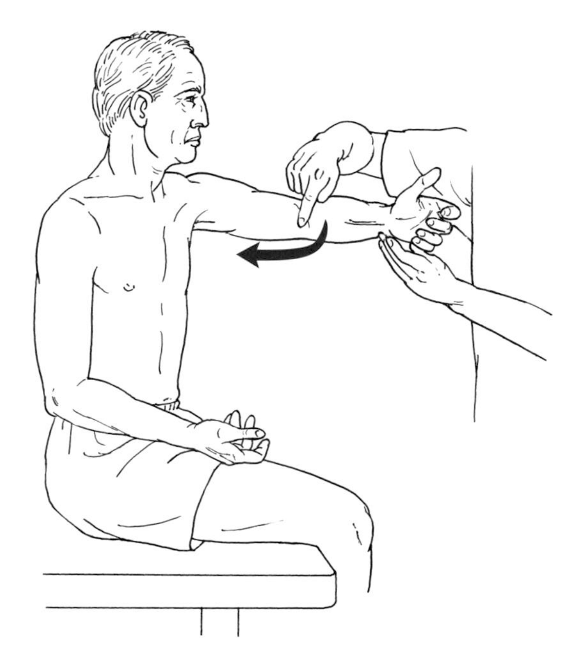

FIGURE 5-114

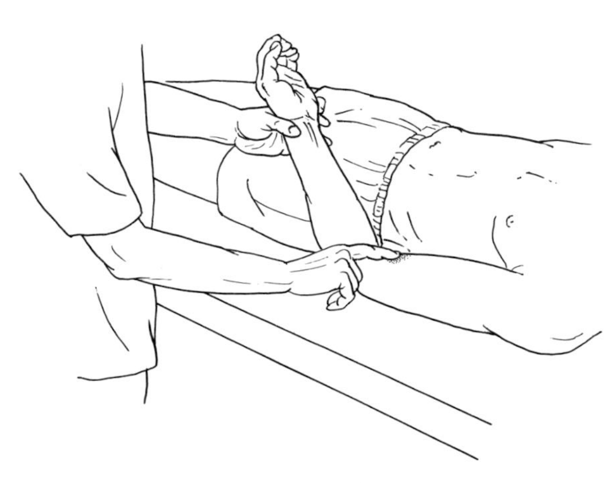

FIGURE 5-115

Grade 2 (Poor) Continued

Position of Therapist:

All Three Flexors: Standing in front of patient and supporting abducted arm under the elbow and wrist if necessary (see Figure 5-114). Palpate the tendon of the biceps in the antecubital space (see Figure 5-115). On the arm, the muscle fibers may be felt on the anterior surface of the middle two thirds with the short head lying medial to the long head.

Palpate the brachialis in the distal arm medial to the tendon of the biceps. Palpate the brachioradialis on the lateral surface of the neutrally positioned forearm, where it forms the lateral border of the cubital fossa (Figure 5-116).

Test: Patient attempts to flex the elbow.

Instructions to Patient: "Try to bend your elbow."

Grading

Grade 2 (Poor): Completes range of motion (in each of the muscles tested).

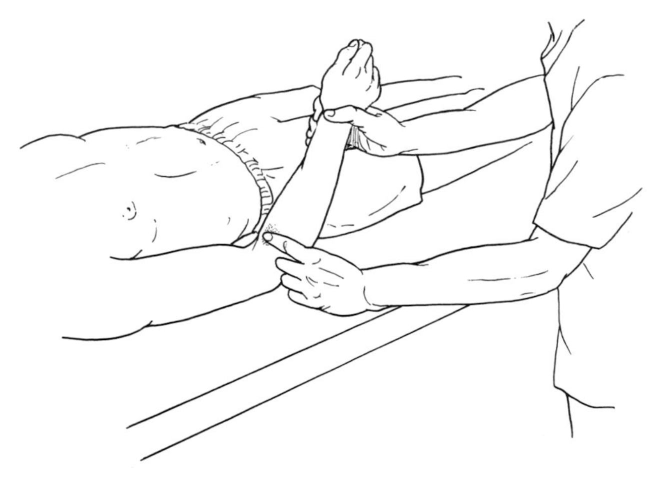

FIGURE 5-116

Grade 1 (Trace) and Grade 0 (Zero)

Positions of Patient and Therapist: Supine for all three muscles with therapist standing at test side (see Figure 5-116). All other aspects are the same as for the Grade 2 test.

Test: Patient attempts to bend elbow with hand supinated, pronated, and in midposition.

Grading

Grade 1 (Trace): Examiner can palpate a contractile response in each of the three muscles for which a Trace grade is given.

Grade 0 (Zero): No palpable contractile activity.

Helpful Hints

- The patient's wrist flexor muscles should remain relaxed throughout the test because strongly contracting wrist flexors may assist in elbow flexion. Recall that the wrist flexors originate above the elbow joint axis on the distal humerus.
- If the sitting position is contraindicated for any reason, all tests for these muscles may be performed in the supine position, but in this case manual resistance should be evaluated using Grade 3 test criteria.

(Triceps brachii)

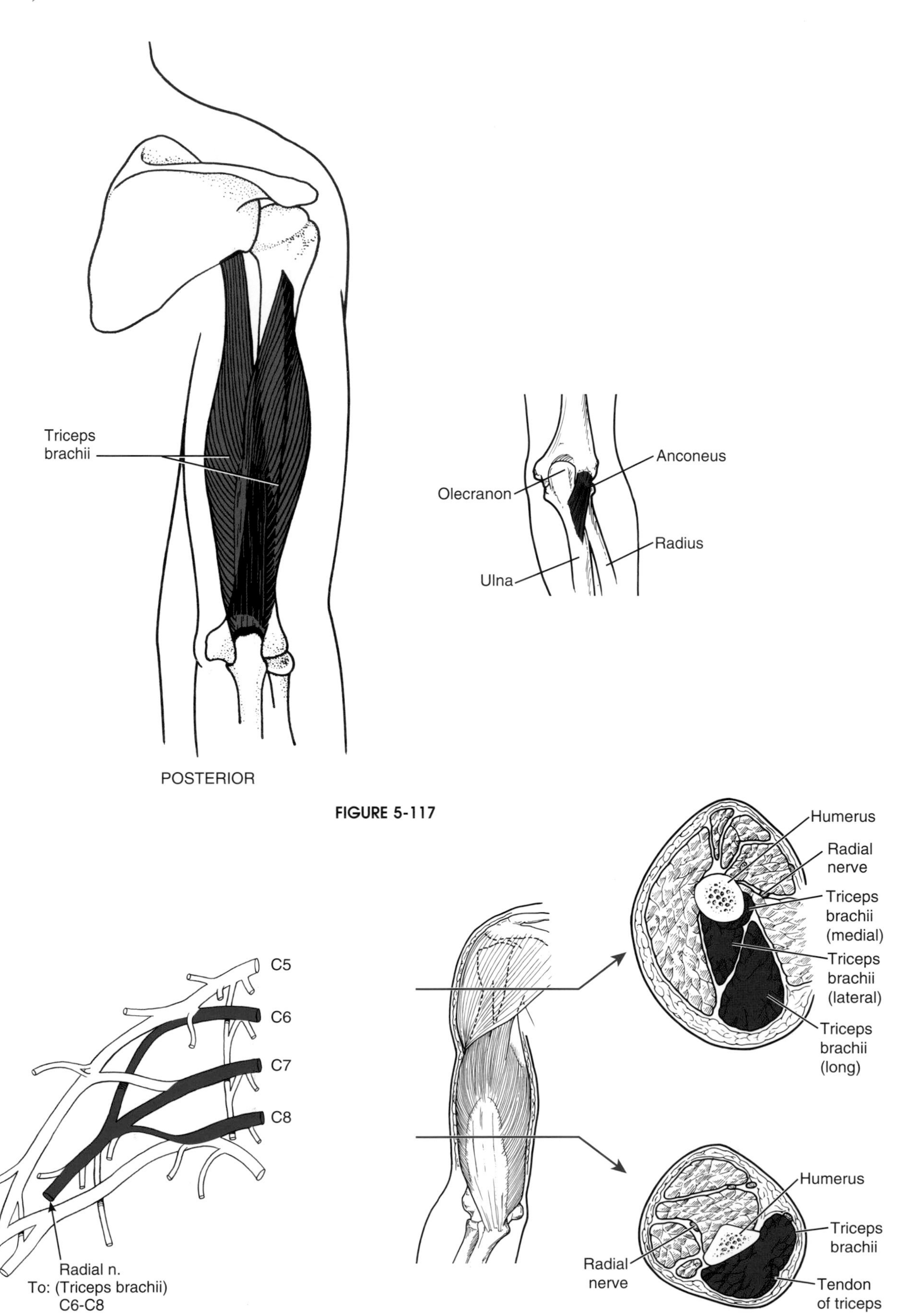

FIGURE 5-117

FIGURE 5-118

FIGURE 5-119 Arrows indicates level of cross sections.

(Triceps brachii)

Range of Motion
150° to 0°

Table 5-14 ELBOW EXTENSION

I.D.	Muscle	Origin	Insertion
142	Triceps brachii		All heads have a common tendon to:
	Long head	Scapula (infraglenoid tuberosity and capsule of glenohumeral joint)	Ulna (olecranon process, upper surface)
	Lateral head	Humerus (shaft: oblique ridge, posterior surface) Lateral intermuscular septum	Blends with antebrachial fascia Capsule of elbow joint
	Medial head	Humerus (shaft: entire length of posterior surface) Medial and lateral intermuscular septa	
Other			
144	Anconeus		See Plate 4

ELBOW EXTENSION

(Triceps brachii)

Grade 5 (Normal), Grade 4 (Good), and Grade 3 (Fair)

Position of Patient: Prone on table. The patient starts the test with the arm in 90° of abduction and the forearm flexed and hanging vertically over the side of the table (Figure 5-120).

Position of Therapist: For the prone patient, the therapist provides support just above the elbow. The other hand is used to apply downward resistance on the dorsal surface of the forearm (Figure 5-121 illustrates end position).

Test: Patient extends elbow to end of available range or until the forearm is horizontal to the floor. Do not allow the patient to hyperextend or lock elbow when providing resistance.

Instructions to Patient: "Straighten your elbow. Hold it. Don't let me bend it."

Grading

Grade 5 (Normal): Completes available range and holds firmly against maximal resistance.

Grade 4 (Good): Completes available range against strong resistance, but there is a "give" to the resistance at the end range.

Grade 3 (Fair): Completes available range with no manual resistance (Figure 5-122).

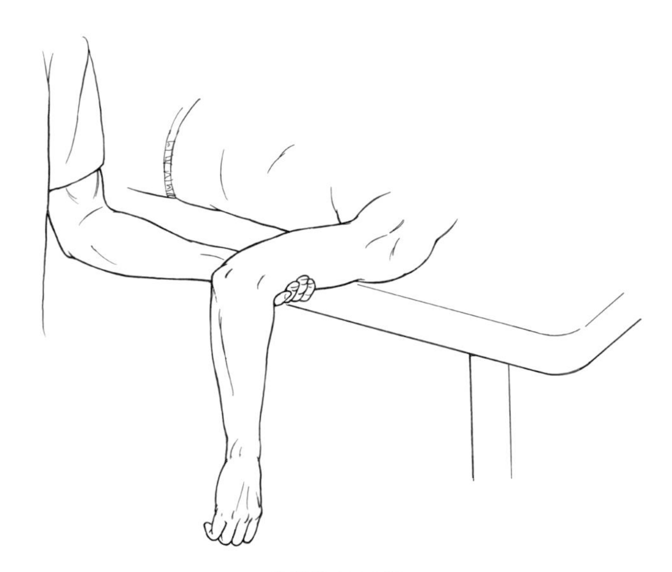

FIGURE 5-120

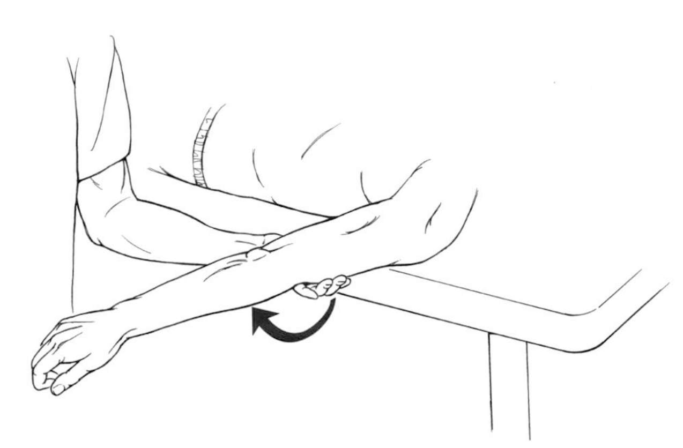

FIGURE 5-122

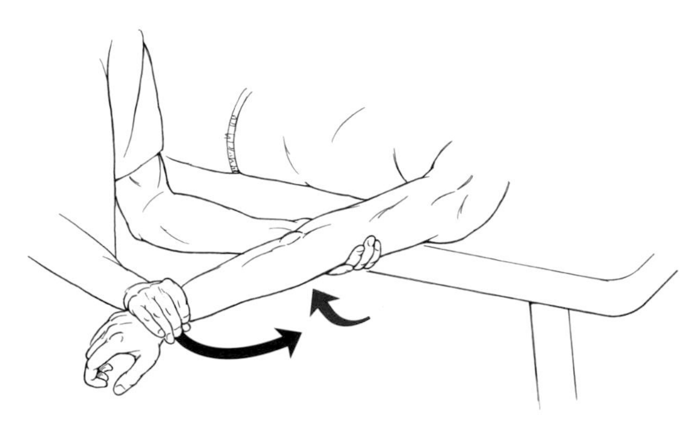

FIGURE 5-121

Grade 2 (Poor), Grade 1 (Trace), and Grade 0 (Zero)

Position of Patient: Short sitting. The arm is abducted to 90° with the shoulder in neutral rotation and the elbow flexed to about 45°. The entire limb is horizontal to the floor (Figure 5-123).

Position of Therapist: Standing at test side of patient. For the Grade 2 test, support the limb at the elbow. For a Grade 1 or 0 test, support the limb under the forearm and palpate the triceps on the posterior surface of the arm just proximal to the olecranon process (Figure 5-124).

Test: Patient attempts to extend the elbow.

Instructions to Patient: "Try to straighten your elbow."

Grading

Grade 2 (Poor): Completes available range in the absence of gravity.

Grade 1 (Trace): Examiner can feel tension in the triceps tendon just proximal to the olecranon (see Figure 5-124) or contractile activity in the muscle fibers on the posterior surface of the arm.

Grade 0 (Zero): No evidence of any muscle activity.

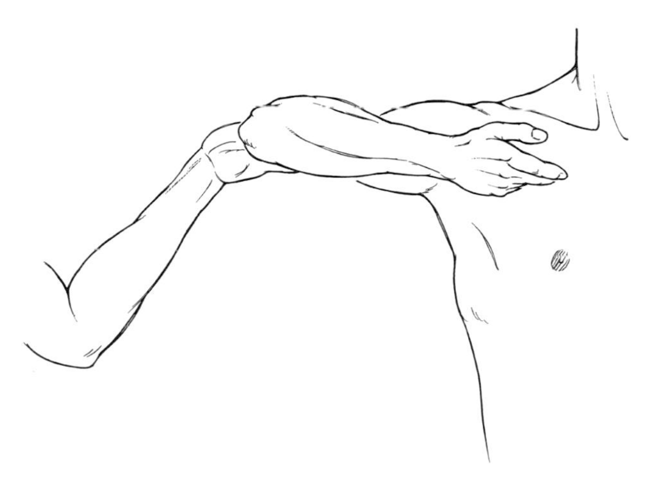

FIGURE 5-123

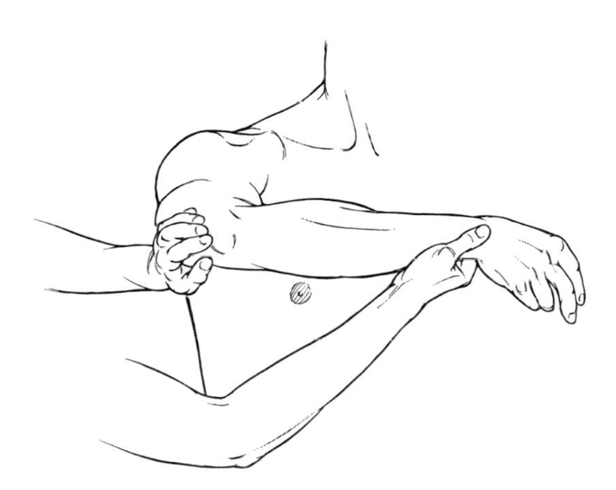

FIGURE 5-124

ELBOW EXTENSION

(Triceps brachii)

Substitutions

- Via external rotation. When the patient is sitting with the arm abducted, elbow extension can be accomplished with a Grade 0 triceps (Figure 5-125). This can occur when the patient externally rotates the shoulder, thus dropping the arm below the forearm. As a result, the elbow literally falls into extension. This can be prevented by using a table or powder board to support the arm.
- Via horizontal adduction. This substitution can accomplish elbow extension and is done purposefully by patients with a cervical cord injury and a Grade 0 triceps. With the distal segment fixed (as when the examiner stabilizes the hand or wrist), the patient horizontally adducts the arm and the thrust pulls the elbow into extension (Figure 5-126). The therapist, therefore, should provide support at the elbow for testing purposes rather than at the wrist.

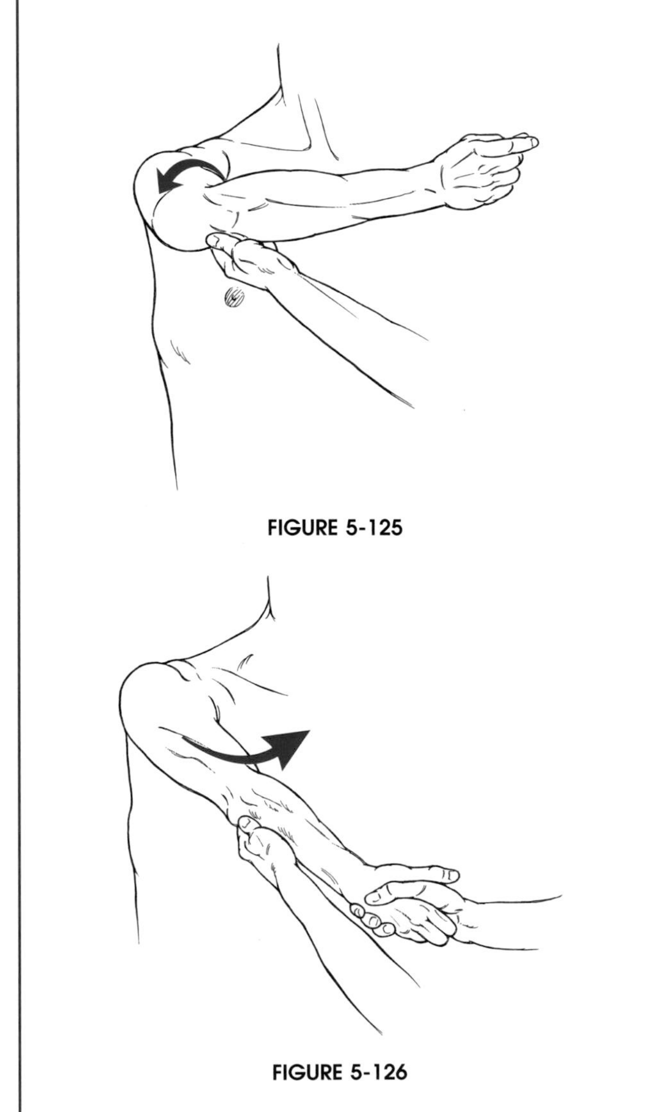

FIGURE 5-125

FIGURE 5-126

Helpful Hints

- The therapist should confirm that muscle activity is seen and felt (i.e., triceps activity is actually present) because patients can become very adept at substituting. In fact, some patients may be taught substitution to accomplish a functional movement, but are not allowed to do so for the purpose of testing.
- Give resistance in Grade 5 and Grade 4 tests with the elbow slightly flexed to avoid enabling the patient to "lock" the elbow joint by hyperextending it.
- Although elbow extension is tested in the prone position, the therapist must be aware that with the shoulder horizontally abducted the two-joint muscle is less effective, and the test grade may be lower than it should be.[1]
- An alternate position for Grades 5, 4, and 3 is with the patient short sitting. The examiner stands behind the patient, supporting the arm in 90° of abduction just above the flexed elbow (Figure 5-127). The patient straightens the elbow against the resistance given at the wrist.

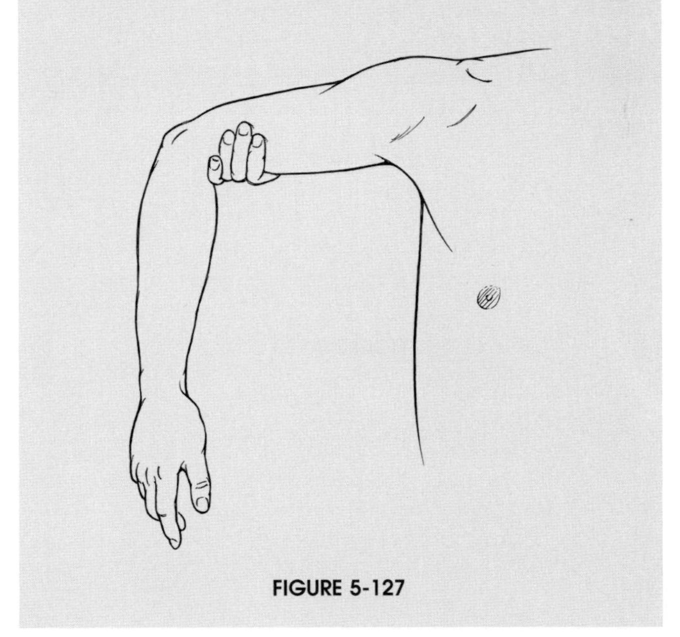

FIGURE 5-127

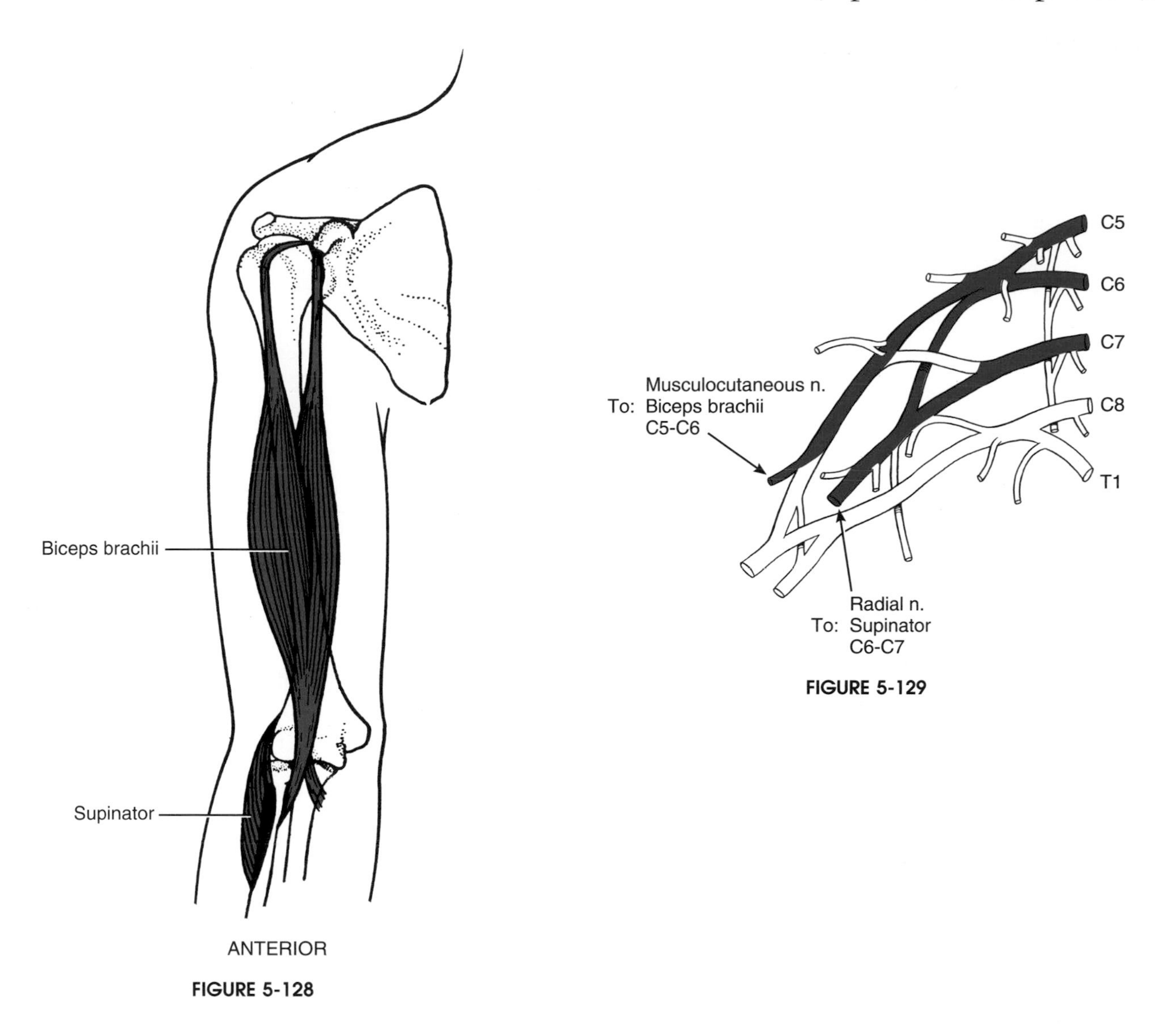

FIGURE 5-128

FIGURE 5-129

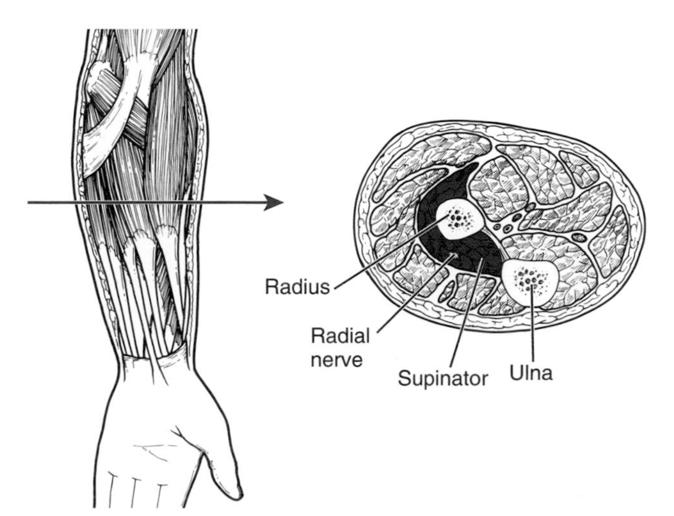

FIGURE 5-130 Arrow indicates level of cross section.

FOREARM SUPINATION

(Supinator and Biceps brachii)

Range of Motion
0° to 80°

Table 5-15 FOREARM SUPINATION

I.D.	Muscle	Origin	Insertion
145	Supinator	Humerus (lateral epicondyle) Ulna (supinator crest) Radial collateral ligament of elbow joint Annular ligament of radioulnar joint Aponeurosis of supinator	Radius (shaft, lateral aspect of proximal 1/3)
140	Biceps brachii		
	Short head	Scapula (coracoid apex)	Radius (radial tuberosity)
	Long head	Scapula (supraglenoid tubercle) Capsule of glenohumeral joint and glenoid labrum	Bicipital aponeurosis See Plate 4

Grade 5 (Normal), Grade 4 (Good), and Grade 3 (Fair)

Position of Patient: Short sitting; arm at side and elbow flexed to 90°; forearm in full pronation to neutral. Alternatively, patient may sit at a table.

Position of Therapist: Standing at side or in front of patient. One hand supports the elbow. Apply resistance with the heel of the hand over the dorsal (extensor) surface at the wrist, being careful not to grip the flexor surface of the forearm (Figure 5-131).

Test: Patient begins in pronation and patient supinates the forearm until the palm faces the ceiling. Therapist resists motion in the direction of pronation. (No resistance is given for Grade 3.)

Alternate Test: Grasp patient's hand as if shaking hands; cradle the elbow and resist via the hand grip (Figure 5-132). This test is used if the patient has Grade 5 or 4 wrist and hand strength.

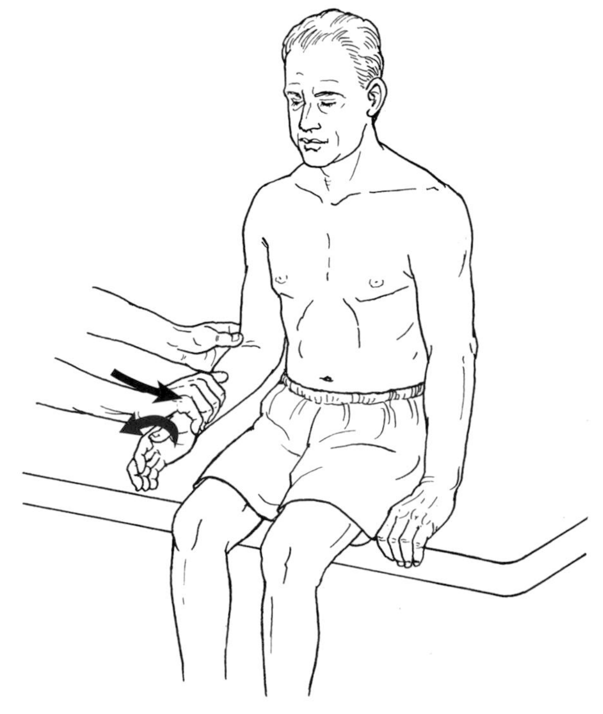

FIGURE 5-131

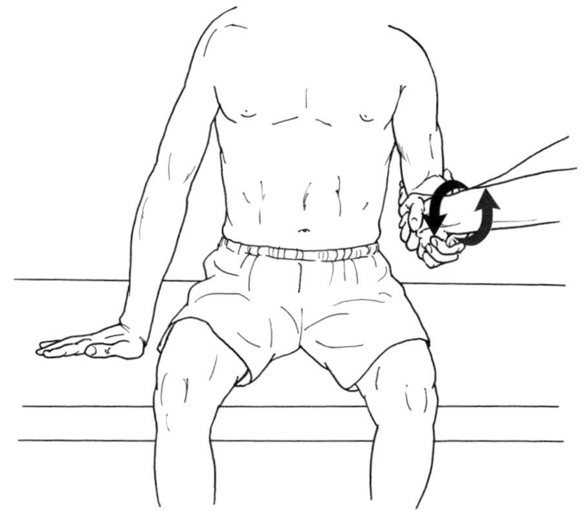

FIGURE 5-132

Grade 5 (Normal), Grade 4 (Good), and Grade 3 (Fair) Continued

Instructions to Patient: "Turn your palm up. Hold it. Don't let me turn it down. Keep your wrist and fingers relaxed."

For Grade 3: "Turn your palm up."

Grading

Grade 5 (Normal): Completes full available range of motion and holds against maximal resistance.

Grade 4 (Good): Completes full range of motion against strong to moderate resistance.

Grade 3 (Fair): Completes available range of motion without resistance (Figure 5-133, showing end range).

Grade 2 (Poor)

Position of Patient: Short sitting with shoulder flexed between 45° and 90° and elbow flexed to 90°. Forearm in neutral.

Position of Therapist: Support the test arm by cupping the hand under the elbow.

Test: Patient supinates forearm (Figure 5-134) through partial range of motion.

Instructions to Patient: "Turn your palm toward your face."

Grading

Grade 2 (Poor): Completes a full range of motion.

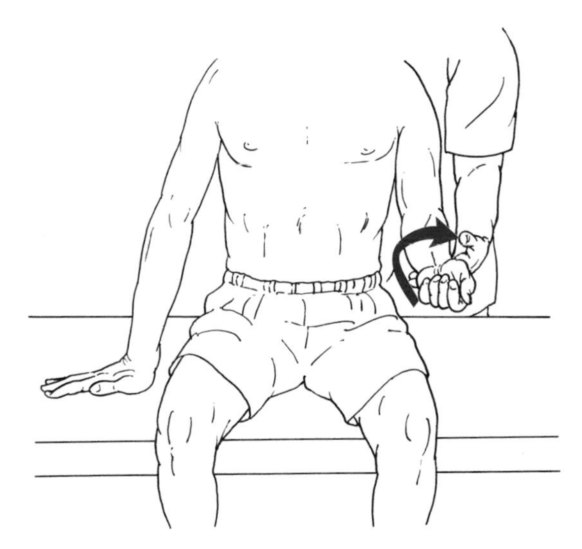

FIGURE 5-133

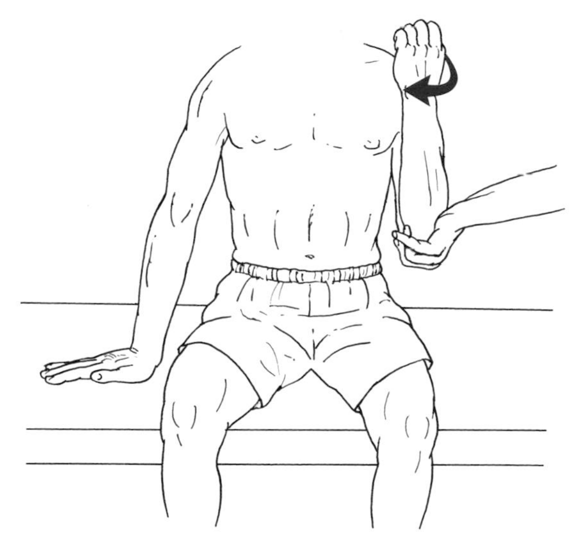

FIGURE 5-134

FOREARM SUPINATION

(Supinator and Biceps brachii)

Grade 1 (Trace) and Grade 0 (Zero)

Position of Patient: Short sitting. Arm and elbow are flexed as for the Grade 3 test.

Position of Therapist: Support the forearm just distal to the elbow. Palpate the supinator distal to the head of the radius on the dorsal aspect of the forearm (Figure 5-135).

Test: Patient attempts to supinate the forearm.

Instructions to Patient: "Try to turn your palm so it faces the ceiling."

Grading

Grade 1 (Trace): Slight contractile activity but no limb movement.

Grade 0 (Zero): No contractile activity.

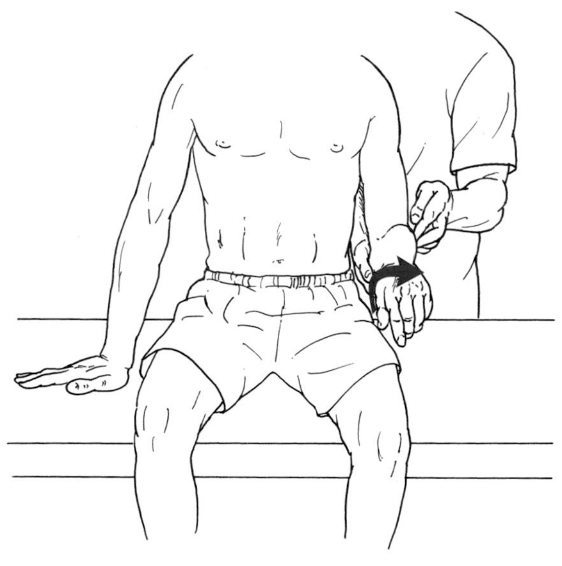

FIGURE 5-135

Substitution

Patient may externally rotate and adduct the arm across the body (Figure 5-136) as forearm supination is attempted. When this occurs, the forearm rolls into supination with no activity of the supinator muscle.

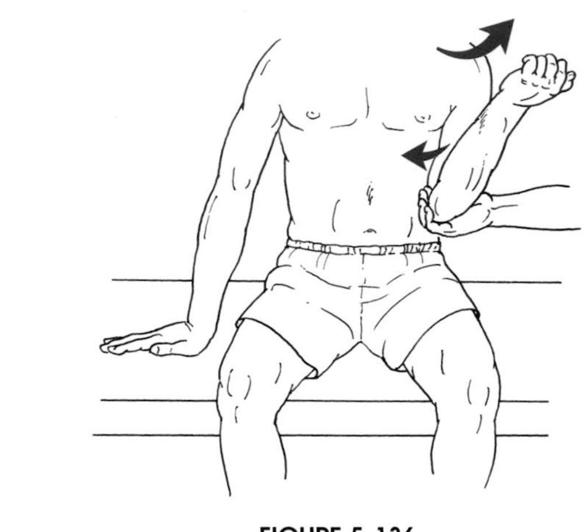

FIGURE 5-136

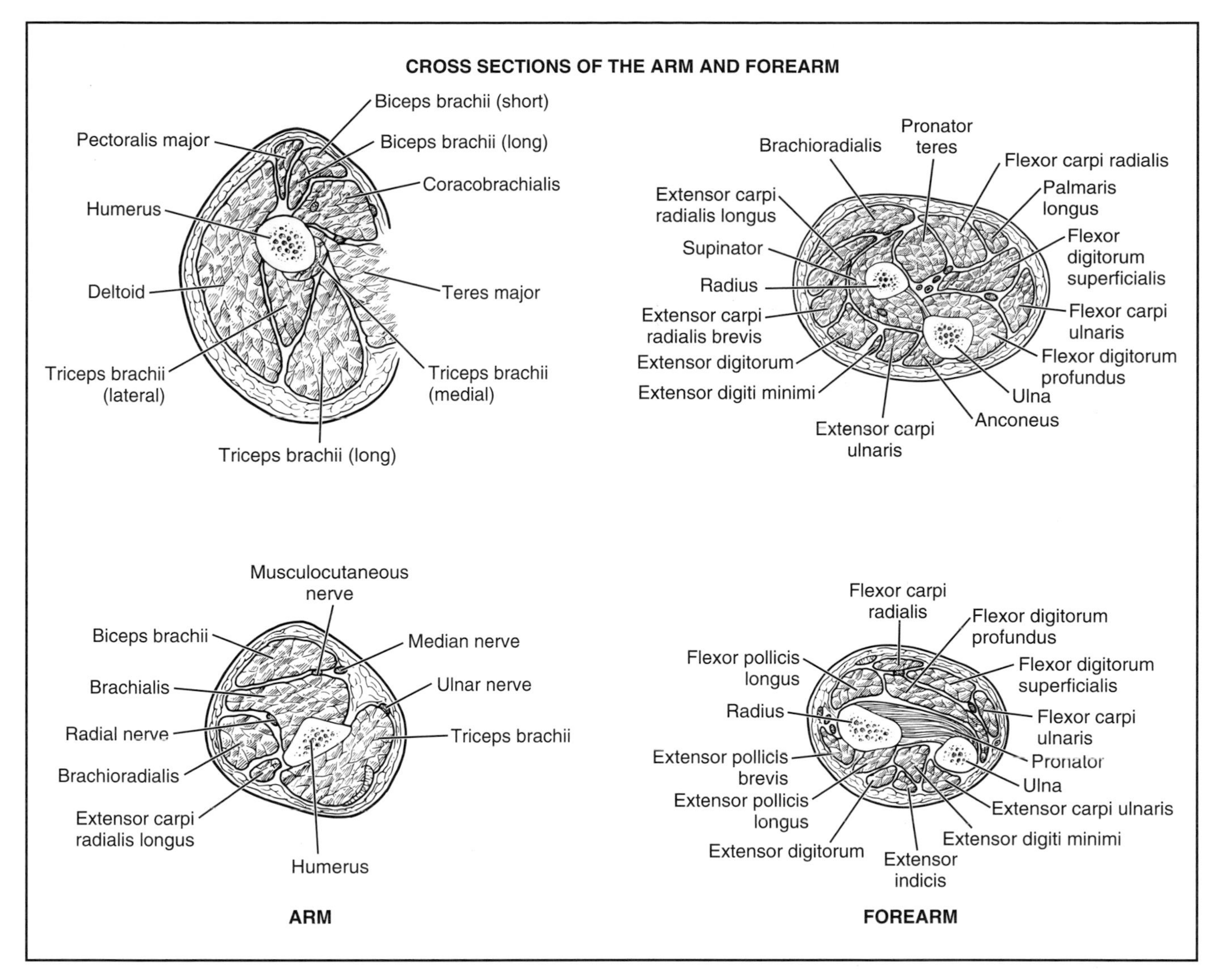
CROSS SECTIONS OF THE ARM AND FOREARM
Biceps brachii (short)
Pectoralis major
Biceps brachii (long)
Coracobrachialis
Humerus
Deltoid
Teres major
Triceps brachii (lateral)
Triceps brachii (medial)
Triceps brachii (long)
Brachioradialis
Pronator teres
Flexor carpi radialis
Extensor carpi radialis longus
Palmaris longus
Supinator
Flexor digitorum superficialis
Radius
Extensor carpi radialis brevis
Flexor carpi ulnaris
Extensor digitorum
Flexor digitorum profundus
Extensor digiti minimi
Ulna
Anconeus
Extensor carpi ulnaris
Musculocutaneous nerve
Biceps brachii
Median nerve
Brachialis
Ulnar nerve
Radial nerve
Triceps brachii
Brachioradialis
Extensor carpi radialis longus
Humerus
ARM
Flexor carpi radialis
Flexor digitorum profundus
Flexor pollicis longus
Flexor digitorum superficialis
Radius
Flexor carpi ulnaris
Extensor pollicis brevis
Pronator
Ulna
Extensor pollicis longus
Extensor carpi ulnaris
Extensor digiti minimi
Extensor digitorum
Extensor indicis
FOREARM

PLATE 4

FOREARM PRONATION

(Pronator teres and Pronator quadratus)

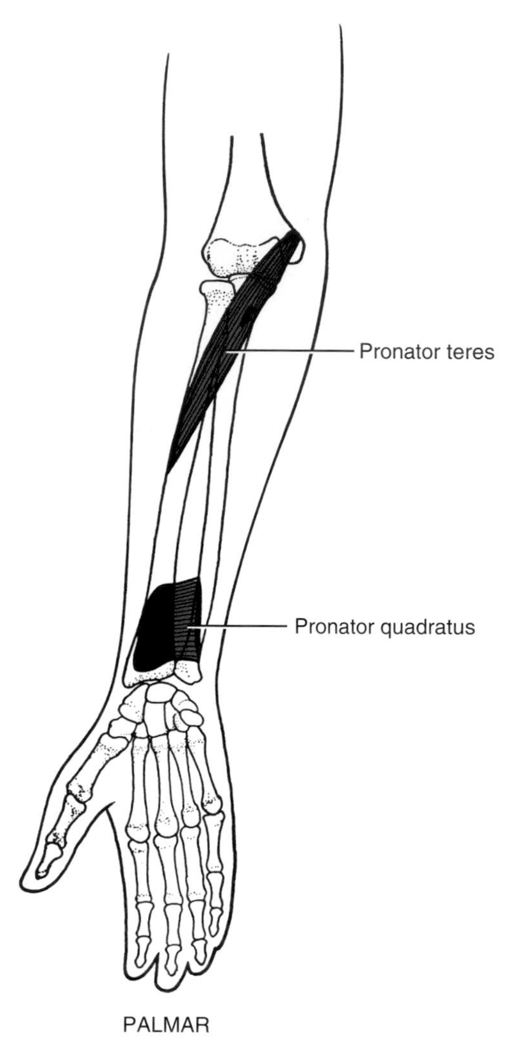

FIGURE 5-137

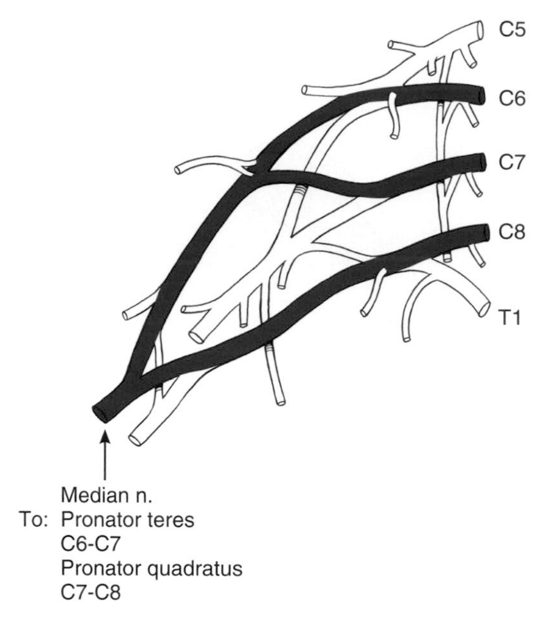

FIGURE 5-138

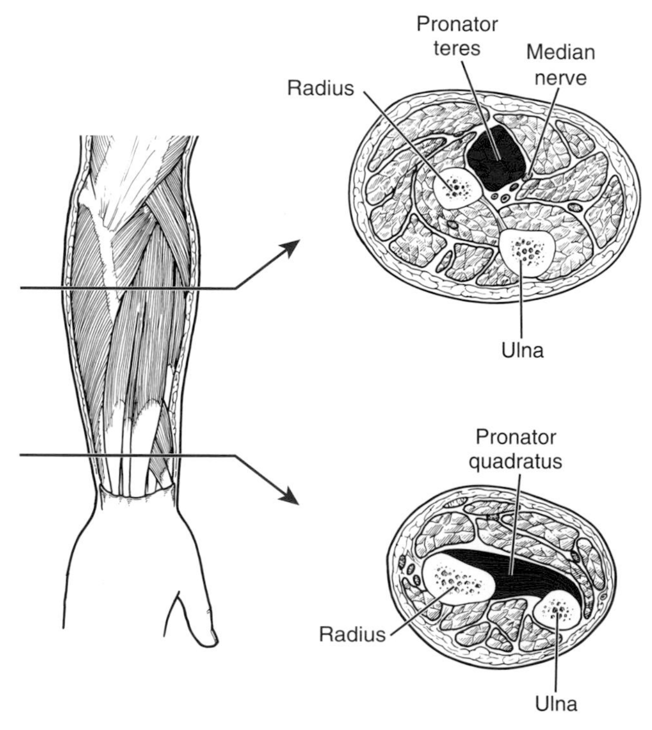

FIGURE 5-139 Arrows indicate level of cross section.

(Pronator teres and Pronator quadratus)

Range of Motion
0° to 80°

Table 5-16 FOREARM PRONATION

I.D.	Muscle	Origin	Insertion
146	Pronator teres		Radius (midshaft, lateral surface)
	Humeral head	Humerus (shaft proximal to medial epicondyle) Common tendon of origin of flexor muscles Intermuscular septum Antebrachial fascia	
	Ulnar head	Ulna (coronoid process, medial) Joins humeral head in common tendon	
147	Pronator quadratus	Ulna (oblique ridge on distal 1/4 of anterior surface) Muscle aponeurosis	Radius (shaft, anterior surface distally; also area above ulnar notch)
Other			
151	Flexor carpi radialis		See Plate 4

Grade 5 (Normal), Grade 4 (Good), and Grade 3 (Fair)

Position of Patient: Short sitting or may sit at a table. Arm at side with elbow flexed to 90° and forearm in supination.

Position of Therapist: Standing at side or in front of patient. Support the elbow. Hand used for resistance applies resistance with hypothenar eminence over radius on the volar (flexor) surface of the forearm at the wrist (Figure 5-140). Avoid pressure on the head of the radius for patient comfort.

Test: Patient pronates the forearm until the palm faces downward. Therapist resists motion at the wrist in the direction of supination for Grades 4 and 5. (No resistance is given for Grade 3.)

Alternate Test: Grasp patient's hand as if to shake hands, cradling the elbow with the other hand and resisting pronation via the hand grip. This alternate test may be used if the patient has Grade 5 or 4 wrist and hand strength.

Instructions to Patient: "Turn your palm down. Hold it. Don't let me turn it up. Keep your wrist and fingers relaxed."

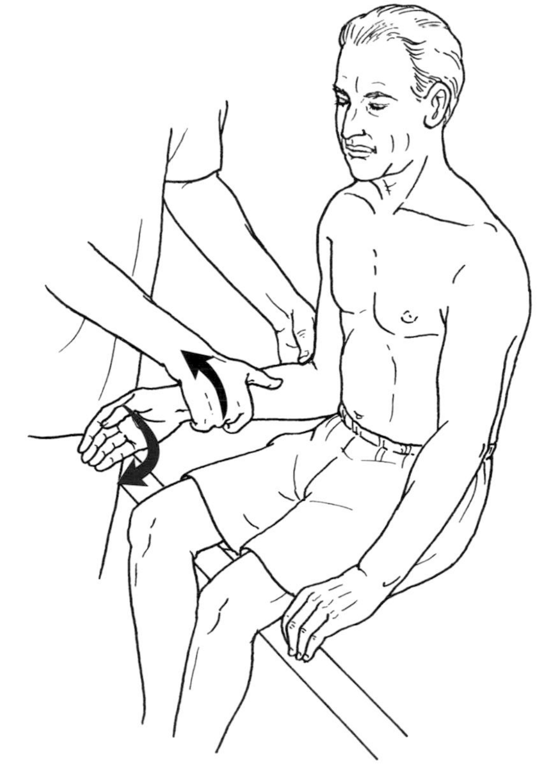

FIGURE 5-140

FOREARM PRONATION

(Pronator teres and Pronator quadratus)

Grade 5 (Normal), Grade 4 (Good), and Grade 3 (Fair) Continued

Grading

Grade 5 (Normal): Completes available range of motion and holds against maximal resistance.

Grade 4 (Good): Completes all available range against strong to moderate resistance.

Grade 3 (Fair): Completes available range without resistance (Figure 5-141), showing end range).

Grade 2 (Poor)

Position of Patient: Short sitting with shoulder flexed between 45° and 90° and elbow flexed to 90°. Forearm in neutral (not illustrated).

Position of Therapist: Support the test arm by cupping the hand under the elbow (Figure 5-142).

Test: Patient pronates forearm.

Instructions to Patient: "Turn your palm facing outward away from your face."

Grading

Grade 2 (Poor): Complete range of motion (see Figure 5-142, which shows end range).

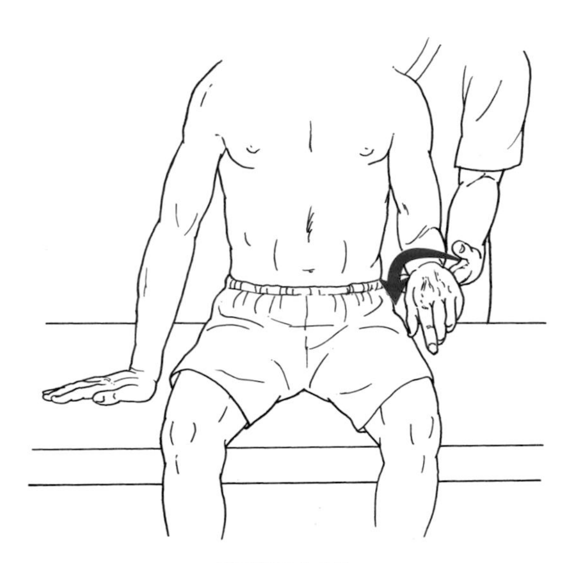

FIGURE 5-141

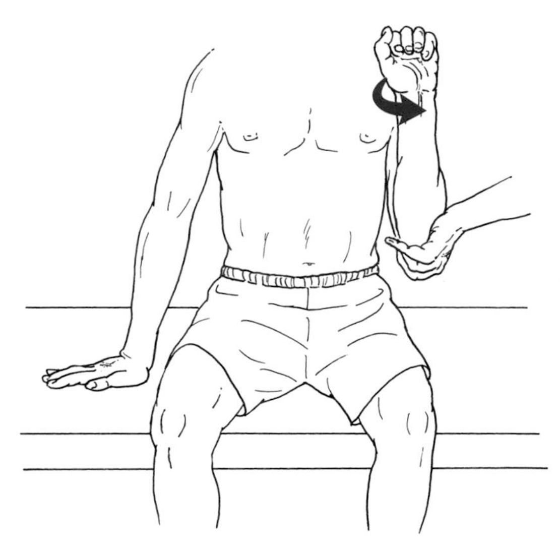

FIGURE 5-142

(Pronator teres and Pronator quadratus)

Grade 1 (Trace) and Grade 0 (Zero)

Position of Patient: Short sitting. Arm is positioned as for the Grade 3 test.

Position of Therapist: Support the forearm just distal to the elbow. The fingers of the other hand are used to palpate the pronator teres over the upper third of the volar (flexor) surface of the forearm on a diagonal line from the medial condyle of the humerus to the lateral border of the radius (Figure 5-143).

Test: Patient attempts to pronate the forearm.

Instructions to Patient: "Try to turn your palm down."

Grading

Grade 1 (Trace): Visible or palpable contractile activity with no motion of the part.

Grade 0 (Zero): No contractile activity.

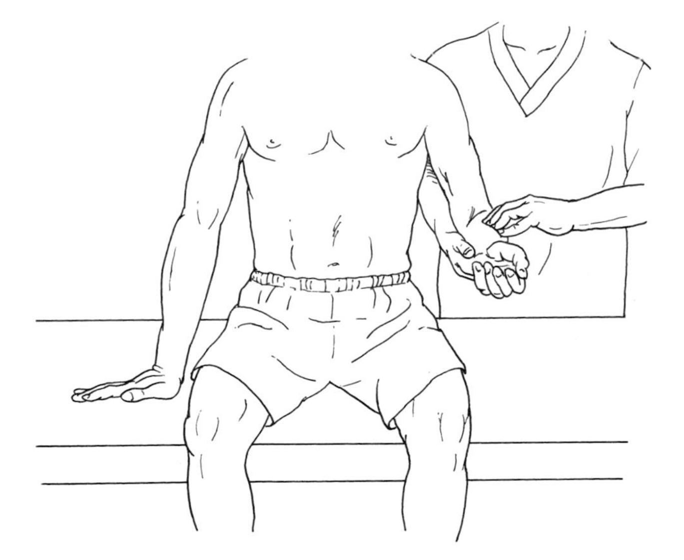

FIGURE 5-143

Substitution

Patient may internally rotate the shoulder or abduct it during attempts at pronation (Figure 5-144). When this occurs, the forearm rolls into pronation without the benefit of activity by the pronator muscles.

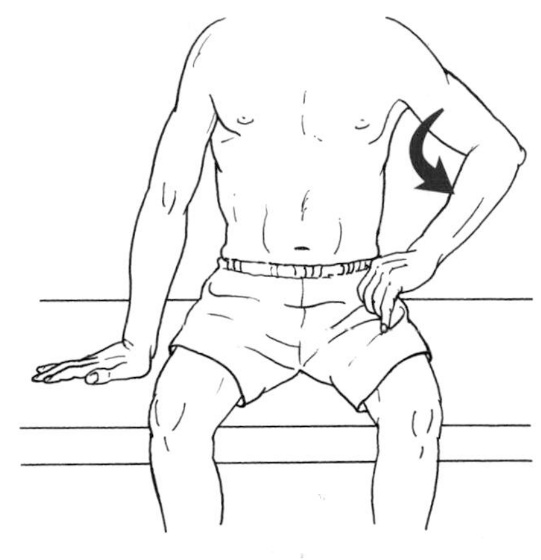

FIGURE 5-144

Helpful Hints

- Nondominant arm elicits 81 to 95% of the force of the dominant arm in forearm rotation.[17]
- Pronation is strongest in position of 45° elbow flexion.[18]
- Men are 63% stronger in pronation and 68% stronger in supination than women, measuring as high as 12.6 to 14.8 Nm.[19]
- In isokinetic studies, women's forearm strength is equal to 5.0 to 5.4 Nm.[19]

Nm., Newton meter.

WRIST FLEXION

(Flexor carpi radialis and Flexor carpi ulnaris)

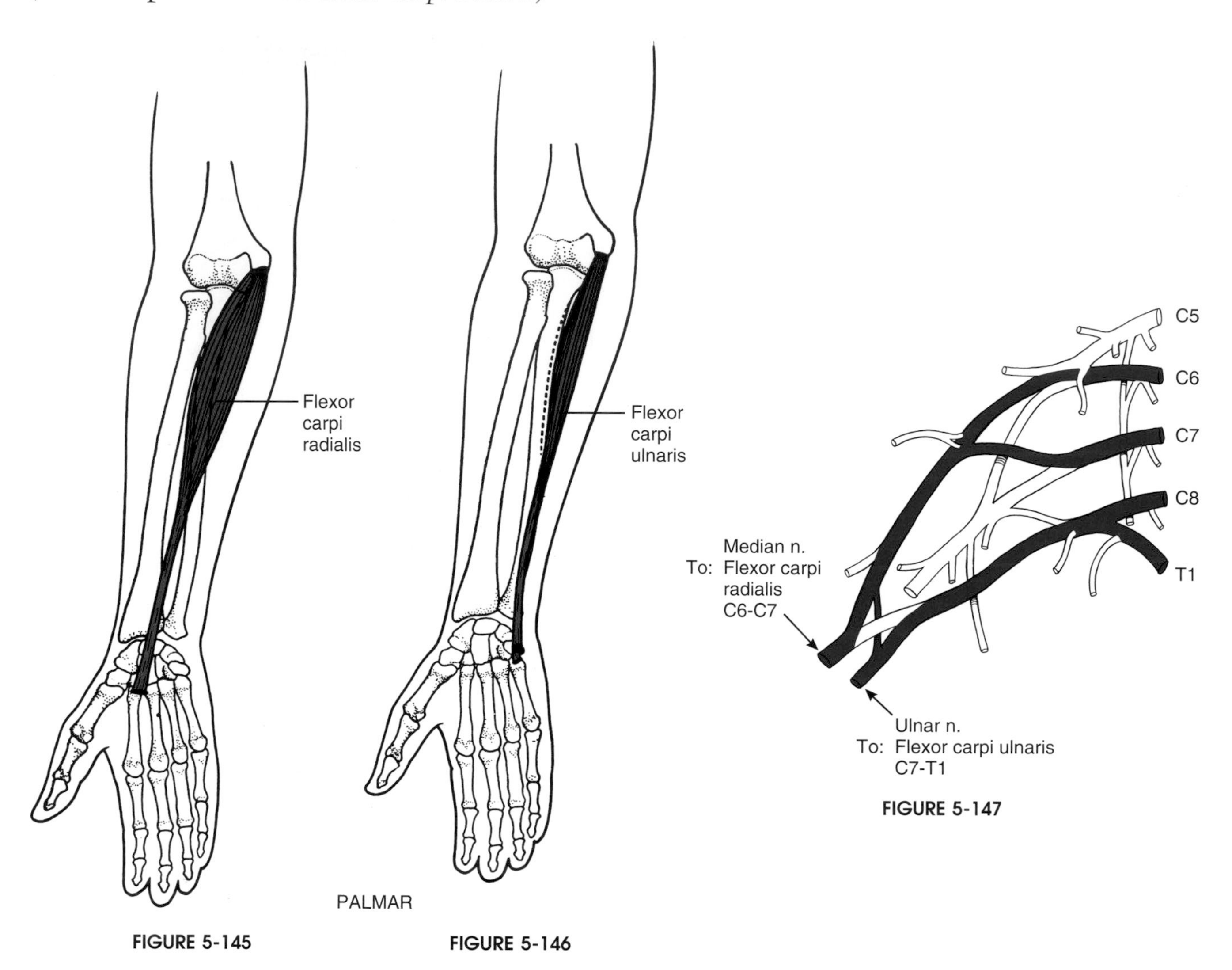

FIGURE 5-145

FIGURE 5-146

FIGURE 5-147

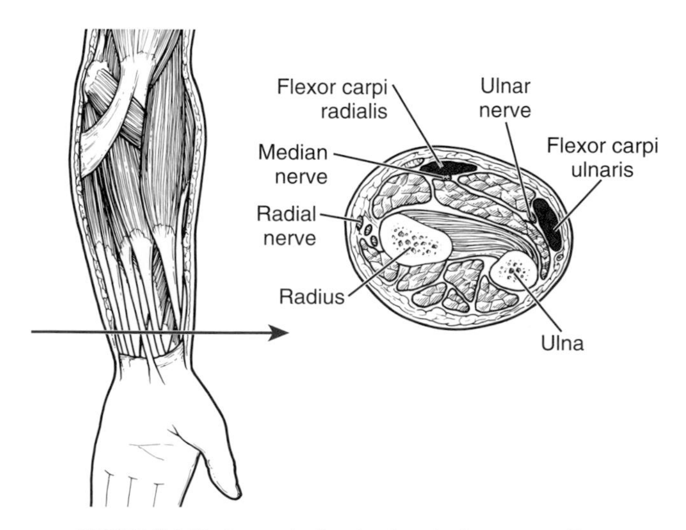

FIGURE 5-148 Arrow indicates level of cross section.

(Flexor carpi radialis and Flexor carpi ulnaris)

Range of Motion
0° to 80°

Table 5-17 WRIST FLEXION

I.D.	Muscle	Origin	Insertion
151	Flexor carpi radialis	Humerus (medial epicondyle via common flexor tendon) Antebrachial fascia Intermuscular septum	2nd and 3rd metacarpals (base, palmar surface)
153	Flexor carpi ulnaris Two heads	Humeral head (medial epicondyle via common flexor tendon) Ulnar head (olecranon, medial margin; shaft, proximal 2/3 posterior via an aponeurosis) Intermuscular septum	Pisiform bone Hamate bone 5th metacarpal, base
Others			
152	Palmaris longus		
156	Flexor digitorum superficialis		
157	Flexor digitorum profundus		
166	Abductor pollicis longus		
169	Flexor pollicis longus		See Plate 4

Grade 5 (Normal) and Grade 4 (Good)

Position of Patient (All Tests): Short sitting. Forearm is supinated (Figure 5-149). Wrist is in neutral position or slightly extended.

Position of Therapist: One hand supports the patient's forearm under the wrist (see Figure 5-149).

Test: Patient flexes the wrist, keeping the digits and thumb relaxed.

To test both wrist flexors: The examiner applies resistance to the palm of the test hand using four fingers or the hypothenar eminence (Figure 5-150). Resistance is given evenly across the hand in a straight-down direction into wrist extension.

To test the flexor carpi radialis: Place the patient's wrist in radial deviation and slight wrist extension. Resistance is applied with the index and long fingers over the 1st and 2nd metacarpal (radial side of the hand) in the direction of extension and ulnar deviation.

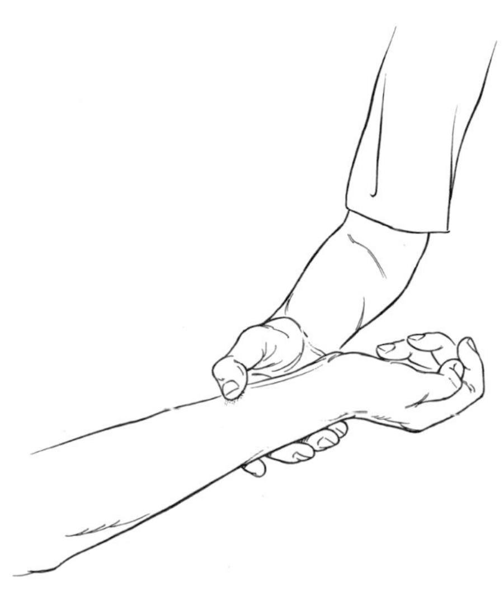

FIGURE 5-149

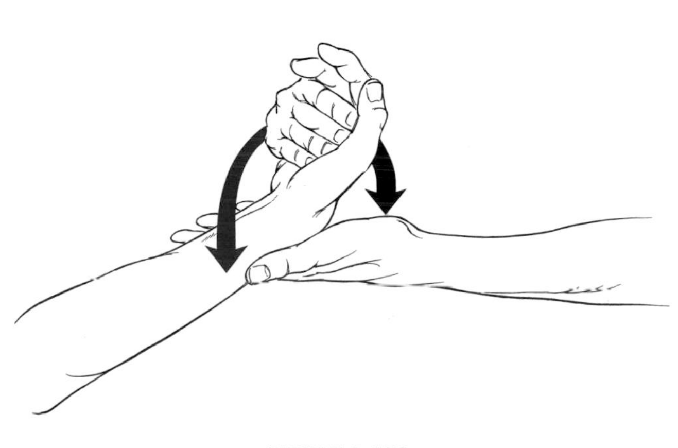

FIGURE 5-150

WRIST FLEXION

(Flexor carpi radialis and Flexor carpi ulnaris)

Grade 5 (Normal) and Grade 4 (Good) Continued

To test the flexor carpi ulnaris: Place the wrist in ulnar deviation and slight wrist extension. Resistance is applied over the 5th metacarpal (ulnar side of the hand) in the direction of extension and radial deviation.

Instructions to Patient (All Tests): "Bend your wrist. Hold it. Don't let me pull it down. Keep your fingers relaxed."

Grading

Grade 5 (Normal): Completes available range of wrist flexion and holds against maximal resistance.

Grade 4 (Good): Completes available range and holds against strong to moderate resistance.

Grade 3 (Fair)

Position of Patient: Starting position with forearm supinated and wrist neutral as in Grades 5 and 4 tests.

Position of Therapist: Support the patient's forearm under the wrist.

Test:

To test both wrist flexors: Patient flexes the wrist straight up without resistance and without radial or ulnar deviation.

To test the flexor carpi radialis: Patient flexes the wrist in radial deviation (Figure 5-151).

To test the flexor carpi ulnaris: Patient flexes the wrist in ulnar deviation (Figure 5-152).

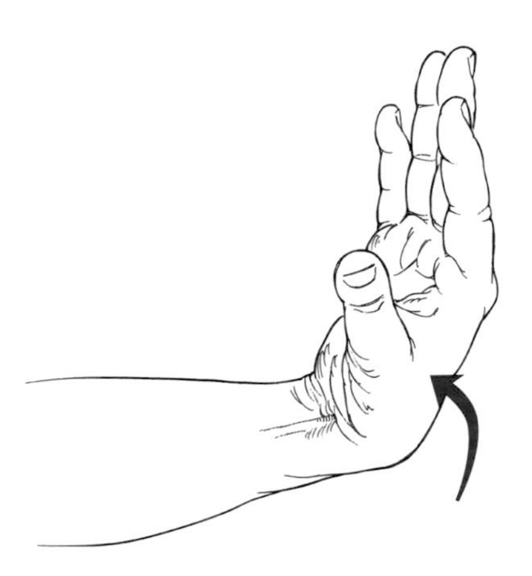

FIGURE 5-151

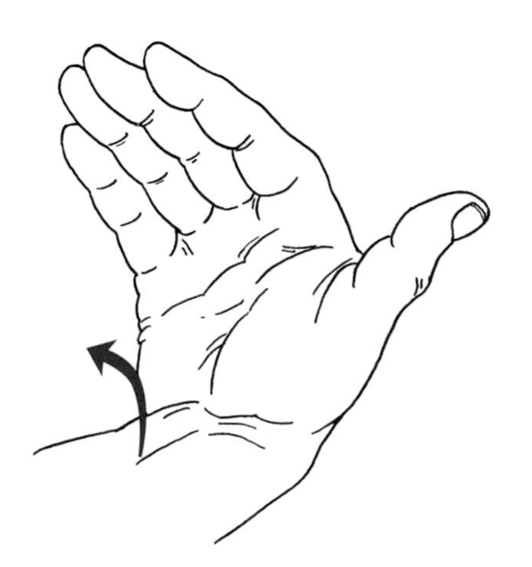

FIGURE 5-152

Grade 3 (Fair) Continued

Instructions to Patient:
For both wrist flexors: "Bend your wrist. Keep it straight with your fingers relaxed."

For flexor carpi radialis: "Bend your wrist leading with the thumb side."

For flexor carpi ulnaris: "Bend your wrist leading with the little finger."

Grading

Grade 3 (Fair) (All Tests): Completes available range without resistance.

Grade 2 (Poor)

Position of Patient: Sitting with elbow supported on table. Forearm in midposition with hand resting on ulnar side (Figure 5-153).

Position of Therapist: Support patient's forearm proximal to the wrist.

Test: Patient flexes wrist with the ulnar surface gliding across or not touching the table (see Figure 5-153). To test the two wrist flexors separately, hold the forearm so that the wrist does not lie on the table and ask the patient to perform the flexion motion while the wrist is in ulnar and then radial deviation.

Instructions to Patient: "Bend your wrist, keeping your fingers relaxed."

Grading

Grade 2 (Poor): Completes available range of wrist flexion with gravity eliminated.

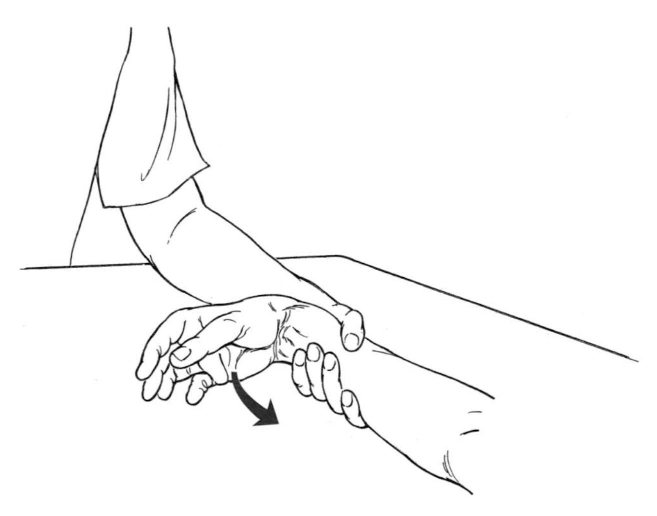

FIGURE 5-153

WRIST FLEXION

(Flexor carpi radialis and Flexor carpi ulnaris)

Grade 1 (Trace) and Grade 0 (Zero)

Position of Patient: Supinated forearm supported on table.

Position of Therapist: Support the wrist in flexion; the index finger of the other hand is used to palpate the appropriate tendons.

Palpate the tendons of the flexor carpi radialis (Figure 5-154) and the flexor carpi ulnaris (Figure 5-155) in separate tests.

The flexor carpi radialis lies on the lateral palmar aspect of the wrist (see Figure 5-150) lateral to the palmaris longus.

The tendon of the flexor carpi ulnaris (see Figure 5-154) lies on the medial palmar aspect of the wrist (at the base of the 5th metacarpal).

Test: Patient attempts to flex the wrist.

Instructions to Patient: "Try to bend your wrist. Relax. Bend it again." Patient should be asked to repeat the test so the examiner can feel the tendons during both relaxation and contraction.

Grading

Grade 1 (Trace): One or both tendons may exhibit visible or palpable contractile activity, but the part does not move.

Grade 0 (Zero): No contractile activity.

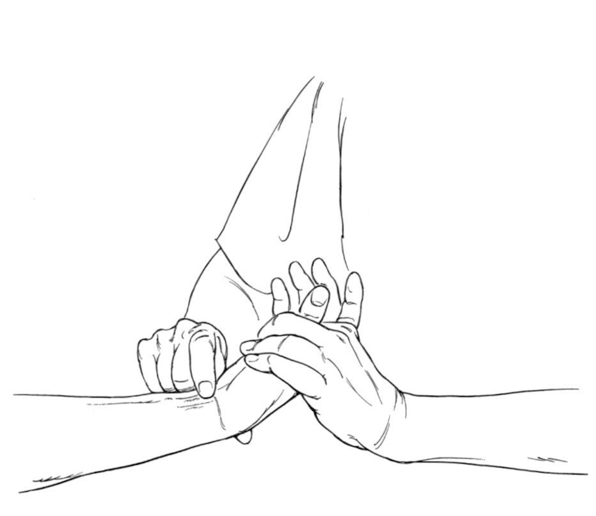

FIGURE 5-154

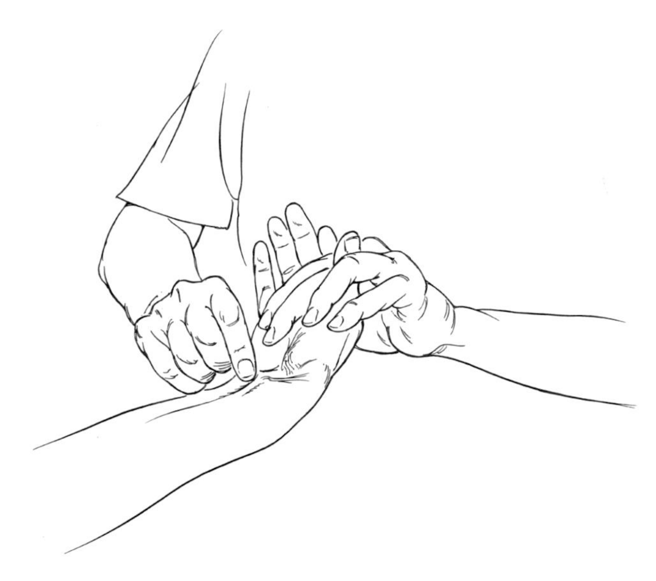

FIGURE 5-155

(Extensor carpi radialis longus, Extensor carpi radialis brevis, and Extensor carpi ulnaris)

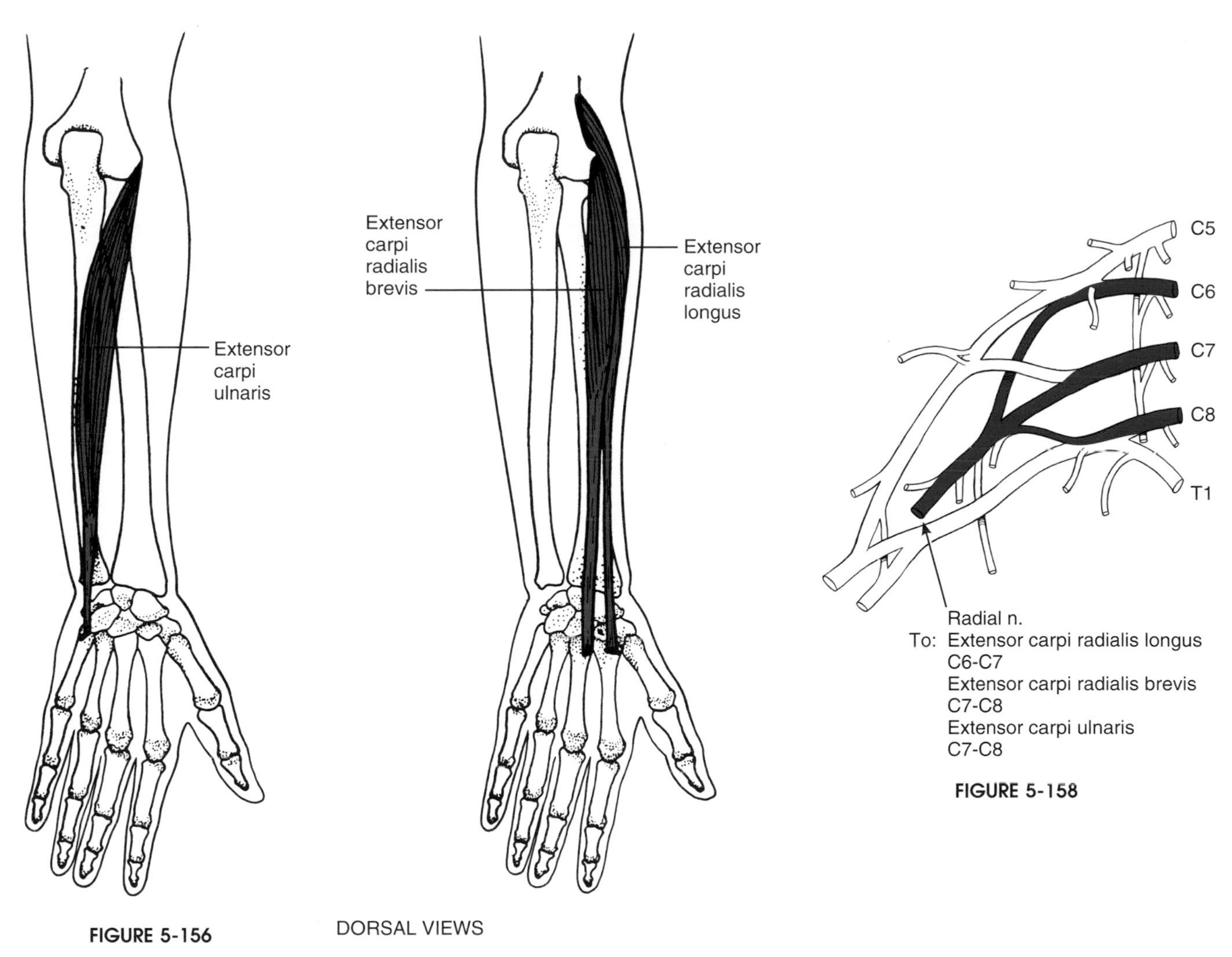

FIGURE 5-156

DORSAL VIEWS

FIGURE 5-157

FIGURE 5-158

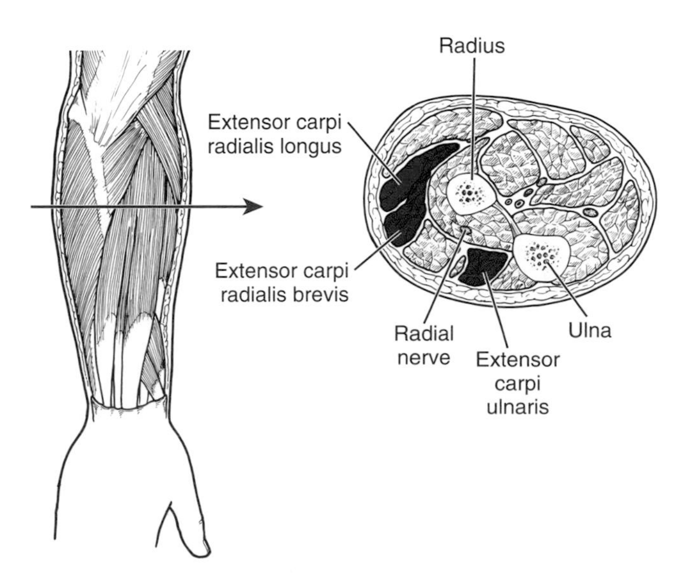

FIGURE 5-159 Arrow indicates level of cross section.

WRIST EXTENSION

(Extensor carpi radialis longus, Extensor carpi radialis brevis, and Extensor carpi ulnaris)

Range of Motion
0° to 70°

Table 5-18 WRIST EXTENSION

I.D.	Muscle	Origin	Insertion
148	Extensor carpi radialis longus	Humerus (lateral supracondylar ridge, distal 1/3) Common forearm extensor tendon Lateral intermuscular septum	2nd metacarpal bone (base on radial side of dorsal aspect)
149	Extensor carpi radialis brevis	Humerus (lateral epicondyle via common forearm extensor tendon) Radial collateral ligament of elbow joint Aponeurosis of muscle	3rd metacarpal bone (base of dorsal surface on radial side) 2nd metacarpal (occasionally)
150	Extensor carpi ulnaris	Humerus (lateral epicondyle via common extensor tendon) Ulna (posterior border by an aponeurosis)	5th metacarpal bone (tubercle on medial side of base)
Others			
154	Extensor digitorum		
158	Extensor digiti minimi		
155	Extensor indicis		See Plate 4

Grade 5 (Normal), Grade 4 (Good), and Grade 3 (Fair)

Position of Patient: Short sitting. Elbow is flexed, forearm is fully pronated, and both are supported on the table.

Position of Therapist: Sitting or standing at a diagonal in front of patient. Support the patient's forearm. The hand used for resistance is placed over the dorsal (extensor) surface of the metacarpals.

To test all three muscles, the patient extends the wrist without deviation. Resistance for Grades 4 and 5 is given in a forward and downward direction over the 2nd to 5th metacarpals (Figure 5-160) with four fingers or hypothenar eminence.

To test the extensor carpi radialis longus and brevis (for extension with radial deviation), resistance is given with two fingers on the dorsal (extensor) surface of the 2nd and 3rd metacarpals (radial side of hand) in the direction of flexion and ulnar deviation.

To test the extensor carpi ulnaris (for extension and ulnar deviation), resistance is given on the dorsal (extensor) surface of the 5th metacarpal (ulnar side of hand) in the direction of flexion and radial deviation.

Test: For the combined test of the three wrist extensor muscles, the patient extends the wrist straight up through the full available range. Do not permit extension of the fingers.

To test the two radial extensors, the patient extends the wrist, leading with the thumb side of the hand. The wrist may be prepositioned in some extension and radial deviation to direct the patient's motion.

To test the extensor carpi ulnaris, the patient extends the wrist, leading with the ulnar side of the hand. The therapist may preposition the wrist in this attitude to direct the movement toward the ulna.

Instructions to Patient: "Bring your wrist up. Hold it. Don't let me push it down." For Grade 3: "Bring your wrist up."

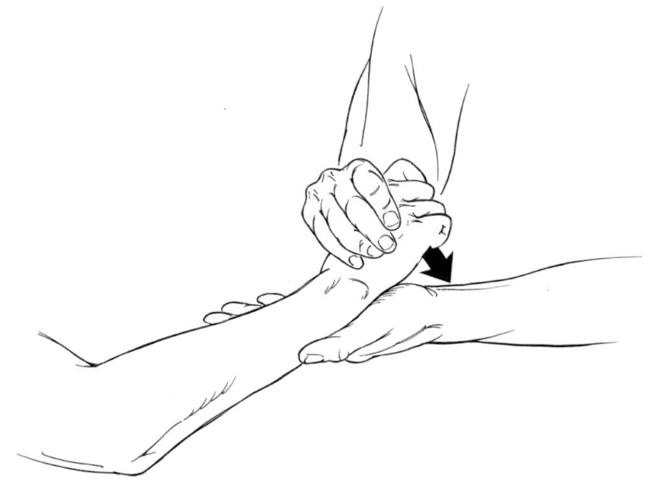

FIGURE 5-160

Grade 5 (Normal), Grade 4 (Good), and Grade 3 (Fair) Continued

Grading

Grade 5 (Normal): Completes full wrist extension (when testing all three muscles) against maximal resistance. Full extension is not required for the tests of radial and ulnar deviation.

Grade 4 (Good): Completes full wrist extension against strong to moderate resistance when all muscles are being tested. When testing the individual muscles, full wrist extension range of motion will not be achieved.

Grade 3 (Fair): Completes full range of motion with no resistance in the test for all three muscles. In the separate tests for the radial and ulnar extensors, the deviation required precludes full range of motion.

Grade 2 (Poor)

Position of Patient: Forearm supported on table in neutral position.

Position of Therapist: Support the patient's wrist. This elevates the hand from the table and removes friction (Figure 5-161).

Test: Patient extends the wrist.

Instructions to Patient: "Bend your wrist back."

Grading

Grade 2 (Poor): Completes full range with gravity eliminated.

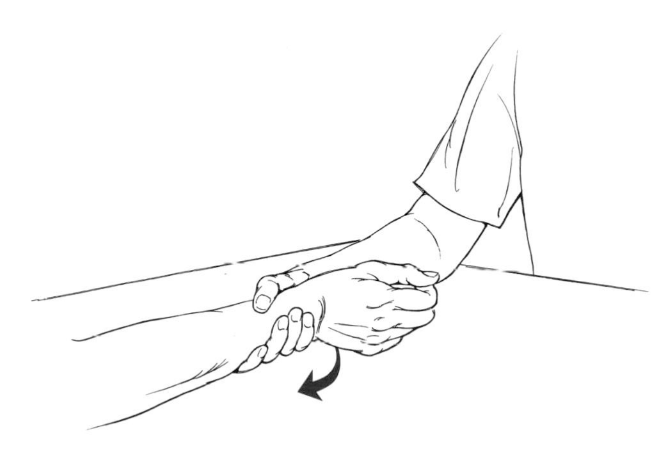

FIGURE 5-161

WRIST EXTENSION

(Extensor carpi radialis longus, Extensor carpi radialis brevis, and Extensor carpi ulnaris)

Grade 1 (Trace) and Grade 0 (Zero)

Position of Patient: Hand and forearm supported on table with hand fully pronated.

Position of Therapist: Support the patient's wrist in extension. The other hand is used for palpation. Use one finger to palpate one muscle in a given test.

Extensor carpi radialis longus: Palpate this tendon on the dorsum of the wrist in line with the 2nd metacarpal (Figure 5-162).

Extensor carpi radialis brevis: Palpate this tendon on the dorsal surface of the wrist in line with the 3rd metacarpal bone (Figure 5-163).

Extensor carpi ulnaris: Palpate this tendon on the dorsal wrist surface proximal to the 5th metacarpal and just distal to the ulnar styloid process (Figure 5-164).

Test: Patient attempts to extend the wrist.

Instructions to Patient: "Try to bring your wrist back."

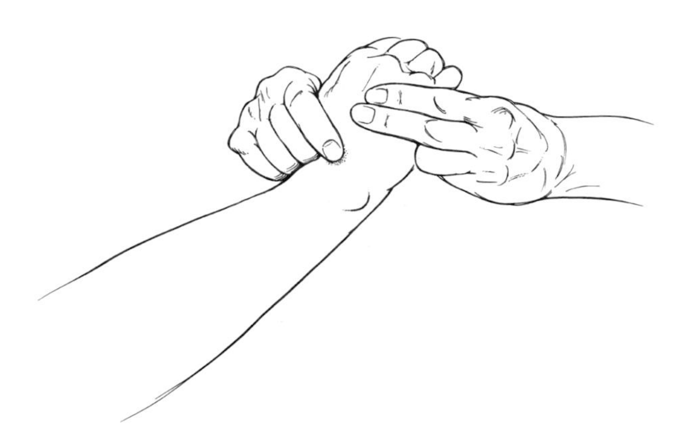

FIGURE 5-162

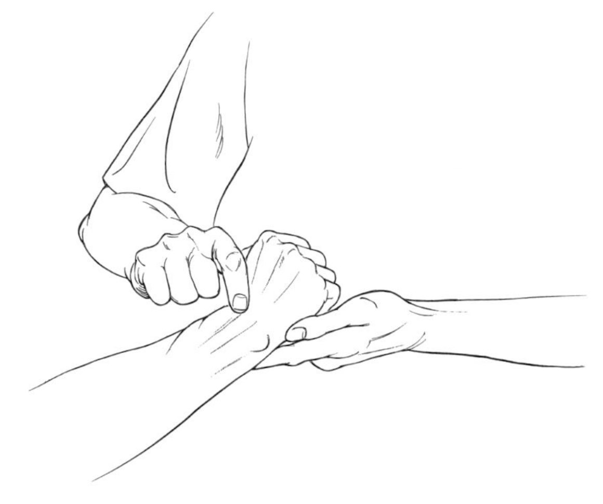

FIGURE 5-163

Grading

Grade 1 (Trace): For any given muscle there is visible or palpable contractile activity, but no wrist motion ensues.

Grade 0 (Zero): No contractile activity.

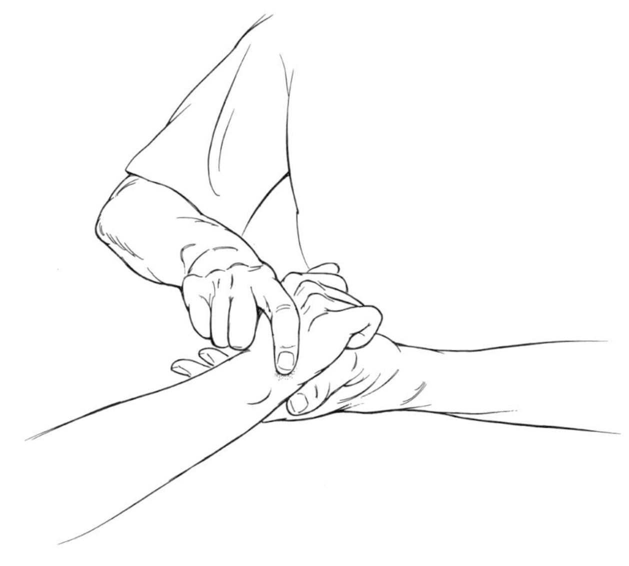

FIGURE 5-164

Substitution

The most common substitution occurs when the finger extensors are allowed to participate. This can be avoided to a large extent by ensuring that the patient's fingers are relaxed and are not permitted to extend.

Helpful Hints

- The radial wrist extensors are considerably stronger than the extensor carpi ulnaris.
- A patient with complete quadriplegia at C5-C6 will have only the radial wrist extensors remaining. Radial deviation during extension is therefore the prevailing extensor motion at the wrist.

Lumbricales
4th
3rd
1st
2nd
PALMAR

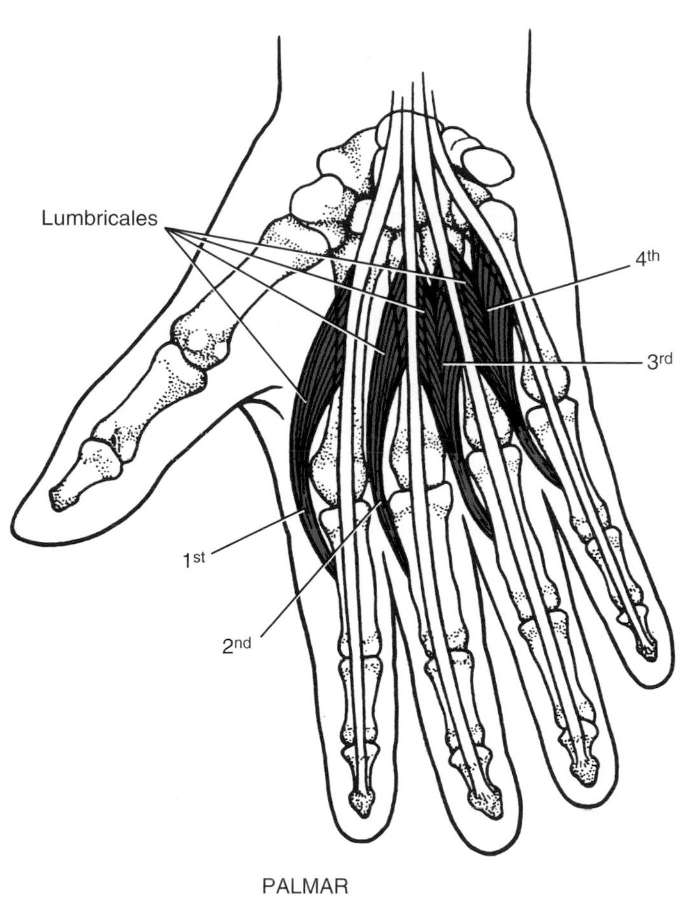

FIGURE 5-165

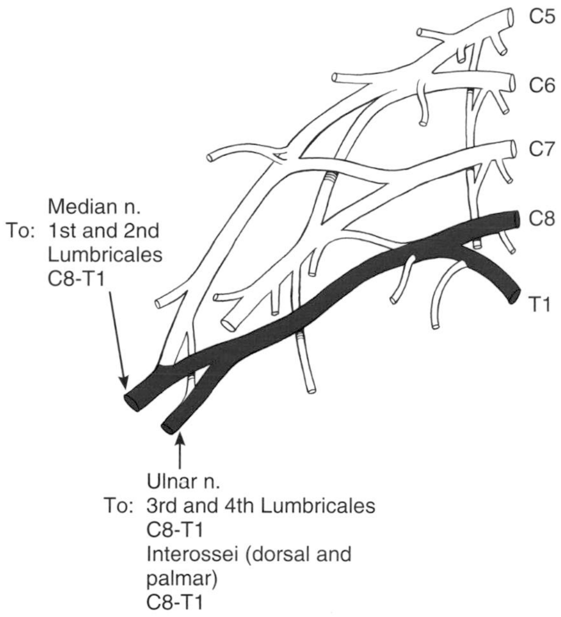

C5
C6
C7
C8
T1
Median n.
To: 1st and 2nd Lumbricales C8-T1
Ulnar n.
To: 3rd and 4th Lumbricales C8-T1
Interossei (dorsal and palmar) C8-T1

FIGURE 5-166

FINGER MP FLEXION

(Interossei and Lumbricales)

Range of Motion
MP joints: 0° to 90°

Table 5-19 MP FLEXION OF FINGERS

I.D.	Muscle	Origin	Insertion
163	Lumbricales (4 in number)	Tendons of flexor digitorum profundus:	Extensor digitorum expansion Each muscle runs distally to the *radial* side of its corresponding digit, attaches to the dorsal digital expansion
	1st lumbrical	Index finger (radial side, palmar surface)	1st lumbrical to index finger
	2nd lumbrical	Middle finger (radial side, palmar surface)	2nd lumbrical to long finger
	3rd lumbrical	Middle and ring fingers (double heads from adjacent sides of tendons)	3rd lumbrical to ring finger
	4th lumbrical	Ring and little fingers (adjacent sides of tendons)	4th lumbrical to little finger
164	Dorsal interossei (four bipennate muscles) 1st dorsal interosseus (often named *Abductor indicis*)	Metacarpal bones (each muscle arises by two heads from adjacent sides of metacarpals between which each lies)	All: dorsal expansion Proximal phalanges (bases)
		1st dorsal: between thumb and index finger	1st dorsal: index finger (radial side)
		2nd dorsal: between index and long finger	2nd dorsal: long finger (radial side)
		3rd dorsal: between long and ring fingers	3rd dorsal: long finger (ulnar side)
		4th dorsal: between ring and little fingers	4th dorsal: ring finger (ulnar side)
165	Palmar interossei three muscles (a 4th muscle often is described)	Metacarpal bones 2, 4, and 5. (muscles lie on palmar surfaces of metacarpals rather than between them) No palmar interosseous on long finger All muscles lie on aspect of metacarpal facing the long finger.	All: Dorsal expansion Proximal phalanges
		1st palmar: 2nd metacarpal (ulnar side)	1st palmar: index finger (ulnar side)
		2nd palmar: 4th metacarpal (radial side)	2nd palmar: ring finger (radial side)
		3rd palmar: 5th metacarpal (radial side)	3rd palmar: little finger (radial side)
Others			
156	Flexor digitorum superficialis		
157	Flexor digitorum profundus		
160	Flexor digiti minimi brevis		
161	Opponens digiti minimi		

Grade 5 (Normal), Grade 4 (Good), and Grade 3 (Fair)

Position of Patient: Short sitting or supine with forearm in supination. Wrist is maintained in neutral. The metacarpophalangeal (MP) joints should be fully extended; all interphalangeal (IP) joints are flexed (Figure 5-167).

Position of Therapist: Stabilize the metacarpals proximal to the MP joint. Resistance is given on the palmar surface of the proximal row of phalanges in the direction of MP extension (Figure 5-168).

Test: Patient simultaneously flexes the MP joints and extends the IP joints. Fingers may be tested separately. Do not allow fingers to curl; they must remain extended.

Instructions to Patient: "Uncurl your fingers while flexing your knuckles. Hold it. Don't let me straighten your knuckles." The final position is a right angle at the MP joints. Demonstrate motion to patient and insist on practice to get the motions performed correctly and simultaneously.

Grading

Grade 5 (Normal): Patient completes simultaneous MP flexion and finger extension and holds against maximal resistance. Resistance is given to fingers individually because of the variant strength of the different interossei and lumbricales. The interossei and lumbricales also have different innervations.

Grade 4 (Good): Patient completes range of motion against moderate to strong resistance.

Grade 3 (Fair): Patient completes both motions correctly and simultaneously without resistance.

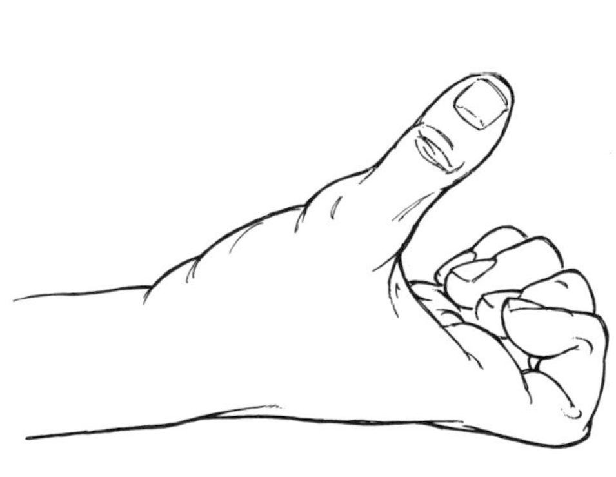

FIGURE 5-167

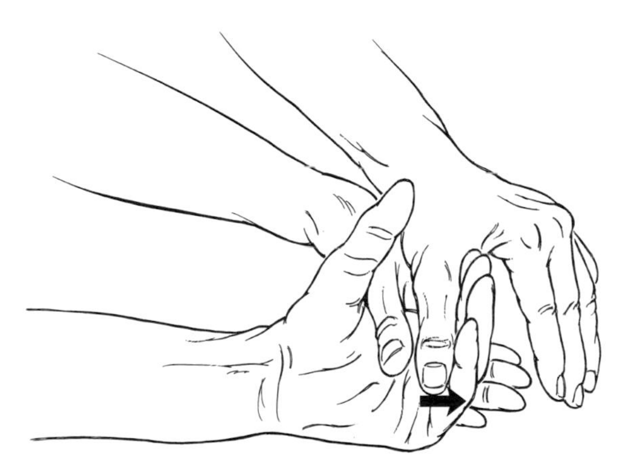

FIGURE 5-168

FINGER MP FLEXION

(Interossei and Lumbricales)

Grade 2 (Poor), Grade 1 (Trace), and Grade 0 (Zero)

Position of Patient: Forearm and wrist in midposition to remove influence of gravity. MP joints are fully extended; all IP joints are flexed.

Position of Therapist: Stabilize metacarpals.

Test: Patient attempts to flex MP joints through full available range while extending IP joints (Figure 5-169).

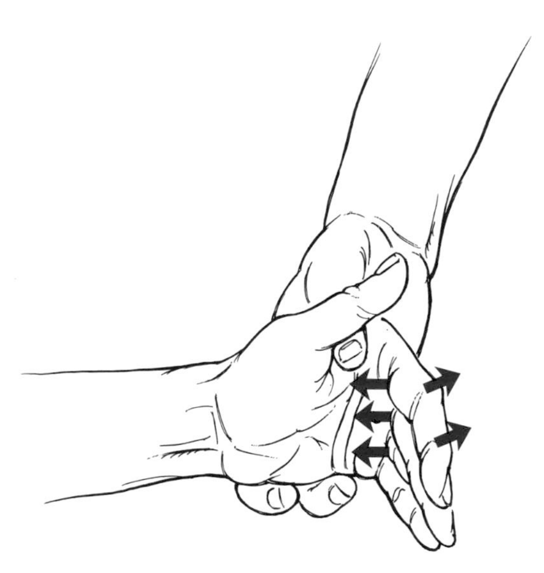

FIGURE 5-169

Instructions to Patient: "Try to uncurl your fingers while bending your knuckles." Demonstrate motion to patient and allow practice.

Grading

Grade 2 (Poor): Completes full range of motion in gravity-eliminated position.

Grade 1 (Trace): Except in the hand that is markedly atrophied, the palmar interossei and lumbricales cannot be palpated. A grade of 1 is given for minimal motion.

Grade 0 (Zero): A grade of zero is given in the absence of any movement.

Substitution

The long finger flexors may substitute for the lumbricales. To avoid this pattern, make sure that the patient's IP joints fully extend.

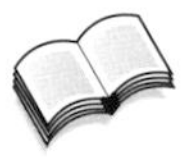

Hand Testing Requires Judgment and Experience

When evaluating the muscles of the hand, care must be taken to use graduated resistance that takes into consideration the relatively small mass of the muscles. In general, the examiner should not use the full thrust of the fist, wrist, or arm but rather one or two fingers to resist hand motions.

The degree of resistance offered to hand muscles is an issue, particularly when testing a postoperative hand. Similarly, the amount of motion allowed or encouraged should be monitored. Sudden or excessive excursions could "tear out" a surgical reconstruction.

Applying resistance in a safe fashion requires experience in assessing hand injuries or repair and a large amount of clinical judgment to avoid dislodging a tendon transfer or other surgical reconstruction. The neophyte examiner would be wise to err in the direction of caution.

Considerable practice in testing normal hands and comparing injured hands with their normal contralateral sides should provide some of the necessary judgment with which to approach the fragile hand.

This text remains true to the principles of testing in the ranges of 5, 4, and 3 with respect to gravity. It is admitted, however, that the influence of gravity on the fingers is inconsequential, so the gravity and antigravity positions are not considered in valid muscle tests of the hand.

FINGER PROXIMAL PHALANGES (PIP) AND DISTAL PHALANGES (DIP) FLEXION

(Flexor digitorum superficialis and Flexor digitorum profundus)

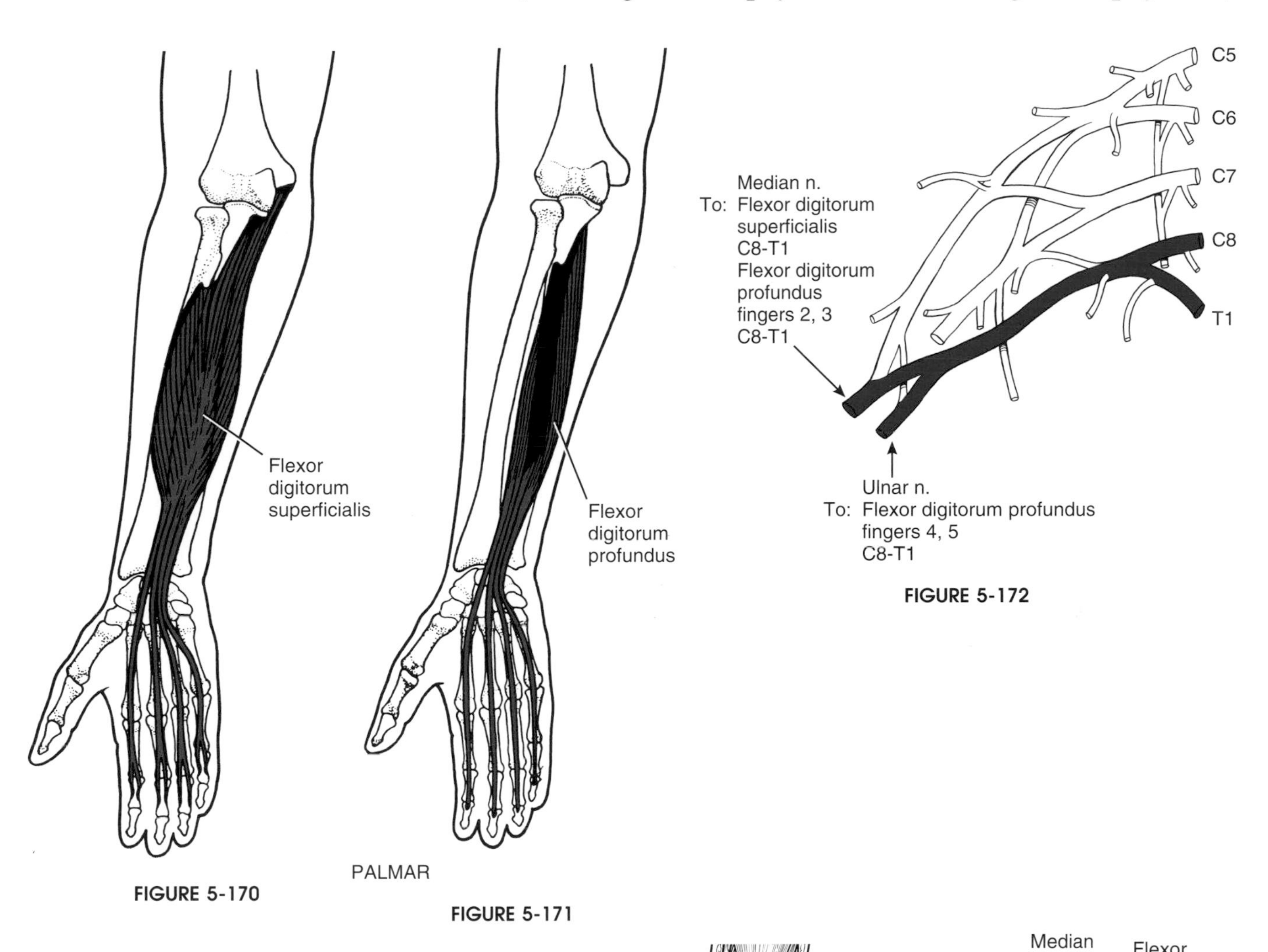

FIGURE 5-170

FIGURE 5-171

FIGURE 5-172

FIGURE 5-173 Arrow indicates level of cross section.

FINGER PROXIMAL PHALANGES (PIP) AND DISTAL PHALANGES (DIP) FLEXION

(Flexor digitorum superficialis and Flexor digitorum profundus)

Range of Motion
PIP joints: 0° to 100° DIP joints: 0° to 90°

Table 5-20 PIP AND DIP FINGER FLEXION

I.D.	Muscle	Origin	Insertion
156	Flexor digitorum superficialis (2 heads)	Humero-ulnar head: humerus (medial epicondyle via common flexor tendon) Ulna (medial collateral ligament of elbow joint); coronoid process (medial side) Intermuscular septum *Radial head:* radius (oblique line on anterior shaft)	Four tendons arranged in 2 pairs Superficial pair: middle and ring fingers (sides of middle phalanges) Deep pair: index and little fingers (sides of middle phalanges)
157	Flexor digitorum profundus	Ulna (proximal 3/4 of anterior and medial shaft; medial coronoid process) Interosseous membrane (ulnar)	Four tendons to digits 2-5 (distal phalanges, at base of palmar surface)

Grade 5 (Normal), Grade 4 (Good), and Grade 3 (Fair)

Position of Patient: Forearm supinated, wrist in neutral. Finger to be tested is in slight flexion at the MP joint (Figure 5-174).

Position of Therapist: Hold all fingers (except the one being tested) in extension at all joints (see Figure 5-174). Isolation of the index finger may not be complete. The other hand is used to resist the head (distal end) of the middle phalanx of the test finger in the direction of extension (not illustrated).

Test: Each of the four fingers is tested separately. Patient flexes the PIP joint without flexing the DIP joint. Do not allow motion of any joints of the other fingers.

Flick the terminal end of the finger being tested with the thumb to make certain that the flexor digitorum profundus is not active; that is, the DIP joint goes into extension. The distal phalanx should be floppy.

Instructions to Patient: "Bend your index [then long, ring, and little] finger; hold it. Don't let me straighten it. Keep your other fingers relaxed."

Grading

Grade 5 (Normal): Completes range of motion and holds against maximal finger resistance.

Grade 4 (Good): Completes range against moderate resistance.

Grade 3 (Fair): Completes range of motion with no resistance (Figure 5-175).

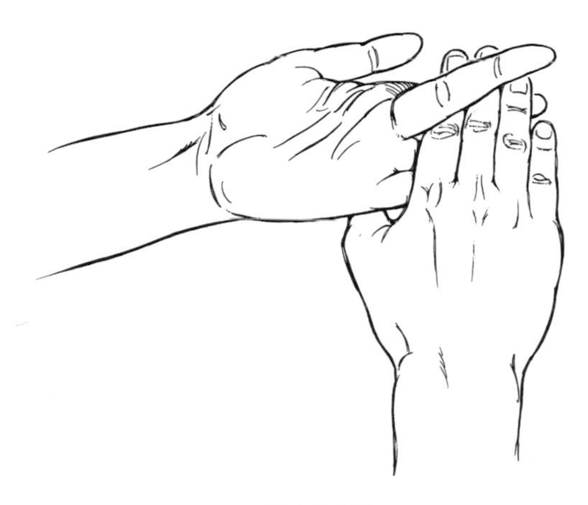

FIGURE 5-174

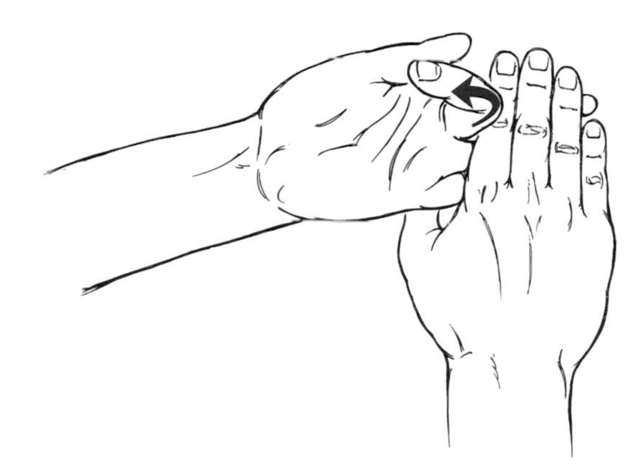

FIGURE 5-175

PIP TESTS

(Flexor digitorum superficialis)

Grade 2 (Poor), Grade 1 (Trace), and Grade 0 (Zero)

Position of Patient: Forearm is in midposition to eliminate the influence of gravity on finger flexion.

Position of Therapist: Same as for Grades 5, 4, and 3.
Palpate the flexor digitorum superficialis on the palmar surface of the wrist between the palmaris longus and the flexor carpi ulnaris (Figure 5-176).

Test: Patient flexes the PIP joint.

Instructions to Patient: "Bend your middle finger." (Select other fingers individually.)

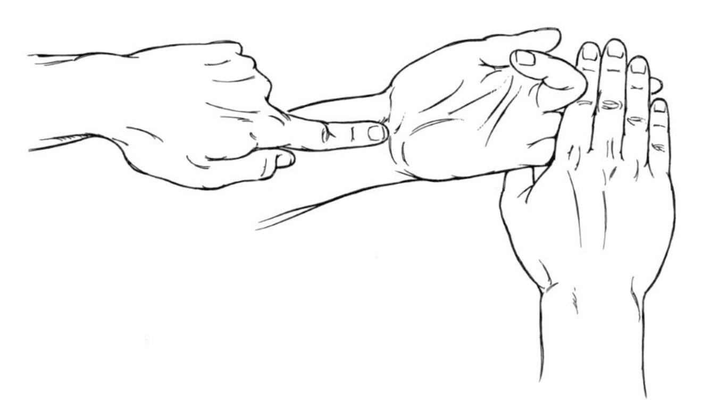

FIGURE 5-176

Grading

Grade 2 (Poor): Completes range of motion.

Grade 1 (Trace): Palpable or visible contractile activity, which may or may not be accompanied by a flicker of motion.

Grade 0 (Zero): No contractile activity.

Substitutions

- The major substitution for this motion is offered by the flexor digitorum profundus, and this will occur if the DIP joint is allowed to flex.
- If the wrist is allowed to extend, tension increases in the long finger flexors, and may result in passive flexion of the IP joints. This is referred to as a "tenodesis" action.
- Relaxation of IP extension will result in passive IP flexion.

Helpful Hint

Many people cannot isolate the little finger. When this is the case, test the little and ring fingers at the same time.

Grade 5 (Normal), Grade 4 (Good), and Grade 3 (Fair)

Position of Patient: Forearm in supination, wrist in neutral, and proximal PIP joint in extension.

Position of Therapist: Stabilize the middle phalanx in extension by grasping it on either side (Figure 5-177). Resistance is provided on the distal phalanx in the direction of extension (not illustrated).

Test: Test each finger individually. Patient flexes distal phalanx of each finger.

Instructions to Patient: "Bend the tip of your finger. Hold it. Don't let me straighten it."

Grading

Grade 5 (Normal): Completes available range against a carefully assessed maximal level of resistance (see page 168).

Grade 4 (Good): Completes maximal available range against some resistance.

Grade 3 (Fair): Completes maximum available range with no resistance (see Figure 5-177).

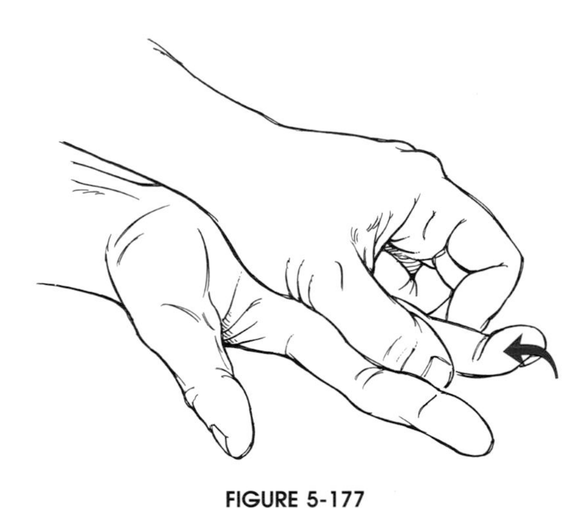

FIGURE 5-177

Grade 2 (Poor), Grade 1 (Trace), and Grade 0 (Zero)

All aspects of testing these grades are the same as those used for the higher grades except that the position of the forearm is in neutral to eliminate the influence of gravity.

Grades are assigned as for the PIP tests.

The tendon of the flexor digitorum profundus can be palpated on the palmar surface of the middle phalanx of each finger.

Substitutions

- The wrist must be kept in a neutral position and must not be allowed to extend to rule out the tenodesis effect of the wrist extensors.
- Don't be fooled if the patient extends the DIP joint and then relaxes, which can give the impression of active finger flexion.

FINGER MP EXTENSION

(Extensor digitorum, Extensor indicis, Extensor digiti minimi)

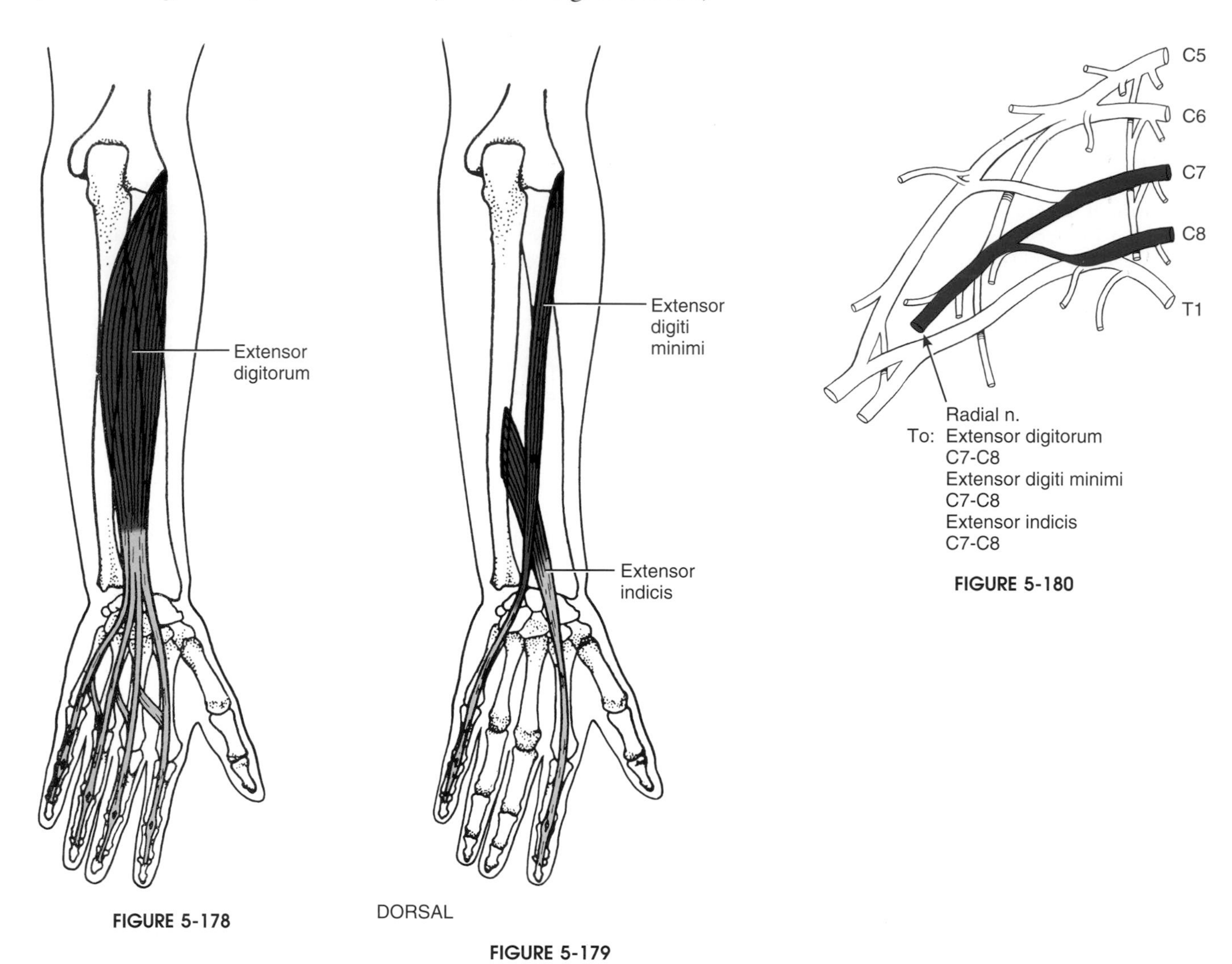

FIGURE 5-178

FIGURE 5-179

FIGURE 5-180

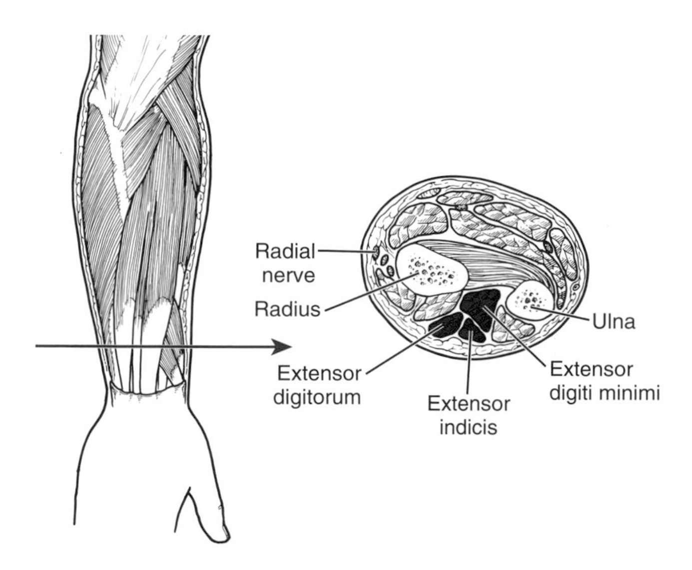

FIGURE 5-181 Arrow indicates level of cross section.

(Extensor digitorum, Extensor indicis, Extensor digiti minimi)

Range of Motion
0° to 45°

Table 5-21 MP FINGER EXTENSION

I.D.	Muscle	Origin	Insertion
154	Extensor digitorum	Humerus (lateral epicondyle via common extensor tendon) Intermuscular septum Antebrachial fascia	Via 4 tendons to digits 2-5 (via the extensor expansion, to dorsum of middle and distal phalanges; one tendon to each finger)
155	Extensor indicis	Ulna (posterior surface of shaft) Interosseous membrane	2nd digit (via tendon of extensor digitorum into extensor hood)
158	Extensor digiti minimi	Humerus (lateral epicondyle via common extensor tendon) Intermuscular septa	5th digit (extensor hood)

Grade 5 (Normal), Grade 4 (Good), and Grade 3 (Fair)

Position of Patient: Forearm in pronation, wrist in neutral. MP and IP joints are in relaxed flexion posture.

Position of Therapist: Stabilize the wrist in neutral. Place the index finger of the resistance hand across the dorsum of all proximal phalanges just distal to the MP joints. Give resistance in the direction of flexion.

Test:

Extensor digitorum: Patient extends MP joints (all fingers simultaneously), allowing the IP joints to be in slight flexion (Figure 5-182).

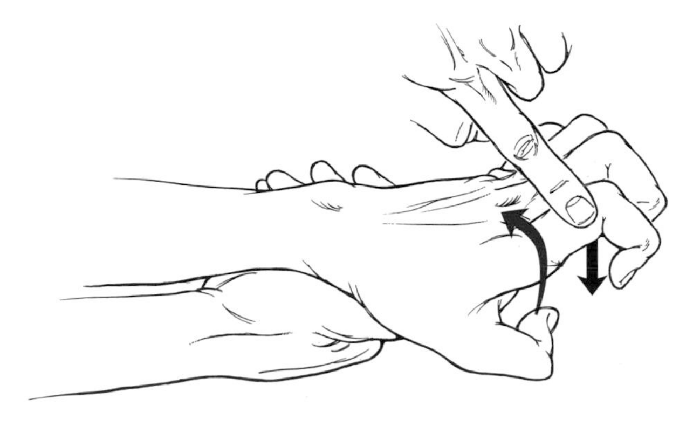

FIGURE 5-182

Extensor indicis: Patient extends the MP joint of the index finger.

Extensor digiti minimi: Patient extends the MP joint of the 5th digit.

Instructions to Patient: "Bend your knuckles back as far as they will go." Demonstrate motion to patient and instruct to copy.

Grading

Grade 5 (Normal): Completes active extension range of motion with appropriate level of strong resistance.

Grade 4 (Good): Completes active range with some resistance.

Grade 3 (Fair): Completes active range with no resistance.

FINGER MP EXTENSION

(Extensor digitorum, Extensor indicis, Extensor digiti minimi)

Grade 2 (Poor), Grade 1 (Trace), and Grade 0 (Zero)

Procedures: Test is the same as that for Grades 5, 4, and 3 except that the forearm is in the midposition.

The tendons of the extensor digitorum (n = 4), the extensor indicis (n = 1), and the extensor digiti minimi (n = 1) are readily apparent on the dorsum of the hand as they course in the direction of each finger.

Grading

Grade 2 (Poor): Completes range.

Grade 1 (Trace): Visible tendon activity but no joint motion.

Grade 0 (Zero): No contractile activity.

Substitution

Flexion of the wrist will produce IP extension through a tenodesis action.

Helpful Hints

- MP extension of the fingers is not a strong motion, and only slight resistance is required to "break" the end position.
- It is usual for the active range of motion to be considerably less than the available passive range. In this test, therefore, the "full available range" is not used, and the active range is accepted.
- Another way to check whether there is functional extensor strength in the fingers is to "flick" the proximal phalanx of each finger downward; if the finger rebounds, it is functional.

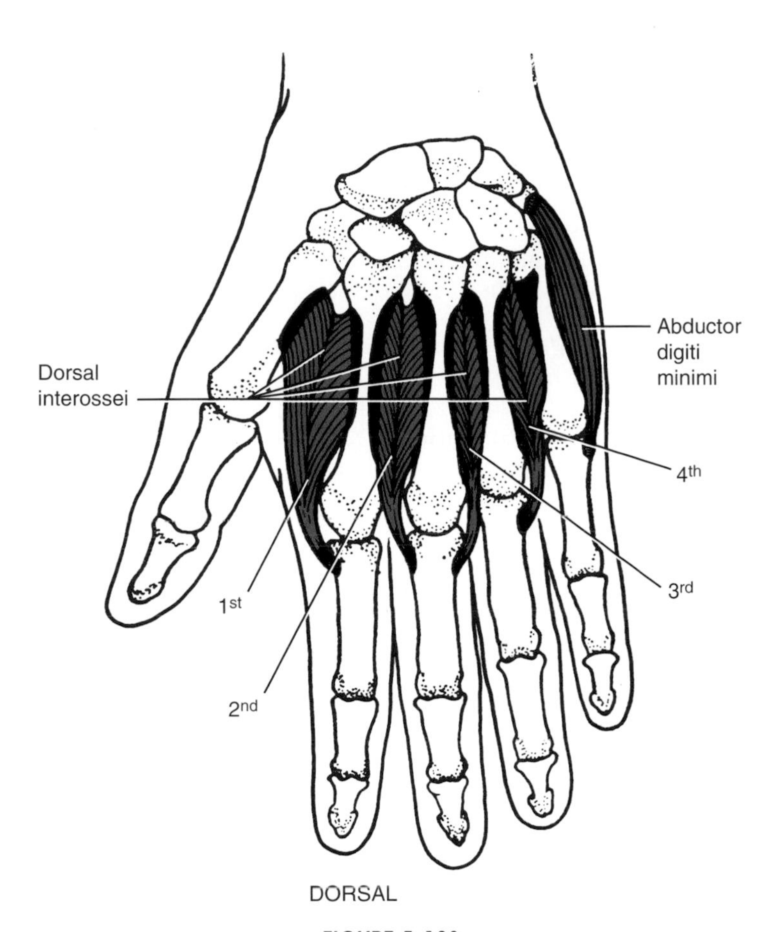

FIGURE 5-183

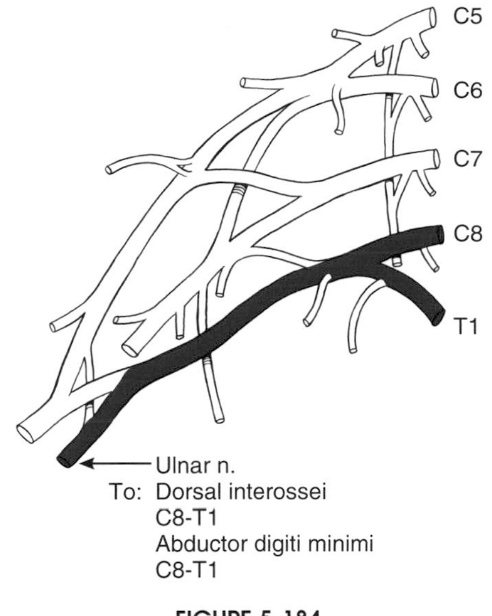

FIGURE 5-184

Range of Motion
0° to 20°

Table 5-22 FINGER ABDUCTION

I.D.	Muscle	Origin	Insertion
164	Dorsal interossei Four bipennate muscles (1st dorsal interosseous, often named *Abductor indicis*)	Metacarpal bones (each muscle arises by 2 heads from adjacent sides of metacarpals between which each lies)	All: dorsal extensor expansion: proximal phalanges (bases)
	1st dorsal: between thumb and index finger	1st dorsal: index finger (radial side)	
	2nd dorsal: between index and long finger	2nd dorsal: long finger (radial side)	
	3rd dorsal: between long and ring fingers	3rd dorsal: long finger (ulnar side)	
	4th dorsal: between ring and little finger	4th dorsal: ring finger (ulnar side)	
159	Abductor digiti minimi	Pisiform bone Tendon of flexor carpi ulnaris Pisohamate ligament	5th digit (base of proximal phalanx, ulnar side) Dorsal expansion of extensor digiti minimi
Others			
154	Extensor digitorum (no action on long finger)		
158	Extensor digiti minimi (little finger)		

FINGER ABDUCTION

(Dorsal interossei)

Grade 5 (Normal) and Grade 4 (Good)

Position of Patient: Forearm pronated, wrist in neutral. Fingers start in extension and adduction. MP joints in neutral and avoid hyperextension.

Position of Therapist: Support the wrist in neutral. The fingers of the other hand are used to give resistance on the distal phalanx, on the radial side of the finger and the ulnar side of the adjacent finger (i.e., they are squeezed together). The direction of resistance will cause any pair of fingers to approximate (Figure 5-185).

Test: Abduction of fingers (individual tests):

Dorsal Interossei:

Abduction of ring finger toward little finger
Abduction of middle finger toward ring finger
Abduction of middle finger toward index finger
Abduction of index finger toward thumb

The long (middle) finger (digit 3, finger 2) will move one way when tested with the index finger and the opposite way when tested with the ring finger (see Figure 5-183), which shows a dorsal interosseus on either side). When testing the little finger with the ring finger, the abductor digiti minimi is being tested along with the 4th dorsal interosseus.

Abductor digiti minimi: Patient abducts 5th digit away from ring finger.

Instructions to Patient: "Spread your fingers. Hold them. Don't let me push them together."

Grading

Grade 5 (Normal) and Grade 4 (Good): Neither the dorsal interossei nor the abductor digiti minimi will tolerate much resistance. Grading between a 5 and a 4 muscle is a judgment call based on possible comparison with the contralateral side as well as on clinical experience. Figure 5-186 illustrates the test for 2nd and 4th dorsal interossei.

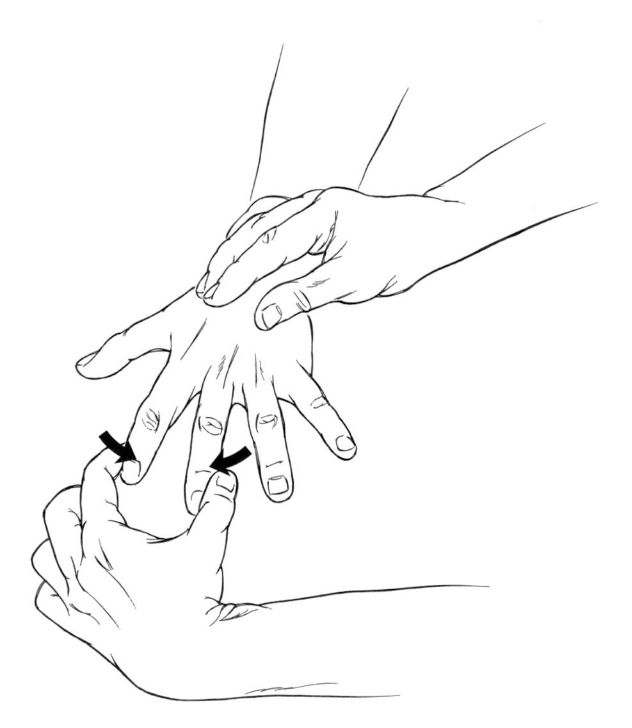

FIGURE 5-185

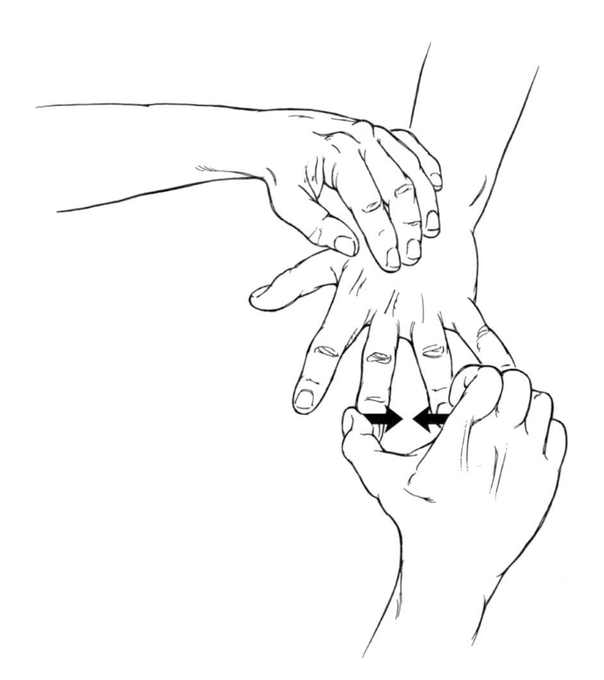

FIGURE 5-186

Grade 3 (Fair)

Grade 3 (Fair): Patient can abduct any given finger. Remember that the long finger has two dorsal interossei and therefore must be tested as it moves away from the midline in both directions (Figure 5-187).

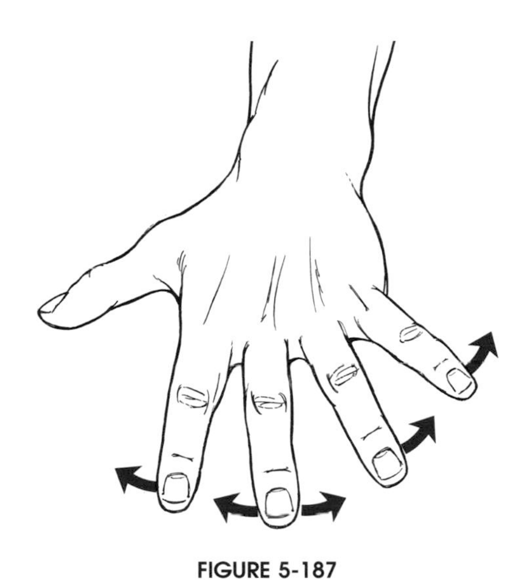

FIGURE 5-187

Grade 2 (Poor), Grade 1 (Trace), and Grade 0 (Zero)

Procedures and Grading: Same as for higher grades in this test. A Grade 2 should be assigned if the patient can complete only a partial range of abduction for any given finger. The only dorsal interosseus that is readily palpable is the first at the base of the proximal phalanx (Figure 5-188).

The abductor digiti minimi is palpable on the ulnar border of the hand.

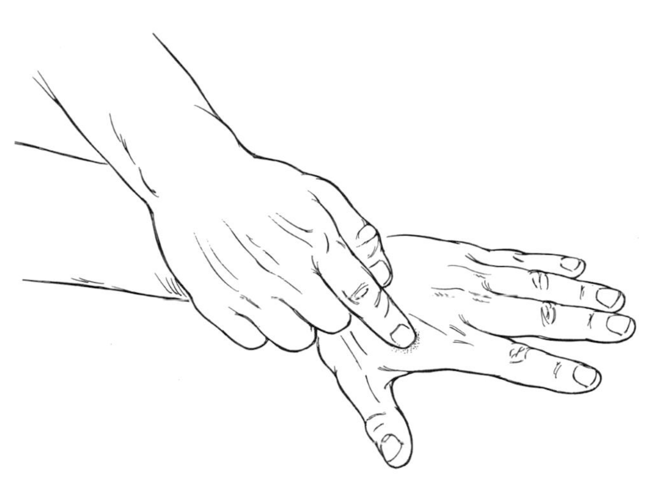

FIGURE 5-188

Helpful Hint

Provide resistance for a Grade 5 test by flicking each finger toward adduction; if the finger tested rebounds, the grade is 5.

FINGER ADDUCTION

(Palmar interossei)

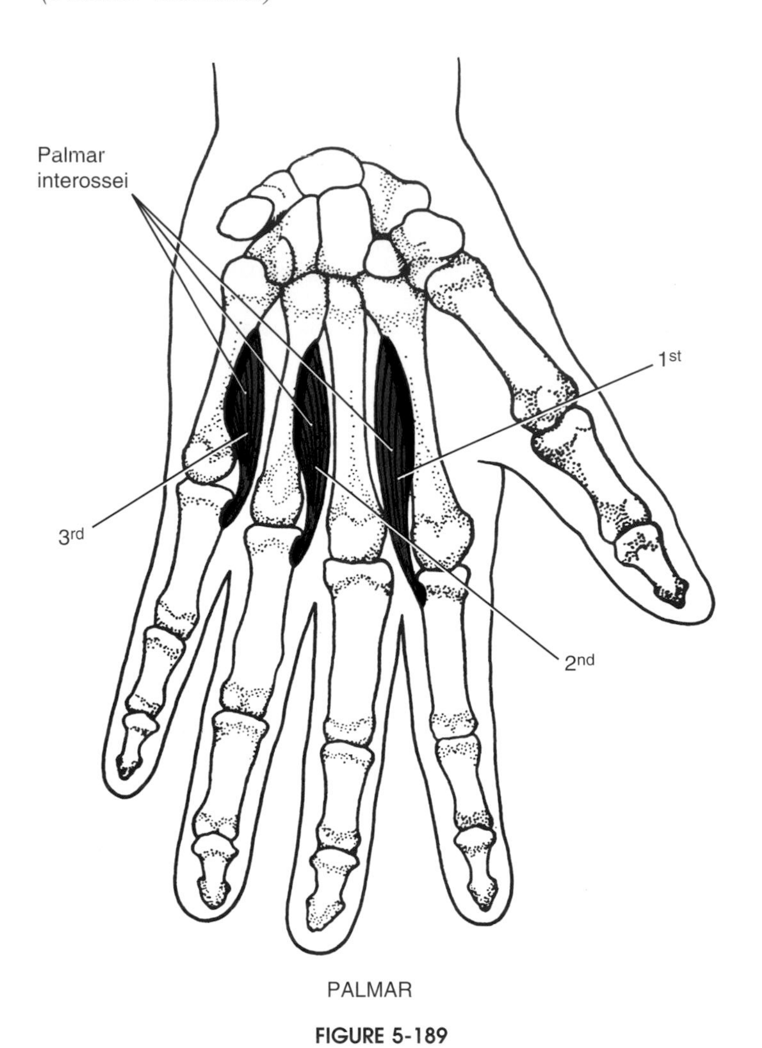

FIGURE 5-189

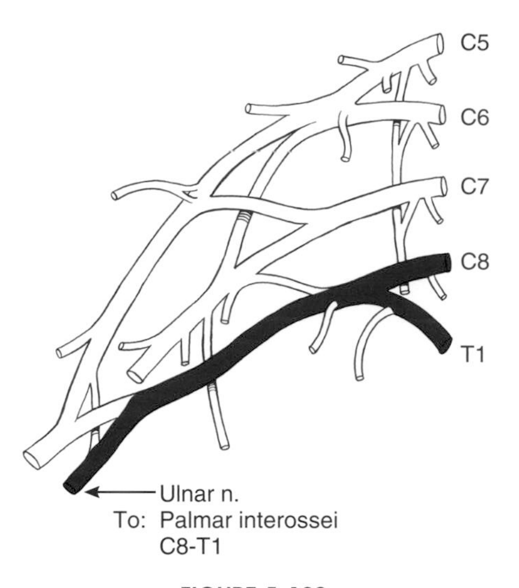

FIGURE 5-190

Range of Motion
20° to 0°

Table 5-23 FINGER ADDUCTION

I.D.	Muscle	Origin	Insertion
165	Palmar interossei, 3 muscles (a 4th muscle often is described)	Metacarpal bones 2, 4, and 5 Muscles lie on palmar surfaces of metacarpals rather than between them. No palmar interosseous on long finger All muscles lie on aspect of a metacarpal facing the long finger	All: dorsal extensor expansion
		1st palmar: 2nd metacarpal (ulnar side)	1st palmar: index finger (proximal phalanx, ulnar side)
		2nd palmar: 4th metacarpal (radial side)	2nd palmar: ring finger (proximal phalanx, radial side)
		3rd palmar: 5th metacarpal (radial side)	3rd palmar: little finger (proximal phalanx, radial side)
Other			
155	Extensor indicis		

Grade 5 (Normal) and Grade 4 (Good)

Position of Patient: Forearm pronated (palm down), wrist in neutral, and fingers extended and adducted. MP joints are neutral; avoid flexion.

Position of Therapist: Examiner grasps the middle phalanx on each of two adjoining fingers (Figure 5-191). Resistance is given in the direction of abduction for each finger tested. The examiner is trying to "pull" the fingers apart. Each finger should be resisted separately.

Test: Adduction of fingers (individual tests):

Adduction of little finger toward ring finger
Adduction of ring finger toward long finger
Adduction of index finger toward long finger
Adduction of thumb toward index finger

Occasionally there is a 4th palmar interosseus (not illustrated in Figure 5-189) that some consider a separate muscle from the adductor pollicis. In any event, the two muscles cannot be clinically separated.

Because the middle finger (also called the long finger, digit 3, or finger 2) has no palmar interosseus, it is not tested in adduction.

Instructions to Patient: "Hold your fingers together. Don't let me spread them apart."

Grading

Grade 5 (Normal) and Grade 4 (Good): These muscles are notoriously weak in the sense of not tolerating much resistance. Distinguishing between Grades 5 and 4 is an exercise in futility, and the grade awarded will depend on the amount of the examiner's experience with normal hands.

Grade 3 (Fair): Patient can adduct fingers toward middle finger but cannot hold against resistance (Figure 5-192).

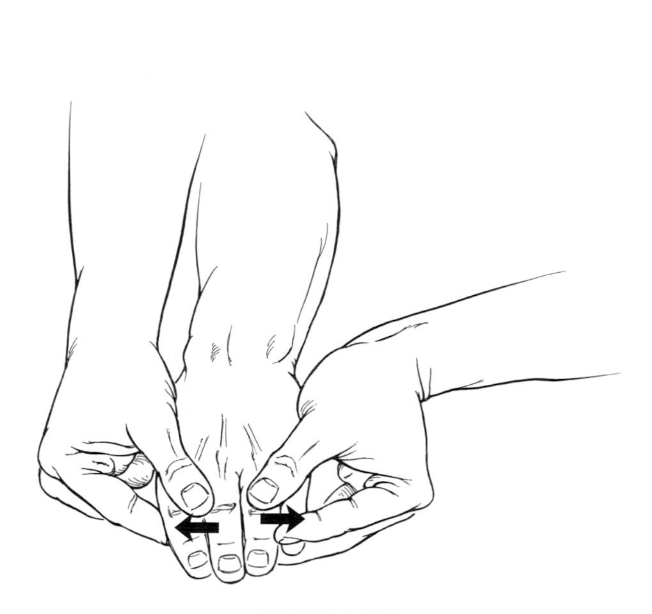

FIGURE 5-191

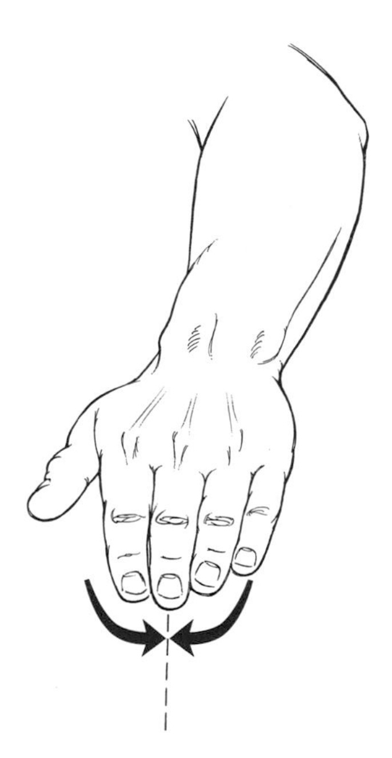

FIGURE 5-192

FINGER ADDUCTION

(Palmar interossei)

Grade 2 (Poor), Grade 1 (Trace), and Grade 0 (Zero)

Procedures: Same as for Grades 5, 4, and 3.

For Grade 2, the patient can adduct each of the fingers tested through a partial range of motion. The test for Grade 2 is begun with the fingers abducted.

Palpation of the palmar interossei is rarely feasible. By placing the examiner's finger against the side of a finger to be tested, the therapist may detect a slight outward motion for a muscle less than Grade 2.

Substitution

Caution must be used to ensure that finger flexion does not occur because the long finger flexors can contribute to adduction.

Helpful Hint

The fingers can be judged quickly by grasping the distal phalanx and flicking the finger in the direction of abduction. If the finger rebounds or snaps back, that interosseous is functional.

(Flexor pollicis brevis and Flexor pollicis longus)

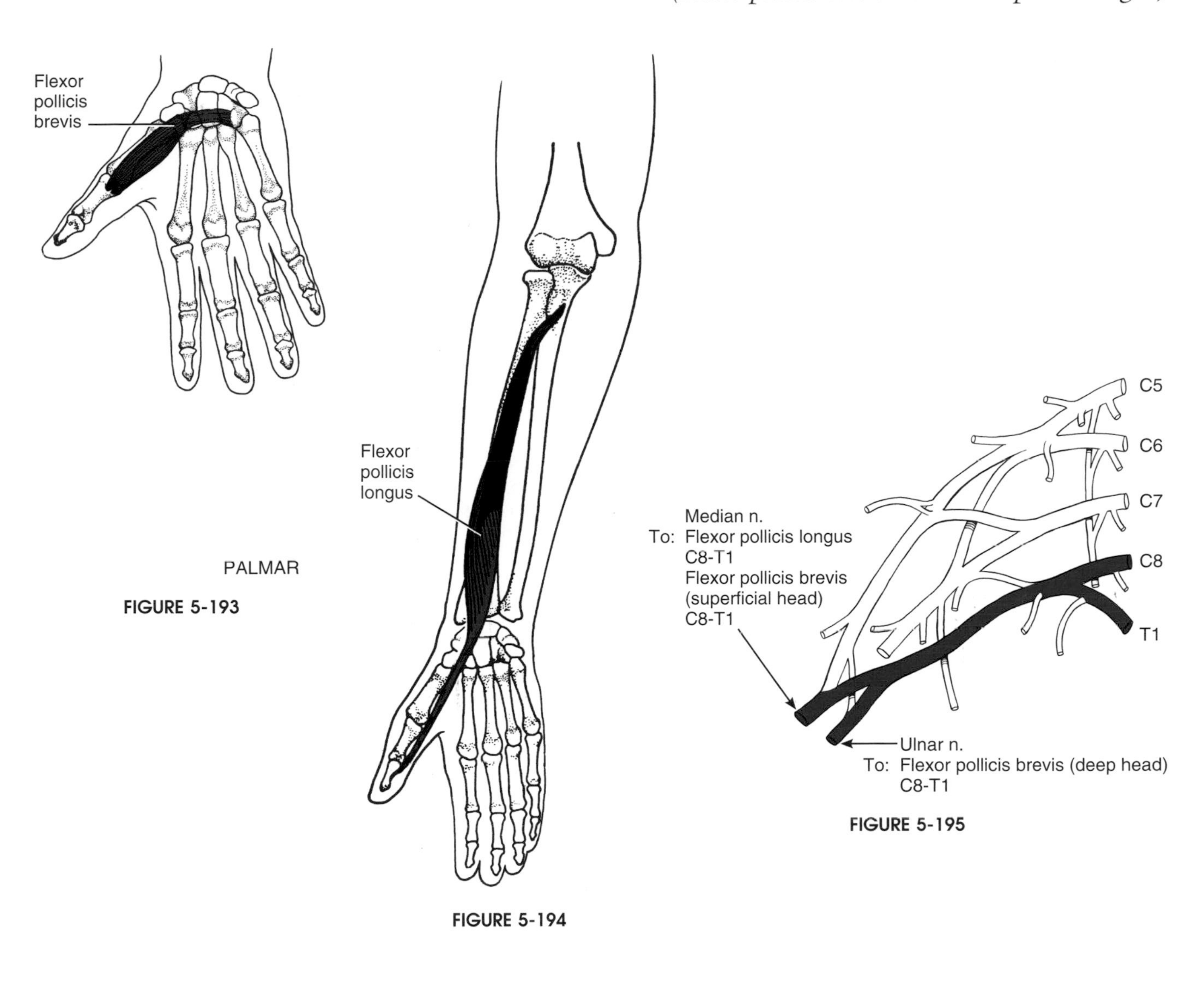

FIGURE 5-193

FIGURE 5-194

FIGURE 5-195

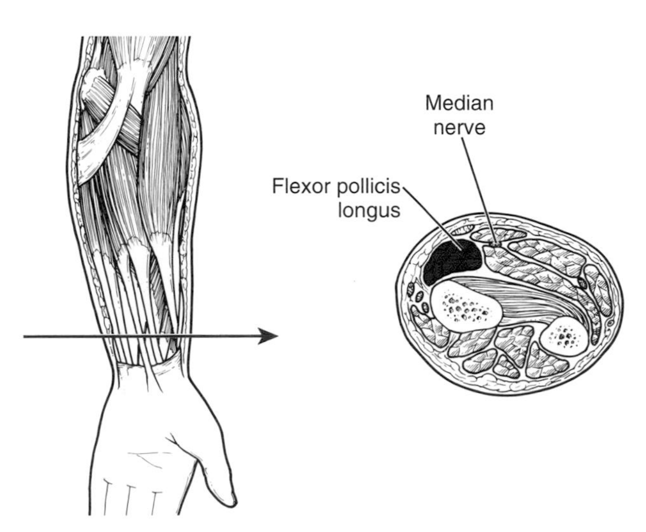

FIGURE 5-196 Arrow indicates level of cross section.

THUMB MP AND IP FLEXION

(Flexor pollicis brevis and Flexor pollicis longus)

Range of Motion
MP flexion: 0° to 50°
IP flexion: 0° to 80°

Table 5-24 THUMB MP AND IP FLEXION

I.D.	Muscle	Origin	Insertion
MP Flexion			
170	Flexor pollicis brevis Superficial head (often blended with opponens pollicis)	Flexor retinaculum (distal) Trapezoid bone (tubercle, distal)	Thumb (base of proximal phalanx, radial side)
	Deep head	Trapezium bone Capitate bone Palmar ligaments of distal carpal bones	
IP Flexion			
169	Flexor pollicis longus	Radius (anterior surface of middle 1/2) and adjacent Interosseous membrane Ulna (coronoid process, lateral border (variable)) Humerus (medial epicondyle (variable))	Thumb (base of distal phalanx, palmar surface)

Grade 5 (Normal) to Grade 0 (Zero)

Position of Patient: Forearm in supination, wrist in neutral. Carpometacarpal (CMC) joint is at 0°; IP joint is at 0°. Thumb in adduction, lying relaxed and adjacent to the 2nd metacarpal (Figure 5-197)

Position of Therapist: Stabilize the 1st metacarpal firmly to avoid any wrist or CMC motion. The other hand gives one-finger resistance to MP flexion on the proximal phalanx in the direction of extension (Figure 5-198).

Test: Patient flexes the MP joint of the thumb, keeping the IP joints straight (see Figure 5-198).

Instructions to Patient: "Bring your thumb across the palm of your hand. Keep the thumb in touch with your palm. Don't bend the end joint. Hold it. Don't let me pull it back."

Demonstrate thumb flexion and have patient practice the motion.

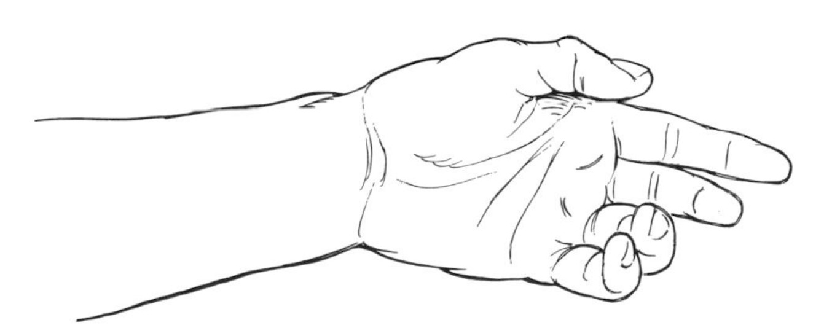

FIGURE 5-197

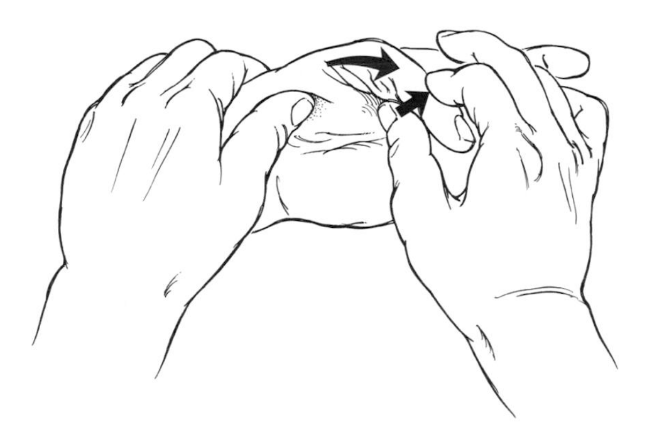

FIGURE 5-198

Grading

Grade 5 (Normal): Completes range of motion against maximal thumb resistance.

Grade 4 (Good): Tolerates strong to moderate resistance.

Grade 3 (Fair): Completes full range of motion with perhaps a slight amount of resistance because gravity is eliminated.

Grade 2 (Poor): Completes range of motion.

Grade 1 (Trace): Palpate the muscle by initially locating the tendon of the flexor pollicis longus in the thenar eminence (Figure 5-199). Then palpate the muscle belly of the flexor pollicis brevis on the ulnar side of the longus tendon in the thenar eminence.

Grade 0 (Zero): No visible or palpable contractile activity.

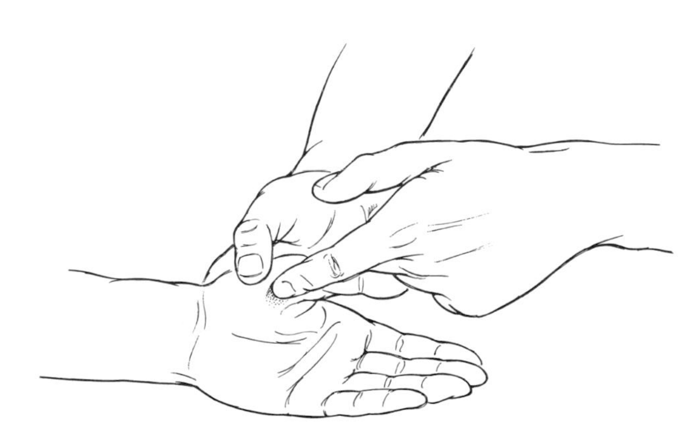

FIGURE 5-199

Substitution by Flexor Pollicis Longus

The long thumb flexor can substitute but only after flexion of the IP joint begins. To avoid this substitution, do not allow flexion of the distal joint of the thumb.

THUMB IP FLEXION TESTS

(Flexor pollicis longus)

Grade 5 (Normal) to Grade 0 (Zero)

Position of Patient: Forearm supinated with wrist in neutral and MP joint of thumb in extension.

Position of Therapist: Stabilize the MP joint of the thumb firmly in extension by grasping the patient's thumb across that joint. Give resistance with the other hand against the palmar surface of the distal phalanx of the thumb in the direction of extension (Figure 5-200).

Test: Patient flexes the IP joint of the thumb.

Instructions to Patient: "Bend the end of your thumb. Hold it. Don't let me straighten it."

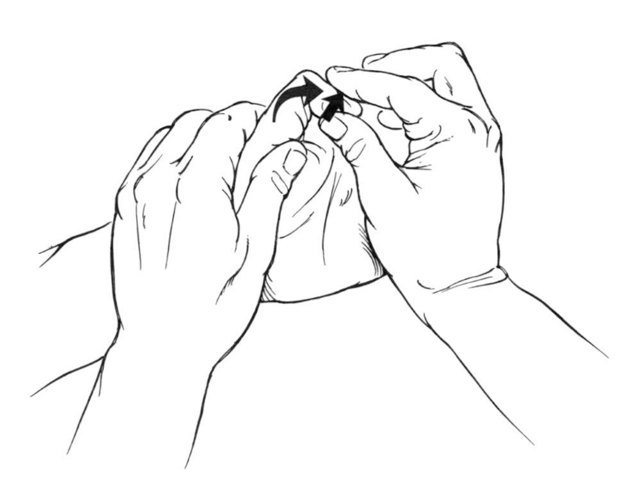

FIGURE 5-200

Grading

Grade 5 (Normal) and Grade 4 (Good): Patient tolerates maximal finger resistance from examiner for Grade 5. This muscle is very strong, and a Grade 4 muscle will tolerate strong resistance. Full range always should be completed.

Grade 3 (Fair): Completes a full range of motion with minimal resistance because gravity is eliminated.

Grade 2 (Poor): Completes range of motion.

Grade 1 (Trace) and Grade 0 (Zero): Palpate the tendon of the flexor pollicis longus on the palmar surface of the proximal phalanx of the thumb. Palpable activity is graded 1; no activity is graded 0.

Substitution

Do not allow the distal phalanx of the thumb to extend at the beginning of the test. If the distal phalanx is extended and then relaxes, the examiner may think active flexion has occurred.

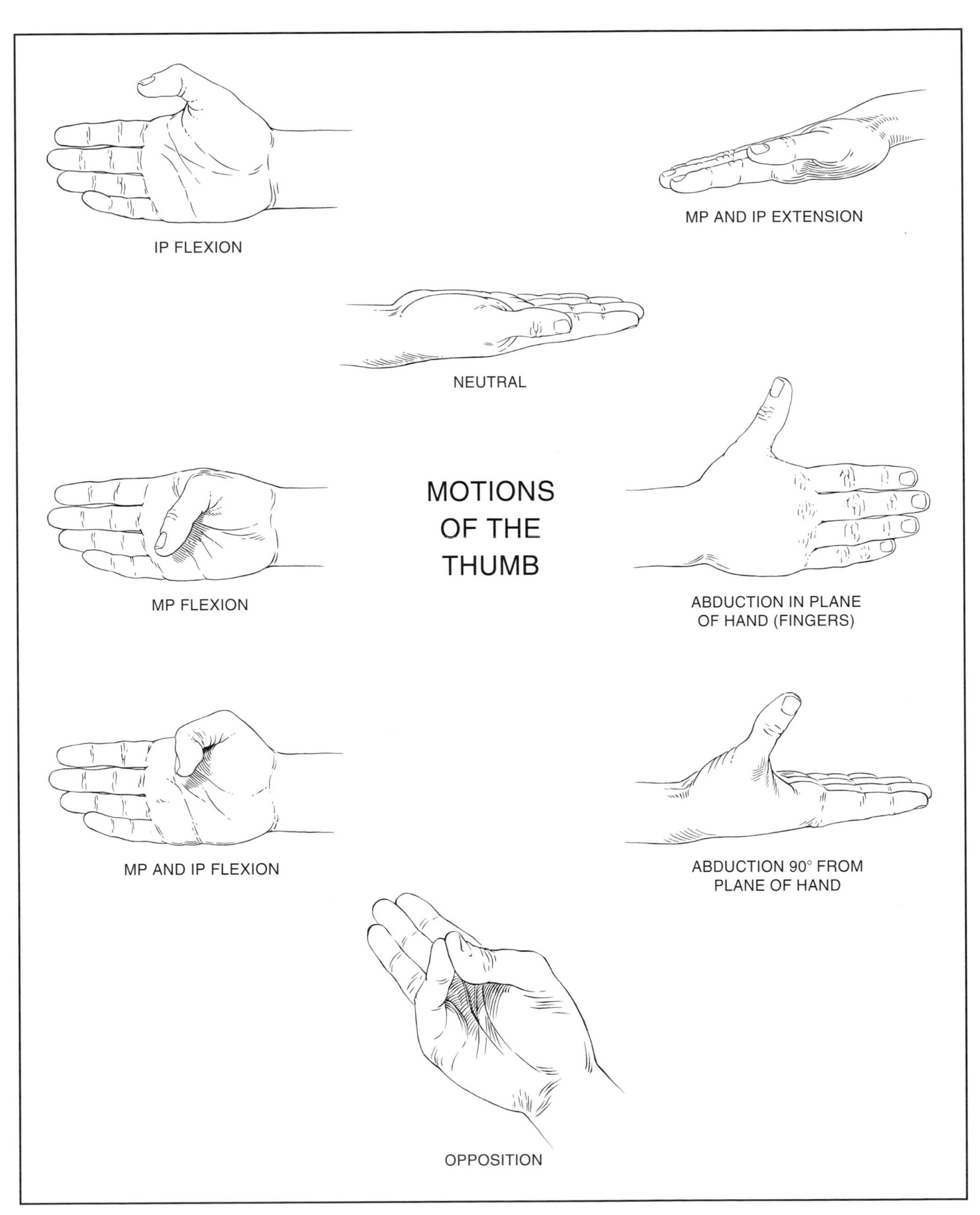
IP FLEXION
MP AND IP EXTENSION
NEUTRAL
MOTIONS OF THE THUMB
MP FLEXION
ABDUCTION IN PLANE OF HAND (FINGERS)
MP AND IP FLEXION
ABDUCTION 90° FROM PLANE OF HAND
OPPOSITION

PLATE 5

THUMB MP AND IP EXTENSION

(Extensor pollicis brevis and Extensor pollicis longus)

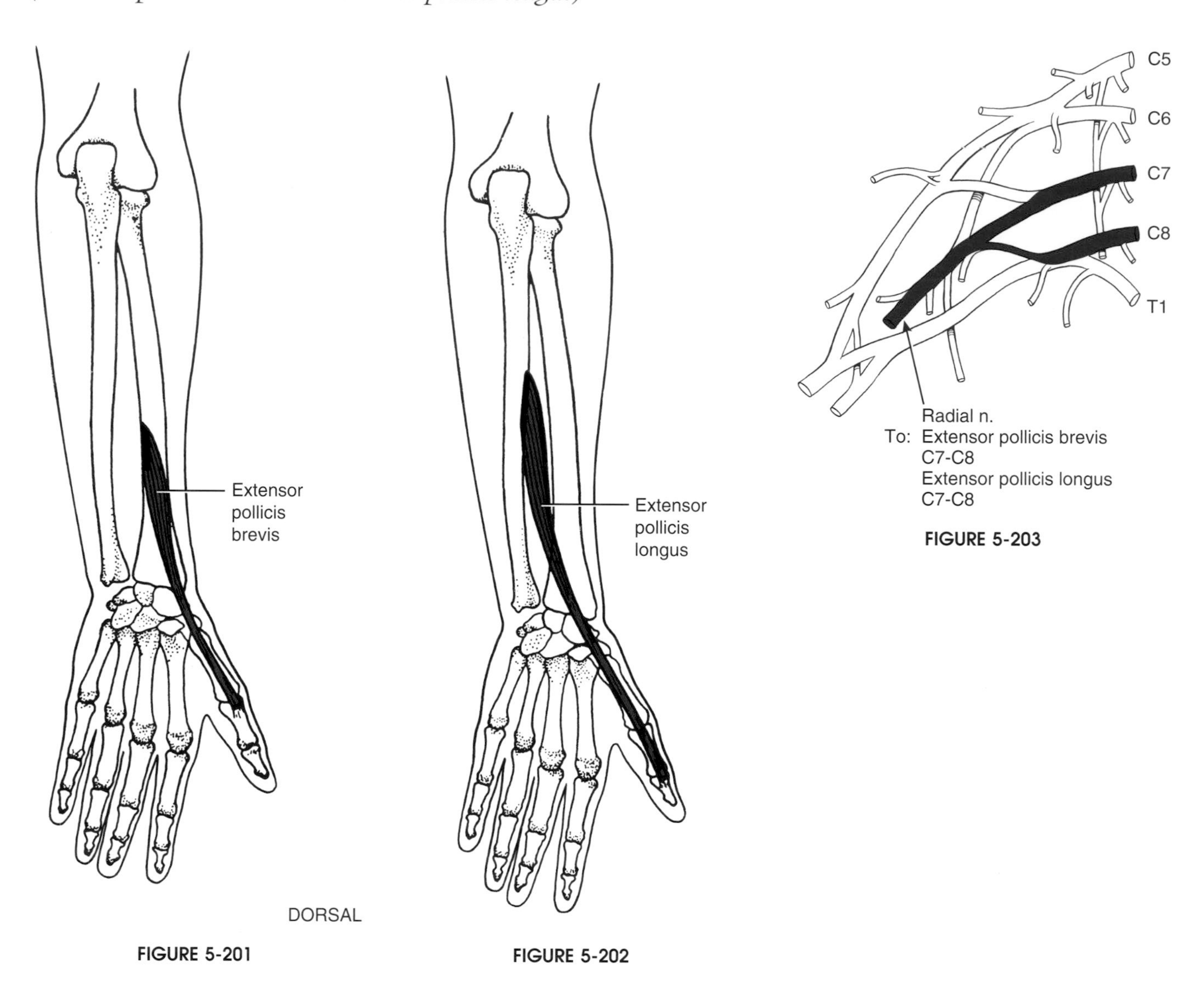

FIGURE 5-201

FIGURE 5-202

FIGURE 5-203

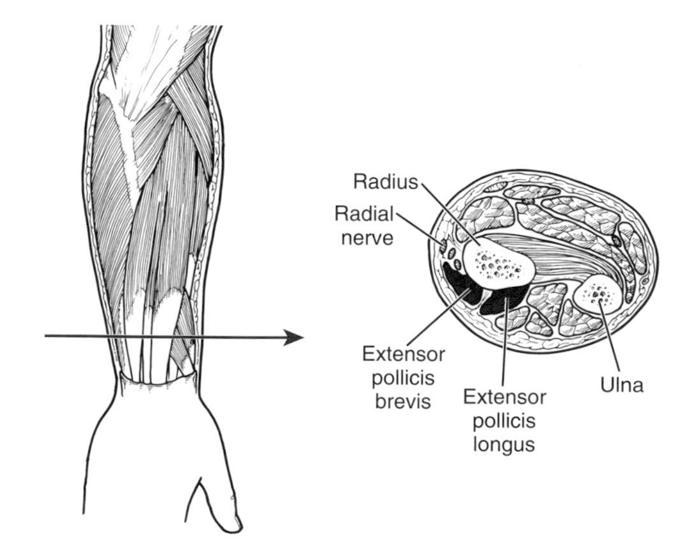

FIGURE 5-204 Arrow indicates level of cross section.

THUMB MP AND IP EXTENSION

(Extensor pollicis brevis and Extensor pollicis longus)

Range of Motion
MP extension: 50° to 0°
IP extension: 80° to 0°

Table 5-25 THUMB MP AND IP EXTENSION

I.D.	Muscle	Origin	Insertion
MP Extension			
168	Extensor pollicis brevis (radiomedial wall of "anatomical snuffbox")	Radius (posterior surface) Adjacent interosseous membrane	Thumb (proximal phalanx, base, dorsolateral surface)
IP Extension			
167	Extensor pollicis longus (ulnar wall of "anatomical snuffbox")	Ulna (shaft, middle 1/3 on posterior-lateral surface) Adjacent interosseous membrane	Thumb (base of distal phalanx)

The extensor pollicis brevis is an inconstant muscle that often blends with the extensor pollicis longus, in which event it is not possible to separate the brevis from the longus by clinical tests, and the test for the longus prevails.

THUMB MP EXTENSION TESTS

(Extensor pollicis brevis)

Grade 5 (Normal) to Grade 0 (Zero)

Position of Patient: Forearm in midposition and wrist in neutral; CMC and IP joints of the thumb are relaxed and in slight flexion. The MP joint of the thumb is in abduction and flexion.

Position of Therapist: Stabilize the first metacarpal firmly, allowing motion to occur only at the MP joint (Figure 5-205). Resistance is provided with the other hand on the dorsal surface of the proximal phalanx in the direction of flexion. This normally is not a strong muscle.

Test: Patient extends the MP joint of the thumb while keeping the IP joint slightly flexed.

Instructions to Patient: "Bring your thumb up so it points toward the ceiling; don't move the end joint. Hold it. Don't let me push it down."

Grading

Grade 5 (Normal) and Grade 4 (Good): Only the experienced examiner can accurately distinguish between Grades 5 and 4. Resistance should be applied carefully and slowly because this usually is a weak muscle.

Grade 3 (Fair): Patient moves proximal phalanx of the thumb through full range of extension with some resistance.

Grade 2 (Poor): Patient moves proximal phalanx through partial range of motion.

Grade 1 (Trace): The tendon of the flexor pollicis brevis is palpated (Figure 5-206) at the base of the first metacarpal, where it lies between the tendons of the abductor pollicis and the extensor pollicis longus.

Grade 0 (Zero): No contractile activity.

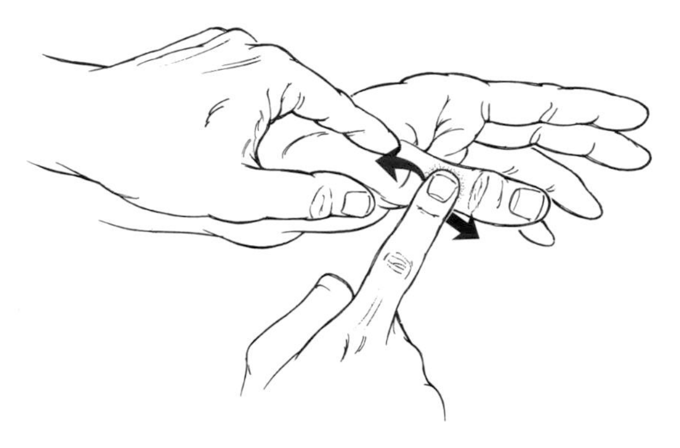

FIGURE 5-205

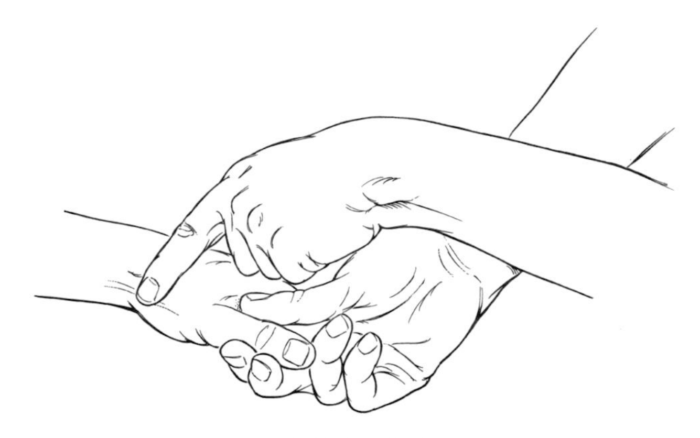

FIGURE 5-206

Substitution

Extension of the IP joint of the thumb with CMC adduction in addition to extension of the MP joint indicates substitution by the extensor pollicis longus.

THUMB IP EXTENSION TESTS

(Extensor pollicis longus)

Grade 5 (Normal), Grade 4 (Good), and Grade 3 (Fair)

Position of Patient: Forearm in midposition, wrist in neutral with ulnar side of hand resting on the table. Thumb relaxed in a flexion posture.

Position of Therapist: Use the table to support the ulnar side of the hand and stabilize the proximal phalanx of the thumb (Figure 5-207). Apply resistance over the 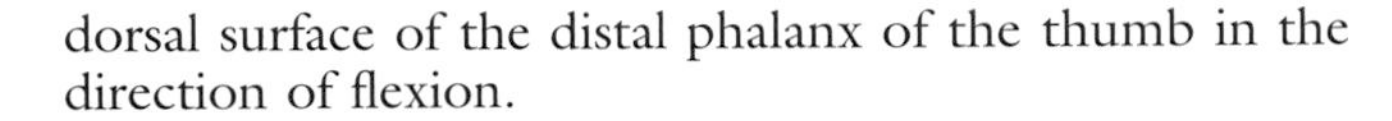 dorsal surface of the distal phalanx of the thumb in the direction of flexion.

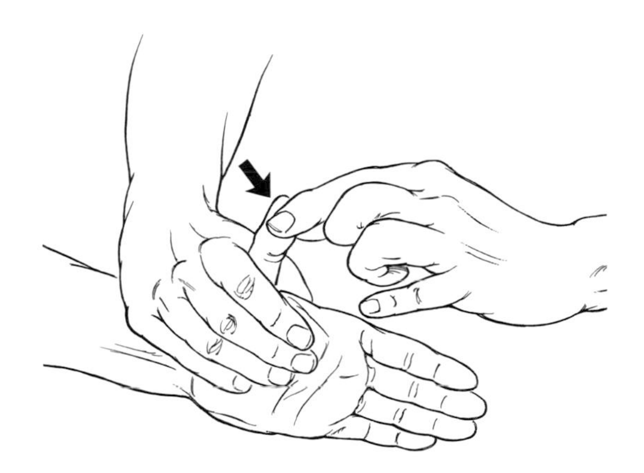

FIGURE 5-207

Test: Patient extends the IP joint of the thumb.

Instructions to Patient: "Straighten the end of your thumb. Hold it. Don't let me push it down."

Grading

Grade 5 (Normal) and Grade 4 (Good): Completes full range of motion. This is not a strong muscle, so resistance must be applied accordingly. The distinction between Grades 5 and 4 is based on comparison with the contralateral normal hand and, barring that, extensive experience in testing the hand.

Grade 3 (Fair): Completes full range of motion with no resistance.

THUMB IP EXTENSION TESTS

(Extensor pollicis longus)

Grade 2 (Poor), Grade 1 (Trace), and Grade 0 (Zero)

Position of Patient: Forearm in pronation with wrist in neutral and thumb in relaxed flexion posture to start.

Position of Therapist: Stabilize the wrist over its dorsal surface. Stabilize the fingers by gently placing the other hand across the fingers just below the MP joints (Figure 5-208).

Test: Patient extends distal joint of the thumb (see Figure 5-208).

Instructions to Patient: "Straighten the end of your thumb."

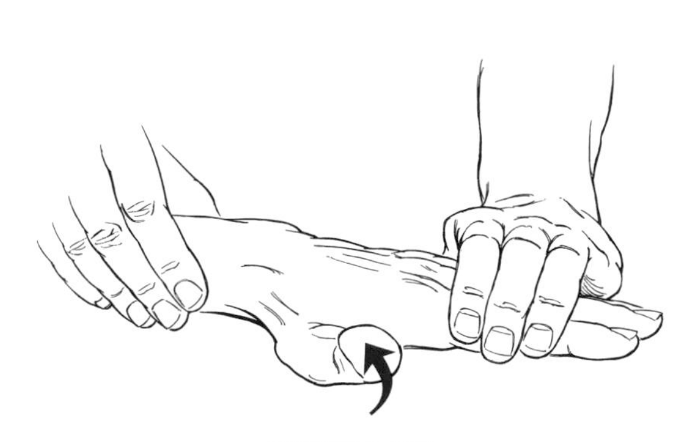

FIGURE 5-208

Grading

Grade 2 (Poor): Thumb completes range of motion.

Grade 1 (Trace): Palpate the tendon of the extensor pollicis longus on the ulnar side of the "anatomical snuff-box" or, alternatively, on the dorsal surface of the proximal phalanx (Figure 5-209).

Grade 0 (Zero): No contractile activity.

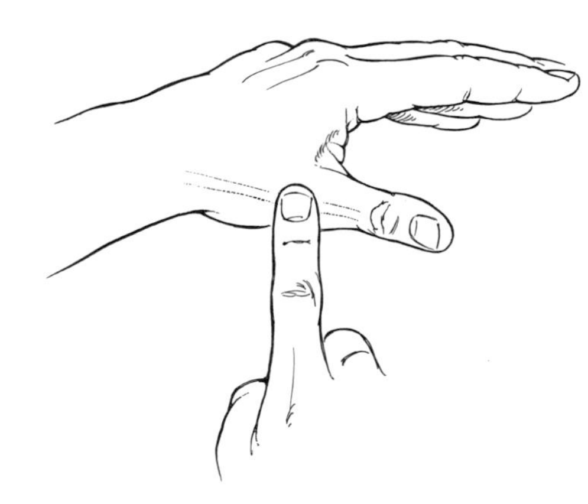

FIGURE 5-209

Substitution

The muscles of the thenar eminence (abductor pollicis brevis, flexor pollicis brevis, and adductor pollicis) can extend the IP joint by flexing the CMC joint (an extensor tenodesis).

Helpful Hints

- Continued action by the extensor pollicis longus will extend the MP and CMC joints.
- A quick way to assess the functional status of the long thumb extensor is to flick the distal phalanx into flexion; if the finger rebounds or snaps back, it is a useful muscle.

THUMB ABDUCTION

(Abductor pollicis longus and Abductor pollicis brevis)

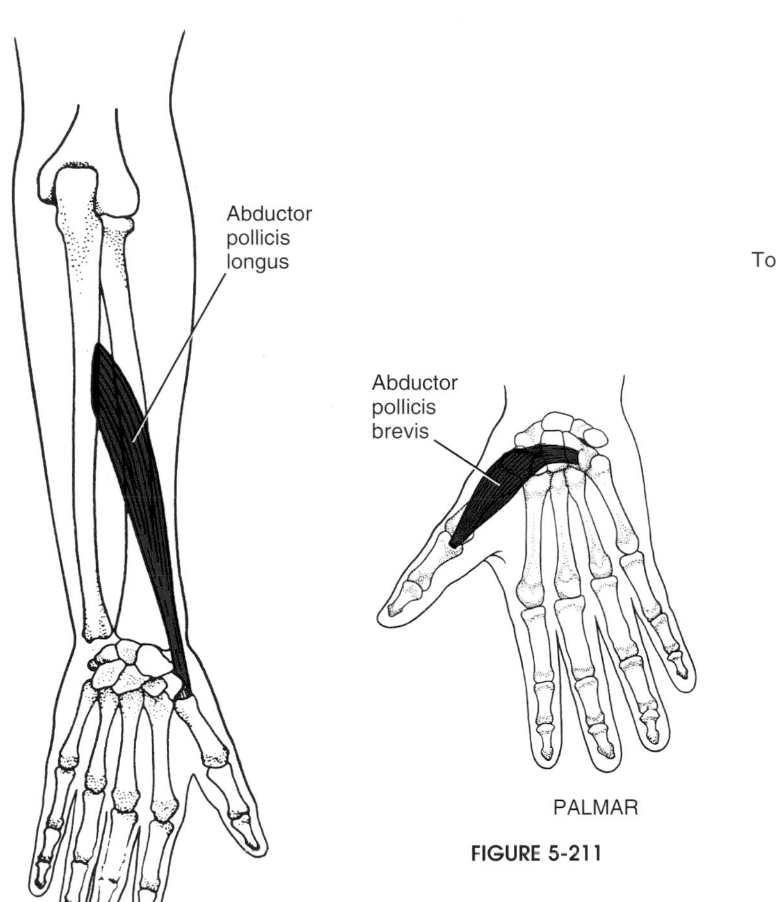

FIGURE 5-210

FIGURE 5-211

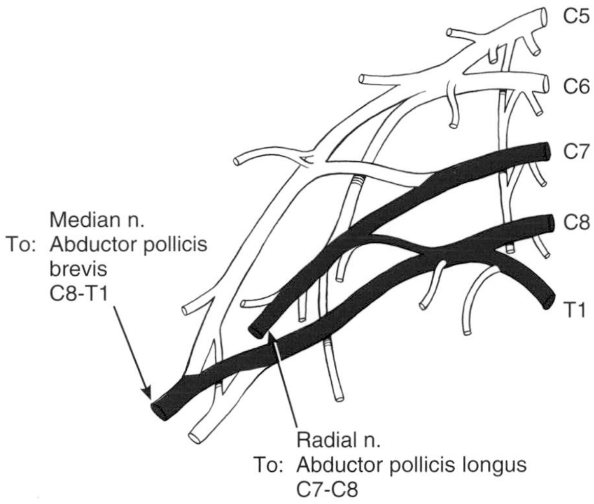

FIGURE 5-212

Range of Motion
0° to 70°

Table 5-26 THUMB ABDUCTION

I.D.	Muscle	Origin	Insertion
166	Abductor pollicis longus (radiolateral wall of "anatomical snuffbox")	Ulna (posterior surface laterally) Radius (shaft, middle 1/3 of posterior aspect) Interosseous membrane	Thumb: 1st metacarpal (radial side of base) Trapezium bone
171	Abductor pollicis brevis	Flexor retinaculum Scaphoid bone (tubercle) Trapezium bone (tubercle) Tendon of abductor pollicis longus	Medial fibers: Thumb (base of proximal phalanx, radial side) Lateral fibers: Extensor expansion of thumb
Others			
152	Palmaris longus		
168	Extensor pollicis brevis		
172	Opponens pollicis		

Grade 5 (Normal) to Grade 0 (Zero)

Position of Patient: Forearm supinated and wrist in neutral; thumb relaxed in adduction.

Position of Therapist: Stabilize the metacarpals of the four fingers and the wrist (Figure 5-213). Resistance is given on the distal end of the 1st metacarpal in the direction of adduction.

Test: Patient abducts the thumb away from the hand in a plane parallel to the finger metacarpals.

Instructions to Patient: "Lift your thumb straight up." Demonstrate motion to the patient.

Grading

Grade 5 (Normal) and Grade 4 (Good): Completes full range of motion against resistance. Distinguishing Grades 5 and 4 may be difficult.

Grade 3 (Fair): Completes full range of motion with no resistance.

Grade 2 (Poor): Completes partial range of motion.

Grade 1 (Trace): Palpate tendon of the abductor pollicis longus at the base of the first metacarpal on the radial side of the extensor pollicis brevis (Figure 5-214). It is the most lateral tendon at the wrist.

Grade 0 (Zero): No contractile activity.

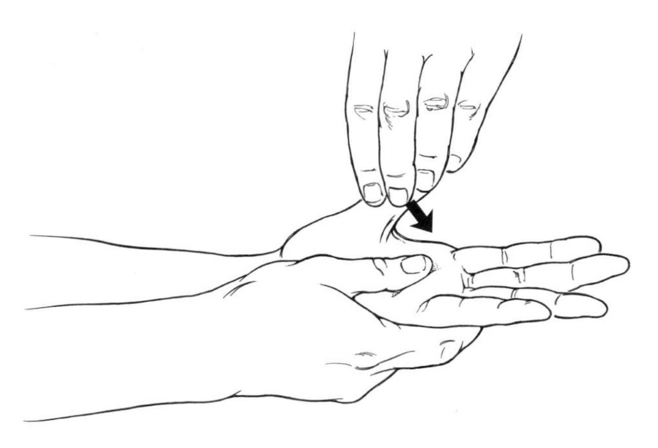

FIGURE 5-213

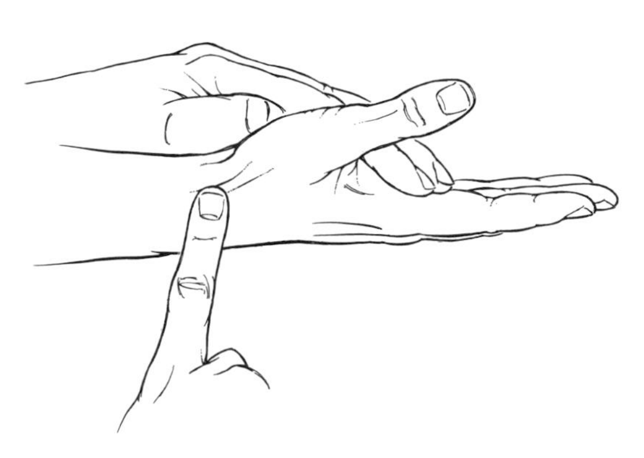

FIGURE 5-214

Substitution

The extensor pollicis brevis can substitute for the abductor pollicis longus. If the line of pull is toward the dorsal surface of the forearm (extensor pollicis brevis), substitution is occurring.

Helpful Hints

- If the abductor pollicis longus is stronger than the brevis, the thumb will deviate toward the radial side of the hand.
- If the abductor pollicis brevis is stronger, deviation will be toward the ulnar side.

Grade 5 (Normal), Grade 4 (Good), and Grade 3 (Fair)

Position of Patient: Forearm in supination, wrist in neutral, and thumb relaxed in adduction.

Position of Therapist: Stabilize the metacarpals (Figure 5-215) by placing the examiner's hand across the patient's palm with the thumb on the dorsal surface of the patient's hand (somewhat like a handshake but maintaining the patient's wrist in neutral). Apply resistance to the lateral aspect of the proximal phalanx of the thumb in the direction of adduction.

Test: Patient abducts the thumb in a plane perpendicular to the palm. Observe wrinkling of the skin over the thenar eminence and watch for the tendon of the palmaris longus to "pop out."

Instructions to Patient: "Lift your thumb vertically until it points to the ceiling." Demonstrate motion to the patient.

Grading

Grade 5 (Normal): Completes full range of motion with maximal finger resistance.

Grade 4 (Good): Tolerates moderate resistance.

Grade 3 (Fair): Completes full range of motion with no resistance.

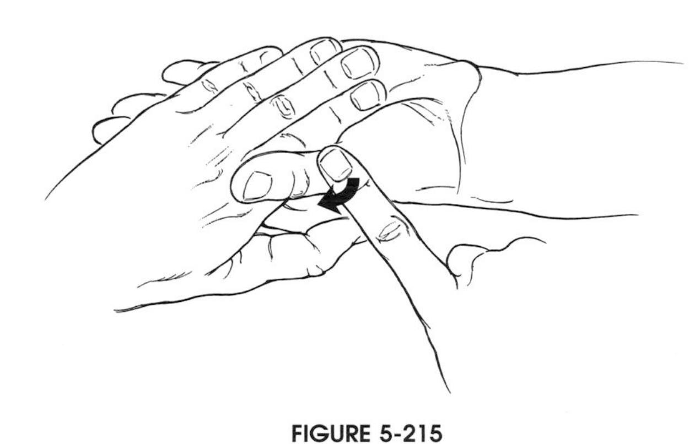

FIGURE 5-215

Grade 2 (Poor), Grade 1 (Trace), and Grade 0 (Zero)

Position of Patient: Forearm in midposition, wrist in neutral, and thumb relaxed in adduction.

Position of Therapist: Stabilize wrist in neutral.

Test: Patient abducts thumb in a plane perpendicular to the palm.

Instructions to Patient: "Try to lift your thumb so it points at the ceiling."

Grading

Grade 2 (Poor): Completes partial range of motion.

Grade 1 (Trace): Palpate the belly of the abductor pollicis brevis in the center of the thenar eminence, medial to the opponens pollicis (Figure 5-216).

Grade 0 (Zero): No contractile activity.

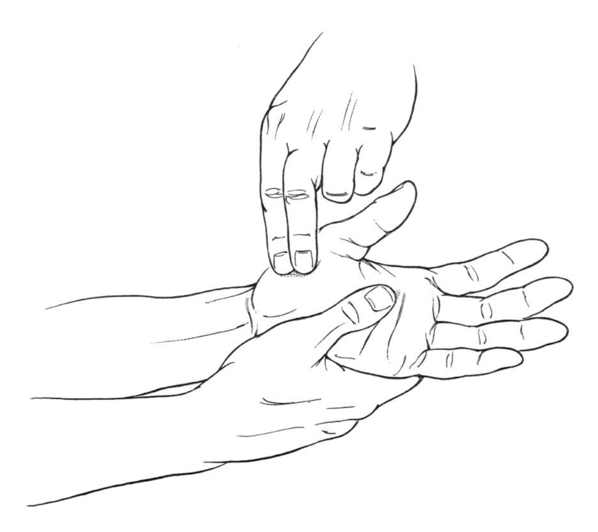

FIGURE 5-216

Substitution

If the plane of motion is not perpendicular, but toward the radial side of the hand, the substitution may be by the abductor pollicis longus.

THUMB ADDUCTION

(Adductor pollicis)

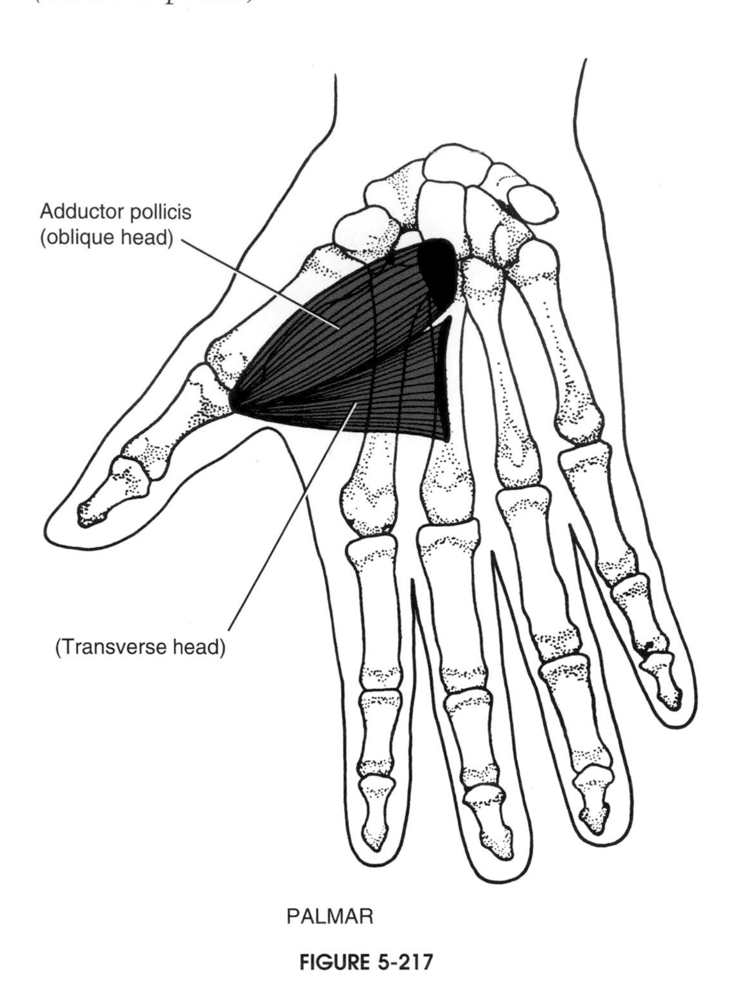

FIGURE 5-217

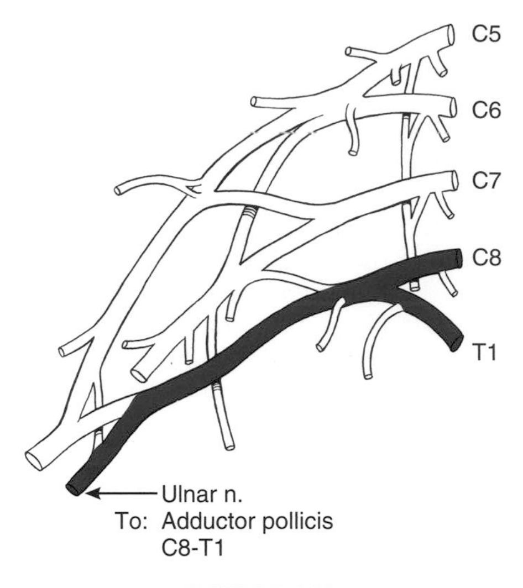

FIGURE 5-218

Range of Motion
70° to 0°

Table 5-27 THUMB ADDUCTION

I.D.	Muscle	Origin	Insertion
173	Adductor pollicis		Thumb (proximal phalanx, ulnar side of base)
	Oblique head	Capitate bone 2nd and 3rd metacarpals (bases) Palmar ligaments of carpal bones Sheath of tendon of flexor carpi radialis	
	Transverse head	3rd metacarpal bone (palmar surface of distal 2/3)	
Other			
164	1st dorsal interosseus		

(Adductor pollicis)

Grade 5 (Normal), Grade 4 (Good), and Grade 3 (Fair)

Position of Patient: Forearm in pronation, wrist in neutral, and thumb relaxed and hanging down in abduction.

Position of Therapist: Stabilize the metacarpals of the four fingers by grasping the patient's hand around the ulnar side (Figure 5-219). Resistance is given on the medial side of the proximal phalanx of the thumb in the direction of abduction.

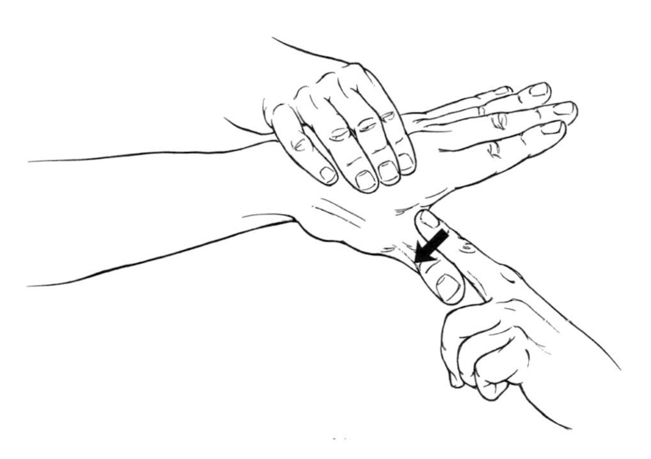

FIGURE 5-219

Test: Patient adducts the thumb by bringing the 1st metacarpal up to the 2nd metacarpal. Alternatively, place a sheet of paper between the thumb and the 2nd metacarpal (palmar pinch) and ask the patient to hold it while you try to pull the paper away.

Instructions to Patient: "Bring your thumb up to your index finger." Demonstrate motion to the patient.

Grading

Grade 5 (Normal) and Grade 4 (Good): Completes full range of motion and holds against maximal resistance. Patient can resist rigidly (Grade 5), or the muscle yields (Grade 4).

Grade 3 (Fair): Completes full range of motion with no resistance.

THUMB ADDUCTION

(Adductor pollicis)

Grade 2 (Poor) and Grade 1 (Trace)

Position of Patient: Forearm in midposition, wrist in neutral resting on table, and thumb in abduction.

Position of Therapist: Stabilize wrist on the table, and use a hand to stabilize the finger metacarpals (Figure 5-220).

Test: Patient moves thumb horizontally in adduction. The end position is shown in Figure 5-220.

Instructions to Patient: "Return your thumb to its place next to your index finger." Demonstrate motion to patient.

Grading

Grade 2 (Poor): Completes full range of motion.

Grade 1 (Trace): Palpate the adductor pollicis on the palmar side of the web space of the thumb by grasping the web between the index finger and thumb (Figure 5-221). The adductor lies between the first dorsal interosseus and the first metacarpal bone. This muscle is difficult to palpate, and the therapist may have to ask the patient to perform a palmar pinch to assist in its location.

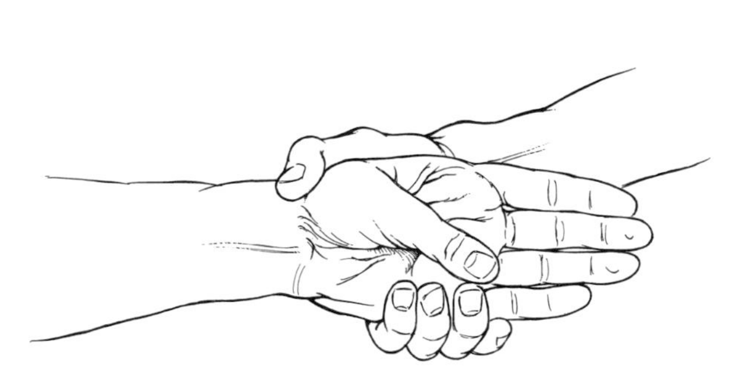

FIGURE 5-220

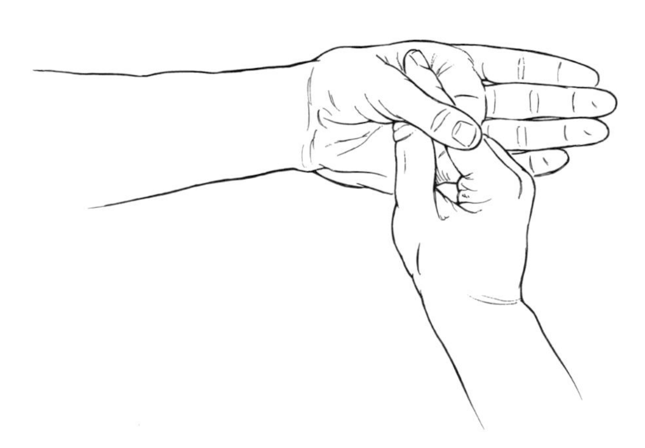

FIGURE 5-221

Substitutions

- The flexor pollicis longus and the flexor pollicis brevis will flex the thumb, drawing it across the palm. These muscles should be kept inactive during the adduction test.
- The extensor pollicis longus may attempt to substitute for the thumb adductor, in which case the CMC joint will extend.

(Opponens pollicis and Opponens digiti minimi)

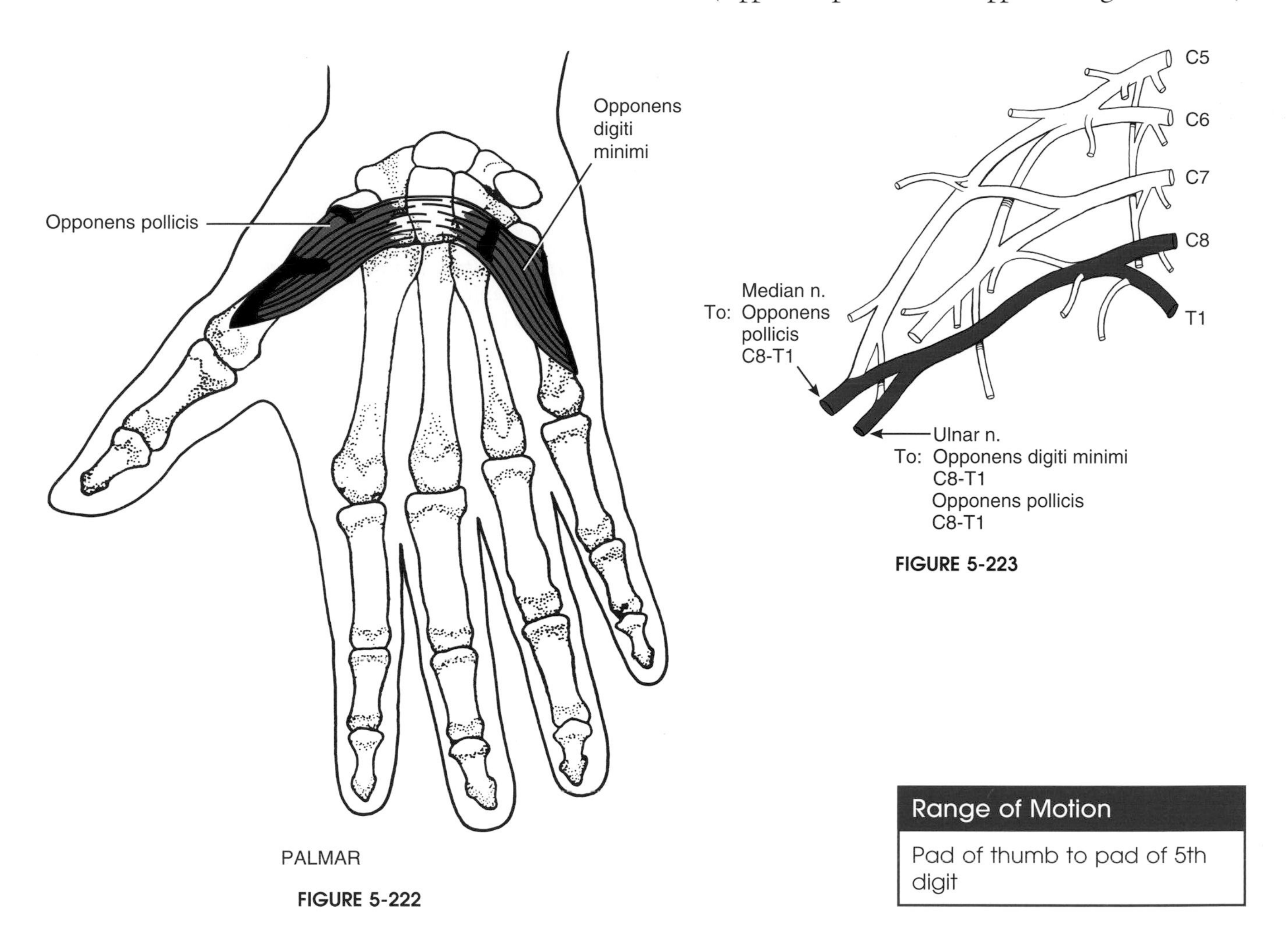

FIGURE 5-222

FIGURE 5-223

Range of Motion

Pad of thumb to pad of 5th digit

Table 5-28 OPPOSITION (THUMB TO LITTLE FINGER)

I.D.	Muscle	Origin	Insertion
172	Opponens pollicis	Trapezium bone (tubercle) Flexor retinaculum	1st metacarpal (entire length of lateral border and adjoining lateral half of palmar surface)
161	Opponens digiti minimi	Hamate (hook) Flexor retinaculum	5th metacarpal (whole length of ulnar margin and adjacent palmar surface)
Others			
171	Abductor pollicis brevis		
170	Flexor pollicis brevis		

OPPOSITION (THUMB TO LITTLE FINGER)

(Opponens pollicis and Opponens digiti minimi)

This motion is a combination of abduction, flexion, and medial rotation of the thumb (Figure 5-224).

The two muscles in thumb-to-fifth-digit opposition (opponens pollicis and opponens digiti minimi) should not be tested together and also should be graded separately.

Grade 5 (Normal) to Grade 0 (Zero)

Position of Patient: Forearm is supinated, wrist in neutral, and thumb in adduction with MP and IP flexion.

Position of Therapist: Stabilize the hand by holding the wrist on the dorsal surface. The examiner may prefer the hand to be stabilized on the table.

Opponens pollicis: Apply resistance for the opponens pollicis at the head of the 1st metacarpal in the direction of lateral rotation, extension, and adduction (see Figure 5-224).

Opponens digiti minimi: Give resistance for the opponens digiti minimi on the palmar surface of the 5th metacarpal in the direction of medial rotation (flattening the palm) (Figure 5-225).

Test: Patient raises the thumb away from the palm and rotates it so that its distal phalanx opposes the distal phalanx of the little finger. Such apposition must be pad to pad and not tip to tip. Opposition also can be evaluated by asking the patient to hold an object between the thumb and little finger (in opposition), which the examiner tries to pull away.

Instructions to Patient: "Bring your thumb to your little finger and touch the two pads, forming the letter 'O' with your thumb and little finger." Demonstrate motion to the patient and require practice.

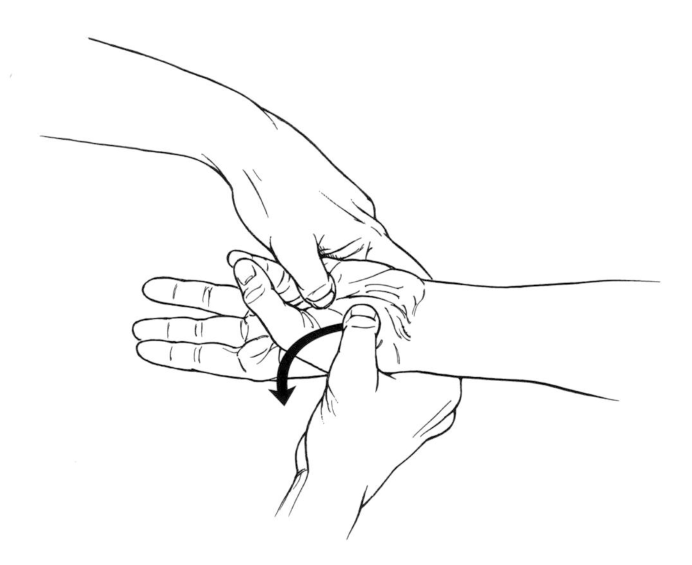

FIGURE 5-224

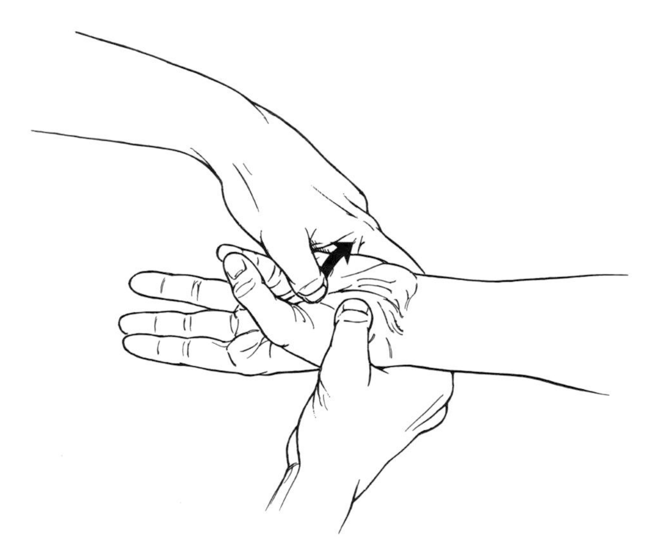

FIGURE 5-225

Grade 5 (Normal) to Grade 0 (Zero) Continued

Grading

Grade 5 (Normal): Completes the full motion correctly against maximal thumb resistance.

Grade 4 (Good): Completes the range against moderate resistance.

Grade 3 (Fair): Moves thumb and 5th digit through full range of opposition with no resistance.

Grade 2 (Poor): Moves through range of opposition. (The two opponens muscles are evaluated separately.)

Grade 1 (Trace): Palpate the opponens pollicis along the radial shaft of the 1st metacarpal (Figure 5-226). It lies lateral to the abductor pollicis brevis. During Grades 5 and 4 contractions, the examiner will have difficulty in palpating the opponens pollicis because of nearby muscles. In Grade 3 muscles and below, the weaker contractions do not obscure palpation.

Palpate the opponens digiti minimi on the hypothenar eminence on the radial side of the 5th metacarpal (Figure 5-227). Be careful not to cover the muscle with the finger or thumb used for palpation lest any contractile activity be missed.

Grade 0 (Zero): No contractile activity.

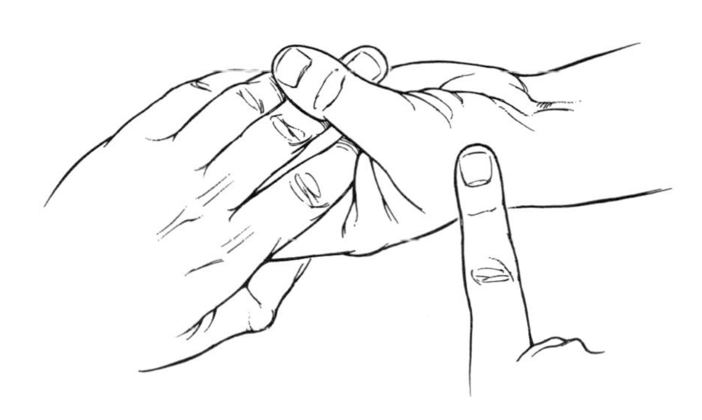

FIGURE 5-226

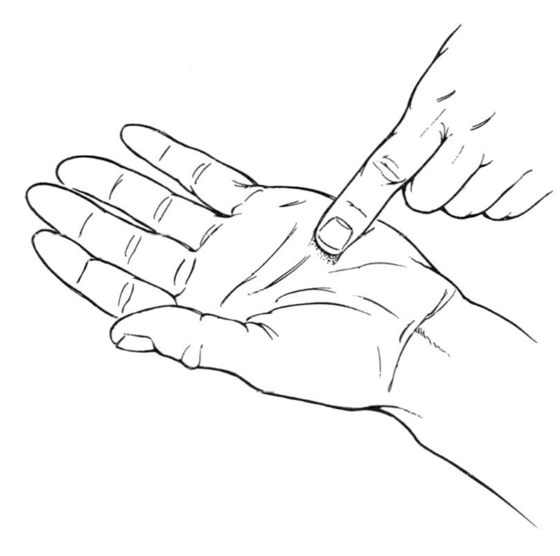

FIGURE 5-227

Substitutions

- The flexor pollicis longus and the flexor pollicis brevis can draw the thumb across the palm toward the little finger. If such motion occurs in the plane of the palm, it is not opposition; contact will be at the tips, not the pads, of the digits.
- Thc abductor pollicis brevis may substitute, but the rotation component of the motion will not be present.

REFERENCES

Cited References

1. Kendall FP, McCreary EK, Provance PG, et al. Muscles: Testing and Function with Posture and Pain. 5th ed. Baltimore, MD: Lippincott, Williams & Wilkins; 2005: 297-305.
2. Cleland J, Koppenhaver S. Netter's Orthopedic Clinical Examination: An Evidence-based Approach. 2nd ed. Philadelphia, PA: Saunders; 2010.
3. Smith J, Padgett DJ, Kaufman KR, et al. Rhomboid muscle electromyography activity during 3 different manual muscle tests. Arch Phys Med Rehabil. 2004;85:987-992.
4. De Freias V, Vitti M, Furlani J. Electromyographic study of levator scapulae and rhomboideus major muscles in movements of the shoulder and arm. Electromyogr Clin Neurophysiol. 1980;20:205-216.
5. Hegedus EJ, Goode A, Campbell S, et al. Physical examination tests of the shoulder: a systematic review with meta-analysis of individual tests. Br J Sports Med. 2008;42: 80-92.
6. Holtby R, Razmjou H. Validity of the supraspinatus test as a single clinical test in diagnosing patients with rotator cuff pathology. J Orthop Sports Phys Ther. 2004;34: 194-200.
7. Ruckstuhl H, Krzycki J, Petrou N, et al. Shoulder abduction moment arms in three clinically important positions. J Shoulder Elbow Surg. 2009;18:632-638.
8. Kashiwaguchi S, Endo K, Matsuura T, et al. The most effective exercise for strengthening the supraspinatus muscle. Evaluation by magnetic resonance imaging. Am J Sports Med. 2002;30:374-381.
9. Wattanaprakornkul D, Halaki M, Boettcher C, et al. A comprehensive analysis of muscle recruitment patterns during shoulder flexion: an electromyographic study. Clin Anat. 2011;24:619-626.
10. Wickham J, Pizzari T, Stansfeld K, et al. Quantifying 'normal' shoulder muscle activity during abduction. J Electromyogr Kinesiol. 2010;20:212-222.
11. Wilk KE, Arrigo CA, Andrews JR. Current concepts: the stabilizing structures of the glenohumeral joint. J Orthop Sports Phys Ther. 1997;25:364-379.
12. Reinold MM, Wilk KE, Fleisig GS, et al. Electromyographic analysis of the rotator cuff and deltoid musculature during common shoulder external rotation exercises. J Orthop Sports Phys Ther. 2004;34:385-394.
13. Boettcher CE, Ginn KA, Cathers I. Which is the optimal exercise to strengthen the supraspinatus? Med Sci Sports Exerc. 2009;41:1979-1983.
14. Kronberg M, Németh G, Bröstrom LA. Muscle activity and coordination in the normal shoulder. Clin Orthop Rel Res. 1990;257:76-85.
15. Gerber C, Krushall RJ. Isolated rupture of the subscapularis tendon. Results of operative repair. J Bone Joint Surg Am. 1996;78:5-23.
16. Tokish JM, Decker MJ, Ellis HB, et al. The belly-press test for the physical examination of the subscapularis muscle: electromyographic validation in comparison to the lift-off test. J Shoulder Elbow Surg. 2003;12:427-430.
17. Matsuoka J, Berger R, Berglund LJ, et al. An analysis of symmetry of torque strength of the forearm under resisted forearm rotation in normal subjects. J Hand Surg. 2006; 31:801-805.
18. O'Sullivan LW, Gallwey TJ. Upper-limb surface electromyography at maximum supination and pronation torques: the effect of elbow and forearm angle. J Electromyogr Kinesiol. 2002;12:275-285.
19. Wong CK, Moskovitz N. New assessment of forearm strength: reliability and validity. Am J Occup Ther. 2010; 64:809-813.

Other Readings

Bagg SD, Forrest WJ. Electromyographic study of scapular rotation during arm abduction in the scapular plane. Am J Phys Med. 1986;65:111-124.

Basmajian JV, Travill J. Electromyography of the pronator muscles in the forearm. Anat Rec. 1961;139:45-49.

Basmajian JV. Muscles and Movements: A Basis for Human Kinesiology. 2nd ed. New York: Kriger; 1977.

Basmajian JV, DeLuca CJ. Muscles Alive. 5th ed. Baltimore, MD: Williams & Wilkins; 1985.

Bearn JG. An electromyographic study of the trapezius, deltoid, pectoralis major, biceps and triceps muscles during static loading of the upper limb. Anat Rec. 1961;140:103-108.

Bharihoke VB, Gupta M. Muscular attachments along the medial border of the scapula. Surg Radiol Anat. 1986;8: 1-13.

Catton WT, Gray JE. Electromyographic study of the action of the serratus anterior in respiration. J Anat. 1951;85:412.

Chang L, Blair WF. The origin and innervation of the adductor pollicis muscle. J Anat. 1985;140:381-388.

Close JR, Kidd CC. The functions of the muscles of the thumb, the index and long fingers. J Bone Joint Surg. 1969;51-A: 1601.

Decker MJ, Tokish JM, Ellis HB, et al. Subscapularis muscle activity during selected rehabilitation exercises. Am J Sports Med. 2003;31:126-134.

Ekstrom RA, Donatelli RA, Soderberg GL. Surface electromyographic analysis of exercises for the trapezius and serratus anterior muscles. J Orthop Sports Phys Ther. 2003;33: 247-258.

Greis PE, Kuhn JE, Schultheis J, et al. Validation of the lift-off test and analysis of subscapularis activity during maximal internal rotation. Am J Sports Med. 1996;24:589-593.

Inman VT, Saunders JB de CM, Abbott LC. Observations on the function of the shoulder joint. J Bone Joint Surg. 1944;26:1-30.

Jonsson B, Hagberg M. Effect of different working heights on the deltoid muscle. Scand J Rehab Med (Suppl). 1974;3: 26-32.

Kasai T, Chiba S. True nature of the muscular arch of the axilla and its nerve supply. Kaibogaku Zasshi. 1977;25:657-669.

Kido T, Itoi E, Lee SB, et al. Dynamic stabilizing function of the deltoid muscle in shoulders with anterior instability. Am J Sports Med. 2003;31:399-403.

Levy AS, Kelly BT, Lintner SA, et al. Function of the long head of the biceps at the shoulder: electromyographic analysis. J Shoulder Elbow Surg. 2001;10:250-255.

Lewis OJ. The comparative morphology of M. flexor accessorius and the associated flexor tendons. J Anat. 1962;96: 321-333.

Liu F, Carlson L, Watson HK. Quantitative abductor pollicis brevis strength testing; reliability and normative values. J Hand Surg. 2000;25A:752-759.

Long C. Intrinsic-extrinsic control of the fingers: electromyographic studies. J Bone Joint Surg. 1968;50-A:973-984.

Long C, Brown ME. Electromyographic kinesiology of the hand: muscles moving the long finger. J Bone Joint Surg. 1964;46-A:1683-1706.

Malanga GA, Jenp Y, Growney ES, et al. EMG analysis of shoulder positioning in testing and strengthening the supraspinatus. Med Sci Sports Exerc. 1996;28:661-664.

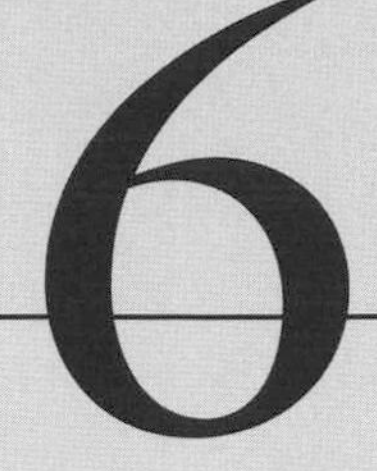

CHAPTER 6

Testing the Muscles of the Lower Extremity

HIP FLEXION

(Psoas major and Iliacus)

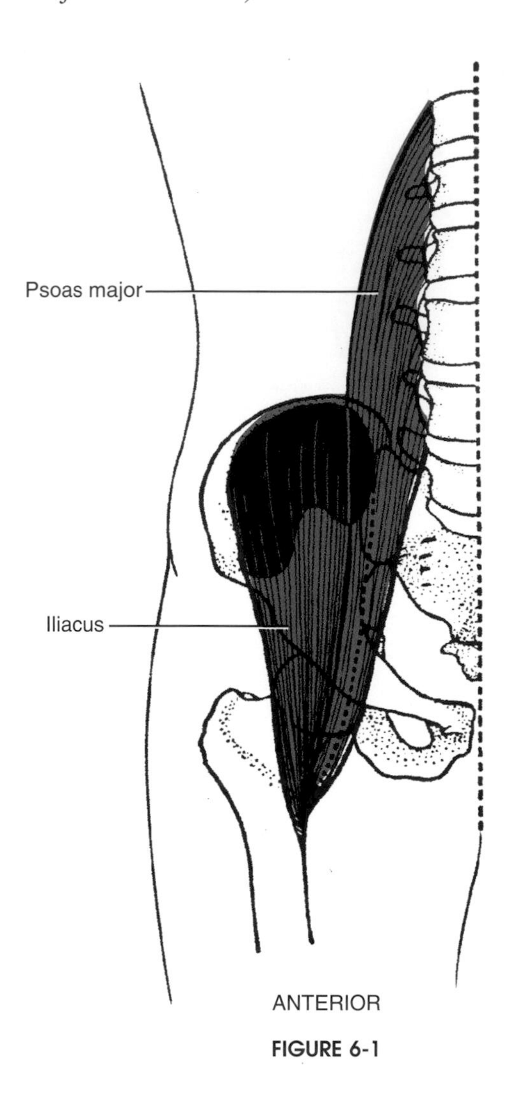

FIGURE 6-1

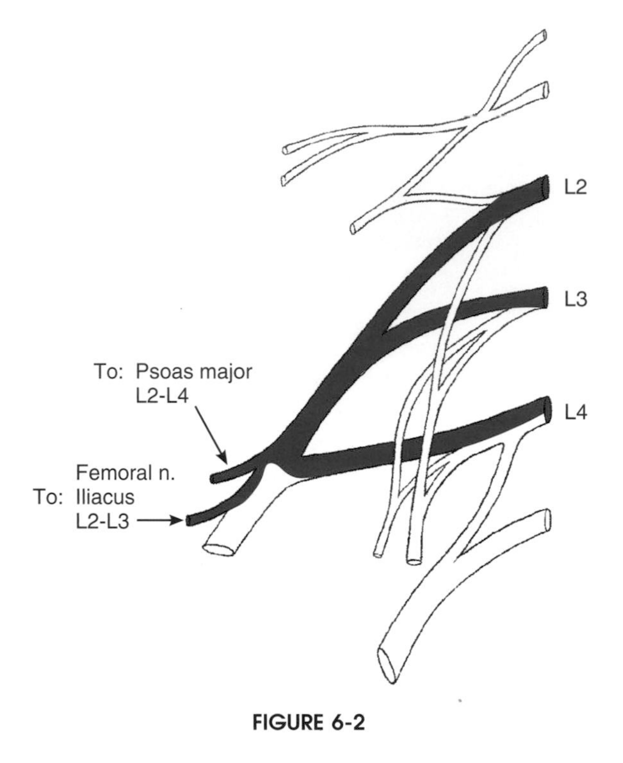

FIGURE 6-2

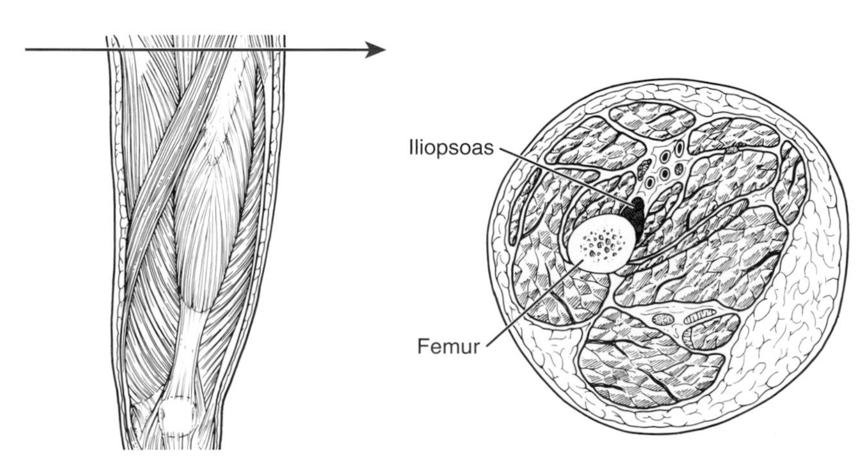

FIGURE 6-3 Arrow indicates level of cross section.

HIP FLEXION

(Psoas major and Iliacus)

Range of Motion
0° to 120°

Table 6-1 HIP FLEXION

I.D.	Muscle	Origin	Insertion
174	Psoas major	L1-L5 vertebrae (transverse processes) T12-L5 vertebral bodies (sides) and their intervertebral discs	Femur (lesser trochanter)
176	Iliacus	Iliac fossa (upper 2/3) Iliac crest (inner lip) Sacroiliac and iliolumbar ligaments Sacrum (upper lateral surface)	Femur (lesser trochanter; joins tendon of psoas major) Femoral shaft below lesser trochanter
Others			
196	Rectus femoris		
195	Sartorius		
185	Tensor fasciae latae		
177	Pectineus		
180	Adductor brevis		
179	Adductor longus		
181	Adductor magnus (superior fibers)		
183	Gluteus medius (anterior)		

HIP FLEXION

(Psoas major and Iliacus)

Grade 5 (Normal), Grade 4 (Good), and Grade 3 (Fair)

Position of Patient: Short sitting with thighs fully supported on table and legs hanging over the edge. Patient may use arms to provide trunk stability by grasping table edge or with hands on table at each side (Figure 6-4).

Position of Therapist: Standing next to limb to be tested. Contoured hand to give resistance over distal thigh just proximal to the knee joint (see Figure 6-4).

Test: Patient flexes hip to end of range, clearing the table and maintaining neutral rotation, holding that position against the therapist's resistance, which is given in a downward direction toward the floor.

Instructions to Patient: "Lift your leg off the table and don't let me push it down."

Grading

Grade 5 (Normal): Thigh clears table. Patient tolerates maximal resistance.

Grade 4 (Good): Hip flexion holds against strong to moderate resistance. There may be some "give" at the end position.

Grade 3 (Fair): Patient completes test range and holds the position without resistance (Figure 6-5).

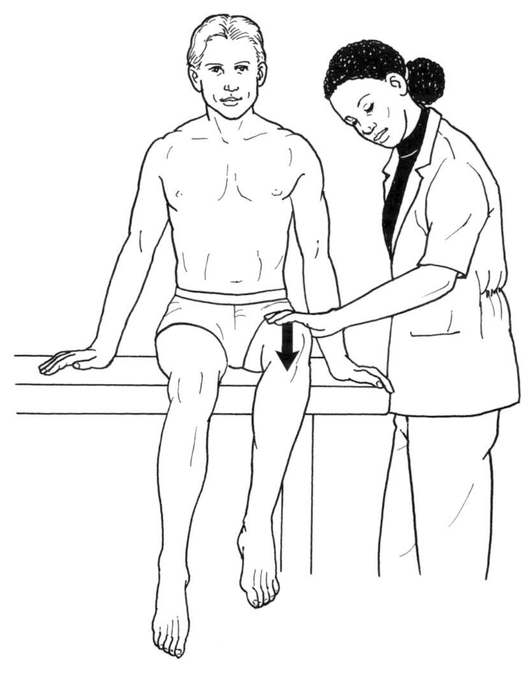

FIGURE 6-4

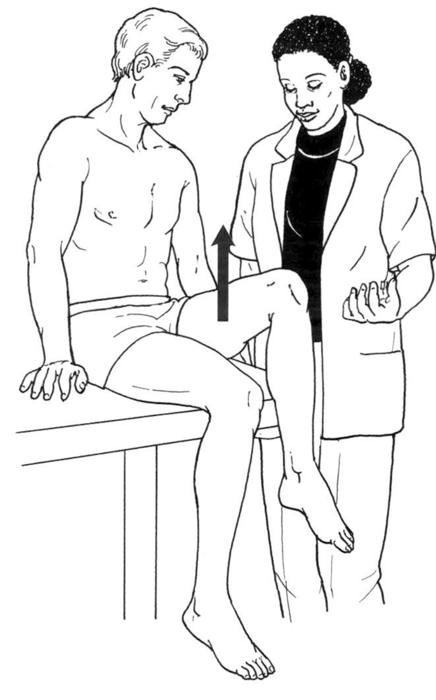

FIGURE 6-5

Helpful Hint

The position of the pelvis influences the action of the hip flexors. An anterior or posterior pelvic tilt influences the length tension of the hip flexors, thereby making them appear stronger or weaker. To eliminate the influence of the pelvis, the pelvis and spine should be in neutral as in Figure 6-4.

Grade 2 (Poor)

Position of Patient: Side-lying with limb to be tested uppermost and supported by therapist (Figure 6-6). Trunk in neutral alignment. Lowermost limb may be flexed for stability. A powder board may also be used to decrease friction.

Position of Therapist: Standing behind patient. Cradle test limb in one arm with hand support under the knee. Opposite hand maintains trunk alignment at hip (see Figure 6-6).

Test: Patient flexes supported hip. Knee is permitted to flex to prevent hamstring tension.

Instructions to Patient: "Bring your knee up toward your chest."

Grading

Grade 2 (Poor): Patient completes the range of motion in side-lying position.

Grade 1 (Trace) and Grade 0 (Zero)

Position of Patient: ***Supine:*** Test limb supported by therapist under calf with hand behind knee (Figure 6-7).

Position of Therapist: Standing at side of limb to be tested. Test limb is supported under calf with hand behind knee. Free hand palpates the muscle just distal to the inguinal ligament on the medial side of the sartorius (see Figure 6-7).

Test: Patient attempts to flex hip.

Instructions to Patient: "Try to bring your knee up to your nose."

Grading

Grade 1 (Trace): Palpable contraction but no visible movement.

Grade 0 (Zero): No palpable contraction of muscle.

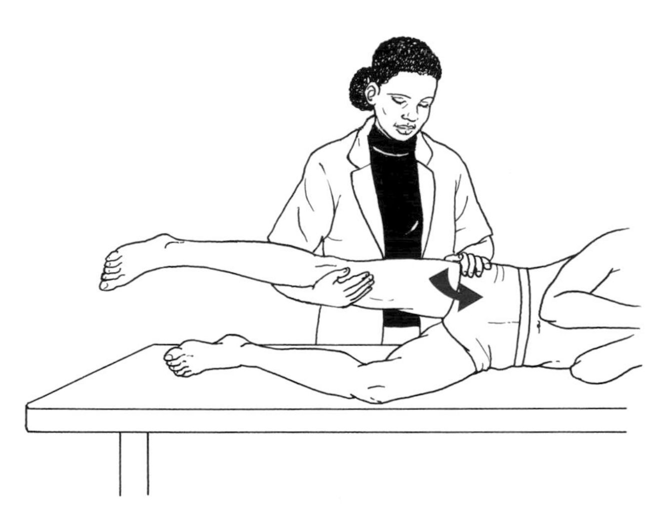

FIGURE 6-6

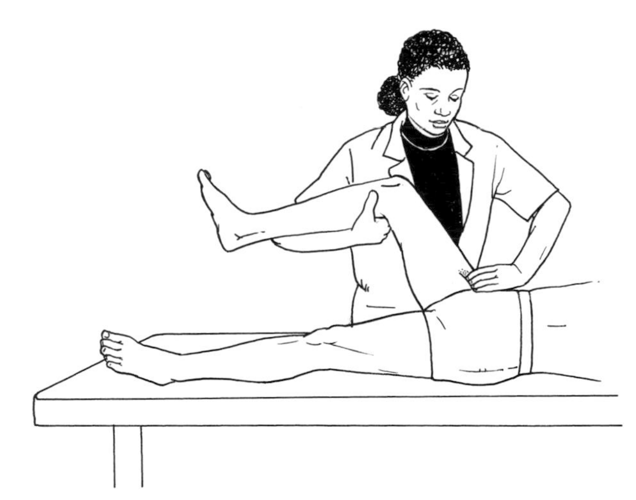

FIGURE 6-7

HIP FLEXION

(Psoas major and Iliacus)

Substitutions

- Use of the sartorius will result in external rotation and abduction of the hip. The sartorius, because it is superficial, will be seen and can be palpated along its entire length (Figure 6-8).
- If the tensor fasciae latae substitutes for the hip flexors, internal rotation and abduction of the hip will result. The tensor may be seen and palpated at its origin on the anterior superior iliac spine (ASIS).

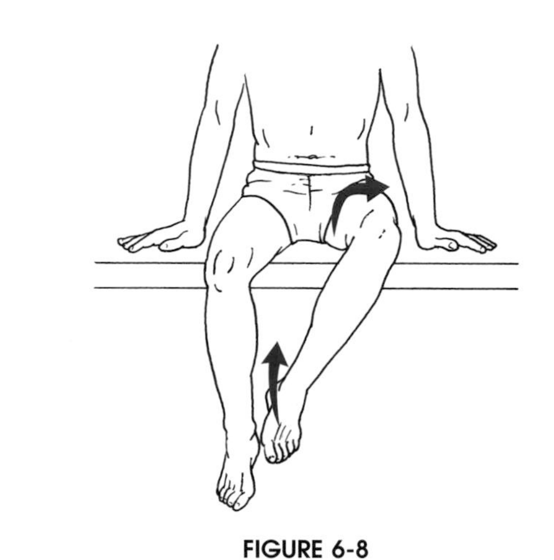

FIGURE 6-8

Helpful Hint

The hip flexors are rather small muscles and therefore do not provide a lot of force, especially as compared with the quadriceps or gluteus maximus. Therefore a negative break test is rarely achieved if using a straight arm technique. This is why Figure 6-4 shows the therapist with a bent arm while providing resistance. Experience is necessary to appreciate what constitutes a normal level of resistance.

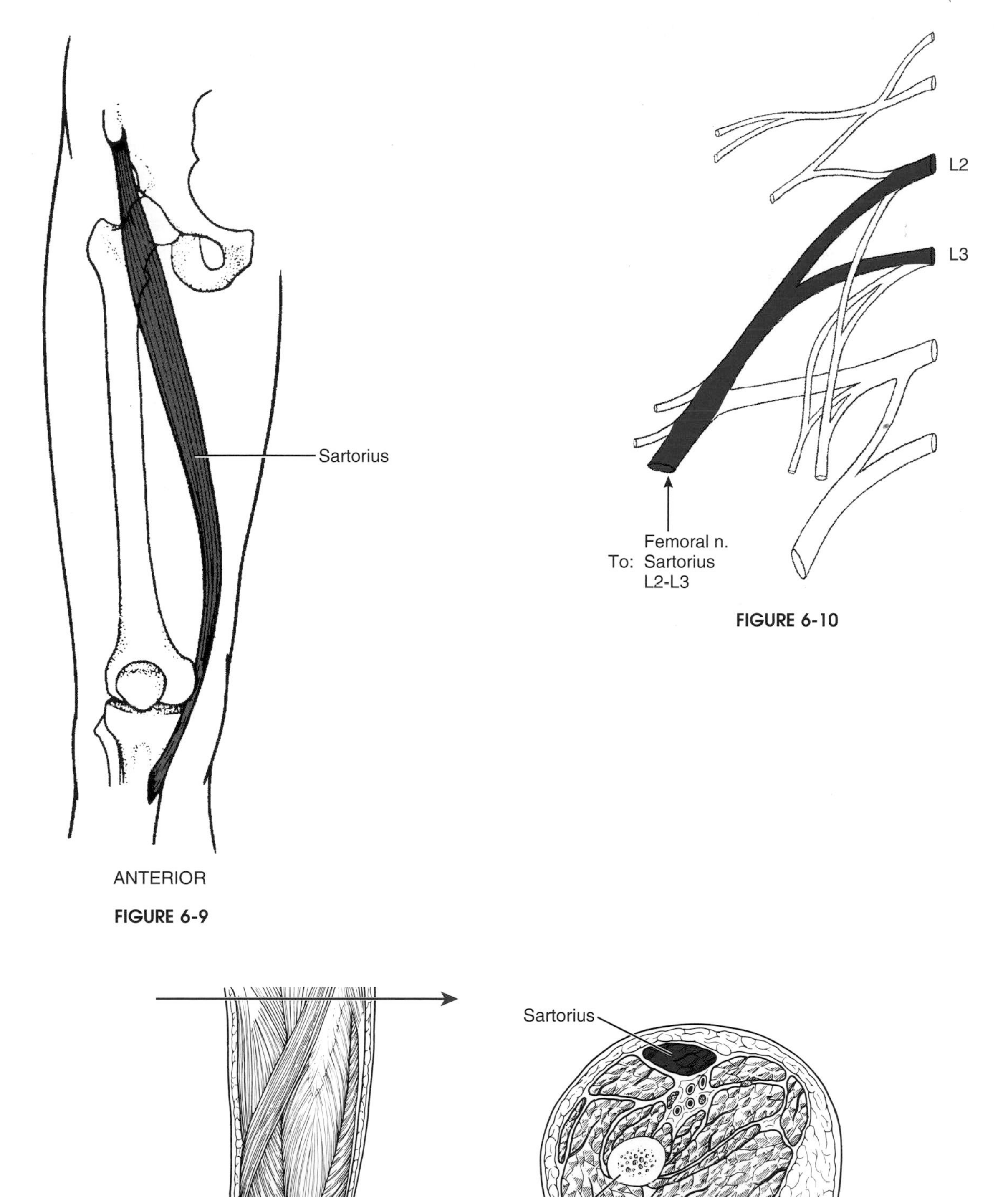

FIGURE 6-9

FIGURE 6-10

FIGURE 6-11 Arrow indicates level of cross section.

HIP FLEXION, ABDUCTION, AND EXTERNAL ROTATION WITH KNEE FLEXION

(Sartorius)

Range of Motion

Because this is a two-joint muscle, no specific range-of-motion value can be assigned solely to the sartorius.

Table 6-2 HIP FLEXION, ABDUCTION, AND EXTERNAL ROTATION

I.D.	Muscle	Origin	Insertion
195	Sartorius	Ilium (anterior superior iliac spine (ASIS)) Iliac notch below ASIS	Tibia (shaft, proximal medial surface) Capsule of knee joint (via slip) Medial side fascia of leg
Others			
Hip and knee flexors			
Hip external rotators			
Hip abductors			

Grade 5 (Normal), Grade 4 (Good), and Grade 3 (Fair)

Position of Patient: Short sitting with thighs supported on table and legs hanging over side. Arms may be used for support.

Position of Therapist: Standing lateral to the leg to be tested. Place one hand on the lateral side of knee; the other hand grasps the medial-anterior surface of the distal leg (Figure 6-12).

Hand at knee resists hip flexion and abduction (down and inward direction) in the Grades 5 and 4 tests. Hand at the ankle resists hip external rotation and knee flexion (up and outward) in Grades 5 and 4 tests. No resistance for Grade 3 test.

Test: Patient flexes, abducts, and externally rotates the hip and flexes the knee (see Figure 6-12).

Instructions to Patient: Therapist may demonstrate the required motion passively and then ask the patient to repeat the motion, or the therapist may place the limb in the desired end position.

"Hold it! Don't let me move your leg or straighten your knee."

Alternate instruction: "Slide your heel up the shin of your other leg."

Grading

Grade 5 (Normal): Holds end point against maximal resistance.

Grade 4 (Good): Tolerates moderate to heavy resistance.

Grade 3 (Fair): Completes movement and holds end position but takes no resistance (Figure 6-13).

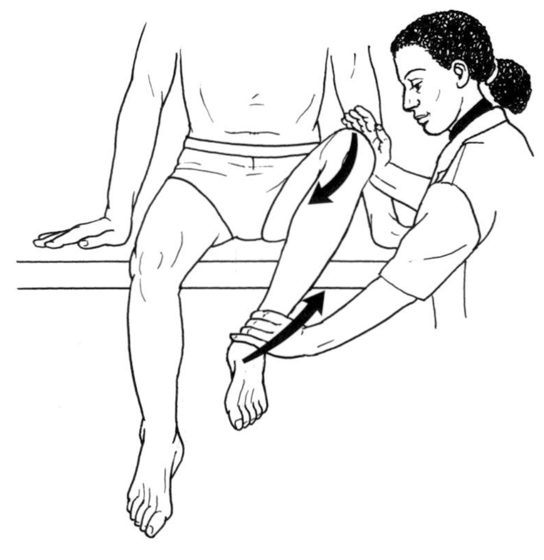

FIGURE 6-12

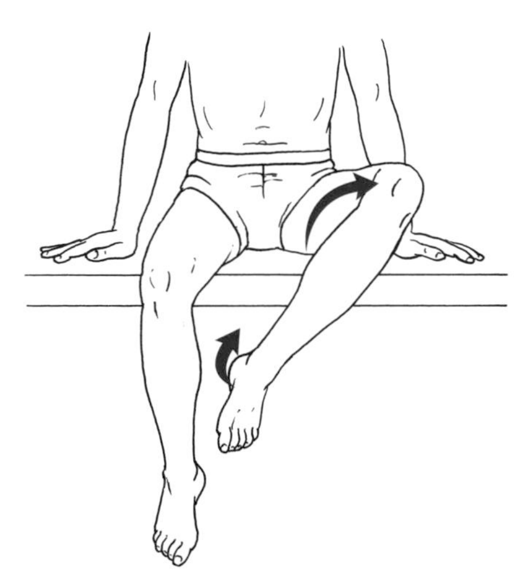

FIGURE 6-13

Grade 2 (Poor)

Position of Patient: Supine. Heel of limb to be tested is placed on contralateral shin (Figure 6-14).

Position of Therapist: Standing at side of limb to be tested. Support limb as necessary to maintain alignment.

Test: Patient slides test heel upward along shin to knee.

Instructions to Patient: "Slide your heel up to your knee."

Grading

Grade 2 (Poor): Completes desired movement.

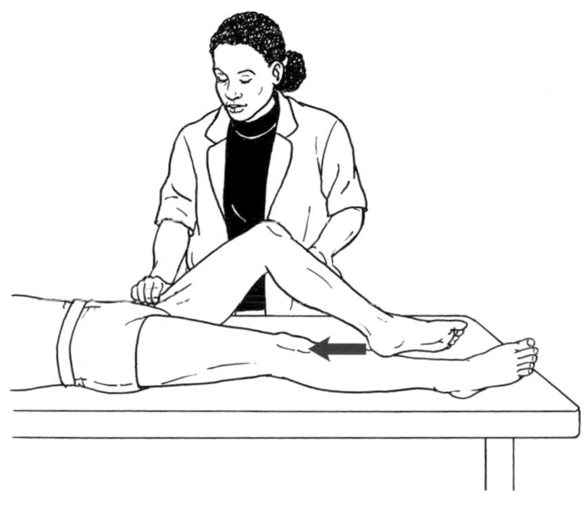

FIGURE 6-14

Grade 1 (Trace) and Grade 0 (Zero)

Position of Patient: Supine.

Position of Therapist: Standing on side to be tested. Cradle test limb under calf with hand supporting limb behind knee. Opposite hand palpates sartorius on medial side of thigh where the muscle crosses the femur (Figure 6-15). Therapist may prefer to palpate near the muscle origin just below the ASIS.

Test: Patient attempts to slide heel up shin toward knee.

Instructions to Patient: "Try to slide your heel up to your knee."

Grading

Grade 1 (Trace): Therapist can detect slight contraction of muscle; no visible movement.

Grade 0 (Zero): No palpable contraction.

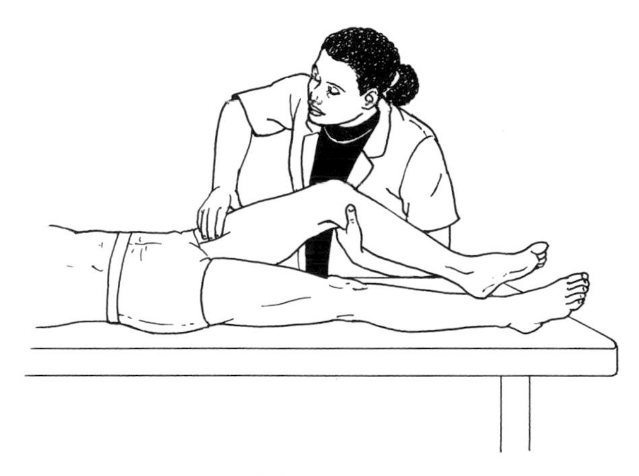

FIGURE 6-15

Helpful Hint

The therapist is reminded that failure of the patient to complete the full range of motion in the Grade 3 test is not an automatic Grade 2. The patient should be tested in the supine position to ascertain whether the correct grade is Grade 2 or less.

Substitution

Substitution by the iliopsoas or the rectus femoris results in pure hip flexion without abduction and external rotation.

HIP EXTENSION

(Gluteus maximus and Hamstrings)

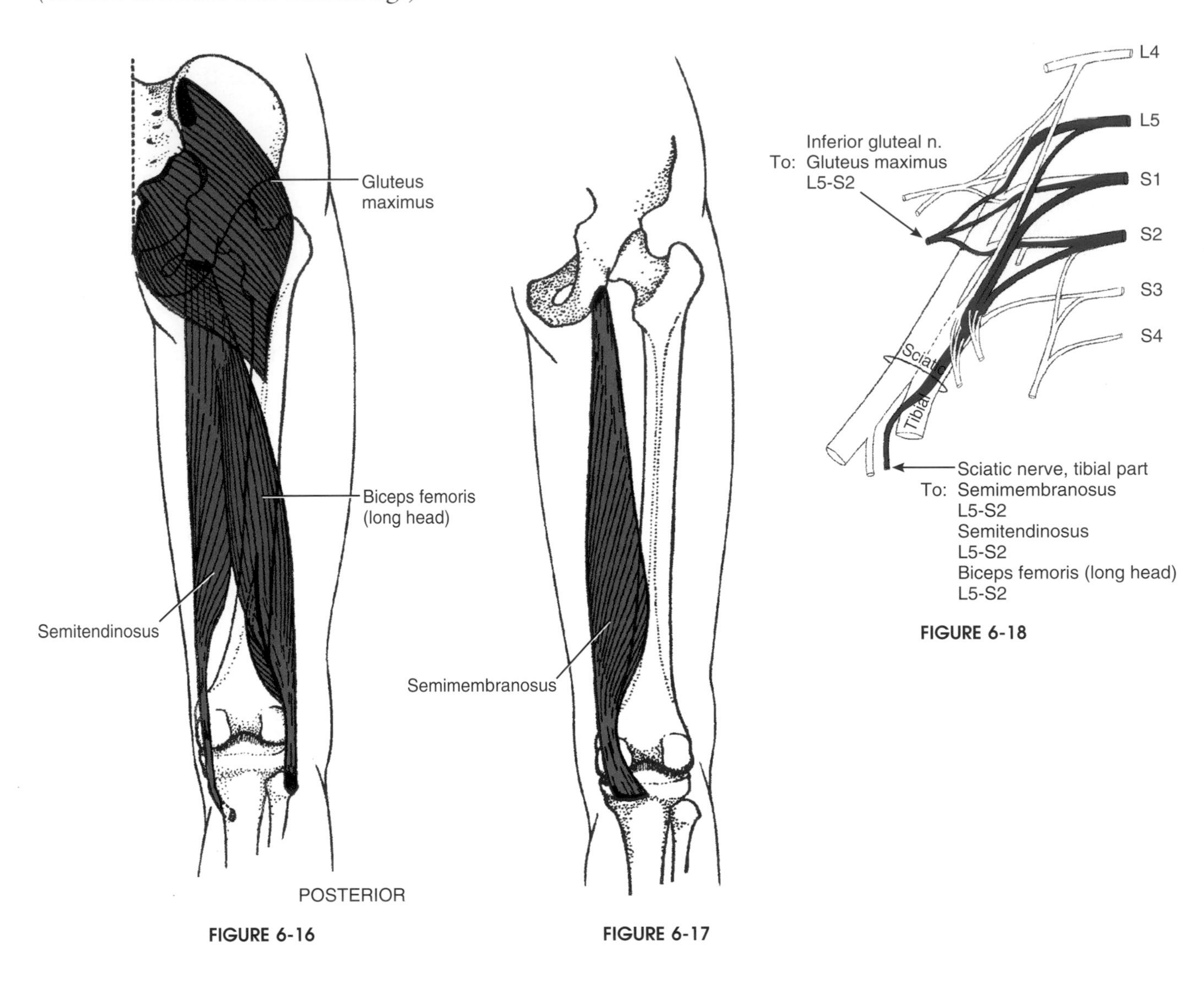

FIGURE 6-16

FIGURE 6-17

FIGURE 6-18

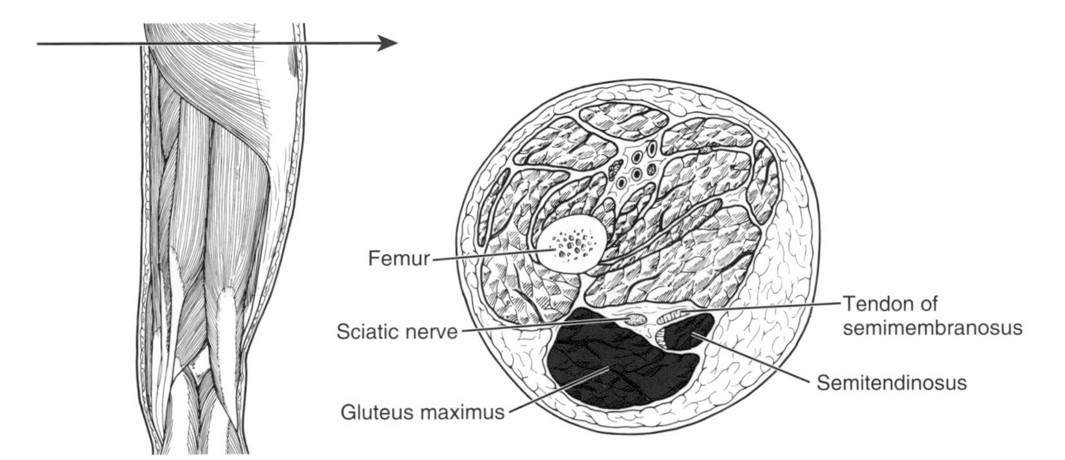

FIGURE 6-19 Arrow indicates level of cross section.

(Gluteus maximus and Hamstrings)

Range of Motion
0° to 20°
Some authors say as low as 0° to 5°.

Table 6-3 HIP EXTENSION

I.D.	Muscle	Origin	Insertion
182	Gluteus maximus	Ilium (posterior gluteal line) Iliac crest (posterior medial) Sacrum (dorsal surface of lower part) Coccyx (side) Sacrotuberous ligament Aponeurosis over gluteus medius	Femur (gluteal tuberosity) Iliotibial tract of fascia lata
193	Semitendinosus	Ischial tuberosity (upper area, inferomedial impression via tendon shared with biceps femoris) Aponeurosis (between the two muscles)	Tibia (proximal medial shaft) Pes anserinus
194	Semimembranosus	Ischial tuberosity (superolateral impression)	Tibia (medial condyle, posterior aspect) Oblique popliteal ligament of knee joint Aponeurosis over distal muscle (variable)
192	Biceps femoris (long head)	Ischial tuberosity (inferomedial impression via tendon shared with semitendinosus) Sacrotuberous ligament	Fibula (head) Tibia (lateral condyle)[1] Aponeurosis
Others			
181	Adductor magnus (inferior)		
183	Gluteus medius (posterior)		

HIP EXTENSION

(Gluteus maximus and Hamstrings)

Grade 5 (Normal), Grade 4 (Good), and Grade 3 (Fair) (Aggregate of all hip extensor muscles)

Position of Patient: Prone. Arms may be overhead or abducted to hold sides of table. (Note: If there is a hip flexion contracture, immediately go to the test described for hip extension modified for hip flexion tightness [see page 216].)

Position of Therapist: Standing at side of limb to be tested at level of pelvis. (Note: Figure 6-20 shows therapist on opposite side to avoid obscuring activity.)

The hand providing resistance is placed on the posterior leg just above the ankle. The opposite hand may be used to stabilize or maintain pelvis alignment in the area of the posterior superior spine of the ilium (see Figure 6-20). This is the most demanding test because the lever arm is longest.

Alternate Position: The hand that gives resistance is placed on the posterior thigh just above the knee (Figure 6-21). This is a less demanding test. Optimal resistance cannot be applied because of the shorter lever arm and so this test is not recommended.

Test: Patient extends hip through entire available range of motion. Resistance is given straight downward toward the floor. (No resistance is given in the Grade 3 test.)

Instructions to Patient: "Lift your leg off the table as high as you can without bending your knee (see Figure 6-20)."

Grading

Grade 5 (Normal): Patient completes available range and holds test position against maximal resistance.

Grade 4 (Good): Patient completes available range against strong to moderate resistance.

Grade 3 (Fair): Completes range and holds the position without resistance (Figure 6-22).

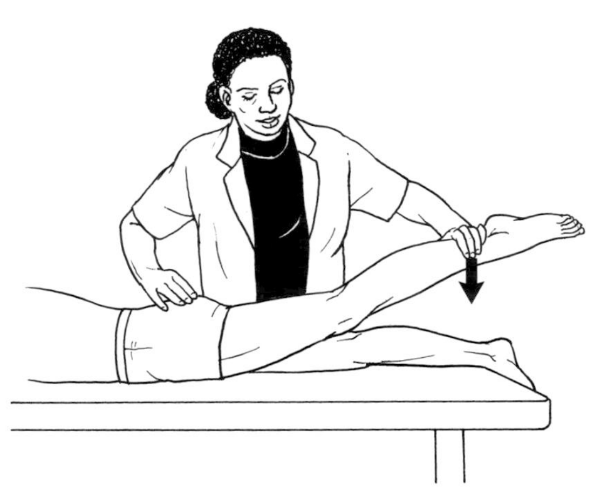

FIGURE 6-20

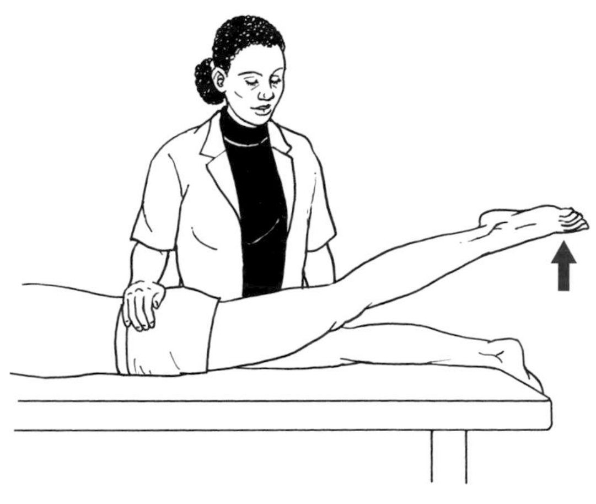

FIGURE 6-22

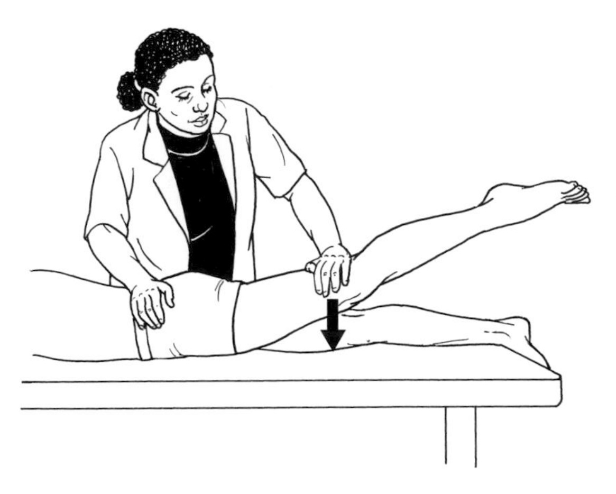

FIGURE 6-21

Helpful Hints

Knowledge of the ranges of motion of the hip is imperative before manual tests of hip strength are conducted. If the therapist does not have a clear idea of hip joint ranges, especially tightness in the hip flexor muscles, test results will be inaccurate. For example, in the presence of a hip flexion contracture, the patient must be standing and leaning over the edge of the table to test hip extension strength. This position (described on page 216) will decrease the influence of the flexion contracture and will allow the patient to move against gravity through the available range. The supine hip extensor test can also be used (see page 218).

Grade 2 (Poor)

Position of Patient: Side-lying with test limb uppermost. Knee straight and supported by therapist. Lowermost limb is flexed for stability.

Position of Therapist: Standing behind patient at thigh level. Therapist supports test limb just below the knee, cradling the leg (Figure 6-23). Opposite hand is placed over the pelvic crest to maintain pelvic and hip alignment.

Test: Patient extends hip through full range of motion.

Instructions to Patient: "Bring your leg back toward me. Keep your knee straight."

Grading

Grade 2 (Poor): Completes range of extension motion in side-lying position.

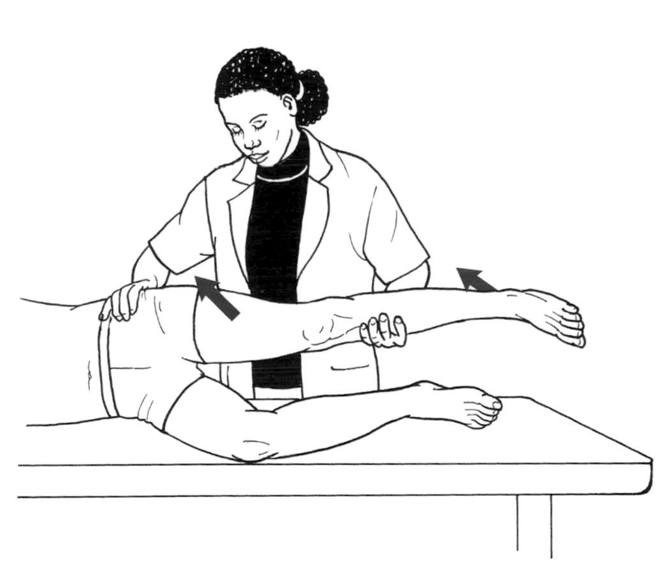

FIGURE 6-23

Grade 1 (Trace) and Grade 0 (Zero)

Position of Patient: Prone.

Position of Therapist: Standing on side to be tested at level of hips. Palpate hamstrings (deep into tissue with fingers) at the ischial tuberosity (Figure 6-24). Palpate the gluteus maximus with deep finger pressure over the center of the buttocks and also over the upper and lower fibers.

Test: Patient attempts to extend hip in prone position or tries to squeeze buttocks together.

Instructions to Patient: "Try to lift your leg from the table." OR "Squeeze your buttocks together."

Grading

Grade 1 (Trace): Palpable contraction of either hamstrings or gluteus maximus but no visible joint movement. Contraction of gluteus maximus will result in narrowing of the gluteal crease.

Grade 0 (Zero): No palpable contraction.

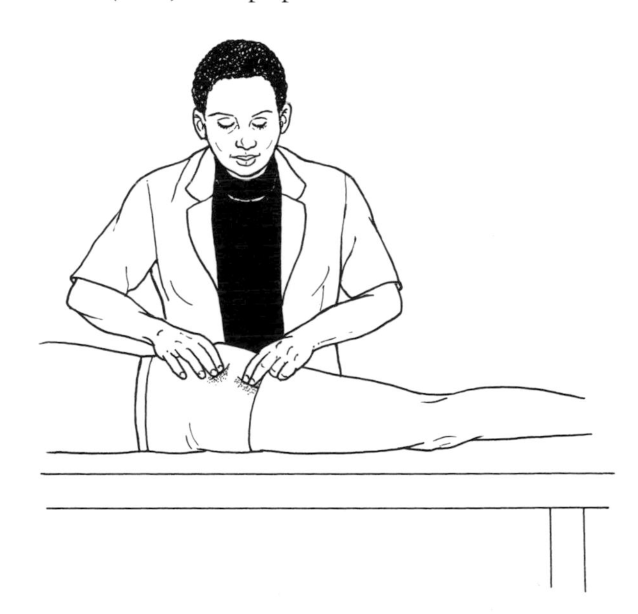

FIGURE 6-24

Helpful Hints

- Because of the strength of the gluteus maximus, it is imperative that the therapist achieve an optimal position for himself or herself, such as using a straight arm technique to apply as much force as the muscle can bear. See hip extensor test to isolate the gluteus maximus on page 214.
- The therapist should be aware that the hip extensors are among the most powerful muscles in the body, and most therapists will not be able to "break" a Grade 5 hip extension. Care should be taken not to overgrade a Grade 4 muscle.
- Care should be taken so that the patient does not rotate the trunk to increase motion or create added force production. Having the patient turn his or her head to the opposite side will help prevent trunk rotation.
- Be aware that isolating the hamstrings (page 240) may be a better indicator of hamstring strength.

(Gluteus maximus and Hamstrings)

HIP EXTENSION TEST TO ISOLATE GLUTEUS MAXIMUS

Grade 5 (Normal), Grade 4 (Good), and Grade 3 (Fair)

Position of Patient: Prone with knee flexed to 90°. (Note: In the presence of a hip flexion contracture, do not use this test but refer to the test for hip extension modified for hip flexion tightness [see page 216].)

Position of Therapist: Standing at the side to be tested at the level of the pelvis. (Note: The therapist in the illustration is shown on the wrong side to avoid obscuring test positions.) Hand for resistance is contoured over the posterior thigh just above the knee. The opposite hand may stabilize or maintain the alignment of the pelvis (Figure 6-25).

For the Grade 3 test, the knee may need to be supported in flexion (by cradling at the ankle).

Test: Patient extends hip through available range, maintaining knee flexion. Resistance is given in a new straight downward direction (toward floor).

Instructions to Patient: "Lift your foot to the ceiling." OR "Lift your leg, keeping your knee bent."

Grading

Grade 5 (Normal): Completes available range of motion and holds end position against maximal resistance.

Grade 4 (Good): Limb position can be held against heavy to moderate resistance.

Grade 3 (Fair): Completes available range of motion and holds end position but takes no resistance (Figure 6-26).

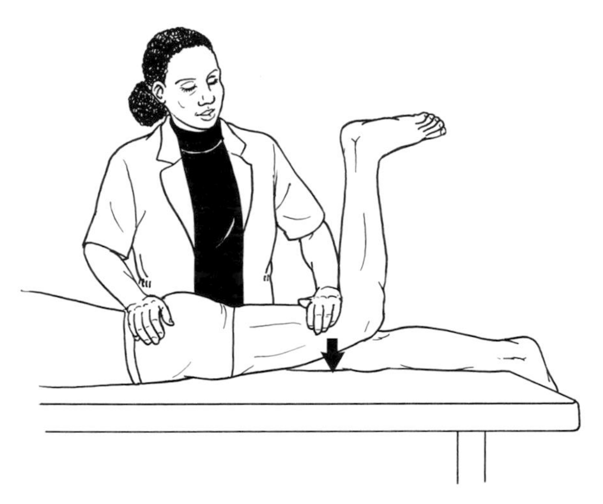

FIGURE 6-25

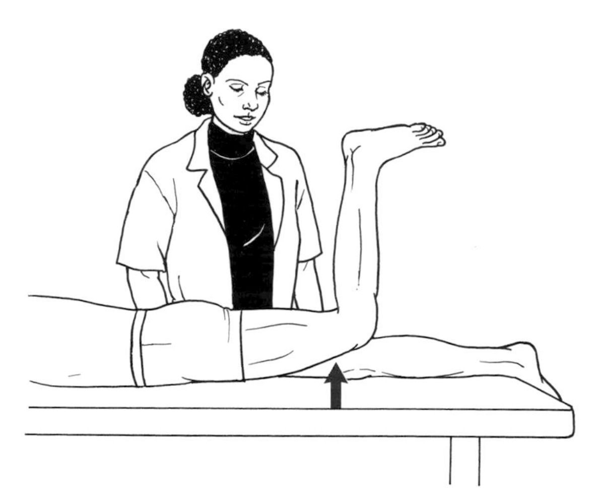

FIGURE 6-26

Grade 2 (Poor)

Position of Patient: Side-lying with test limb uppermost. Knee is flexed and supported by therapist. Lowermost hip and knee should be flexed for stability (Figure 6-27).

Position of Therapist: Standing behind the patient at thigh level. (Note: The therapist in the illustration is shown on the wrong side to avoid obscuring test positions.) Therapist cradles uppermost leg with forearm and hand under the flexed knee. Other hand is on pelvis to maintain postural alignment.

Test: Patient extends hip with supported knee flexed.

Instructions to Patient: "Move your leg back toward me."

Grading

Grade 2 (Poor): Completes available range of motion in side-lying position.

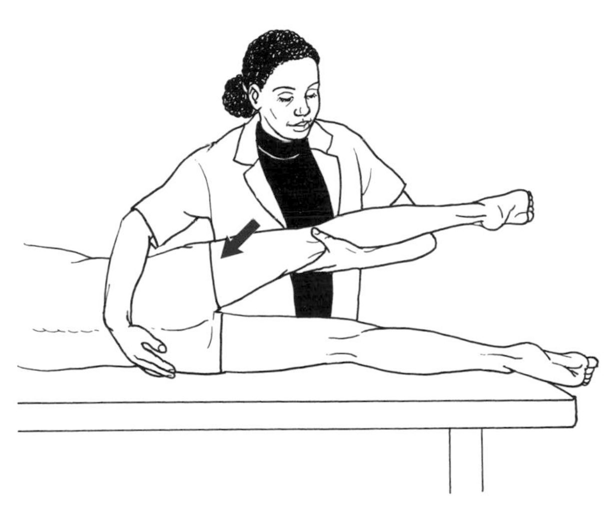

FIGURE 6-27

Grade 1 (Trace) and Grade 0 (Zero)

This test is identical to the Grades 1 and 0 tests for aggregate hip extension (see Figure 6-24). The patient is prone and attempts to extend the hip or squeeze the buttocks together while the therapist palpates the gluteus maximus.

Helpful Hints

- Hip extension range is less when the knee is flexed because of tension in the rectus femoris. A diminished range may be observed, therefore, in tests that isolate the gluteus maximus.
- Often, cramping will occur when the patient contracts the hamstrings during this test. The authors have found that flexing the knee to 70° or applying resistance in the middle of the muscle belly during the test will decrease the likelihood of a cramp.

HIP EXTENSION TESTS MODIFIED FOR HIP FLEXION TIGHTNESS

Grade 5 (Normal), Grade 4 (Good), and Grade 3 (Fair)

Position of Patient: Patient stands with hips flexed and places torso prone on the table (Figure 6-28). The arms are used to "hug" the table for support. The knee of the non-test limb should be flexed to allow the test limb to rest on the floor at the start of the test.

Position of Therapist: Standing at side of limb to be tested. (Note: Figure 6-28 shows the therapist on the opposite side to avoid obscuring test positions.) The hand used to provide resistance is contoured over the posterior thigh just above the knee. The opposite hand stabilizes the pelvis laterally to maintain hip and pelvis posture (see Figure 6-25).

Test: Patient extends hip through available range, but hip extension range is less when the knee is flexed. Keeping the knee in extension will test all hip extensor muscles; with the knee flexed, the isolated gluteus maximus will be evaluated.

Resistance is applied downward (toward floor) and forward.

Instructions to Patient: "Lift your foot off the floor as high as you can."

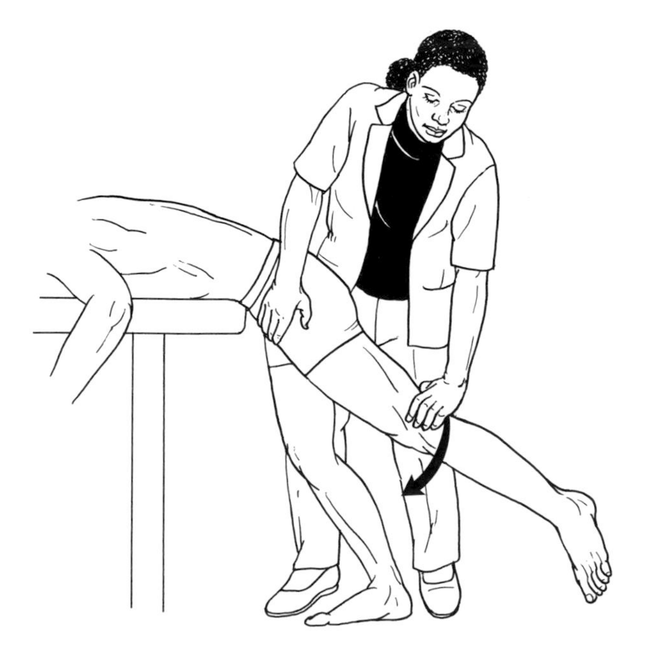

FIGURE 6-28

Grading

Grade 5 (Normal): Completes available range of hip extension. Holds end position against maximal resistance.

Grade 4 (Good): Completes available range of hip extension. (Note: Because of the intrinsic strength of these muscles, weakened extensor muscles frequently are overgraded.) Limb position can be held against heavy to moderate resistance.

Grade 3 (Fair): Completes available range and holds end position without resistance.

Grade 2 (Poor), Grade 1 (Trace), and Grade 0 (Zero)

Do not test the patient with hip flexion contractures and weak extensors (less than Grade 3) in the standing position. Position the patient side-lying on the table. Conduct the test as described for the aggregate of extensor muscles (see page 212) or for the isolated gluteus maximus (see page 214).

Helpful Hint

The modified hip extensor test is the preferred test for people who are not able or are unwilling to lay prone. This test may elicit a greater effort than the alternate supine hip extensor test.

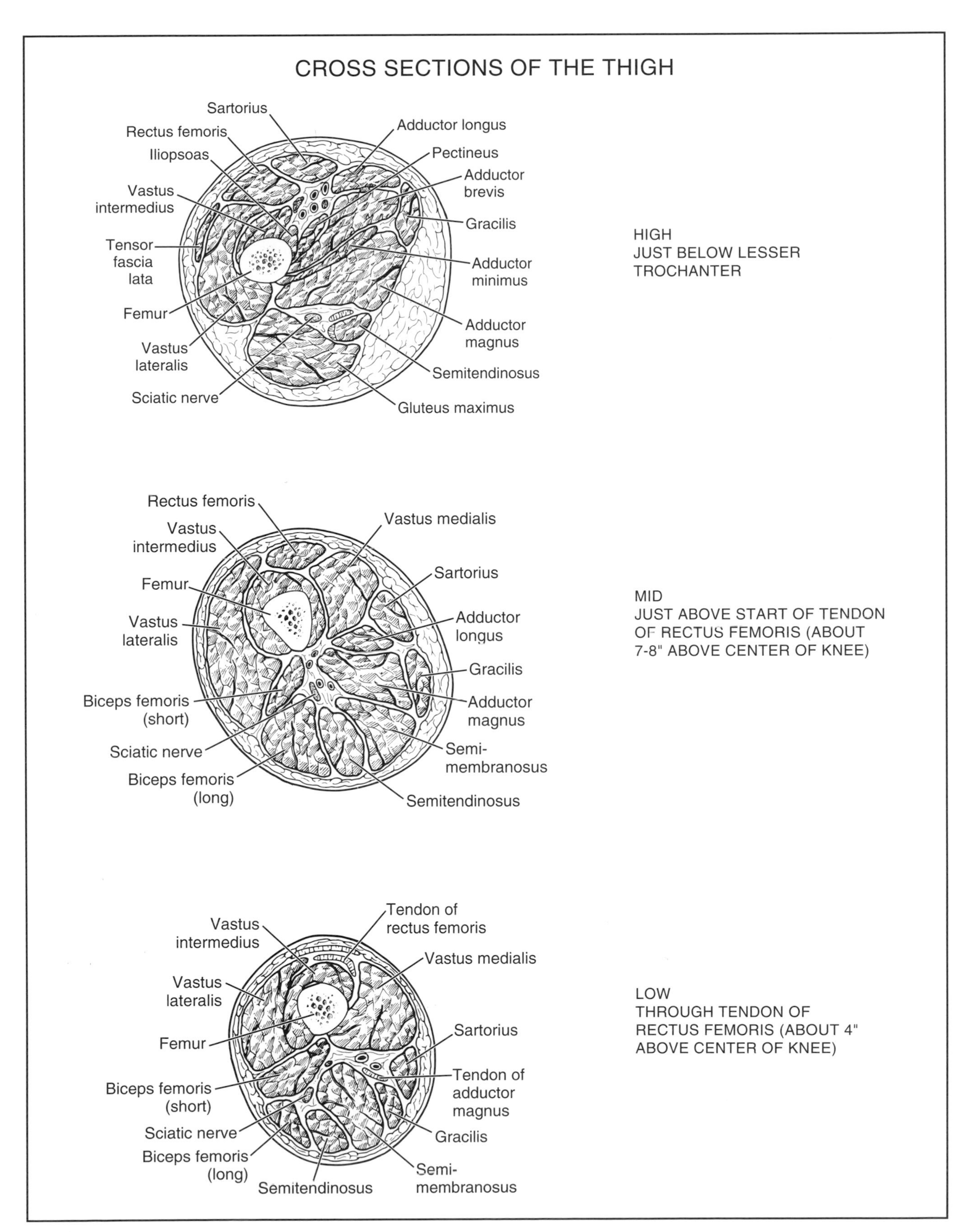
CROSS SECTIONS OF THE THIGH
Sartorius
Rectus femoris
Iliopsoas
Vastus intermedius
Tensor fascia lata
Femur
Vastus lateralis
Sciatic nerve
Adductor longus
Pectineus
Adductor brevis
Gracilis
Adductor minimus
Adductor magnus
Semitendinosus
Gluteus maximus
HIGH
JUST BELOW LESSER TROCHANTER
Rectus femoris
Vastus intermedius
Femur
Vastus lateralis
Biceps femoris (short)
Sciatic nerve
Biceps femoris (long)
Vastus medialis
Sartorius
Adductor longus
Gracilis
Adductor magnus
Semi-membranosus
Semitendinosus
MID
JUST ABOVE START OF TENDON OF RECTUS FEMORIS (ABOUT 7-8" ABOVE CENTER OF KNEE)
Vastus intermedius
Vastus lateralis
Femur
Biceps femoris (short)
Sciatic nerve
Biceps femoris (long)
Semitendinosus
Tendon of rectus femoris
Vastus medialis
Sartorius
Tendon of adductor magnus
Gracilis
Semi-membranosus
LOW
THROUGH TENDON OF RECTUS FEMORIS (ABOUT 4" ABOVE CENTER OF KNEE)

PLATE 6

HIP EXTENSION

(Gluteus maximus and Hamstrings)

SUPINE HIP EXTENSION TEST

An alternate hip extensor test is the supine hip extension test. This supine test may be substituted to eliminate change of patient position. Grades 5, 4, 3, and 2 have been validated in this position (n = 44 subjects) by measuring maximum hip extension torques recorded via a strain gauge dynamometer.[2]

Grade 5 (Normal), Grade 4 (Good), Grade 3 (Fair), and Grade 2 (Poor)

Position of Patient: Supine with heels off end of table. Arms folded across chest or abdomen. (Do not allow patient to push into table with upper extremities.) The patient's hip range should be measured to assure approximately 35 inches (approximately 65° of flexion). This is the distance the leg should be lifted during the test (Figure 6-29).

Position of Therapist: Standing at end of table. Both hands are cupped under the heel (Figure 6-30). The therapist should be in a position to resist this typically very strong muscle.

Test: Patient presses heel into therapist's cupped hands, attempting to maintain full extension of the limb as the therapist raises the limb approximately 35 inches from the table. No instructions are given for the opposite leg except to relax.

Instructions to Patient: "Don't let me lift your leg from the table. Keep your hip locked tight."

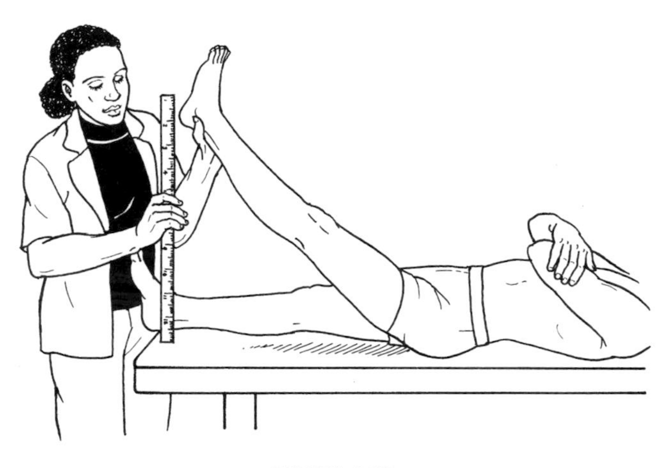

FIGURE 6-29

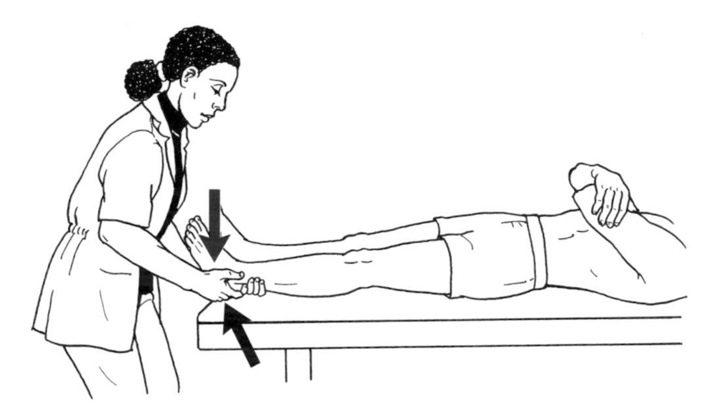

FIGURE 6-30

Grade 5 (Normal), Grade 4 (Good), Grade 3 (Fair), and Grade 2 (Poor) Continued

Grading

Grade 5 (Normal): Hip locks in neutral (full extension) throughout this test. Pelvis and back elevate as one locked unit as the therapist raises the limb (Figure 6-31). The opposite limb will rise involuntarily, illustrating a locked pelvis.

Grade 4 (Good): Hip flexes before pelvis and back elevate and lock as the limb is raised by the therapist. Hip flexion should not exceed 30° before locking occurs (Figure 6-32). The other leg will rise involuntarily, but will have some hip flexion because the pelvis is not fully locked.

Grade 3 (Fair): Full elevation of the limb to the end of straight-leg raising range (60° of hip flexion) with little or no elevation of the pelvis, demonstrated by the other leg remaining on the table. Therapist feels strong resistance throughout the test (Figure 6-33).

Grade 2 (Poor): Hip flexes fully with only minimal resistance felt (therapist should check to ensure that the resistance felt exceeds the weight of the limb; see Figure 6-33).

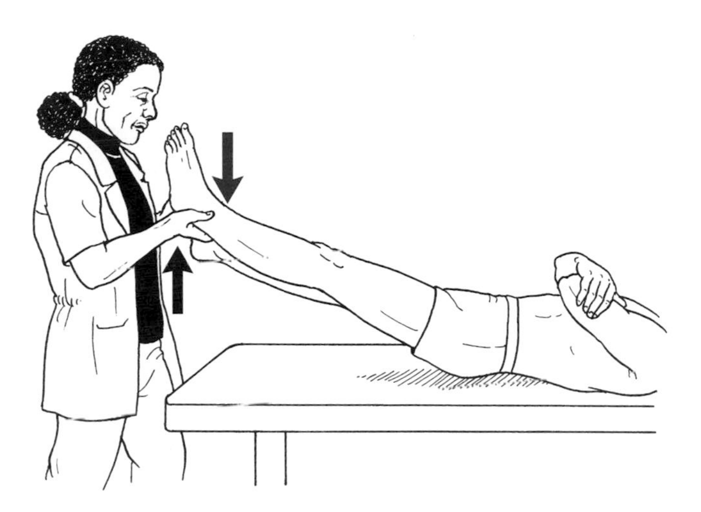

FIGURE 6-31

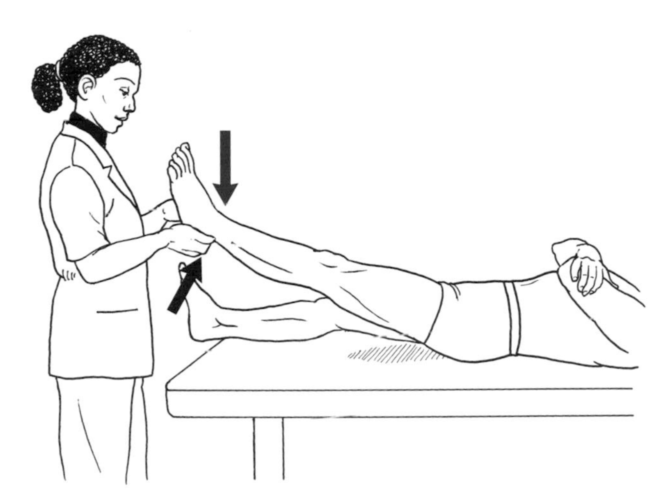

FIGURE 6-33

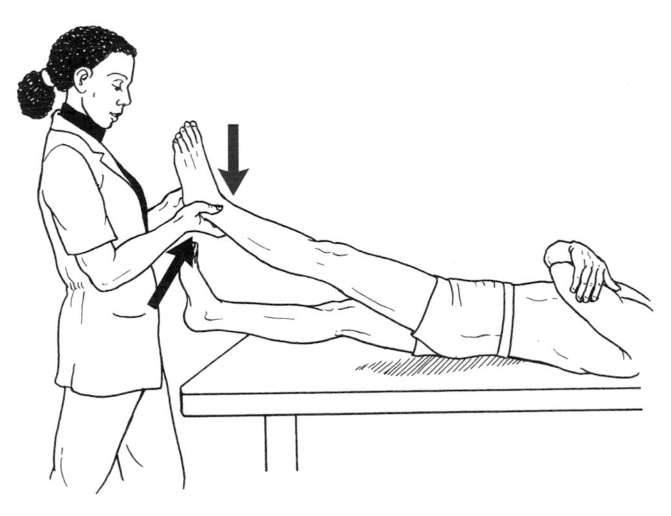

FIGURE 6-32

HIP ABDUCTION

(Gluteus medius and Gluteus minimus)

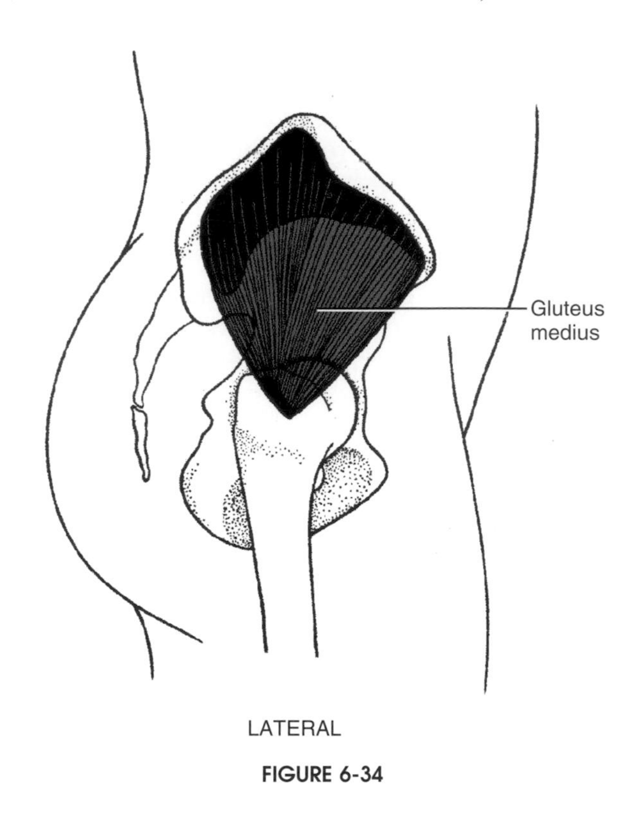

FIGURE 6-34

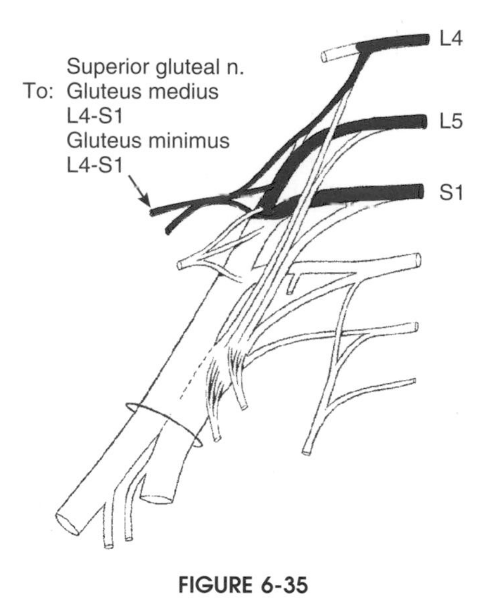

FIGURE 6-35

Range of Motion
0° to 45°

Table 6-4 HIP ABDUCTION

I.D.	Muscle	Origin	Insertion
183	Gluteus medius*	Ilium (outer surface between crest and anterior and posterior gluteal lines) Fascia (over upper part)	Femur (greater trochanter, lateral aspect)
184	Gluteus minimus	Ilium (outer surface between anterior and inferior gluteal lines) Greater sciatic notch	Femur (greater trochanter, anterolateral ridge) Fibrous capsule of hip joint
Others			
182	Gluteus maximus (upper fibers)		
185	Tensor fasciae latae		
187	Obturator internus (thigh flexed)		
189	Gemellus superior (thigh flexed)		
190	Gemellus inferior (thigh flexed)		
195	Sartorius		

*The greatest percentage of maximum voluntary contraction (MVC) in the gluteus medius was recorded during single limb stance when the subject was simultaneously abducting the opposite leg. This finding validates the gluteus medius as a pelvic stabilizer.[3,4]

Grade 5 (Normal), Grade 4 (Good), and Grade 3 (Fair)

Position of Patient: Side-lying with test leg uppermost. Start test with the limb slightly extended beyond the midline and the pelvis rotated slightly forward (Figure 6-36). Lowermost leg is flexed for stability.

Position of Therapist: Standing behind patient. Hand used to give resistance is contoured across the lateral surface of the knee. The hand used to palpate the gluteus medius is just proximal to the greater trochanter of the femur (see Figure 6-36). (No resistance is used in a Grade 3 test.)

To distinguish a Grade 5 from a Grade 4 result, first apply resistance at the ankle and then at the knee (Figure 6-37). Applying resistance at the ankle creates a longer lever arm, thus requiring more patient effort to resist the movement. If the patient cannot hold the limb in the test position with the resistance at the ankle but can at the knee, the grade is Grade 4. The therapist is reminded always to use the same lever in a given test sequence and in subsequent comparison tests.

Test: Patient abducts hip through the complete available range of motion without flexing the hip or rotating it in either direction. Resistance is given in a straight downward direction.

Instructions to Patient: "Lift your leg up in the air. Hold it. Don't let me push it down."

Grading

Grade 5 (Normal): Completes available range and holds end position against maximal resistance.

Grade 4 (Good): Completes available range and holds against heavy to moderate resistance or with resistance given at the knee.

Grade 3 (Fair): Completes range of motion and holds end position without resistance (Figure 6-38).

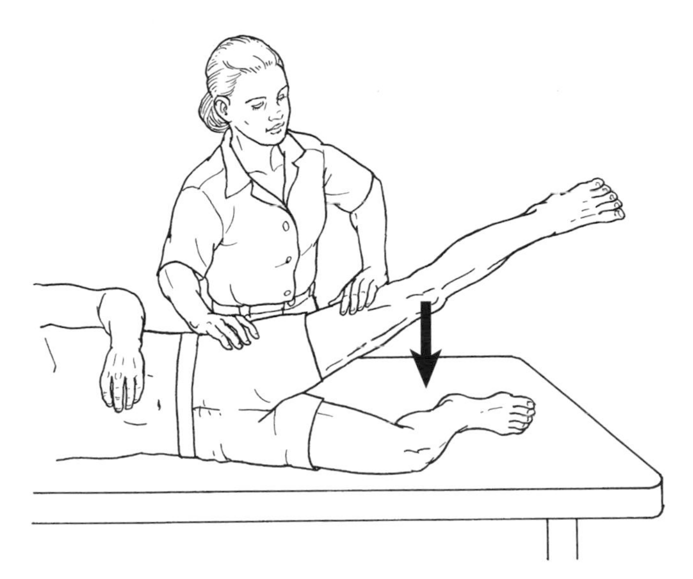

FIGURE 6-36

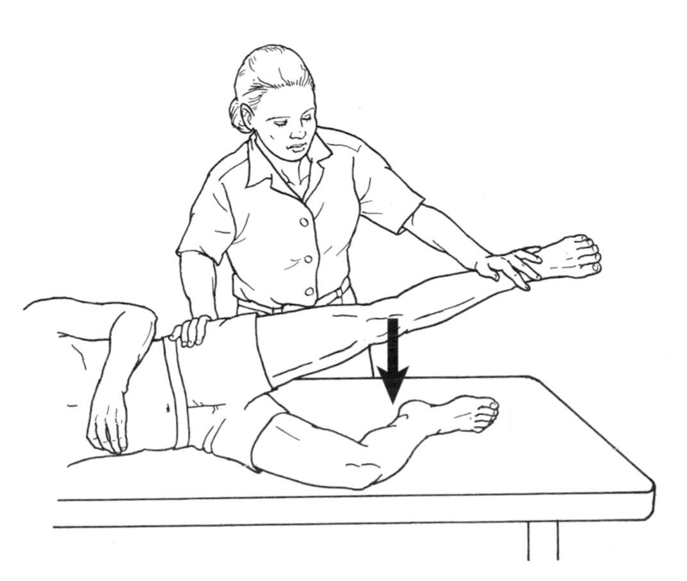

FIGURE 6-37

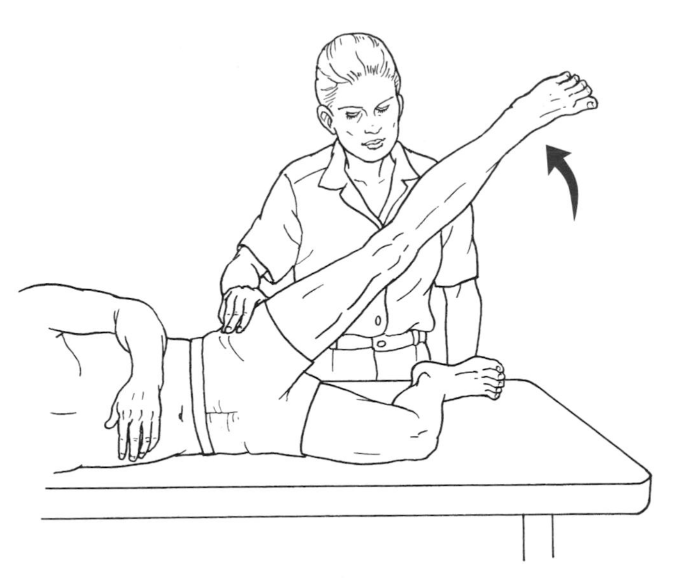

FIGURE 6-38

(Gluteus medius and Gluteus minimus)

Grade 2 (Poor)

Position of Patient: Supine.

Position of Therapist: Standing on side of limb being tested. One hand supports and lifts the limb by holding it under the ankle to raise limb just enough to decrease friction. This hand offers no resistance, nor should it be used to offer assistance to the movement. On some smooth surfaces, such support may not be necessary (Figure 6-39). (Note: Figures 6-39 and 6-40 show therapist on opposite side of patient to avoid obscuring test positions.)

The other hand palpates the gluteus medius just proximal to the greater trochanter of the femur (Figure 6-40).

Test: Patient abducts hip through available range.

Instructions to Patient: "Bring your leg out to the side. Keep your kneecap pointing to the ceiling."

Grading

Grade 2 (Poor): Completes range of motion supine with no resistance and minimal to zero friction.

Grade 1 (Trace) and Grade 0 (Zero)

Position of Patient: Supine.

Position of Therapist: Standing at side of limb being tested at level of thigh. One hand supports the limb under the ankle just above the malleoli. The hand should provide neither resistance nor assistance to movement (see Figure 6-40). Palpate the gluteus medius on the lateral aspect of the hip just above the greater trochanter.

Test: Patient attempts to abduct hip.

Instructions to Patient: "Try to bring your leg out to the side."

Grading

Grade 1 (Trace): Palpable contraction of gluteus medius but no movement of the part.

Grade 0 (Zero): No palpable contraction.

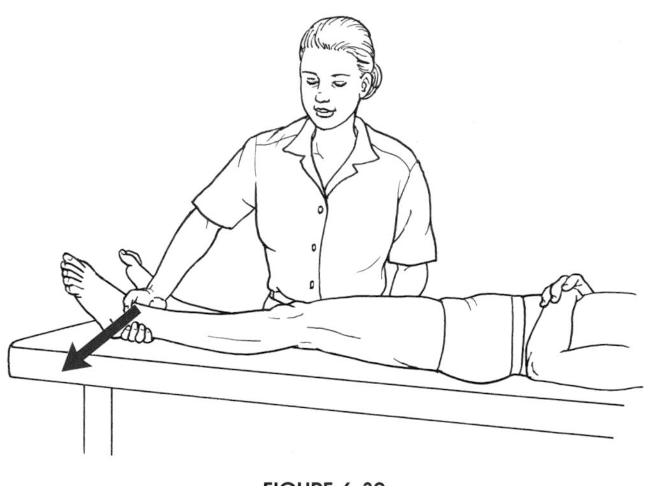

FIGURE 6-39

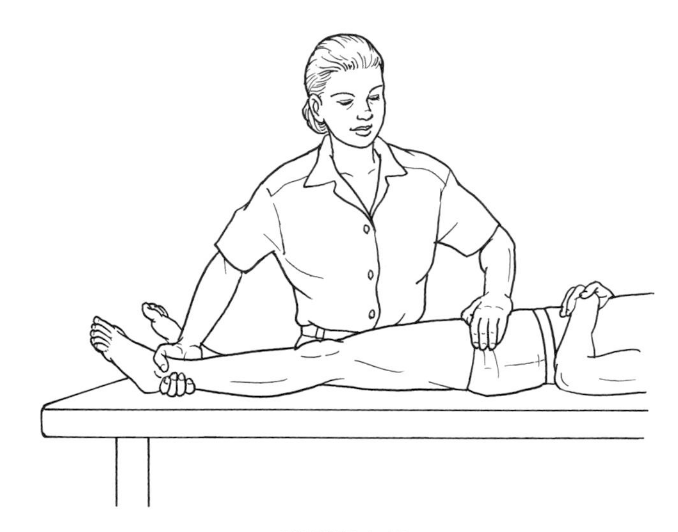

FIGURE 6-40

Substitutions

- Hip-hike substitution: Patient may "hike hip" by approximating pelvis to thorax using the lateral trunk muscles, which move the limb through partial abduction range (Figure 6-41). This movement may be detected by observing the lateral trunk and hip (move clothing aside) and palpating the gluteus medius above the trochanter.
- External rotation and flexion substitution: The patient may try to externally rotate during the motion of abduction (Figure 6-42). This could allow the oblique action of the hip flexors to substitute for the gluteus medius.
- Tensor fasciae latae substitution: If the test is allowed to begin with active hip flexion or with the hip positioned in flexion, there is an opportunity for the tensor fasciae latae to abduct the hip.

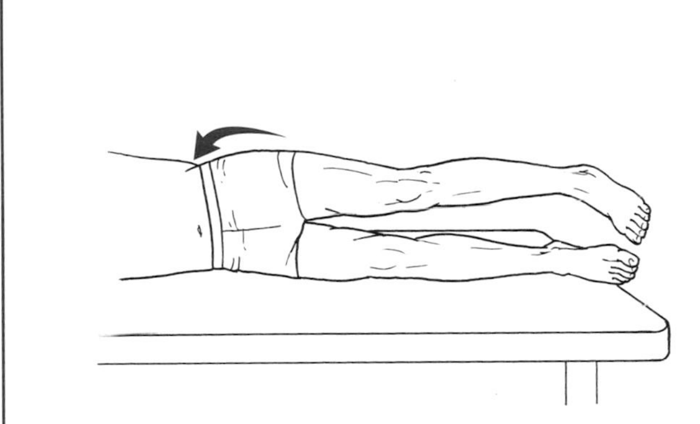
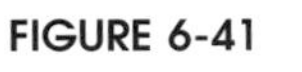

FIGURE 6-41

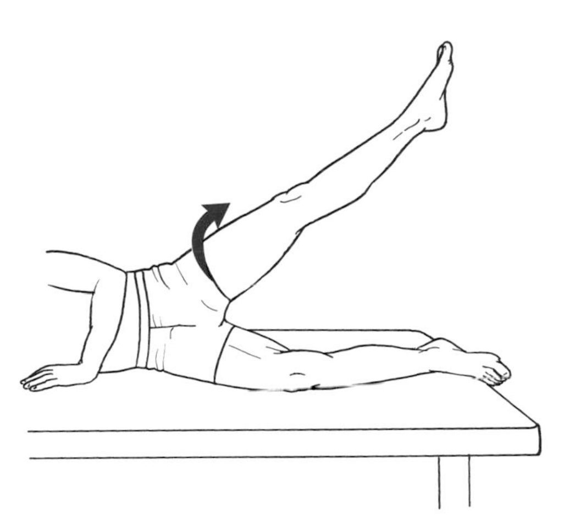

FIGURE 6-42

Helpful Hints

- The therapist should not be able to "break" a Grade 5 muscle (resistance applied at the ankle) and most therapists will not be able to "break" a Grade 4 muscle. A grade of 4 often masks significant weakness because of the intrinsic great strength of these muscles. Giving resistance at the ankle rather than at the knee is helpful in overcoming this problem. However, respect the long lever arm and apply resistance carefully, assessing whether the patient can adequately resist the movement through the long lever arm.
- Do not attempt to palpate contractile activity of muscle through clothing. (This is one of the cardinal principles of manual muscle testing.)
- When the patient is supine, the weight of the opposite limb stabilizes the pelvis. It is not necessary, therefore, to use a hand to manually stabilize the contralateral limb.
- A patient should be able to stand on one leg keeping the pelvis level with a muscle grade of 4 or 5.

HIP ABDUCTION FROM FLEXED POSITION

(Tensor fasciae latae)

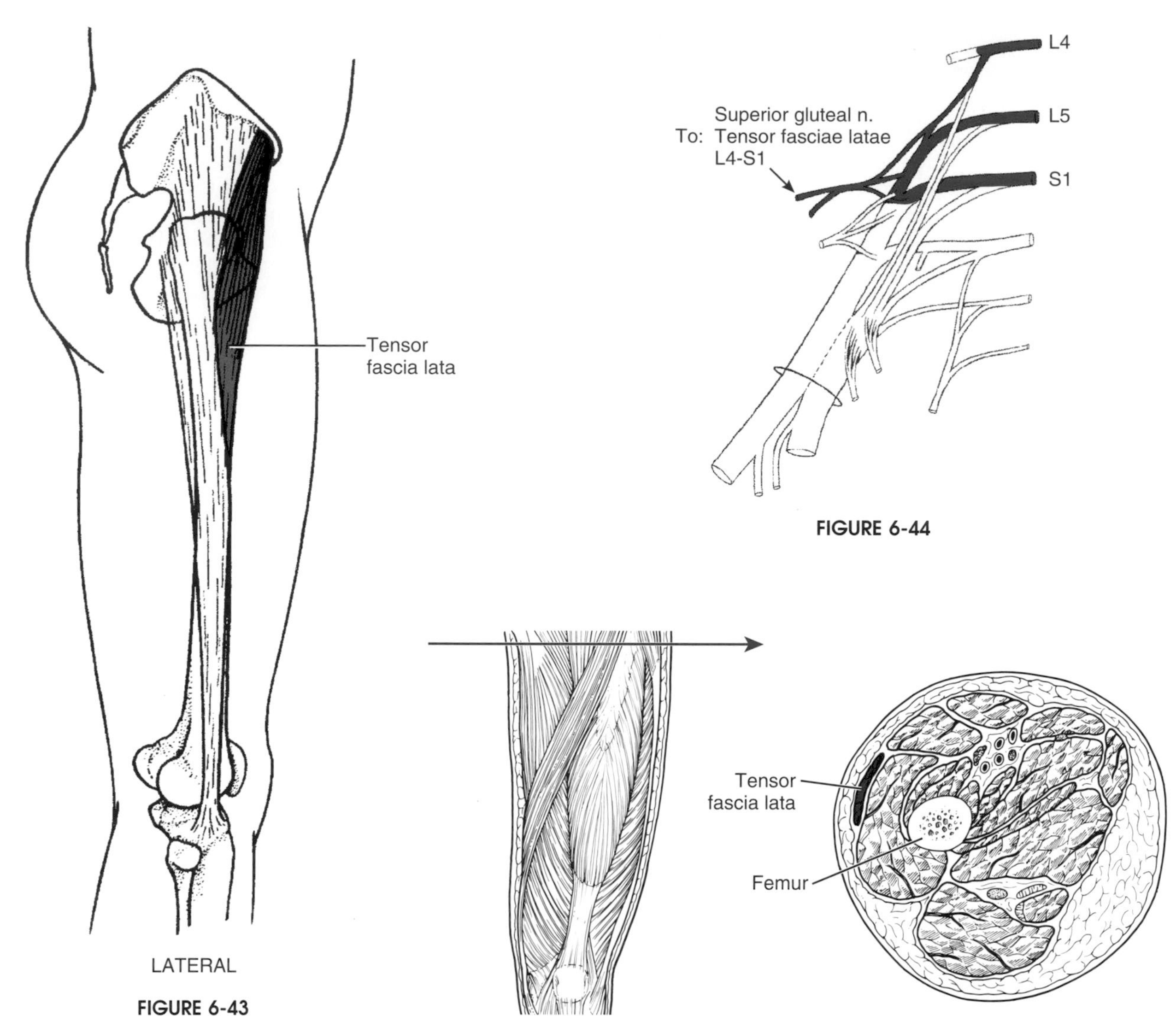

FIGURE 6-43

FIGURE 6-44

FIGURE 6-45 Arrow indicates level of cross section.

Range of Motion

Two-joint muscle. No specific range of motion can be assigned solely to the tensor.

Table 6-5 HIP ABDUCTION FROM FLEXION

I.D.	Muscle	Origin	Insertion
185	Tensor fasciae latae	Iliac crest (outer lip) Fasciae latae (deep) Anterior superior iliac spine (lateral surface)	Iliotibial tract (between its 2 layers, ending 1/3 of the way down)
Others			
183	Gluteus medius		
184	Gluteus minimus		

Grade 5 (Normal), Grade 4 (Good), and Grade 3 (Fair)

Position of Patient: Side-lying. Uppermost limb (test limb) is flexed to 45° and lies across the lowermost limb with the foot resting on the table (Figure 6-46).

Position of Therapist: Standing behind patient at level of pelvis. Hand for resistance is placed on lateral surface of the thigh just above the knee. Hand providing stabilization is placed on the crest of the ilium (Figure 6-47).

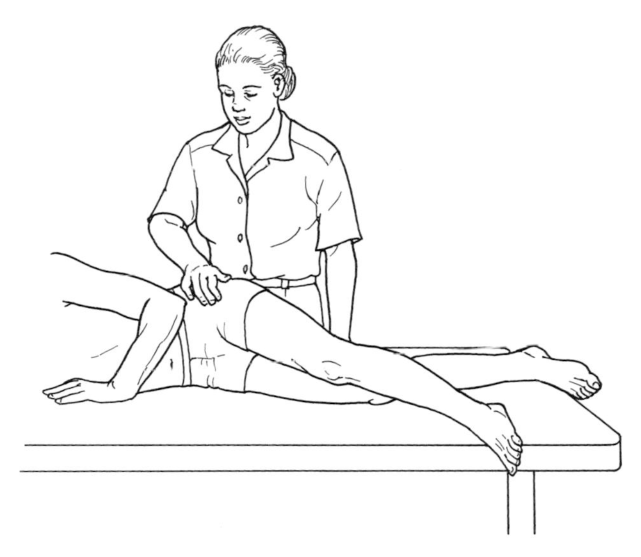

FIGURE 6-46

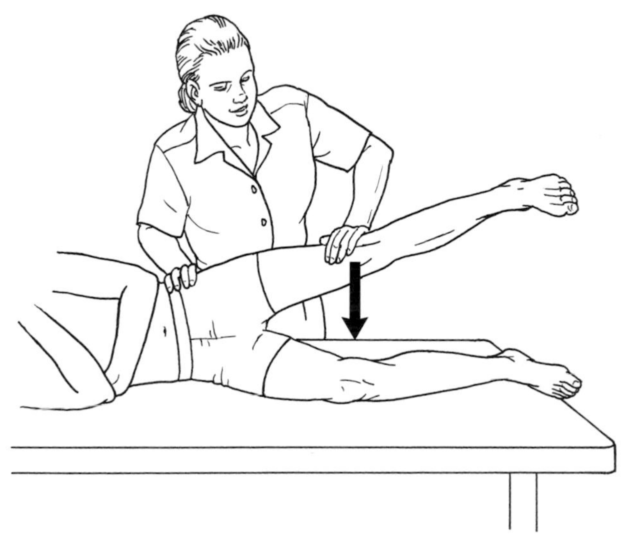

FIGURE 6-47

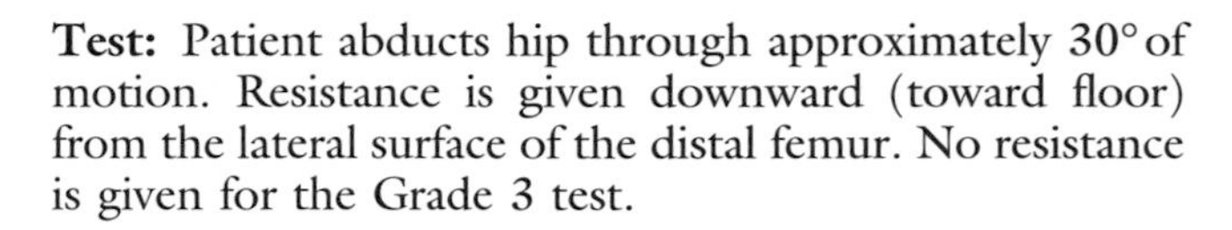

Test: Patient abducts hip through approximately 30° of motion. Resistance is given downward (toward floor) from the lateral surface of the distal femur. No resistance is given for the Grade 3 test.

Instructions to Patient: "Lift your leg and hold it. Don't let me push it down."

Grading

Grade 5 (Normal): Completes available range; holds end position against maximum resistance.

Grade 4 (Good): Completes available range and holds against strong to moderate resistance.

Grade 3 (Fair): Completes movement; holds end position but takes no resistance (Figure 6-48).

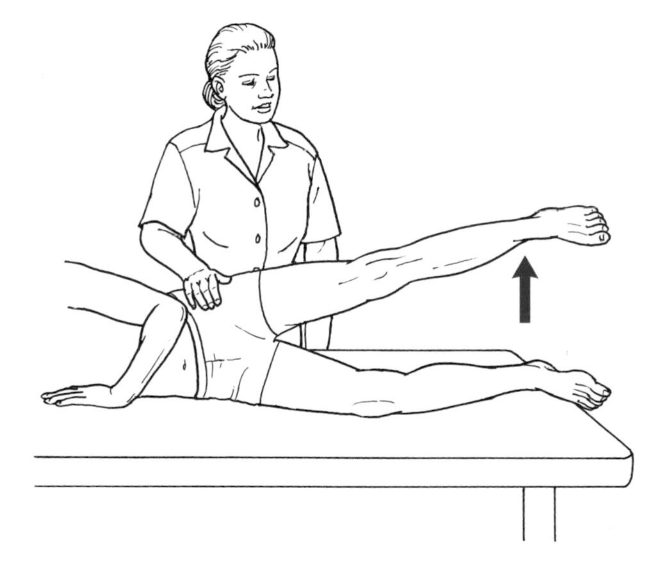

FIGURE 6-48

HIP ABDUCTION FROM FLEXED POSITION

(Tensor fasciae latae)

Grade 2 (Poor)

Position of Patient: Patient is in long-sitting position, supporting trunk with hands placed behind body on table. Trunk may lean backward up to 45° from vertical (Figure 6-49).

Position of Therapist: Standing at side of limb to be tested. (Note: Figure 6-49 deliberately shows therapist on wrong side to avoid obscuring test positions.) One hand supports the limb under the ankle; this hand will be used to reduce friction with the surface as the patient moves but should neither resist nor assist motion.

The other hand palpates the tensor fasciae latae on the proximal anterolateral thigh where it inserts into the iliotibial band.

Test: Patient abducts hip through 30° of range.

Instructions to Patient: "Bring your leg out to the side."

Grading

Grade 2 (Poor): Completes hip abduction motion to 30°.

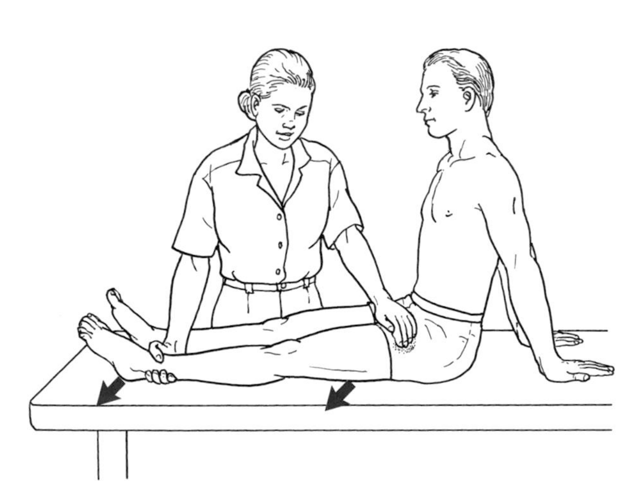

FIGURE 6-49

Grade 1 (Trace) and Grade 0 (Zero)

Position of Patient: Long sitting.

Position of Therapist: One hand palpates the insertion of the tensor at the lateral aspect of the knee. The other hand palpates the tensor on the anterolateral thigh (Figure 6-50).

Test: Patient attempts to abduct hip.

Instructions to Patient: "Try to move your leg out to the side."

Grading

Grade 1 (Trace): Palpable contraction of tensor fibers but no limb movement.

Grade 0 (Zero): No palpable contractile activity.

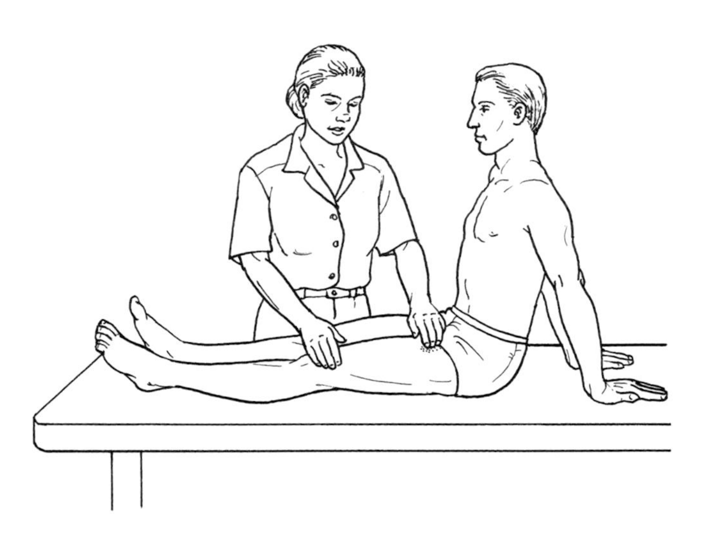

FIGURE 6-50

(Adductors magnus, brevis, and longus; Pectineus and Gracilis)

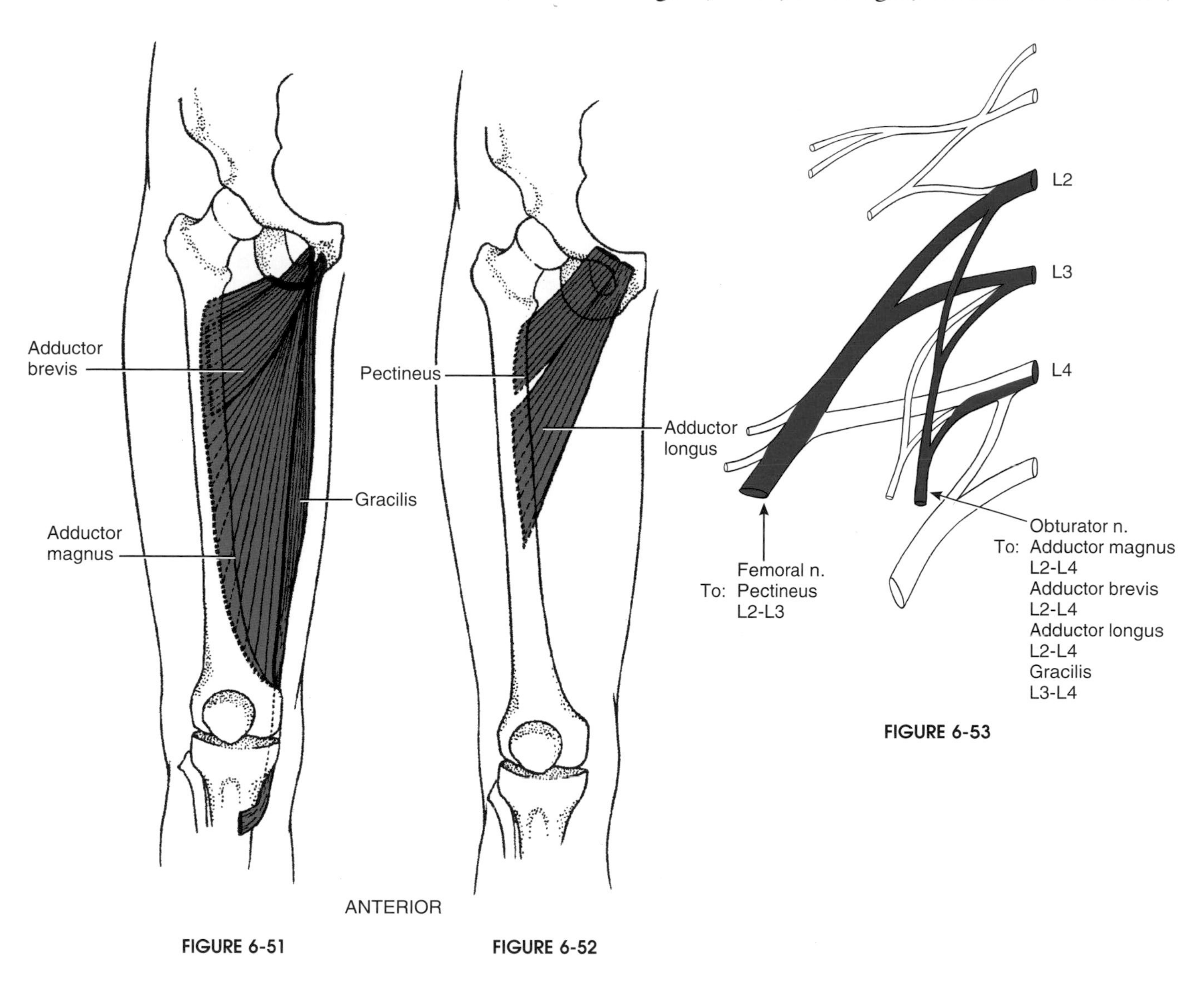

FIGURE 6-51

FIGURE 6-52

FIGURE 6-53

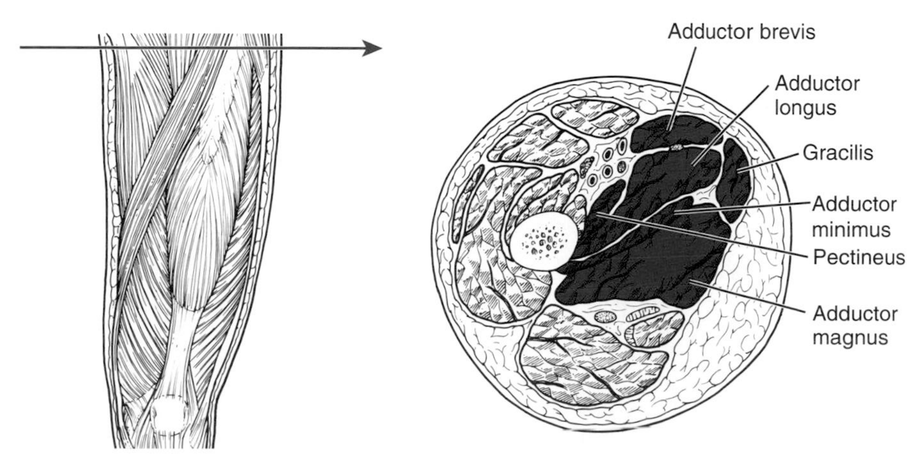

FIGURE 6-54 Arrow indicates level of cross section.

HIP ADDUCTION

(Adductors magnus, brevis, and longus; Pectineus and Gracilis)

Range of Motion
0° to 15°-20°

Table 6-6 HIP ADDUCTION

I.D.	Muscle	Origin	Insertion
181	Adductor magnus	Ischial tuberosity (inferolateral) Ischium (inferior ramus) Pubis (inferior ramus) Fibers from pubic ramus to femur (gluteal tuberosity), often named the *Adductor minimus*	Femur (linea aspera via aponeurosis, medial supracondylar line, and adductor tubercle on medial condyle)
180	Adductor brevis	Pubis (body and inferior ramus)	Femur (via aponeurosis to linea aspera)
179	Adductor longus	Pubis (anterior aspect between crest and symphysis)	Femur (linea aspera via aponeurosis)
177	Pectineus	Pubic pectin Fascia of pectineus	Femur (on a line from lesser trochanter to linea aspera)
178	Gracilis	Pubis (body and inferior ramus) Ischial ramus	Tibia (medial shaft distal to condyle) Pes anserinus Deep fascia of leg
Others			
188	Obturator externus		
182	Gluteus maximus (lower)		

Grade 5 (Normal), Grade 4 (Good), and Grade 3 (Fair)

Position of Patient: Side-lying with test limb (lowermost) resting on the table. Uppermost limb (nontest limb) in 25° of abduction supported by the therapist. The therapist cradles the leg with the forearm, the hand supporting the limb on the medial surface of the knee (Figure 6-55). Alternatively, the upper limb can be placed on a padded stool approximately 9 to 12 inches high.

Position of Therapist: Standing behind patient at knee level. The hand giving resistance to the test limb (lowermost limb) is placed on the medial surface of the distal femur, just proximal to the knee joint. Resistance is directed straight downward toward the table (Figure 6-56).

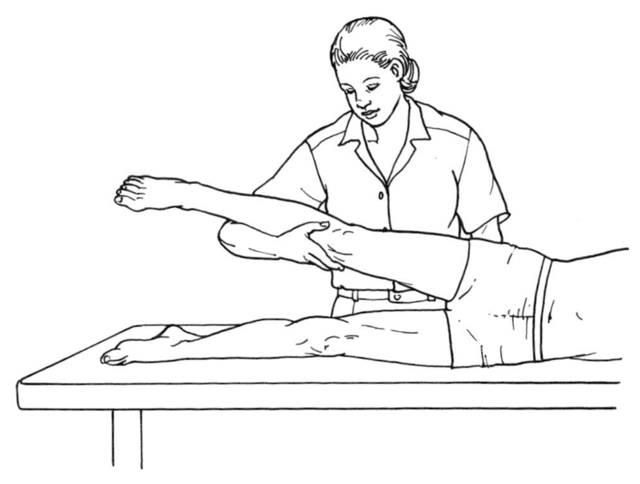

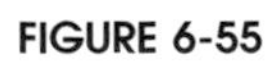
FIGURE 6-55

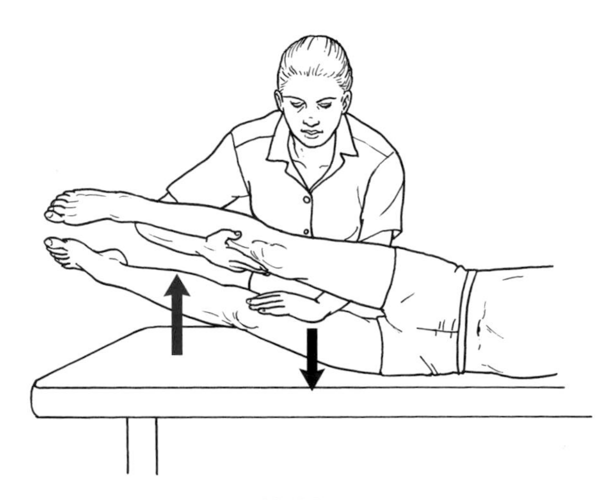

FIGURE 6-56

Grade 5 (Normal), Grade 4 (Good), and Grade 3 (Fair) Continued

Test: Patient adducts hip until the lower limb contacts the upper one.

Instructions to Patient: "Lift your bottom leg up to your top one. Hold it. Don't let me push it down."

For Grade 3: "Lift your bottom leg up to your top one. Don't let it drop!"

Grading

Grade 5 (Normal): Completes full range; holds end position against maximal resistance.

Grade 4 (Good): Completes full movement but tolerates strong to moderate resistance.

Grade 3 (Fair): Completes full movement; holds end position but takes no resistance (Figure 6-57).

Grade 2 (Poor)

Position of Patient: Supine. The non-test limb is positioned in some abduction to prevent interference with motion of the test limb.

Position of Therapist: Standing at side of test limb at knee level. One hand supports the ankle and elevates it slightly from the table surface to decrease friction as the limb moves across the table (Figure 6-58). The therapist uses this hand neither to assist nor to resist motion. The opposite hand palpates the adductor mass on the inner aspect of the proximal thigh.

Test: Patient adducts hip without rotation. Toes stay pointed toward the ceiling.

Instructions to Patient: "Bring your leg in toward the other one."

Grading

Grade 2 (Poor): Patient adducts limb through full range.

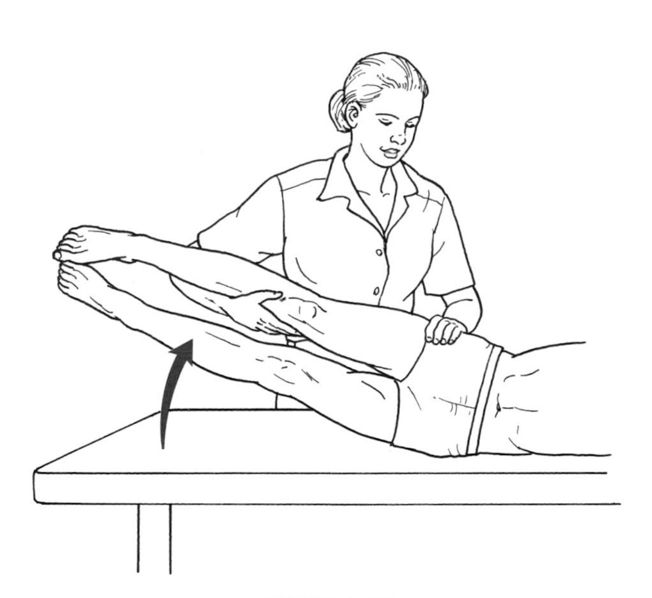

FIGURE 6-57

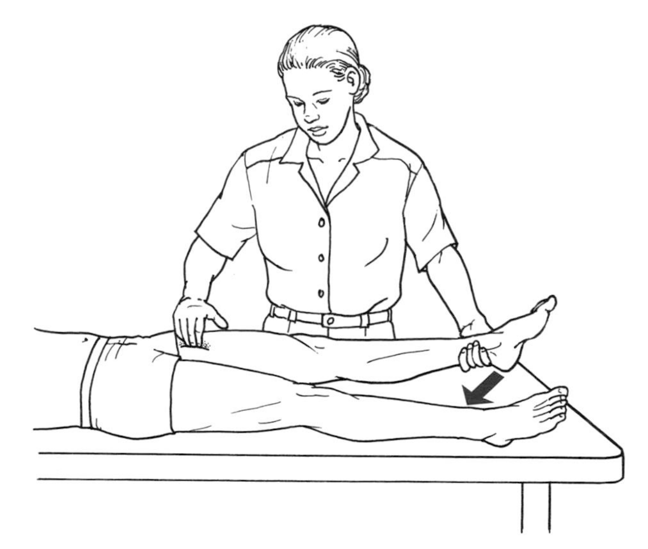

FIGURE 6-58

HIP ADDUCTION

(Adductors magnus, brevis, and longus; Pectineus and Gracilis)

Grade 1 (Trace) and Grade 0 (Zero)

Position of Patient: Supine.

Position of Therapist: Standing on side of test limb. One hand supports the limb under the ankle. The other hand palpates the adductor mass on the proximal medial thigh (Figure 6-59).

Test: Patient attempts to adduct hip.

Instructions to Patient: "Try to bring your leg in."

Grading

Grade 1 (Trace): Palpable contraction, no limb movement.

Grade 0 (Zero): No palpable contraction.

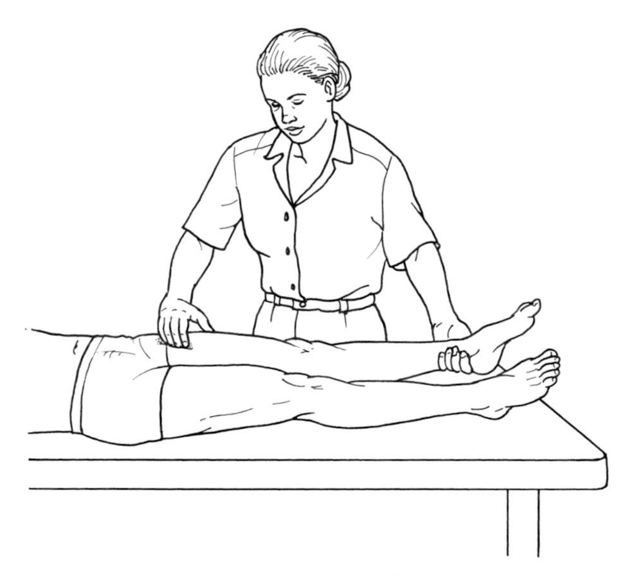

FIGURE 6-59

Substitution

Hip flexor substitution: The patient may attempt to substitute the hip flexors for the adductors by internally rotating the hip (Figure 6-60). The patient will appear to be trying to turn supine from side-lying. Maintenance of true side-lying is necessary for an accurate test.

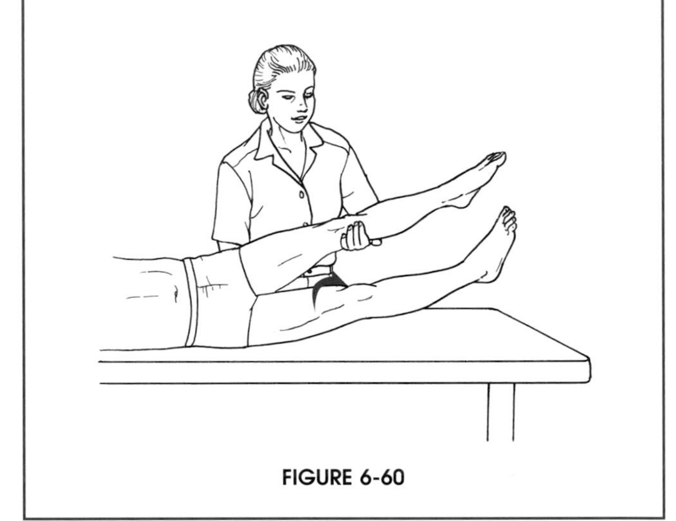

FIGURE 6-60

Helpful Hint

In the supine test position for Grades 2, 1, and 0, the weight of the opposite limb stabilizes the pelvis, so there is no need for manual stabilization of the non-test hip.

(Obturators internus and externus, Gemelli superior and inferior, Piriformis, Quadratus femoris, Gluteus maximus [posterior])

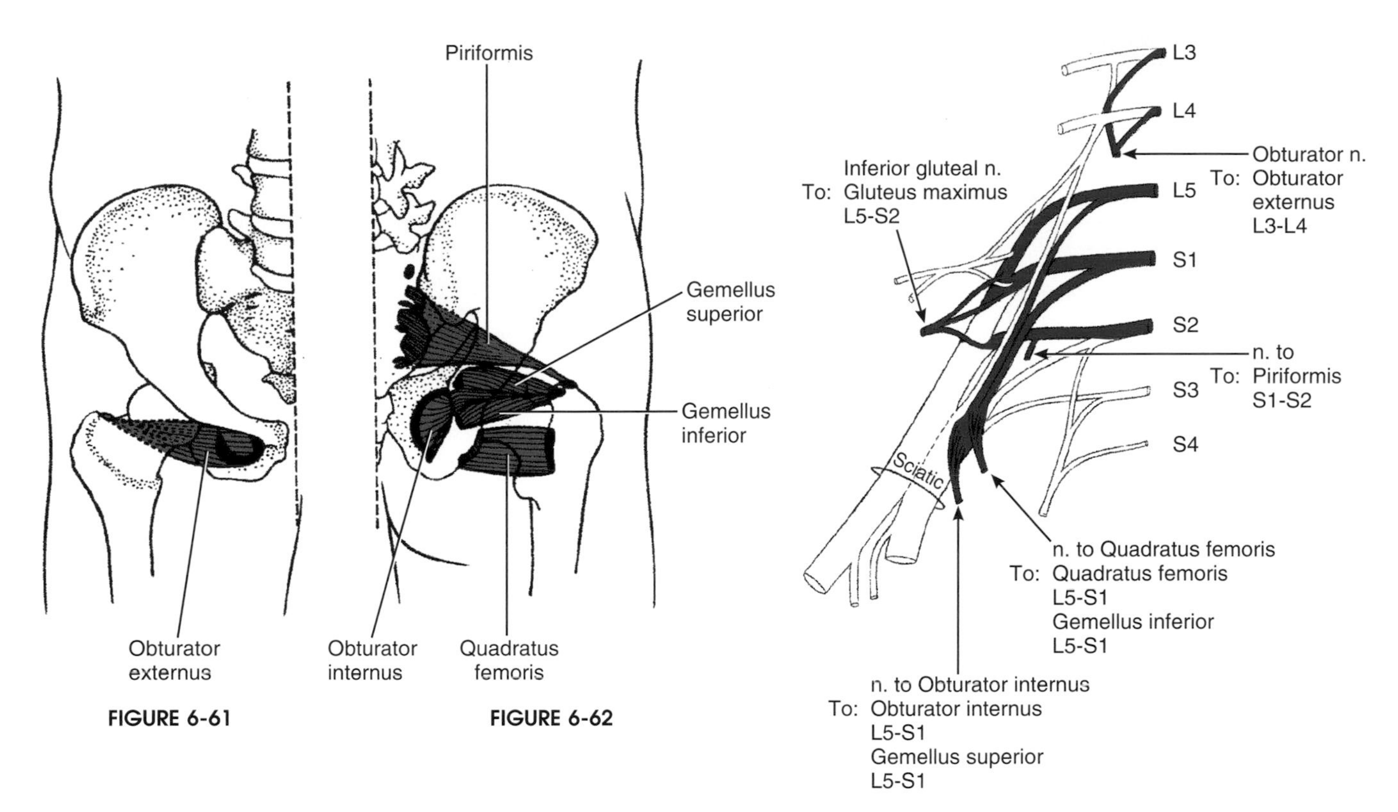

FIGURE 6-61

FIGURE 6-62

FIGURE 6-63

HIP EXTERNAL ROTATION

(Obturators internus and externus, Gemelli superior and inferior, Piriformis, Quadratus femoris, Gluteus maximus [posterior])

Range of Motion
0° to 45°

Table 6-7 HIP EXTERNAL ROTATION

I.D.	Muscle	Origin	Insertion
188	Obturator externus	Obturator membrane (external surface) Ischium (ramus) Pubis (inferior ramus) Pelvis (lesser pelvic cavity, inner surface)	Femur (trochanteric fossa)
187	Obturator internus	Pubis (inferior ramus) Ischium (ramus) Obturator fascia Obturator foramen (margin) Obturator membrane Upper brim of greater sciatic foramen	Femur (greater trochanter, medial) Tendon fuses with gemelli
191	Quadratus femoris (may be absent)	Ischial tuberosity (external aspect)	Femur (quadrate tubercle on trochanteric crest)
186	Piriformis	Sacrum (anterior surface) Ilium (gluteal surface near posterior inferior iliac spine) Sacrotuberous ligament Capsule of sacroiliac joint	Femur (greater trochanter, medial side)
189	Gemellus superior (may be absent)	Ischium (spine, dorsal surface)	Femur (greater trochanter, medial surface) Blends with tendon of obturator internus
190	Gemellus inferior	Ischial tuberosity (upper part)	Femur (greater trochanter, medial surface) Blends with tendon of obturator internus
182	Gluteus maximus	Ilium (posterior gluteal line and crest) Sacrum (dorsal and lower aspects) Coccyx (side) Sacrotuberous ligament Aponeurosis over gluteus medius	Femur (gluteal tuberosity) Iliotibial tract of fascia lata
Others			
195	Sartorius		
192	Biceps femoris (long head)		
183	Gluteus medius (posterior)		
174	Psoas major		
181	Adductor magnus (position-dependent)		
179	Adductor longus		
202	Popliteus (tibia fixed)		

(Obturators internus and externus, Gemelli superior and inferior, Piriformis, Quadratus femoris, Gluteus maximus [posterior])

Grade 5 (Normal), Grade 4 (Good), and Grade 3 (Fair)

Position of Patient: Short sitting. (Trunk may be supported by placing hands flat or fisted at sides of chair or table [Figure 6-64].)

Position of Therapist: Sits on a low stool or kneels beside limb to be tested. The hand that gives resistance is placed on the medial aspect of the ankle just above the malleolus. Resistance is applied as a laterally directed force at the ankle (see Figure 6-64).

The other hand, which will offer counter-pressure, is contoured over the lateral aspect of the distal thigh just above the knee. Stabilization is provided in a medially directed force at the knee counteracting the resistance provided at the ankle. The two forces are applied in counter-directions for this rotary motion (see Figure 6-64).

Test: Patient externally rotates the hip.

Instructions to Patient: "Don't let me turn your leg out."

Grading

Grade 5 (Normal): Holds at end of range against maximal resistance.

Grade 4 (Good): Holds at end of range against strong to moderate resistance.

Grade 3 (Fair): Holds end position but tolerates no resistance (Figure 6-65).

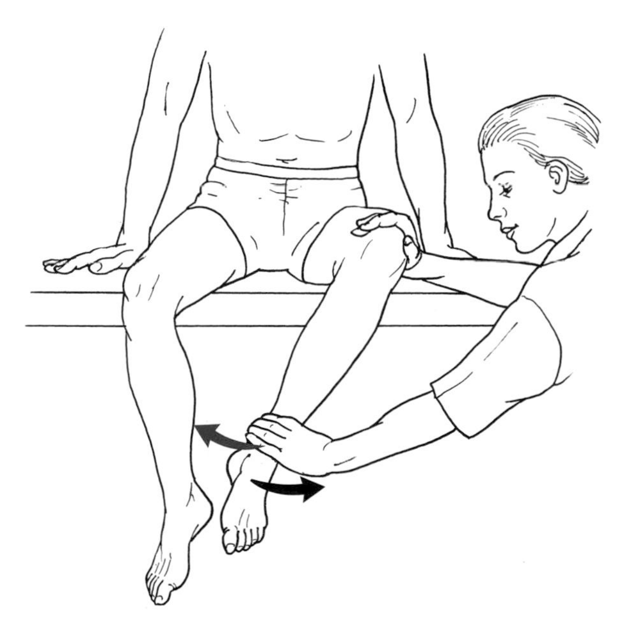

FIGURE 6-64

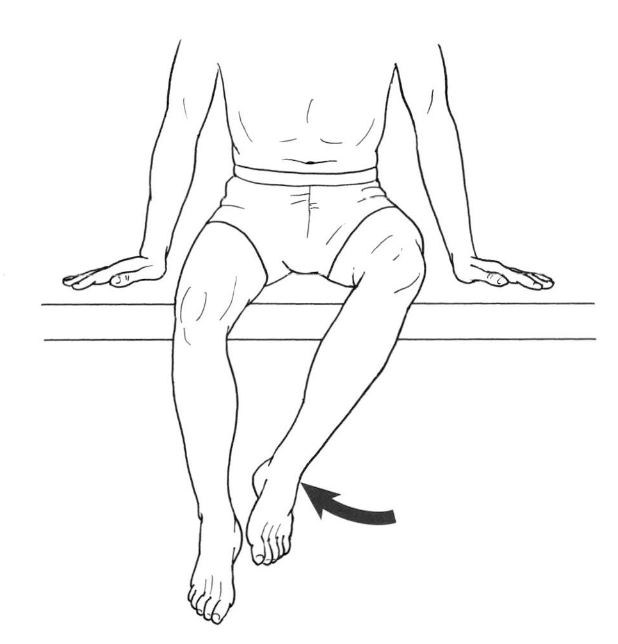

FIGURE 6-65

HIP EXTERNAL ROTATION

(Obturators internus and externus, Gemelli superior and inferior, Piriformis, Quadratus femoris, Gluteus maximus [posterior])

Grade 2 (Poor)

Position of Patient: Supine. Test limb is in internal rotation.

Position of Therapist: Standing at side of limb to be tested. The therapist may need to support the limb in internal rotation since gravity tends to pull the limb into external rotation.

Test: Patient externally rotates hip in available range of motion (Figure 6-66). One hand may be used to maintain pelvic alignment at lateral hip.

Instructions to Patient: "Roll your leg out."

Grading

Grade 2 (Poor): Completes external rotation range of motion. As the hip rolls past the midline, minimal resistance can be offered to offset the assistance of gravity.

Alternate Test for Grade 2: With the patient short sitting, the therapist places the test limb in maximal internal rotation. The patient then is instructed to return the limb actively to the midline (neutral) position against slight resistance. Care needs to be taken to ensure that gravity is not the predominant force. If this motion is performed satisfactorily, the test is assessed as a Grade 2.

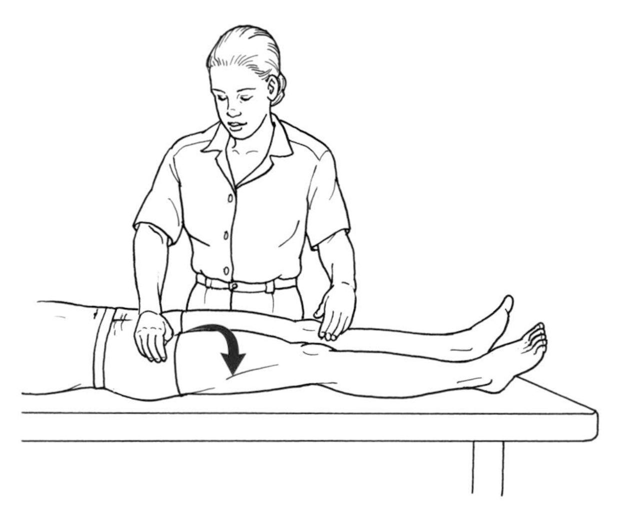

FIGURE 6-66

Grade 1 (Trace) and Grade 0 (Zero)

Position of Patient: Supine with test limb placed in internal rotation.

Position of Therapist: Standing at side of limb to be tested.

Test: Patient attempts to externally rotate hip.

Instructions to Patient: "Try to roll your leg out."

Grading

Grade 1 (Trace) and Grade 0 (Zero): The external rotator muscles, except for the gluteus maximus, are not palpable. If there is any discernible movement (contractile activity), a grade of 1 should be given; otherwise, a grade of 0 is assigned on the principle that whenever uncertainty exists, the lesser grade should be awarded.

Helpful Hints

- There is wide variation in the amount of hip external rotation range of motion that can be considered normal. It is imperative, therefore, that a patient's accurate range (in each test position) be known before manual muscle testing takes place.
- There is greater range of rotation at the hip when the hip is flexed than when it is extended, probably secondary to laxity of hip joint structures.
- In short-sitting tests, the patient should *not* be allowed to use the following motions, lest they add visual distortion and confound the test results:
  a. Lift the contralateral buttock off the table or lean in any direction to lift the pelvis;
  b. Increase flexion of the test knee;
  c. Abduct the test hip.

(Glutei minimus and medius; Tensor fasciae latae)

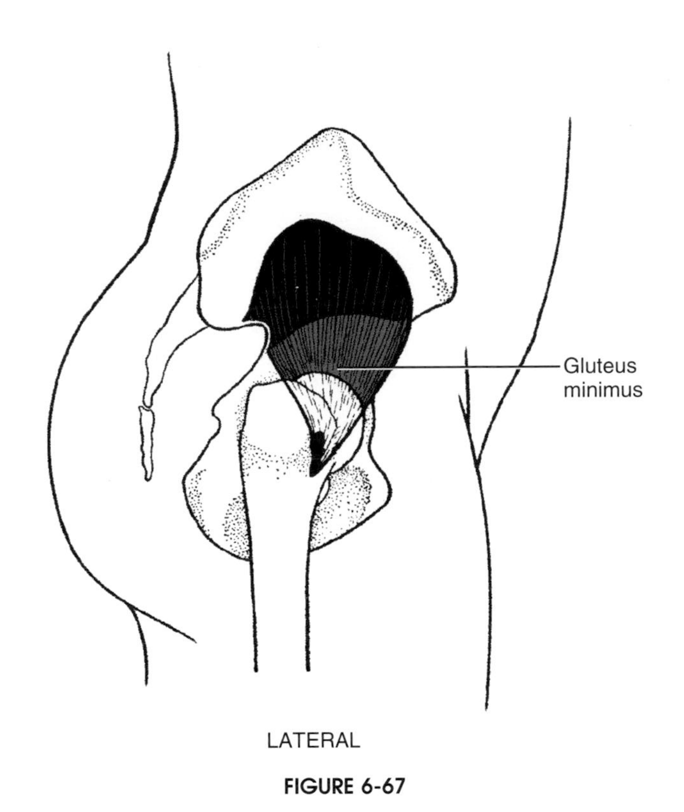

FIGURE 6-67

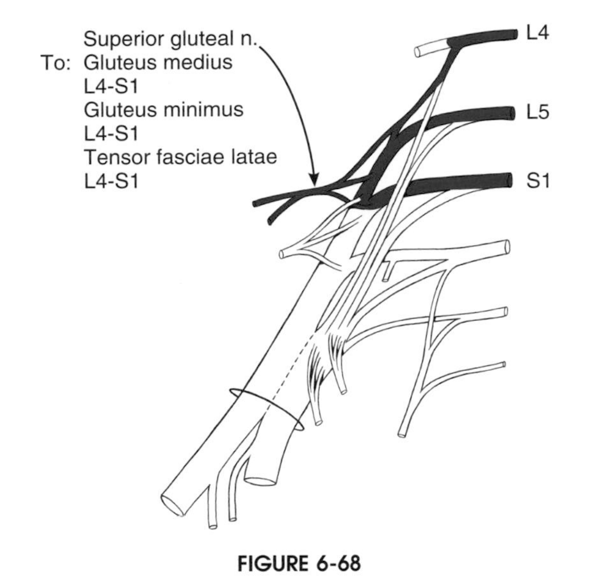

FIGURE 6-68

Range of Motion

0° to 45°

Table 6-8 HIP INTERNAL ROTATION

I.D.	Muscle	Origin	Insertion
184	Gluteus minimus (anterior fibers)	Ilium (outer surface between anterior and inferior gluteal lines) Greater sciatic notch	Femur (greater trochanter, anterior aspect) Fibrous capsule of hip joint
185	Tensor fasciae latae	Iliac crest (outer lip) Fascia lata (deep) Anterior superior iliac spine (lateral surface)	Iliotibial tract (between its two layers ending 1/3 down femur)
183	Gluteus medius (anterior fibers)	Ilium (outer surface between crest and posterior gluteal line) Gluteal fascia	Femur (greater trochanter, lateral surface)
Others			
193	Semitendinosus		
194	Semimembranosus		
181	Adductor magnus (position-dependent)		
179	Adductor longus (position-dependent)		

HIP INTERNAL ROTATION

(Glutei minimus and medius; Tensor fasciae latae)

Grade 5 (Normal), Grade 4 (Good), and Grade 3 (Fair)

Strength at the hip often plays a role in biomechanical alignment at the knee. This is particularly true with weakness of the abductors, external rotators, and hip extensors. Therefore it is critical to consider the role of strength at the hip when knee pain or dysfunction is present.

Position of Patient: Sitting. Arms may be used for trunk support at sides or may be crossed over chest.

Position of Therapist: Sitting or kneeling in front of patient. One hand is placed on the lateral surface of the ankle just above the malleolus (Figure 6-69). Resistance is given (Grades 5 and 4 only) as a medially directed force at the ankle.

The opposite hand, which offers counter-pressure, is contoured over the medial surface of the distal thigh just above the knee. Resistance is applied as a laterally directed force at the knee. Note the counter-directions of the force applied.

Test: The limb should be placed in the end position of full internal rotation for best results (see Figure 6-69).

Grading

Grade 5 (Normal): Holds end position against maximal resistance.

Grade 4 (Good): Holds end position against strong to moderate resistance.

Grade 3 (Fair): Holds end position but takes no resistance (Figure 6-70).

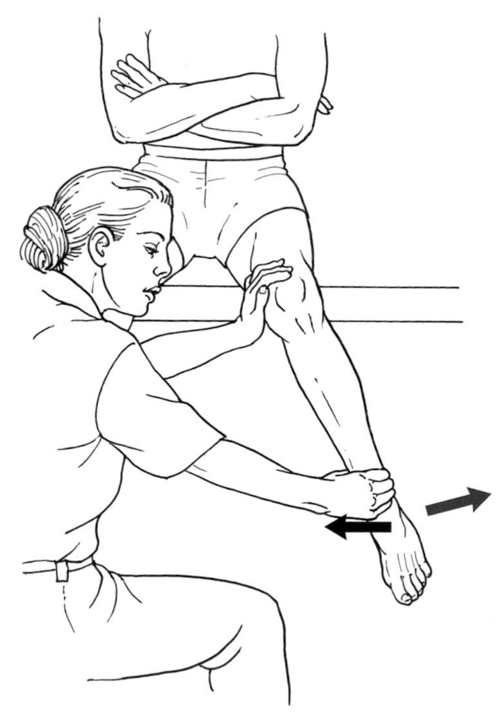

FIGURE 6-69

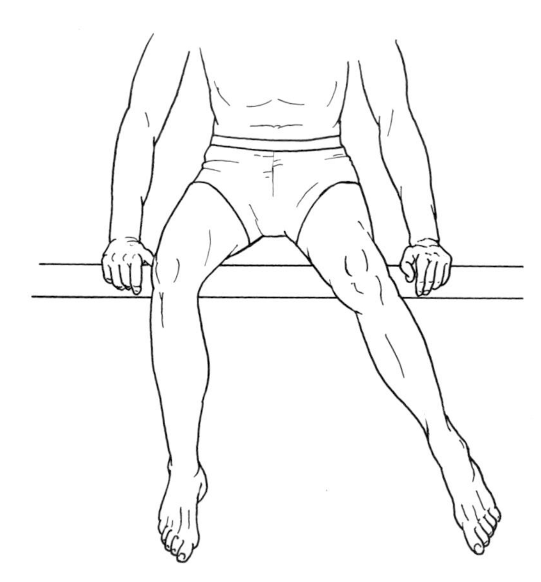

FIGURE 6-70

Grade 2 (Poor)

Position of Patient: Supine. Test limb in partial external rotation.

Position of Therapist: Standing next to test leg. Palpate the gluteus medius proximal to the greater trochanter and the tensor fasciae latae (Figure 6-71) over the anterolateral hip below the ASIS.

Test: Patient internally rotates hip through available range.

Instructions to Patient: "Roll your leg in toward the other one."

Grading

Grade 2 (Poor): Completes the range of motion. As the hip rolls inward past the midline, minimal resistance can be offered to offset the assistance of gravity.

Alternate Test for Grade 2: With patient short sitting, the therapist places the test limb in maximal external rotation. The patient then is instructed to return the limb actively to the midline (neutral) position against slight resistance. Care needs to be taken to ensure that gravity is not the predominant force. If this motion is performed satisfactorily, the test may be assessed a Grade 2.

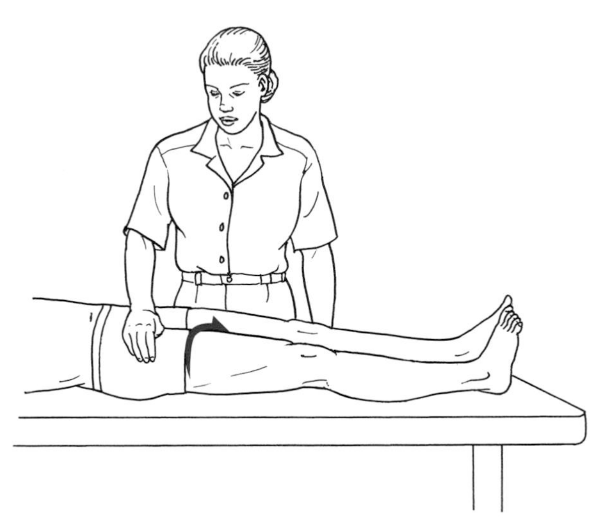

FIGURE 6-71

Grade 1 (Trace) and Grade 0 (Zero)

Position of Patient: Patient supine with test limb placed in external rotation.

Position of Therapist: Standing next to test leg.

Test: Patient attempts to internally rotate hip. One hand is used to palpate the gluteus medius (over the posterolateral surface of the hip above the greater trochanter). The other hand is used to palpate the tensor fasciae latae (on the anterolateral surface of the hip below the ASIS).

Instructions to Patient: "Try to roll your leg in."

Grading

Grade 1 (Trace): Palpable contractile activity in either or both muscles.

Grade 0 (Zero): No palpable contractile activity.

Helpful Hints

- In the short-sitting tests, do not allow the patient to assist internal rotation by lifting the pelvis on the side of the limb being tested.
- Neither should the patient be allowed to extend the knee or adduct and extend the hip during performance of the test. These motions contaminate the test by offering visual distortion to the therapist.
- For the external rotation test, the reader is referred to the second and third Helpful Hints under External Rotation (page 234), which apply here as well.

KNEE FLEXION

(All hamstring muscles)

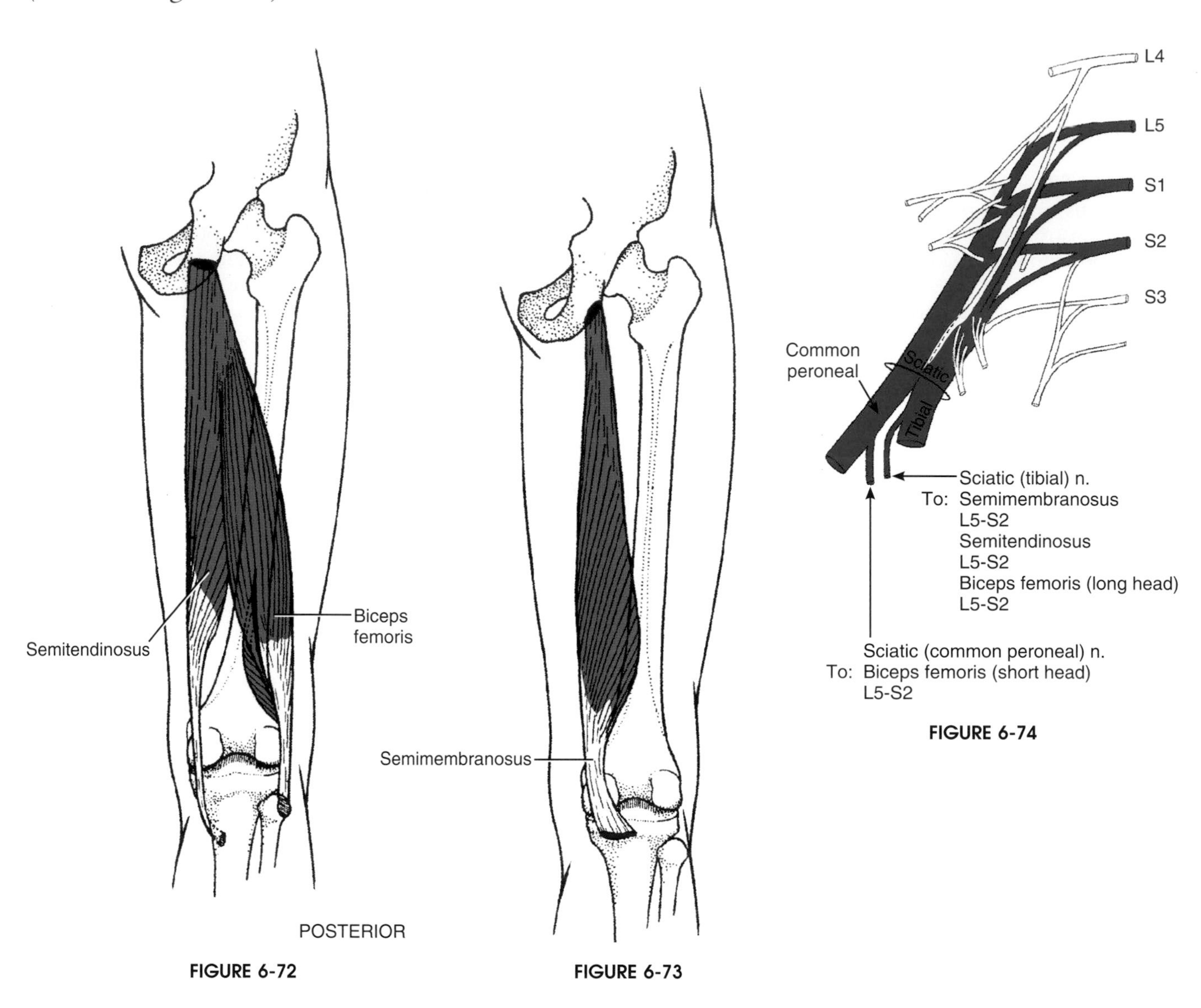

FIGURE 6-72

FIGURE 6-73

FIGURE 6-74

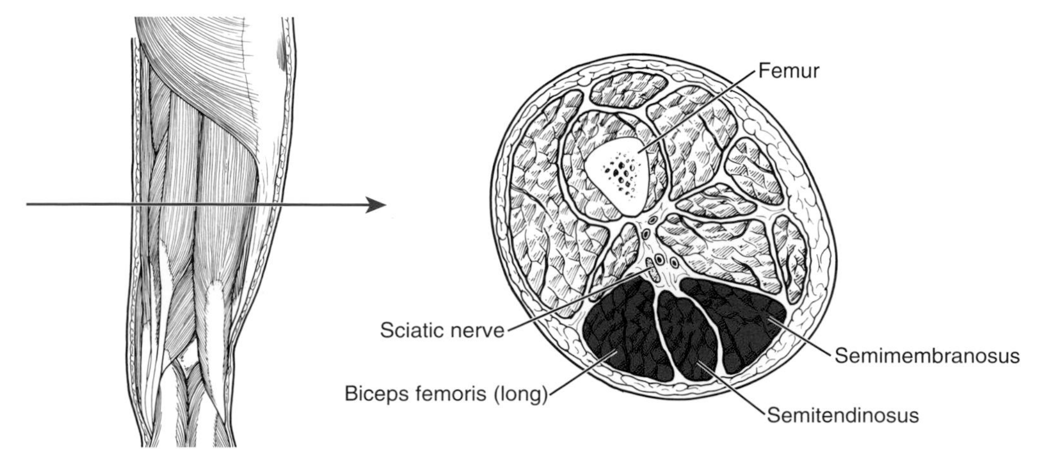

FIGURE 6-75 Arrow indicates level of cross section.

KNEE FLEXION

(All hamstring muscles)

Range of Motion
0° to 135°

Table 6-9 KNEE FLEXION

I.D.	Muscle	Origin	Insertion
192	Biceps femoris		
	Long head	Ischium (tuberosity) Sacrotuberous ligament	Aponeurosis (posterior) Fibula (head, lateral aspect) Fibular collateral ligament
	Short head	Femur (linea aspera and lateral condyle) Lateral intermuscular septum	Tibia (lateral condyle)
193	Semitendinosus	Ischial tuberosity (inferior medial aspect) Tendon via aponeurosis shared with biceps femoris (long)	Tibia (proximal shaft) Pes anserinus Deep fascia of leg
194	Semimembranosus	Ischial tuberosity Sacrotuberous ligament	Distal aponeurosis Tibia (medial condyle) Oblique popliteal ligament of knee joint
Others			
178	Gracilis		
185	Tensor fasciae latae (knee flexed more than 30°)		
195	Sartorius		
202	Popliteus		
205	Gastrocnemius		
207	Plantaris		

(All hamstring muscles)

Grade 5 (Normal), Grade 4 (Good), and Grade 3 (Fair)

There are three basic muscle tests for the hamstrings at Grades 5 and 4. The therapist should test first for the aggregate of the three hamstring muscles (with the foot in midline). Only if there is deviation (or asymmetry) in the movement or a question in the therapist's mind is there a need to test the medial and lateral hamstrings separately.

HAMSTRING MUSCLES IN AGGREGATE

Position of Patient: Prone with limbs straight and toes hanging over the edge of the table. Test may be started in about 45° of knee flexion.

Position of Therapist: Standing next to limb to be tested. (Note: The therapist in the illustration is shown on the wrong side to avoid obscuring test positions.) Hand giving resistance is contoured around the posterior surface of the leg just above the ankle (Figure 6-76). Resistance is applied in the direction of knee extension for Grades 5 and 4.

The other hand is placed over the hamstring tendons on the posterior thigh (optional).

Test: Patient flexes knee while maintaining leg in neutral rotation.

Instructions to Patient: "Bend your knee. Hold it! Don't let me straighten it."

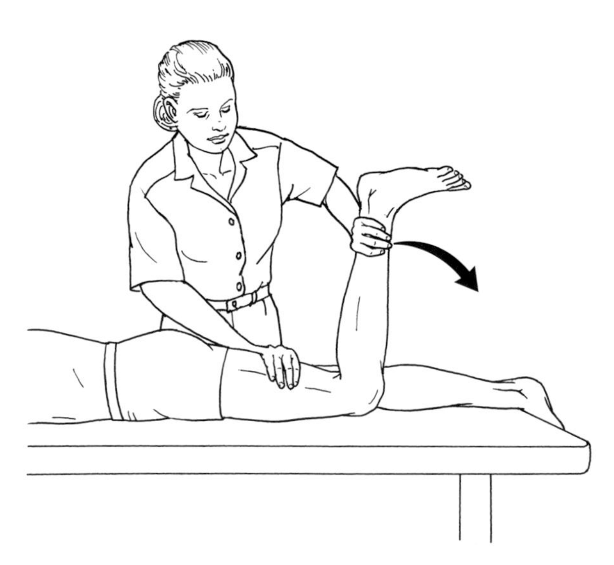

FIGURE 6-76

MEDIAL HAMSTRING TEST (SEMITENDINOSUS AND SEMIMEMBRANOSUS)

Position of Patient: Prone with knee flexed to less than 90°. Leg in internal rotation (toes pointing toward midline).

Position of Therapist: Hand giving resistance grasps the leg at the ankle. Resistance is applied in an oblique direction (down and out) toward knee extension (Figure 6-77).

Test: Patient flexes knee, maintaining the leg in internal rotation (heel toward therapist, toes pointing toward midline).

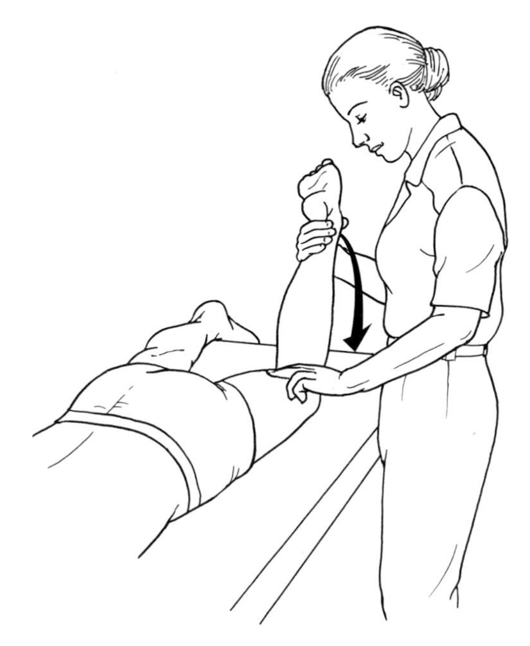

FIGURE 6-77

LATERAL HAMSTRING TEST (BICEPS FEMORIS)

Position of Patient: Prone with knee flexed to less than 90°. Leg is in external rotation (toes pointing laterally).

Position of Therapist: Therapist resists knee flexion at the ankle using a downward and inward force (Figure 6-78).

Test: Patient flexes knee, maintaining leg in external rotation (heel away from therapist, toes pointing toward therapist) (see Figure 6-78).

Grading the Hamstring Muscles (Grades 5 to 3)

Grade 5 (Normal) for All Three Tests: Resistance will be maximal, and the end knee flexion position (approximately 90°) cannot be broken.

Grade 4 (Good) for All Three Tests: End knee flexion position is held against strong to moderate resistance.

Grade 3 (Fair) for All Three Tests: Holds end range position but tolerates no resistance (Figure 6-79).

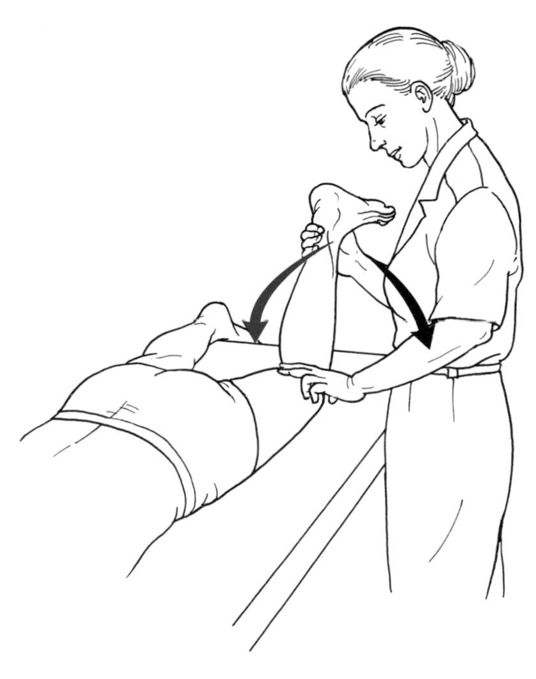

FIGURE 6-78

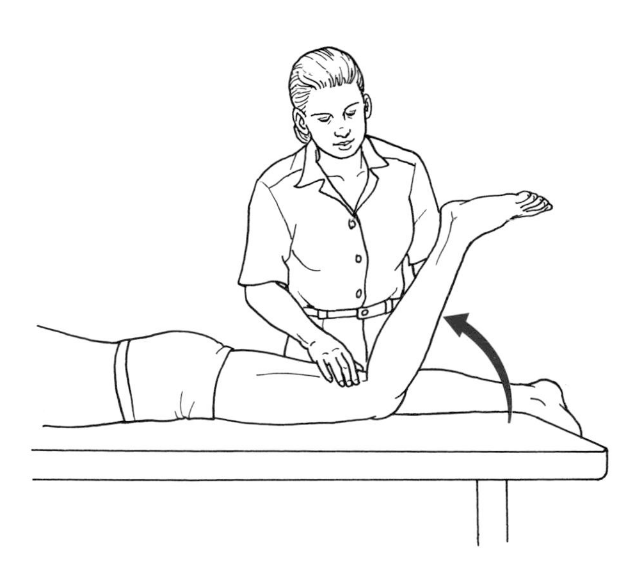

FIGURE 6-79

KNEE FLEXION

(All hamstring muscles)

Grade 2 (Poor)

Position of Patient: Side-lying with test limb (uppermost limb) supported by therapist or on suitable height stool. Lower limb flexed for stability.

Position of Therapist: Standing behind patient at knee level. One arm is used to cradle thigh, providing hand support at medial side of knee. Other hand supports the leg at the ankle just above the malleolus (Figure 6-80).

Test: Patient flexes knee through available range of motion.

Instructions to Patient: "Bend your knee."

Grading

Grade 2 (Poor): Completes available range of motion in side-lying position.

Grade 1 (Trace) and Grade 0 (Zero)

Position of Patient: Prone. Limbs are straight with toes extending over end of table. Knee is partially flexed and supported at ankle by therapist.

Position of Therapist: Standing next to test limb at knee level. One hand supports the flexed limb at the ankle (Figure 6-81). The opposite hand palpates both the medial and the lateral hamstring tendons just above the posterior knee.

Test: Patient attempts to flex knee.

Instructions to Patient: "Try to bend your knee."

Grading

Grade 1 (Trace): Tendons become prominent, but no visible movement occurs.

Grade 0 (Zero): No palpable contraction of the muscles; tendons do not stand out.

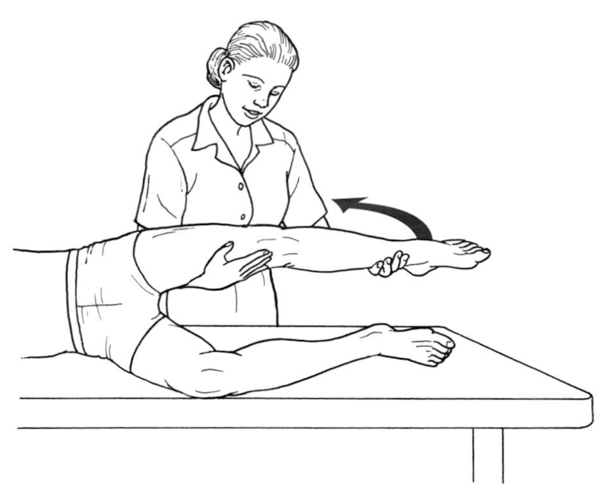

FIGURE 6-80

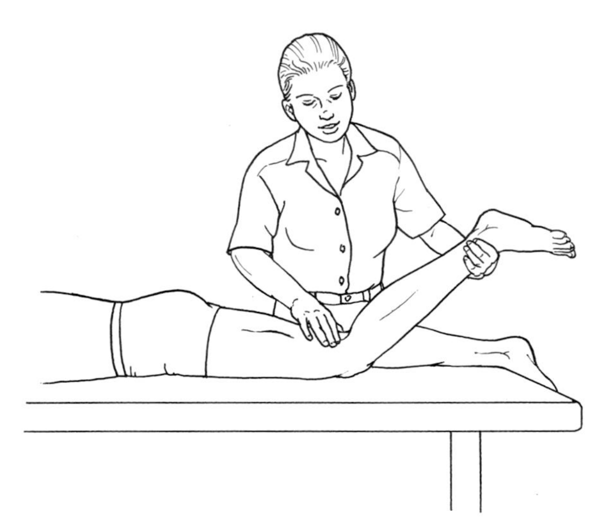

FIGURE 6-81

Substitutions

- Hip flexion substitution: The prone patient may flex the hip to start knee flexion. The buttock on the test side will rise as the hip flexes, and the patient may appear to roll slightly toward supine (Figure 6-82).
- Sartorius substitution: The sartorius may try to assist with knee flexion, but this also causes flexion and external rotation of the hip. Knee flexion when the hip is externally rotated is less difficult because the leg is not raised vertically against gravity.
- Gracilis substitution: Action of the gracilis contributes a hip adduction motion.
- Gastrocnemius substitution: Do not permit the patient to strongly dorsiflex in an attempt to use the tenodesis effect of the gastrocnemius.

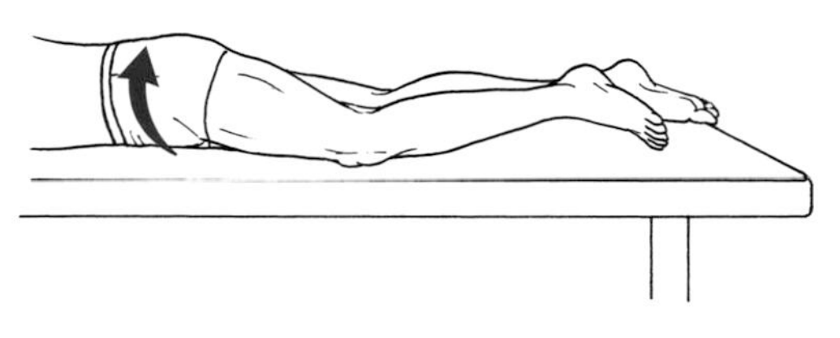

FIGURE 6-82

Helpful Hints

- If the biceps femoris is stronger than the medial hamstrings, the leg will externally rotate during knee flexion. Similarly, if the semitendinosus and semimembranosus are the stronger components, the leg will internally rotate during knee flexion. This is the situation that, when observed, indicates asymmetry and the need to test the medial and lateral hamstrings separately.
- If the hip flexes at the end of the knee flexion range of motion, check for a tight rectus femoris muscle because this tightness will limit the range of knee motion.

KNEE EXTENSION

(Quadriceps femoris)

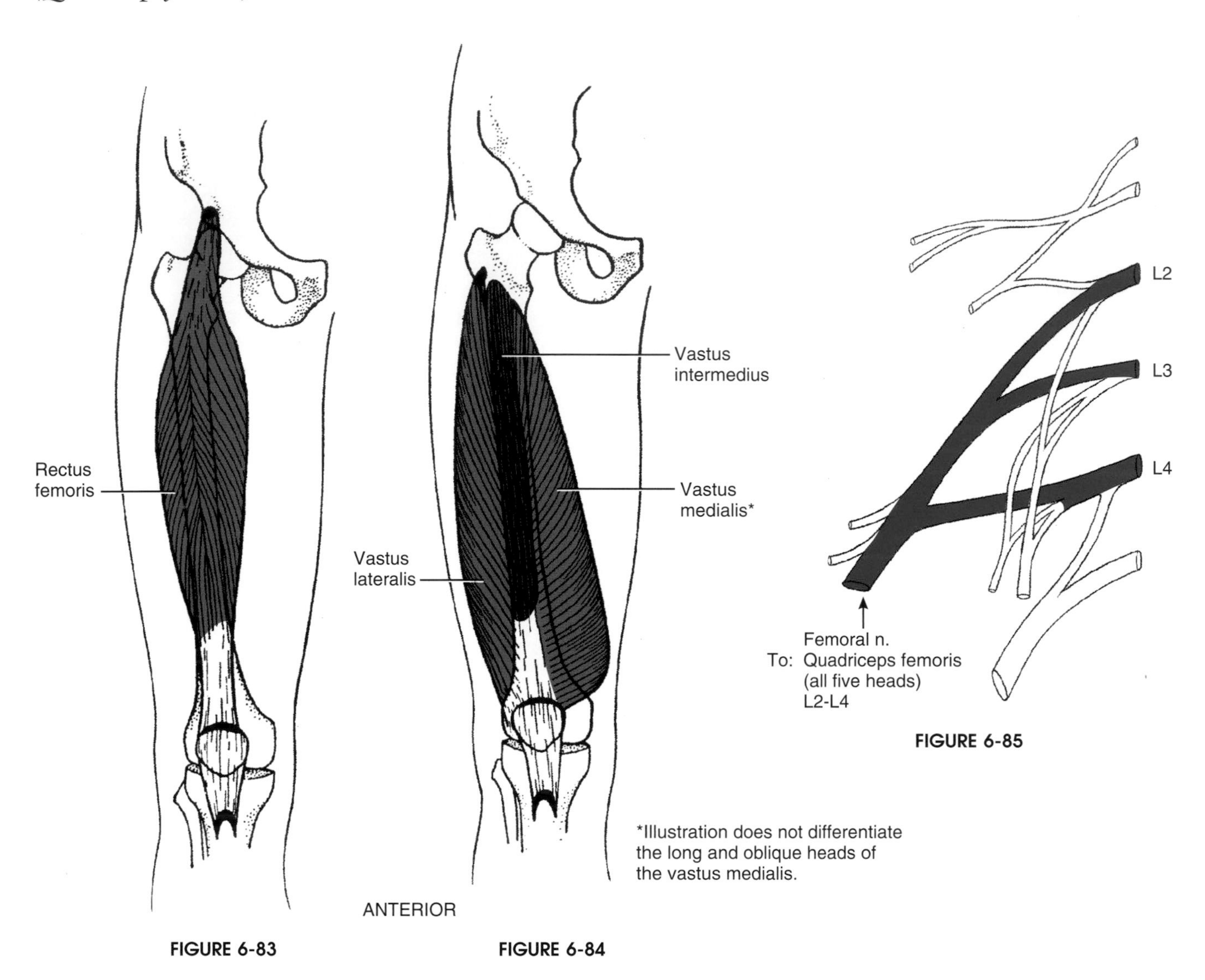

FIGURE 6-83

FIGURE 6-84

FIGURE 6-85

(Quadriceps femoris)

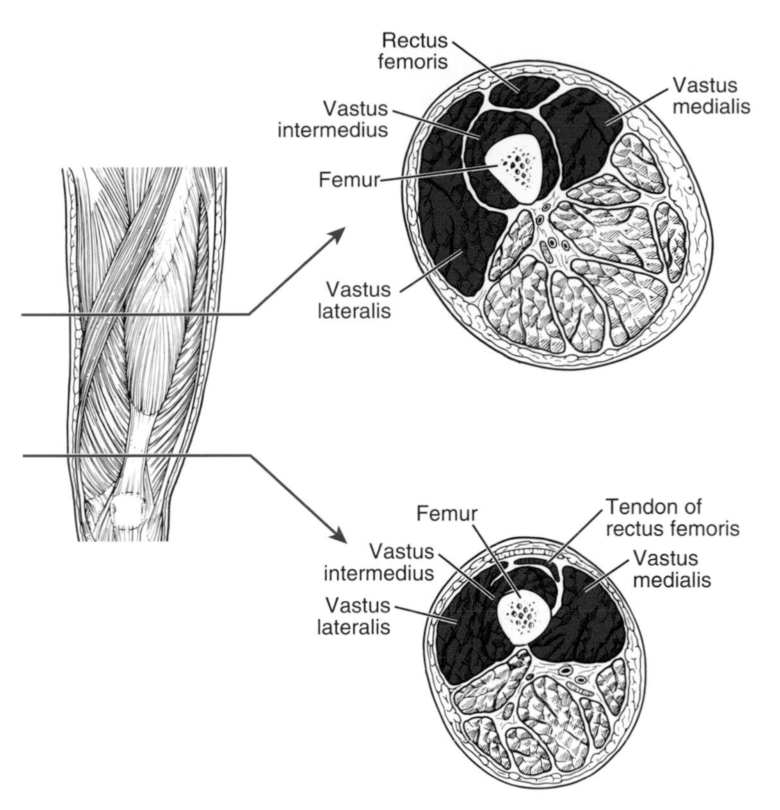

FIGURE 6-86 Arrows indicate level of cross section.

Range of Motion
135° to 0°
May extend 10° beyond 0° in those with hyperextension

Table 6-10 KNEE EXTENSION

I.D.	Muscle	Origin	Insertion
196	Rectus femoris	Ilium (anterior inferior iliac spine) Acetabulum (groove above) Capsule of hip joint Aponeurosis (anterior)	Aponeurosis (posterior) Patella (base via quadriceps tendon) Tibial tuberosity via ligamentum patellae
198	Vastus intermedius	Femur (shaft, upper 2/3 lateral and anterior surfaces) Intermuscular septum (lateral)	Aponeurosis (anterior forming deep quadriceps tendon) Patella (base, lateral aspect) Tibia (lateral condyle) Tibial tuberosity via ligamentum patellae
197	Vastus lateralis	Femur Linea aspera (lateral lip) Greater trochanter (inferior) Intertrochanteric line (via aponeurosis) Gluteal tuberosity (lateral lip) Lateral intermuscular septum	Aponeurosis (deep surface, distal) Patella (base and lateral border via quadriceps tendon) Lateral expansion to capsule of knee joint and iliotibial tract Tibial tuberosity via ligamentum patellae
199	Vastus medialis longus	Femur (linea aspera, medial lip; intertrochanteric line) Origin of vastus medialis oblique Tendon of adductor magnus Intermuscular septum (medial)	Aponeurosis (deep) Patella (medial border) Tibial tuberosity via ligamentum patellae
200	Vastus medialis oblique	Femur: linea aspera (distal); supracondylar line Tendon of adductor magnus Intermuscular septum	Aponeurosis to capsule of knee joint Patella (medial aspect) Quadriceps tendon (medial) Tibial tuberosity via ligamentum patellae
Other			
185	Tensor fasciae latae		

KNEE EXTENSION

(Quadriceps femoris)

The quadriceps femoris muscles are tested together as a functional group. None of the four muscle heads can be separated from any other by manual muscle testing. The rectus femoris may be partially isolated from the other quadriceps during a hip flexion test. At one time, the vastus medialis was thought to be activated during the terminal 15° of knee extension; however, this has been conclusively disproven.[5-7]

Knowledge of the patient's hamstring range of motion is useful before conducting tests for knee extension strength, because tight (shortened) hamstrings will limit knee extension. In short sitting for Grades 5, 4, and 3, the shorter the hamstrings, the greater the backward trunk lean.

Grade 5 (Normal), Grade 4 (Good), and Grade 3 (Fair)

Position of Patient: Short sitting. Place either a wedge or a hand under the patient's distal thigh to cushion it (Figure 6-87). The patient's hands rest on the table on either side of the body for stability or may grasp the table edge. The patient should be allowed to lean backward to relieve hamstring muscle tension. Do not allow the patient to hyperextend the knee because this may lock the knee into position, thus masking weakness.

Position of Therapist: Standing at side of limb to be tested. The palm of the resistance hand is over the anterior surface of the distal leg just above the ankle. For Grades 5 and 4, resistance is applied in a downward direction toward the floor.

Test: Patient extends knee through available range of motion but not beyond 0°.

Instructions to Patient: "Straighten your knee. Hold it! Don't let me bend it."

Helpful Hint

To prevent the patient's pelvis from rising (a common occurrence in a Grade 4 or 5 test), the patient may be secured to the testing surface by a belt or strap.

Grading

Grade 5 (Normal): Holds end position against maximal resistance. Most physical therapists will not be able to break the Grade 5 knee extensors.

Grade 4 (Good): Holds end position against strong to moderate resistance.

Grade 3 (Fair): Completes available range and holds the position without resistance (Figure 6-88).

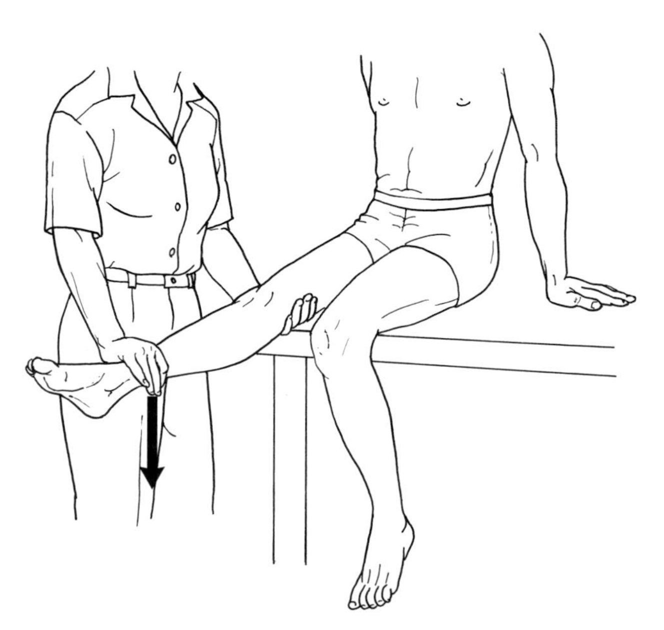

FIGURE 6-87

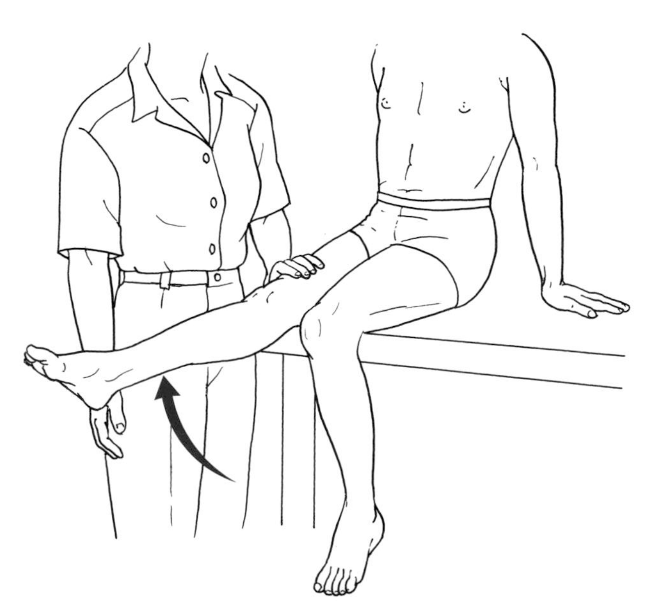

FIGURE 6-88

Grade 2 (Poor)

Position of Patient: Side-lying with test limb uppermost. Lowermost limb may be flexed for stability. Limb to be tested is held in about 90° of knee flexion. The hip should be in full extension.

Position of Therapist: Standing behind patient at knee level. One arm cradles the test limb around the thigh with the hand supporting the underside of the knee (Figure 6-89); alternatively, the test limb may be placed on a powder board. The other hand holds the leg just above the malleolus.

Test: Patient extends knee through the available range of motion. The therapist supporting the limb provides neither assistance nor resistance to the patient's voluntary movement. This is part of the art of muscle testing that must be acquired.

Be alert to activity by the internal rotators (see Substitution, page 248).

Instructions to Patient: "Straighten your knee."

Grading

Grade 2 (Poor): Completes available range of motion.

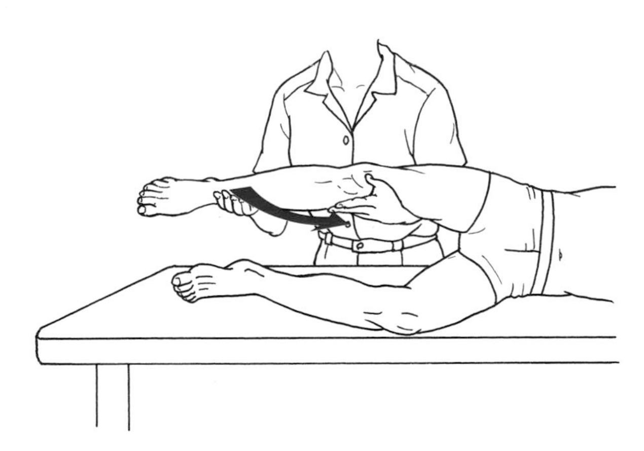

FIGURE 6-89

Grade 1 (Trace) and Grade 0 (Zero)

Position of Patient: Supine.

Position of Therapist: Standing next to limb to be tested at knee level. Hand used for palpation should be on the quadriceps tendon just above the knee with the tendon "held" gently between the thumb and fingers. The therapist also may want to palpate the patellar tendon with two to four fingers just below the knee (Figure 6-90).

Test: Patient attempts to extend knee.

As an alternate test, the therapist may place one hand under the slightly flexed knee; palpate either the quadriceps or the patellar tendon while the patient tries to extend the knee.

Instructions to Patient: "Push the back of your knee down into the table." OR "Tighten your kneecap" (quadriceps setting).

For Alternate Test: "Push the back of your knee down into my hand."

Grading

Grade 1 (Trace): Contractile activity can be palpated in muscle through the tendon. No joint movement occurs.

Grade 0 (Zero): No palpable contractile activity.

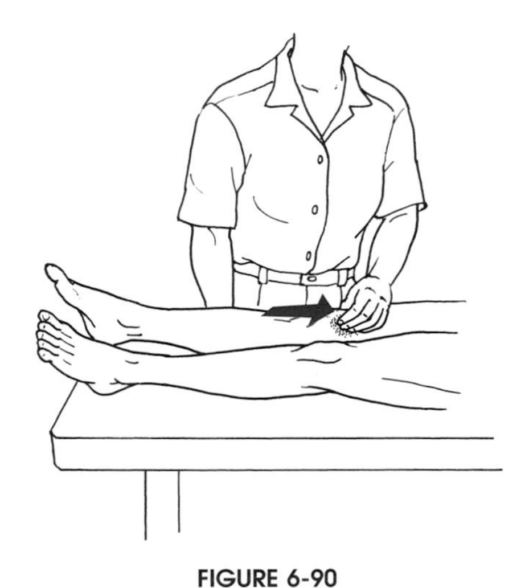

FIGURE 6-90

KNEE EXTENSION

(Quadriceps femoris)

Substitution

When the patient is side-lying (as in the Grade 2 test), he or she may use the hip internal rotators to substitute for the quadriceps, thereby allowing the knee to fall into extension.

Helpful Hints

- To assess functional strength, the quadriceps can be tested by a chair stand test (see description in Chapter 9, page 360) where strength equal to half the body weight is needed to rise from a chair without arms.[8]
- In stair descent, the forces transmitted through the knee are equal to nearly 3×/body weight,[9,10] necessitating a greater magnitude of strength than can be detected in a manual muscle test.
- Alternatively, using quantitative methods such as hand-held muscle dynamometry or a 1-repetition maximum leg press to confirm age and sex appropriate strength should be used when strength is Grades 4 or 5.

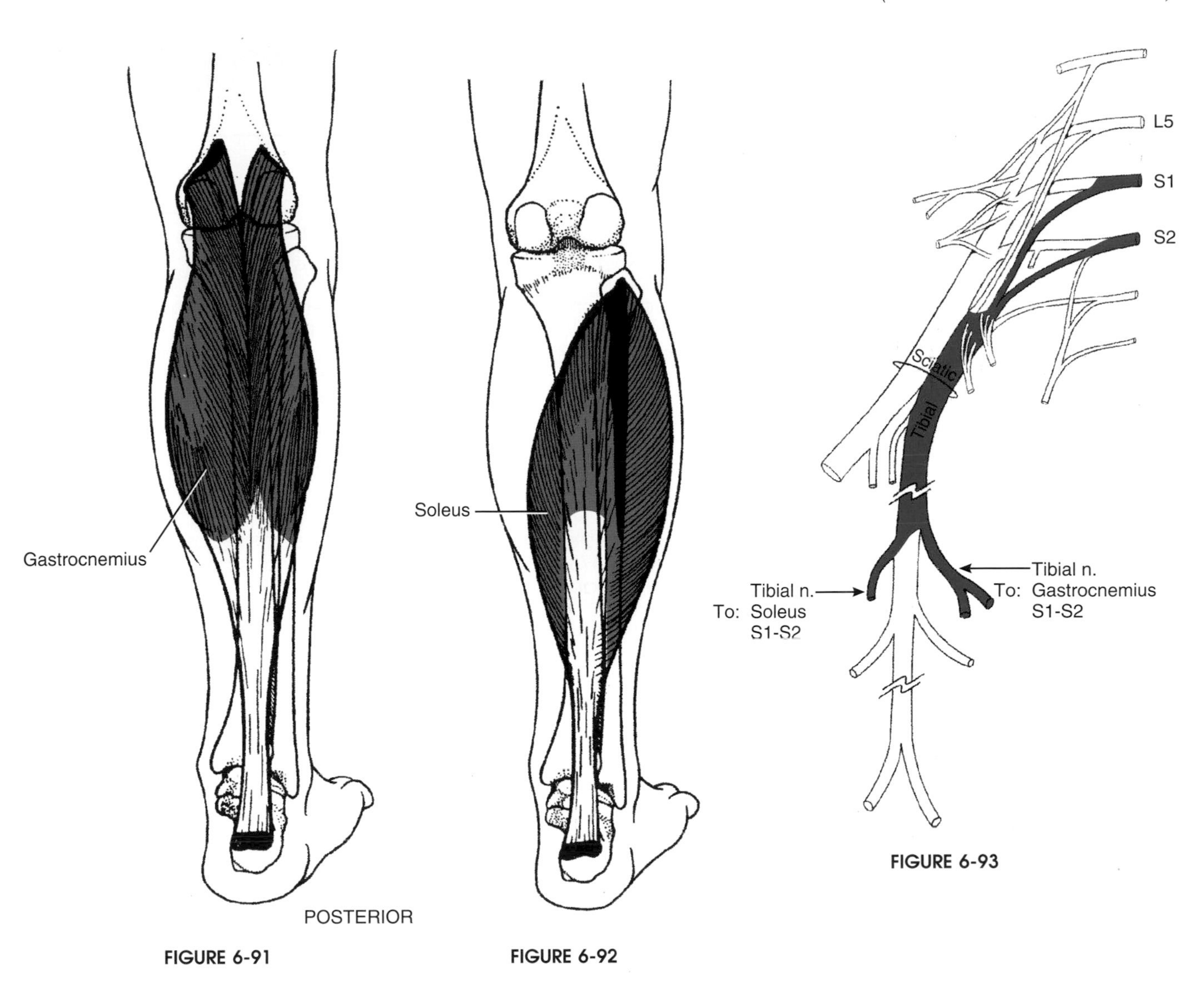

FIGURE 6-91

FIGURE 6-92

FIGURE 6-93

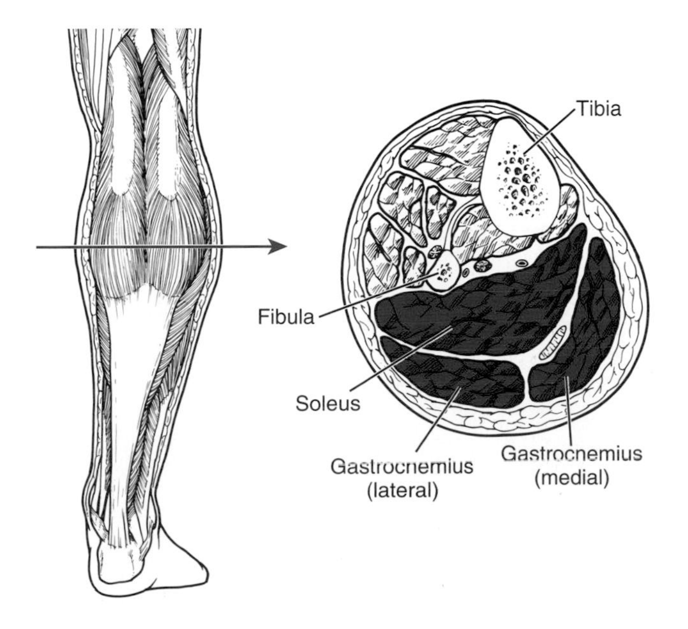

FIGURE 6-94 Arrow indicates level of cross section.

ANKLE PLANTAR FLEXION

(Gastrocnemius and Soleus)

Range of Motion
0° to 45°

Table 6-11 PLANTAR FLEXION

I.D.	Muscle	Origin	Insertion
205	Gastrocnemius		
	Medial head	Femur (medial condyle, popliteal surface) Capsule of knee joint	Anterior aponeurosis Tendo calcaneus (tendon of Achilles) formed when tendon of gastrocnemius joins tendon of soleus)
	Lateral head	Femur (lateral condyle, lateral surface, and supracondylar line) Capsule of knee joint Aponeurosis (posterior)	Calcaneus (posterior)
206	Soleus	Fibula (head, posterior aspect, and proximal 1/3 of shaft) Tibia (soleal line and middle 1/3 of medial shaft) Aponeurosis between tibia and fibula over popliteal vessels Aponeurosis (anterior)	Aponeurosis (posterior; tendinous raphe in midline of muscle) Tendo calcaneus when tendon of soleus joins tendon of gastrocnemius Calcaneus via tendo calcaneus
Others			
204	Tibialis posterior		
207	Plantaris		
208	Peroneus longus		
209	Peroneus brevis		
213	Flexor digitorum longus		
222	Flexor hallucis longus		

If the gastrocnemius-soleus complex is paralyzed, there is negligible capacity for the remaining muscles to contribute to plantar flexion to substitute for the action of plantar flexion.

GASTROCNEMIUS AND SOLEUS TEST

Grade 5 (Normal), Grade 4 (Good), and Grade 3 (Fair)

Position of Patient: Patient stands on dominant limb to be tested with knee extended. Patient is likely to need external support; no more than one or two fingers should be used on a table (or other surface) (Figure 6-95).

Position of Therapist: Standing or sitting with a lateral view of test limb to ascertain height of heel rise.

Test: Patient raises heel from floor consecutively through maximum available range at a rate of one rise every 2 seconds until patient no longer achieves 50% of initial plantar range (Figure 6-96).

Instructions to Patient: Therapist demonstrates correct heel rise to patient. "Stand on your right leg. Go up on your tiptoes. Now down. Try to repeat this as many times as possible, lifting your heel as high as you can." Repeat test for left limb.

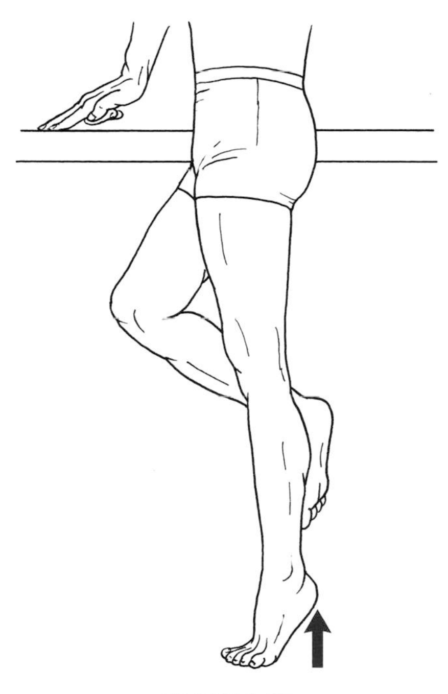

FIGURE 6-95

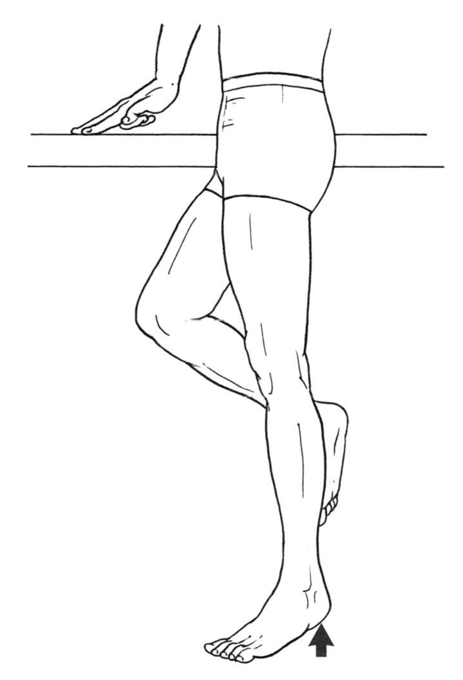

FIGURE 6-96

Grade 5 (Normal), Grade 4 (Good), and Grade 3 (Fair) Continued

Grading

Grade 5 (Normal): Patient successfully completes a minimum of 25 heel rises through full range of motion without a rest between rises and without fatigue.[11] Twenty-five heel rises elicit approximately 60% of the maximum electromyographic activity of the plantar flexors.[11] Lunsford and Perry suggest a "normal" response requires 25 complete heel rises.[12]

In the current standardized tests that have been in use for many years, 25 repetitions is the accepted norm. However, a more recent study suggests that the average number of repetitions in the sample studied is less than 25 repetitions (Table 6-12).[13] The therapist should be aware that strength deficits in the plantar flexors are common, particularly with advancing age, and strength deficits will affect the heel rise portion of the gait cycle and thus reduce gait speed.

Grade 4 (Good): A Grade of 4 is conferred when the patient completes between 2 and 24 correct heel rises at a consistent rate of one rise every 2 seconds using correct form in all repetitions. The criterion for Grade 4 is not well defined.

Grade 3 (Fair): Patient completes one heel rise correctly.

If the patient cannot complete at least one correct full-range heel rise in the standing position, the grade must be less than 3 (Fair). Regardless of any resistance to a nonstanding position for any reason, the patient must be given a grade of less than 3.[11]

Grade 2 (Poor): Patient is not able to lift heel from floor in standing position and must be tested in a non–weight-bearing position (Figure 6-97).

Table 6-12 AVERAGE VALUES OF UNTRAINED SUBJECTS

	Males (by Age)				Females (by Age)			
	Lunsford and Perry[12]	***Jan et al[13]***	***Jan et al[13]***	***Jan et al[13]***	***Lunsford and Perry[12]***	***Jan et al[13]***	***Jan et al[13]***	***Jan et al[13]***
	X = 34.7	21-40	41-60	61-80	X = 29.3	21-40	41-60	61-80
Mean	27.8	22.1	12.1	4.1	28.4	16.1	9.3	2.7
SD	11.5	9.8	6.6	1.9	9.8	6.7	3.6	1.5
Plantar flexion range	X = 24.9 (9.5)	9-46	4-30	0-7	X = 34.6 (10.1)	6-30	5-19	0.5
80th percentile		17	7	2		10	5	1

Grade 2 (Poor)

Position of Patient: Prone with feet off end of table.

Position of Therapist: Standing at end of table in front of foot to be tested. One hand is contoured under and around the test leg just above the ankle (Figure 6-97). Heel and palm of hand giving resistance are placed against the plantar surface at the level of the metatarsal heads.

Test: Patient plantar flexes ankle through the available range of motion. Manual resistance is down and forward toward dorsiflexion.

Grading

Grade 2 (Poor): Patient completes plantar flexion range against resistance.

Grade 2– (Poor–): Patient completes only a partial range of motion.

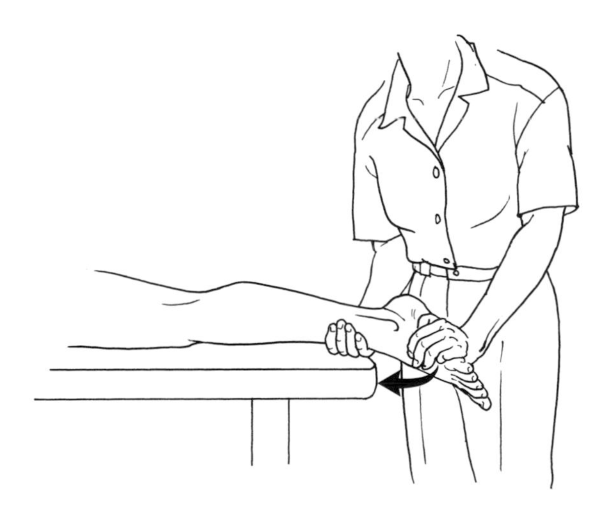

FIGURE 6-97

Grade 1 (Trace) and Grade 0 (Zero)

Position of Patient: Prone with feet off end of table.

Position of Therapist: Standing at end of table in front of foot to be tested. One hand palpates gastrocnemius-soleus activity by monitoring tension in the Achilles tendon just above the calcaneus (Figure 6-98). The muscle bellies of the two muscles also may be palpated (not illustrated).

Test: Patient attempts to plantar flex the ankle.

Instructions to Patient: "Point your toes down, like a ballet dancer."

Grading

Grade 1 (Trace): Tendon reflects some contractile activity in muscle, but no joint motion occurs. Contractile activity may be palpated in muscle bellies. The best location to palpate the gastrocnemius is at midcalf with thumb and fingers on either side of the midline but above the soleus. Palpation of the soleus is best done on the posterolateral surface of the distal calf. In most people with calf strength of Grade 3 or better, the two muscles can be observed and differentiated during plantar flexion testing because their definition is clear.

Grade 0 (Zero): No palpable contraction.

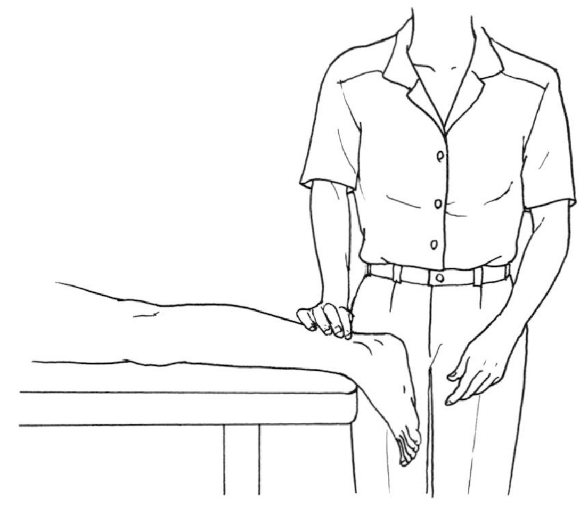

FIGURE 6-98

ANKLE PLANTAR FLEXION

(Gastrocnemius and Soleus)

Substitutions

- By flexor hallucis longus and flexor digitorum longus: When substitution by the toe flexors occurs, their motions will be accompanied by plantar flexion of the forefoot and incomplete movement of the calcaneus (Figure 6-99).
- By peroneus longus and peroneus brevis: These muscles substituting for the gastrocnemius and soleus will pull the foot into eversion.
- By tibialis posterior: The foot will move into inversion during plantar flexion testing if the tibialis posterior substitutes for the primary plantar flexors.
- By tibialis posterior, peroneus longus, and peroneus brevis: Substitution by these three muscles will plantar flex the forefoot instead of the ankle.

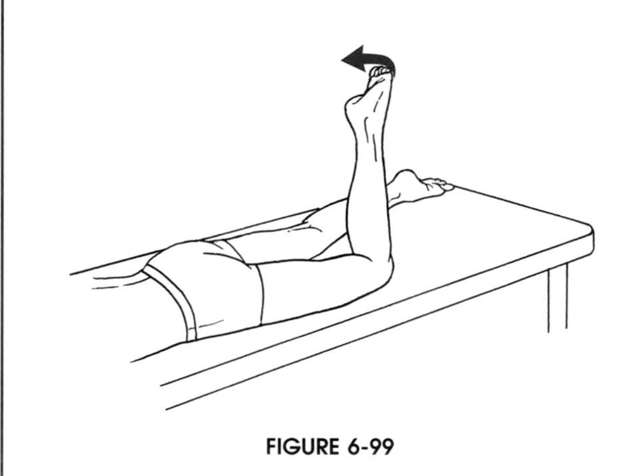

FIGURE 6-99

Helpful Hints

- If for any reason the patient cannot lie prone for Grades 2, 1, or 0, an alternative for any of these tests is to use the supine position for non–weight-bearing testing. The highest grade awarded in this case is a 2.
- If the patient is unable to perform a standing plantar flexion test but has a stable forefoot, a different application of resistance may be used with the patient supine. The resistance is applied against the sole of the foot with the forearm while the heel is cupped with the hand of the same arm and the ankle is forced into dorsiflexion. The highest grade that may be awarded in this case is a 2.
- During standing plantar flexion tests, the tibialis posterior and the peroneus longus and brevis muscles must be Grades 5 or 4 to stabilize the forefoot to attain and hold the tiptoe position.
- Care must be taken to avoid transferring weight through the finger tips used for balance. Therefore it is recommended to place the patient's arms above the head on the wall in front of the patient. However, be sure that the patient maintains a fully erect posture. If the subject leans forward or flexes knee, such posture can bring the heel off the ground, creating a testing artifact.
- In normal plantar flexion, the patient should be able to raise heel 2 inches; thus, when the patient can no longer achieve 1 inch of rise, the test is terminated.

CROSS SECTIONS OF THE LEG

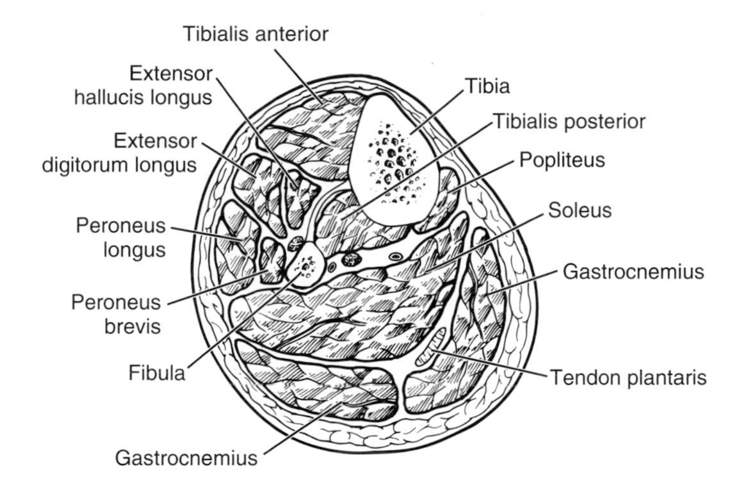

MID LEG
AT UPPER PORTION OF GASTROCNEMIUS AND SOLEUS AT LARGEST CIRCUMFERENCE OF CALF

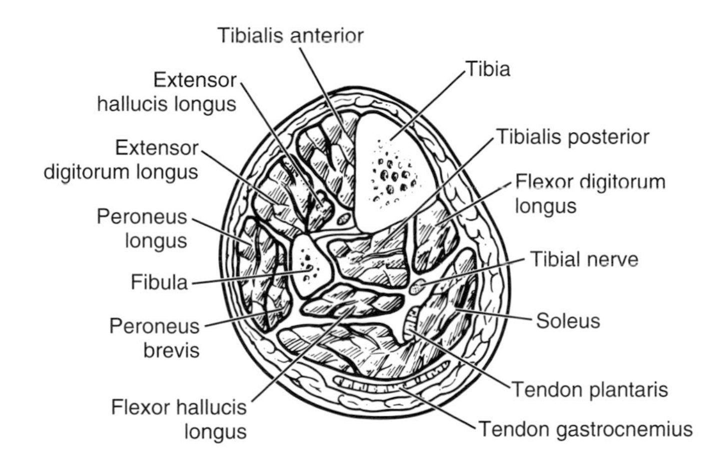

LOWER LEG
NEAR END OF MUSCULAR PORTIONS OF TRICEPS SURAE. GASTROCNEMIUS IS ALL TENDINOUS.

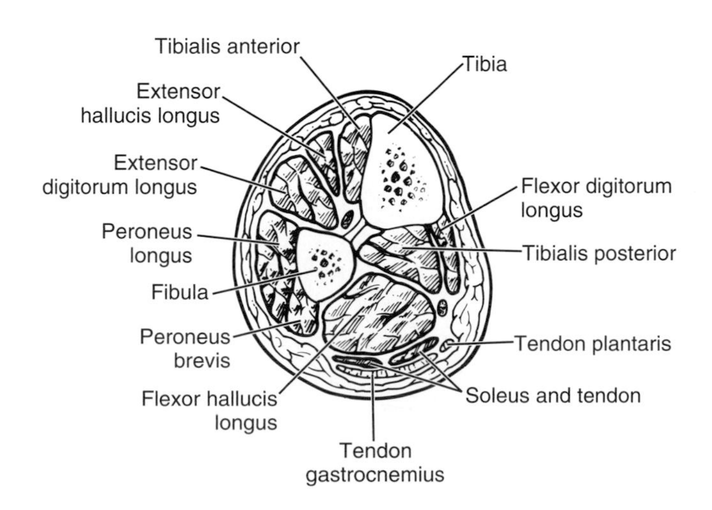

HIGH ANKLE
LOWER LEG WHERE GASTROCNEMIUS, SOLEUS, AND PLANTARIS ARE TENDINOUS

PLATE 7

FOOT DORSIFLEXION AND INVERSION

(Tibialis anterior)

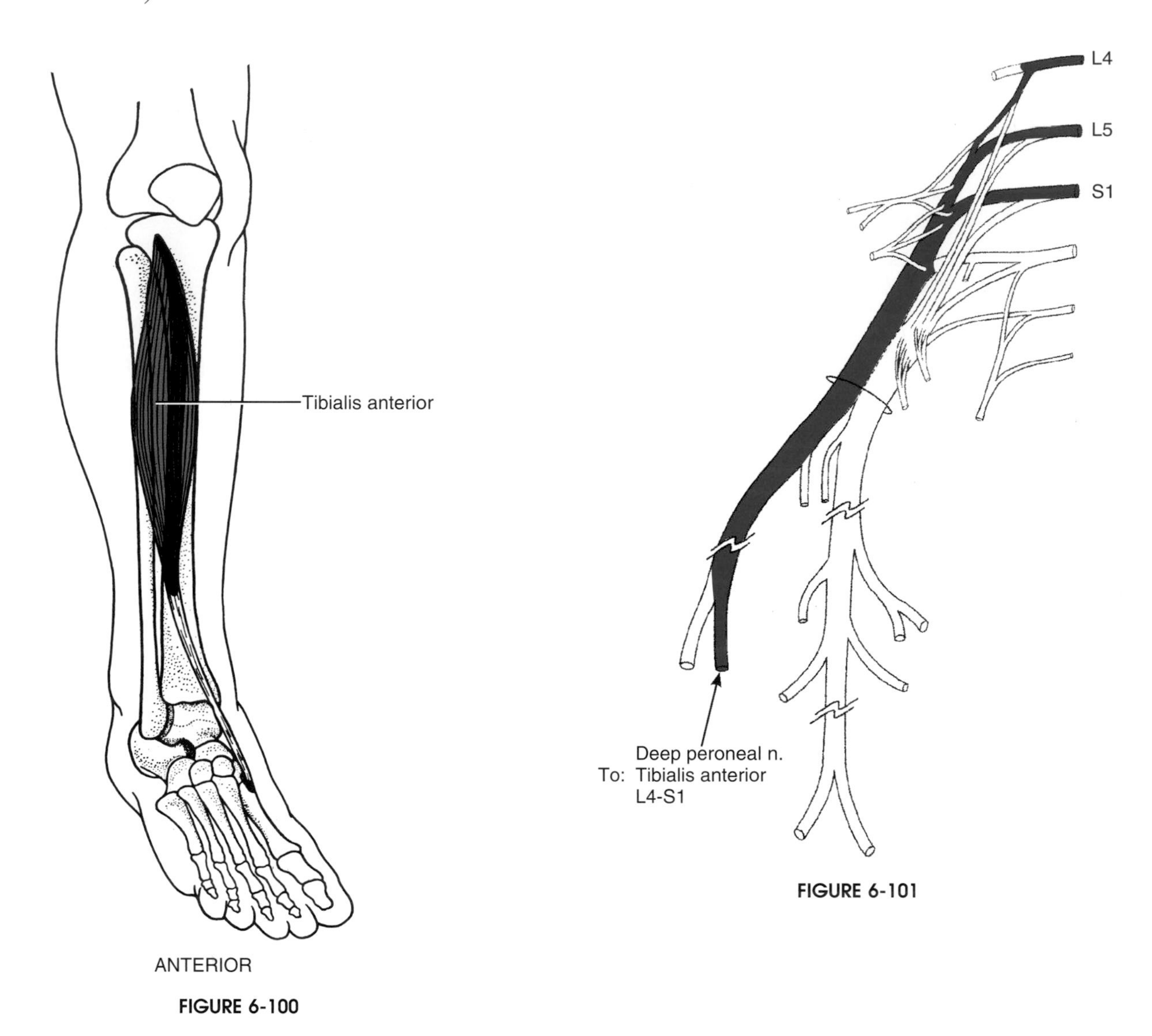

FIGURE 6-100

FIGURE 6-101

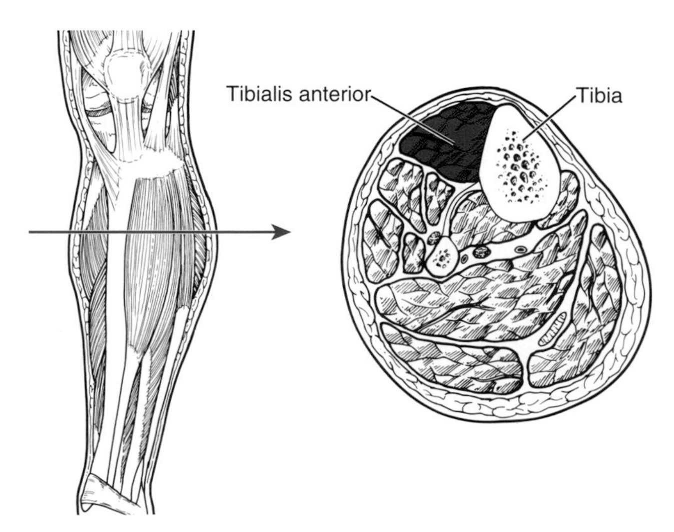

FIGURE 6-102 Arrow indicates level of cross section.

(Tibialis anterior)

Range of Motion
0° to 20°

Table 6-13 FOOT DORSIFLEXION AND INVERSION

I.D.	Muscle	Origin	Insertion
203	Tibialis anterior	Tibia (lateral condyle and proximal 2/3 of lateral shaft) Interosseous membrane Fascia cruris (deep) Intermuscular septum	1st (medial) cuneiform (on medial and plantar surfaces) 1st metatarsal (base)
Others			
210	Peroneus tertius		
211	Extensor digitorum longus		
221	Extensor hallucis longus		

Grades 5 (Normal) to 0 (Zero)

Position of Patient: Sitting. Alternatively, patient may be supine.

Position of Therapist: Sitting on stool in front of patient with patient's heel resting on thigh. One hand is contoured around the posterior leg just above the malleoli for Grades 5 and 4 (Figure 6-103). The hand providing resistance for the same grades is cupped over the dorsomedial aspect of the foot (see Figure 6-103).

Test: Patient dorsiflexes ankle and inverts foot, keeping toes relaxed.

Instructions to Patient: "Bring your foot up and in. Hold it! Don't let me push it down."

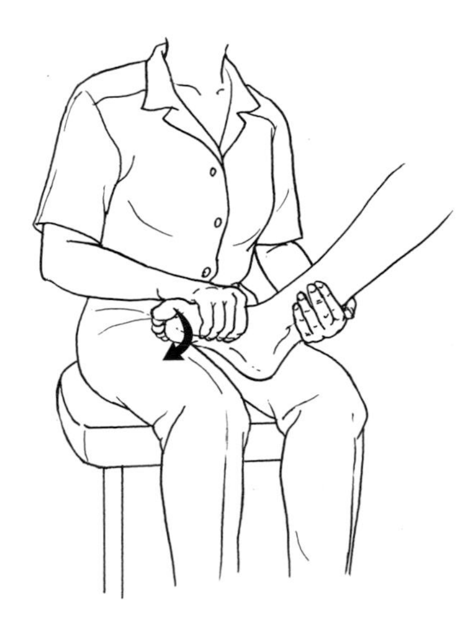

FIGURE 6-103

FOOT DORSIFLEXION AND INVERSION

(Tibialis anterior)

Grades 5 (Normal) to 0 (Zero) Continued

Grading

Grade 5 (Normal): Completes full range and holds against maximal resistance.

Grade 4 (Good): Completes available range against strong to moderate resistance.

Grade 3 (Fair): Completes available range of motion and holds end position without resistance (Figure 6-104).

Grade 2 (Poor): Completes only a partial range of motion.

Grade 1 (Trace): Therapist will be able to detect some contractile activity in the muscle, or the tendon will "stand out." There is no joint movement.

Palpate the tendon of the tibialis anterior on the anteromedial aspect of the ankle at about the level of the malleoli (Figure 6-105, lower hand). Palpate the muscle for contractile activity over its belly just lateral to the "shin" (see Figure 6-105, upper hand).

Grade 0 (Zero): No palpable contraction.

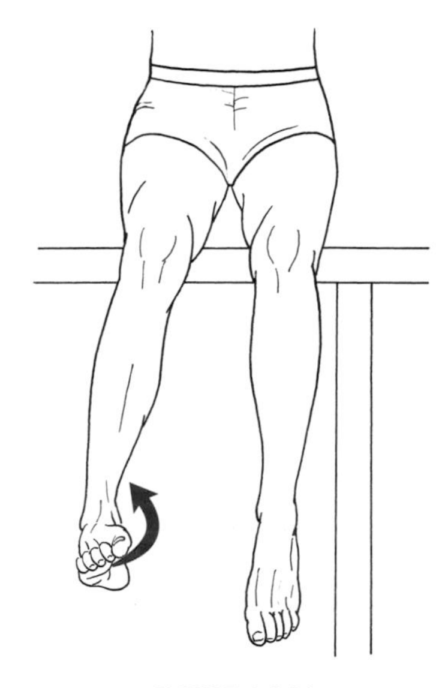

FIGURE 6-104

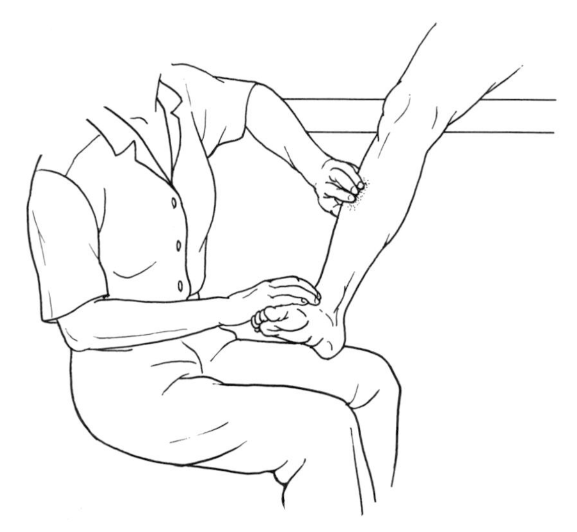

FIGURE 6-105

Substitution

Substitution by the extensor digitorum longus and the extensor hallucis longus muscles results also in toe extension. Instruct the patient, therefore, to keep the toes relaxed so that they are not part of the test movement.

Helpful Hints

- In the sitting and supine positions, make sure the knee is flexed to put the gastrocnemius on slack. If the knee is extended and there is gastrocnemius tightness, the patient will not be able to achieve full dorsiflexion range.
- If the supine position is used in lieu of the sitting position for the Grade 3 test, the therapist should add a degree of difficulty to the test to compensate for the lack of gravity. For example, give mild resistance in the supine position but award no more than a Grade 3.
- In the supine position, to earn a Grade 2 the patient must complete a full range of motion.

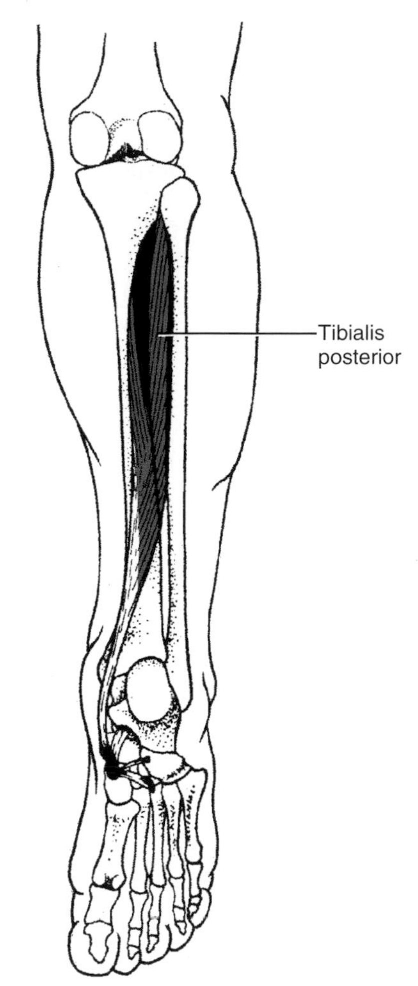

POSTERIOR VIEW OF LEG
PLANTAR VIEW OF FOOT

FIGURE 6-106

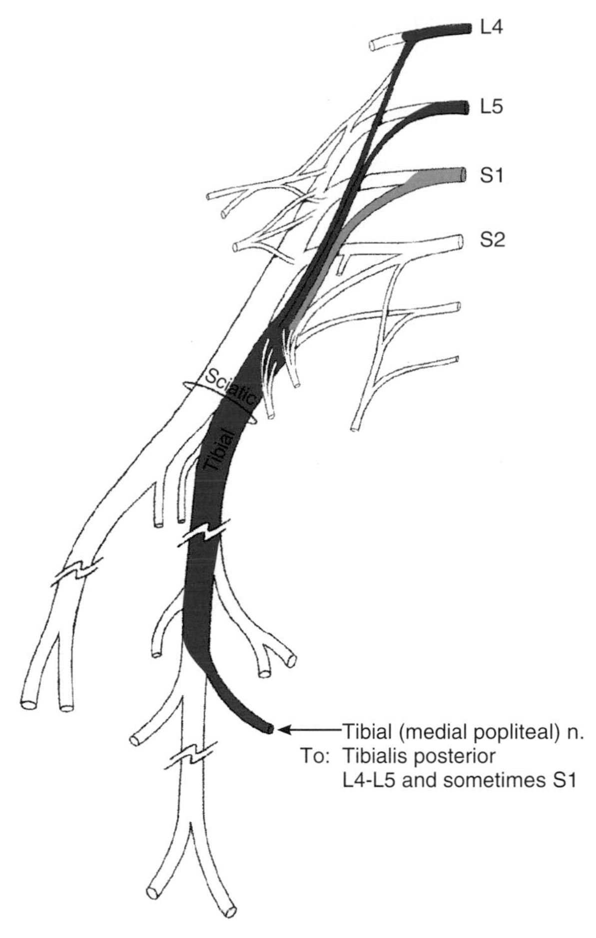

FIGURE 6-107

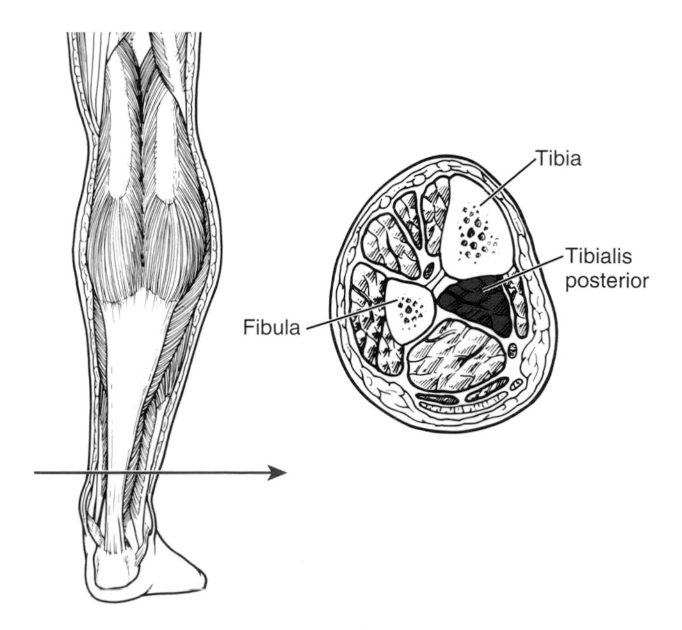

FIGURE 6-108 Arrow indicates level of cross section.

Range of Motion
0° to 35°

FOOT INVERSION

(Tibialis posterior)

Table 6-14 FOOT INVERSION

I.D.	Muscle	Origin	Insertion
204	Tibialis posterior	Tibia (proximal 2/3 of posterior lateral shaft below soleal line) Interosseous membrane (posterior) Fibula (shaft, proximal posterior medial 2/3) Deep transverse fascia Intermuscular septa	Navicular bone (tuberosity) Cuneiform bones Sustentaculum tali (distal) Metatarsals 2–4 (via tendinous band)
Others			
203	Tibialis anterior		
213	Flexor digitorum longus		
222	Flexor hallucis longus		
206	Soleus		
221	Extensor hallucis longus		

Grades 5 (Normal) to 2 (Poor)

Position of Patient: Sitting with ankle in slight plantar flexion.

Position of Therapist: Sitting on low stool in front of patient or on side of test limb. One hand is used to stabilize the ankle just above the malleoli (Figure 6-109). Hand providing resistance is contoured over the dorsum and medial side of the foot at the level of the metatarsal heads. Resistance is directed toward eversion and slight dorsiflexion (forefoot abduction).

Test: Patient inverts foot through available range of motion.

Instructions to Patient: Therapist may need to demonstrate motion. "Turn your foot down and in. Hold it."

Grading

Grade 5 (Normal): The patient completes the full range and holds against maximal resistance.

Grade 4 (Good): The patient completes available range against strong to moderate resistance.

Grade 3 (Fair): The patient will be able to invert the foot through the full available range of motion (Figure 6-110).

Grade 2 (Poor): The patient will be able to complete only a partial range of motion.

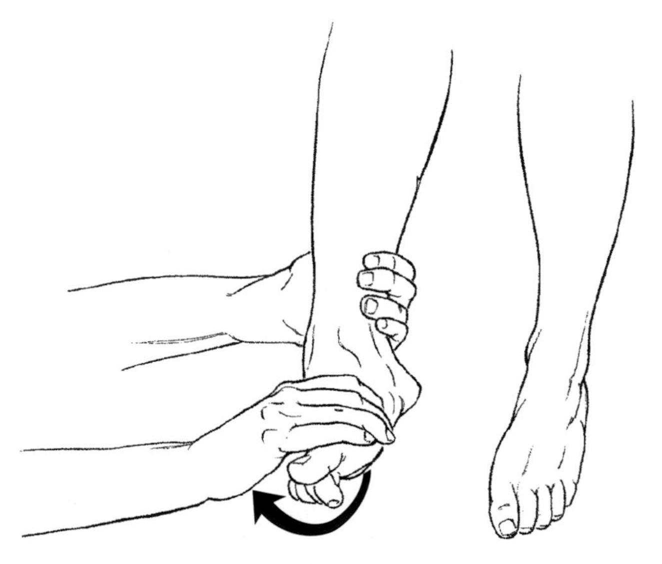

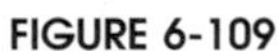

FIGURE 6-109

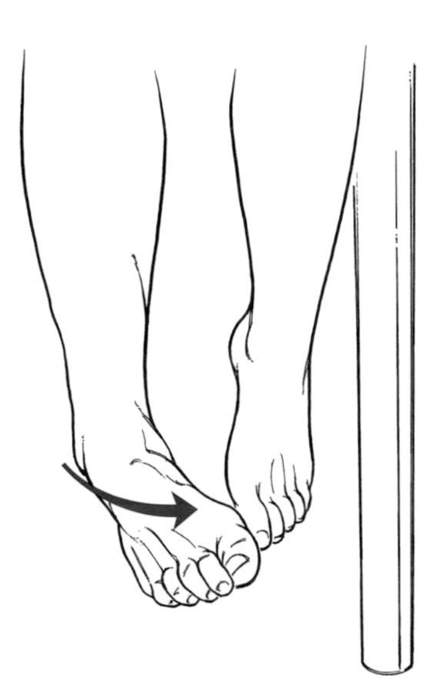

FIGURE 6-110

Grade 1 (Trace) and Grade 0 (Zero)

Position of Patient: Sitting or supine.

Position of Therapist: Sitting on low stool or standing in front of patient. Palpate tendon of the tibialis posterior between the medial malleolus and the navicular bone (Figure 6-111). Alternatively, palpate tendon above the malleolus.

Test: Patient attempts to invert foot.

Instructions to Patient: "Try to turn your foot down and in."

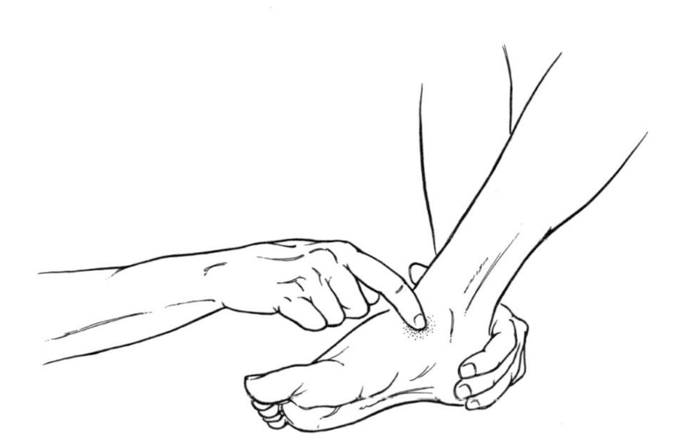

FIGURE 6-111

Grading

Grade 1 (Trace): The posterior tibialis tendon will stand out if there is contractile activity in the muscle. If palpable activity occurs in the absence of movement, the grade is 1.

Grade 0 (Zero): No palpable contraction.

Substitution

Flexors of the toes should remain relaxed to prevent substitution by the flexor digitorum longus and flexor hallucis longus.

FOOT EVERSION WITH PLANTAR FLEXION

(Peroneus longus and Peroneus brevis)

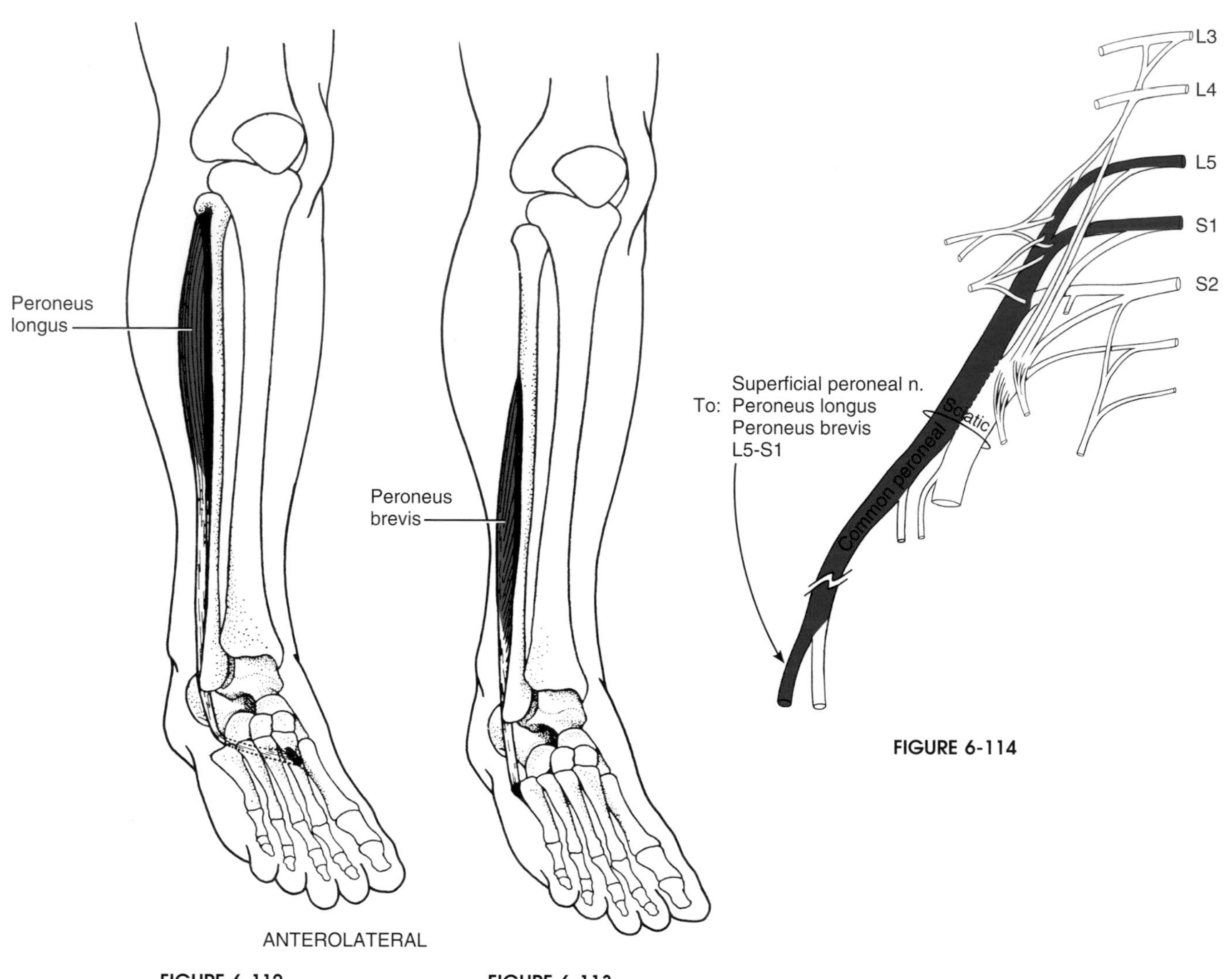

FIGURE 6-112

FIGURE 6-113

FIGURE 6-114

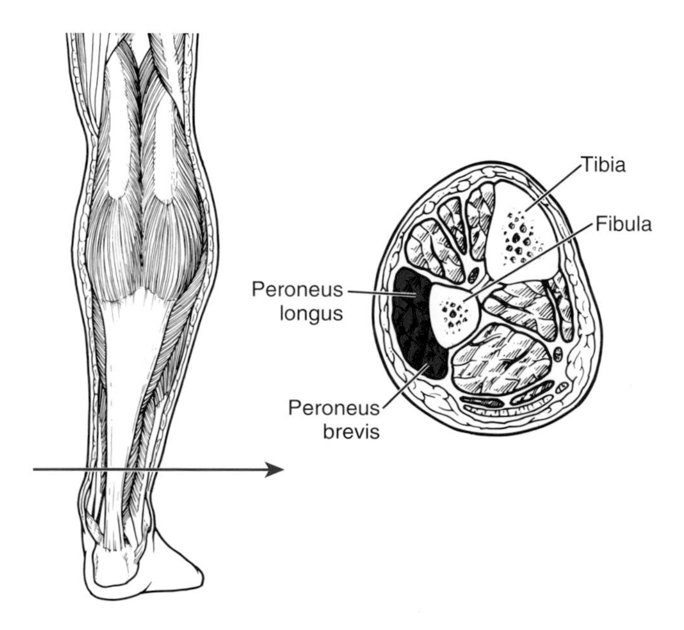

FIGURE 6-115 Arrow indicates level of cross section.

(Peroneus longus and Peroneus brevis)

Range of Motion
0° to 25°

Table 6-15 FOOT EVERSION

I.D.	Muscle	Origin	Insertion
With Plantar Flexion			
208	Peroneus longus	Fibula (head and proximal 2/3 of shaft, lateral aspect) Tibia (lateral condyle, occasionally) Fascia cruris Intermuscular septa	1st metatarsal (base and lateral aspect) Medial cuneiform (base and lateral aspect) Other metatarsals occasionally
209	Peroneus brevis	Fibula (distal and lateral 2/3 of shaft) Crural intermuscular septum	5th metatarsal (tuberosity at base, lateral aspect)
With Dorsiflexion			
211	Extensor digitorum longus	Tibia (lateral condyle on lateral side) Fibula (shaft: upper 3/4 of medial surface) Interosseous membrane (anterior surface) Deep crural fascia and intermuscular septum	Tendon of insertion divides into four tendon slips to dorsum of foot that form an expansion over each toe: Toes 2 to 5: Middle phalanges (PIP joints) of the four lesser toes (intermediate slip to dorsum of base of each) Distal phalanges (two lateral slips to dorsum of base of each)
210	Peroneus tertius	Fibula (distal 1/3 of medial surface) Interosseous membrane (anterior) Intermuscular septum	5th metatarsal (dorsal surface of base; shaft, medial aspect)
Other			
205	Gastrocnemius		

FOOT EVERSION WITH PLANTAR FLEXION

(Peroneus longus and Peroneus brevis)

Grade 5 (Normal) to Grade 2 (Poor)

Position of Patient: Sitting with ankle in neutral position (midway between dorsiflexion and plantar flexion) (Figure 6-116). Test also may be performed with patient supine.

Position of Therapist: Sitting on low stool in front of patient or standing at end of table if patient is supine.

One hand stabilizes the ankle just above the malleoli. Hand giving resistance is contoured around the dorsum and lateral border of the forefoot (see Figure 6-116). Resistance is directed toward inversion and slight dorsiflexion.

Test: Patient everts foot with depression of first metatarsal head and some plantar flexion.

Instructions to Patient: "Turn your foot down and out. Hold it! Don't let me move it in."

Grading

Grade 5 (Normal): Patient completes full range and holds end position against maximal resistance.

Grade 4 (Good): Patient completes available range of motion against strong to moderate resistance.

Grade 3 (Fair): Patient completes available range of eversion but tolerates no resistance (Figure 6-117).

Grade 2 (Poor): The patient will be able to complete only a partial range of eversion motion.

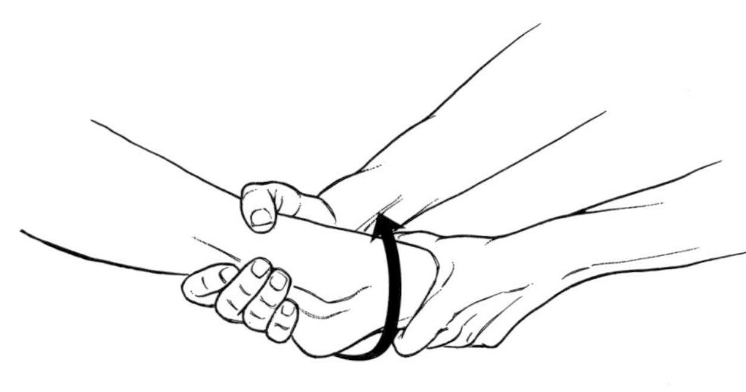

FIGURE 6-116

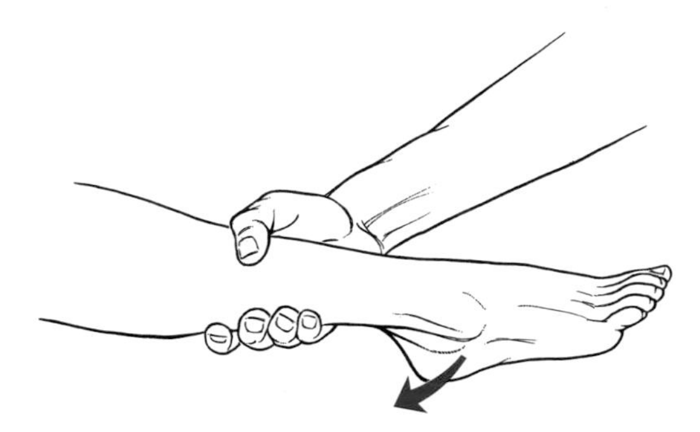

FIGURE 6-117

Grade 1 (Trace) and Grade 0 (Zero)

Position of Patient: Short sitting or supine.

Position of Therapist: Sitting on low stool or standing at end of table. To palpate the peroneus longus, place fingers on the lateral leg over the upper one-third just below the head of the fibula. The tendon of the muscle can be felt posterior to the lateral malleolus but behind the tendon of the peroneus brevis.

To palpate the tendon of the peroneus brevis, place index finger over the tendon as it comes forward from behind the lateral malleolus, proximal to the base of the 5th metatarsal (Figure 6-118). The belly of the peroneus brevis can be palpated on the lateral surface of the distal leg over the fibula.

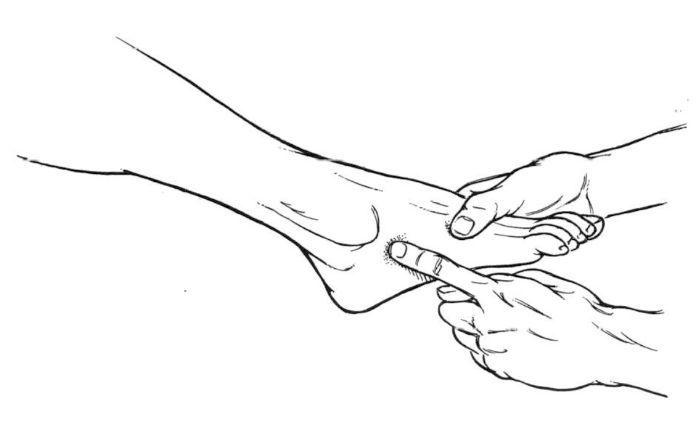

FIGURE 6-118

Grading

Grade 1 (Trace): Palpation will reveal contractile activity in either or both muscles, which may cause the tendon to stand out. No motion occurs.

Grade 0 (Zero): No palpable contractile activity.

Isolation of Peroneus Longus

Give resistance against the plantar surface of the head of the 1st metatarsal in a direction toward inversion and dorsiflexion.

Foot Eversion with Dorsiflexion

If the peroneus tertius is present, it can be tested by asking the patient to evert and dorsiflex the foot. In this motion, however, the extensor digitorum longus participates.

The tendon of the peroneus tertius can be palpated on the lateral aspect of the dorsum of the foot, where it lies lateral to the tendon of the extensor digitorum longus slip to the little toe.

Helpful Hints

- Foot eversion is accompanied by either dorsiflexion or plantar flexion. The toe extensors are the primary dorsiflexors accompanying eversion because the peroneus tertius is not always present.
- The primary motion of eversion with plantar flexion is accomplished by the peroneus brevis because the peroneus longus is primarily a depressor of the 1st metatarsal head rather than an evertor.
- The peroneus brevis cannot be isolated if both peronei are innervated and active.
- If there is a difference in strength between the peroneus longus and the peroneus brevis, the stronger of the two can be ascertained by the relative amount of resistance taken in eversion versus the resistance taken at the 1st metatarsal head. If greater resistance is taken at the 1st metatarsal head, the peroneus longus is the stronger muscle.

HALLUX AND TOE MP FLEXION

(Lumbricales and Flexor hallucis brevis)

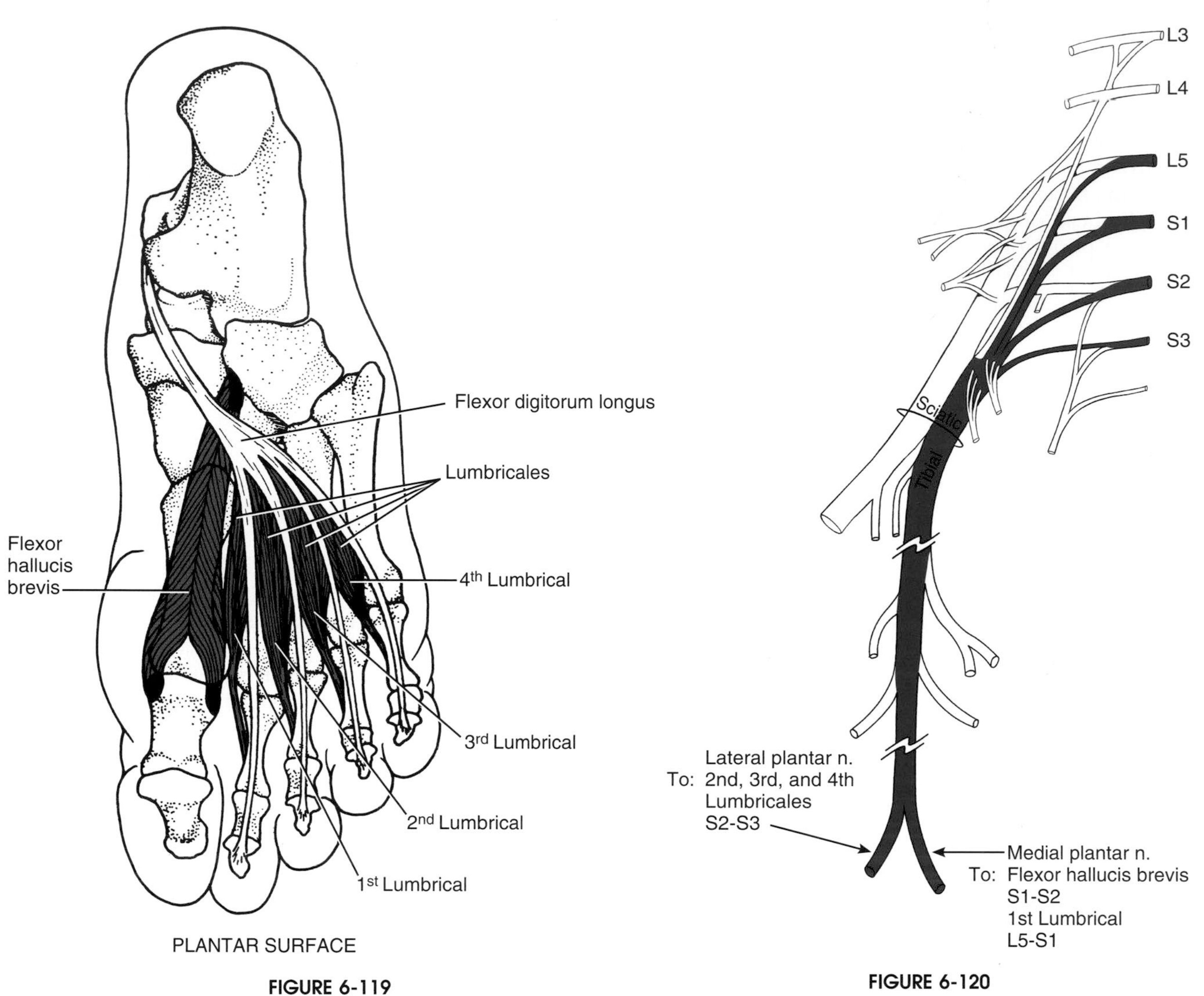

FIGURE 6-119

FIGURE 6-120

Range of Motion
Great toe, 0° to 45°
Lateral four toes, 0° to 40°

Table 6-16 FLEXION OF MP JOINTS OF TOES AND HALLUX

I.D.	Muscle	Origin	Insertion
Toes			
218	Lumbricales	Tendons of flexor digitorum longus near angles of separation 1st lumbrical (by a single head, tendon of flexor digitorum longus bound for toe 2) 2nd–4th lumbricales (arise by dual heads from adjacent sides of tendons of flexor digitorum longus bound for toes 3-5)	All: toes 2-5 (proximal phalanges and dorsal expansions of the tendons of extensor digitorum longus)
Hallux			
223	Flexor hallucis brevis (rises by 2 heads)		
	Lateral head	Cuboid bone (plantar surface) Lateral cuneiform bone	Hallux (proximal phalanx on both sides of base) Blends with adductor hallucis
	Medial head	Medial intermuscular septum Tibialis posterior (tendon)	Hallux (proximal phalanx on both sides of base) Blends with abductor hallucis
Others			
219, 220	Interossei, dorsal and plantar		
216	Flexor digiti minimi brevis		
213	Flexor digitorum longus		
214	Flexor digitorum brevis		
222	Flexor hallucis longus		
224	Abductor hallucis		
225	Adductor hallucis		

HALLUX MP FLEXION *(Flexor hallucis brevis)*

Grades 5 (Normal) to 0 (Zero)

Position of Patient: Sitting (alternate position: supine) with legs hanging over edge of table. Ankle is in neutral position (midway between dorsiflexion and plantar flexion).

Position of Therapist: Sitting on low stool in front of patient. Alternate position: standing at side of table near patient's foot.

Test foot rests on therapist's lap. One hand is contoured over the dorsum of the foot just below the ankle for stabilization (Figure 6-121). The index finger of the other hand is placed beneath the proximal phalanx of the great toe. Alternatively, the tip of the finger (with very short fingernails) is placed up under the proximal phalanx.

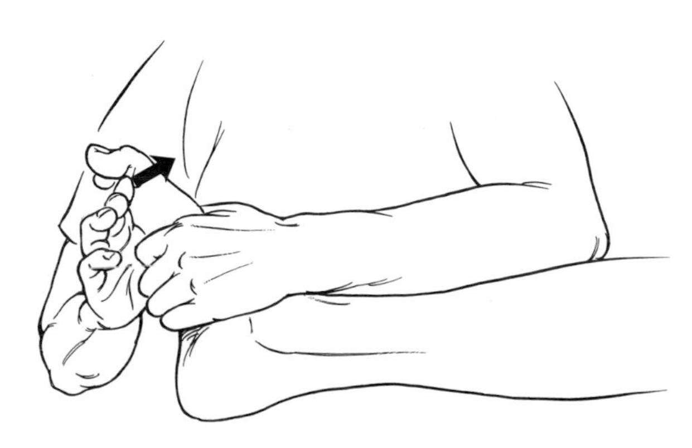

FIGURE 6-121

HALLUX AND TOE MP FLEXION

(Lumbricales and Flexor hallucis brevis)

Grades 5 (Normal) to 0 (Zero) Continued

Test: Patient flexes great toe.

Instructions to Patient: "Bend your big toe over my finger. Hold it. Don't let me straighten it."

Grading

Grade 5 (Normal): Patient completes available range and tolerates strong resistance.

Grade 4 (Good): Patient completes available range and tolerates moderate to mild resistance.

Grade 3 (Fair): Patient completes available range of metatarsophalangeal (MP) flexion of the great toe but is unable to hold against any resistance.

Grade 2 (Poor): Patient completes only partial range of motion.

Grade 1 (Trace): Therapist may note contractile activity but no toe motion.

Grade 0 (Zero): No contractile activity.

Helpful Hints

- The muscle and tendon of the flexor hallucis brevis cannot be palpated.
- When the flexor hallucis longus is not functional, the flexor hallucis brevis will flex the MP joint but without flexion of the interphalangeal (IP) joint. In the opposite condition, when the flexor hallucis brevis is not functional, the IP joint flexes and the metatarsophalangeal joint may hyperextend. (When this condition is chronic, the posture is called hammer toe.)

TOE MP FLEXION *(Lumbricales)*

Grades 5 (Normal) to 0 (Zero)

Position of Patient: Sitting with foot on therapist's lap. Alternate position: supine. Ankle is in neutral (midway between dorsiflexion and plantar flexion).

Position of Therapist: Sitting on low stool in front of patient. Alternate position: standing next to table beside test foot.

One hand provides stabilization (as in test for flexion of the hallux) over the dorsum of the foot (Figure 6-122). The index finger of the other hand is placed under the MP joints of the four lateral toes to provide resistance to flexion.

Test: Patient flexes lateral four toes at the MP joints, keeping the interphalangeal (IP) joints neutral.

Instructions to Patient: "Bend your toes over my finger."

Grading

Grading is the same as that used for the great toe.

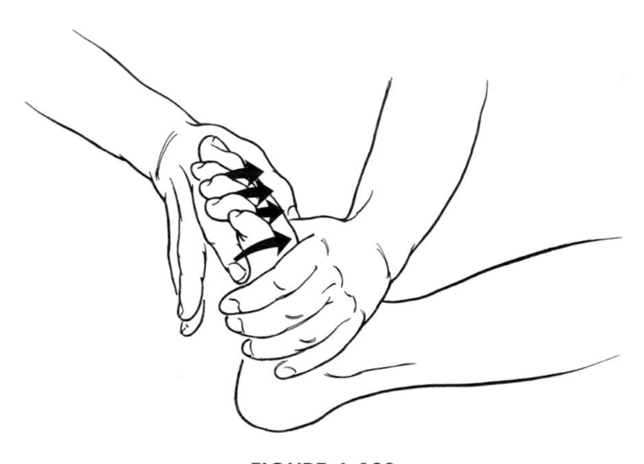

FIGURE 6-122

Helpful Hints

- In actual practice, the great toe and the lateral toes are rarely tested independently. Many patients cannot separate hallux motion from motion of the lateral toes, nor can they separate MP and IP motions.
- The therapist could test each toe separately because the lumbricales are notoriously uneven in strength. This may not, however, be practicable.

(Flexor digitorum longus, Flexor digitorum brevis, Flexor hallucis longus)

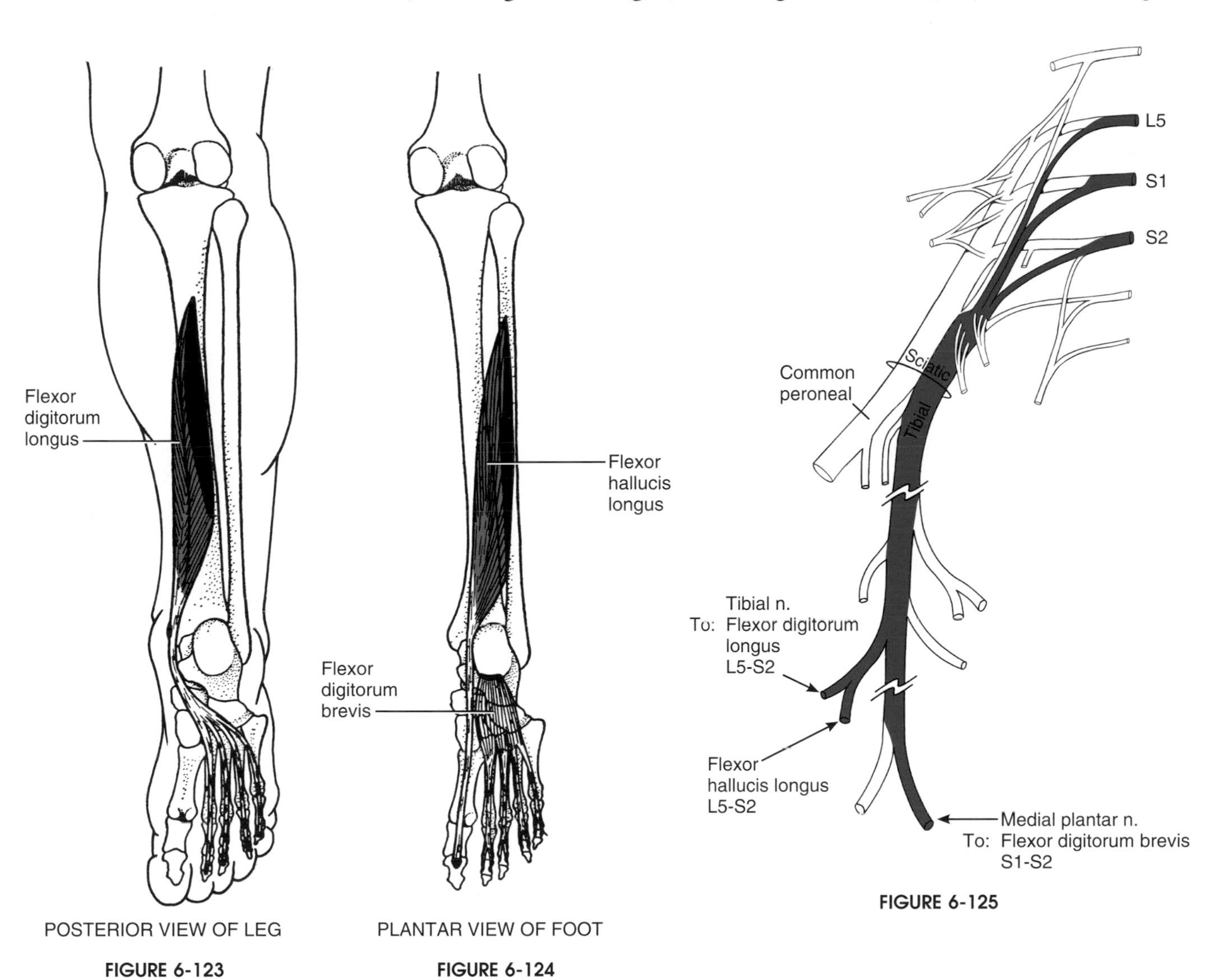

POSTERIOR VIEW OF LEG

FIGURE 6-123

PLANTAR VIEW OF FOOT

FIGURE 6-124

FIGURE 6-125

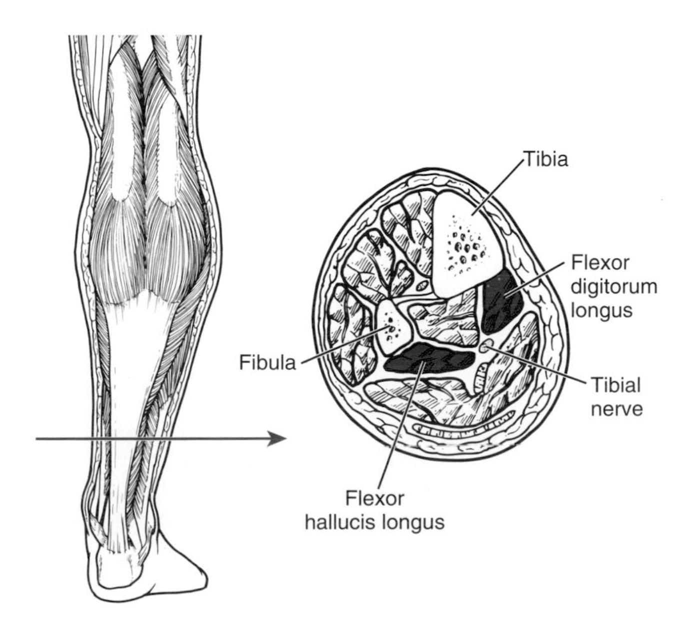

FIGURE 6-126 Arrow indicates level of cross section.

HALLUX AND TOE DIP AND PIP FLEXION

(Flexor digitorum longus, Flexor digitorum brevis, Flexor hallucis longus)

Range of Motion
PIP flexion, four lateral toes: 0° to 35°
DIP flexion, four lateral toes: 0° to 60°
IP flexion of hallux: 0° to 90°

Table 6-17 FLEXION OF IP JOINTS OF HALLUX AND TOES

I.D.	Muscle	Origin	Insertion
DIP, Toes			
213	Flexor digitorum longus	Tibia (shaft, posterior aspect of middle 2/3) Fascia over tibialis posterior	Toes 2–5 (distal phalanges, plantar surfaces and base)
PIP, Toes			
214	Flexor digitorum brevis	Calcaneus (tuberosity, medial process) Plantar aponeurosis Intermuscular septum	Toes 2–5 (by 4 tendons to middle phalanges, both sides)
IP, Hallux			
222	Flexor hallucis longus	Fibula (shaft, 2/3 of posterior aspect) Interosseous membrane Intermuscular septum (posterior crural) Fascia over tibialis posterior	Slip of tendon to flexor digitorum longus Hallux (distal phalanx, base, plantar aspect)
Others			
DIP, Toes			
217	Quadratus plantae		
PIP, Toes			
213	Flexor digitorum longus		

(Flexor digitorum longus, Flexor digitorum brevis, Flexor hallucis longus)

Grades 5 (Normal) to 0 (Zero)

Position of Patient: Sitting with foot on therapist's lap, or supine.

Position of Therapist: Sitting on short stool in front of patient or standing at side of table near patient's foot.

One hand provides stabilization over the anterior foot with the fingers placed across the dorsum of the foot and the thumb under the proximal phalanges (PIP) or distal phalanges (DIP) or under the IP of the hallux (Figure 6-127, Figure 6-128, and Figure 6-129).

The other hand applies resistance using the four fingers or the thumb under the middle phalanges (for 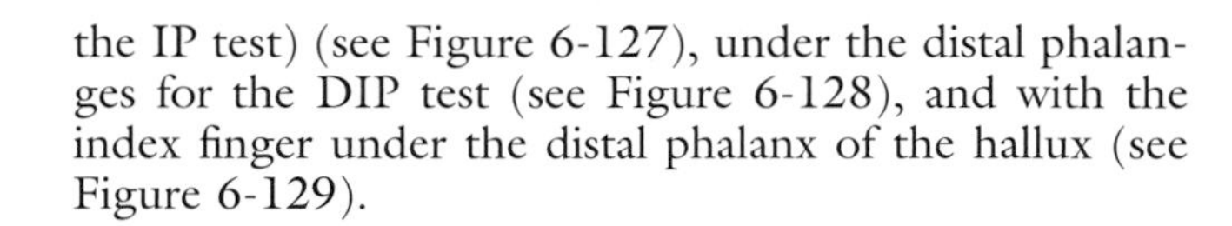the IP test) (see Figure 6-127), under the distal phalanges for the DIP test (see Figure 6-128), and with the index finger under the distal phalanx of the hallux (see Figure 6-129).

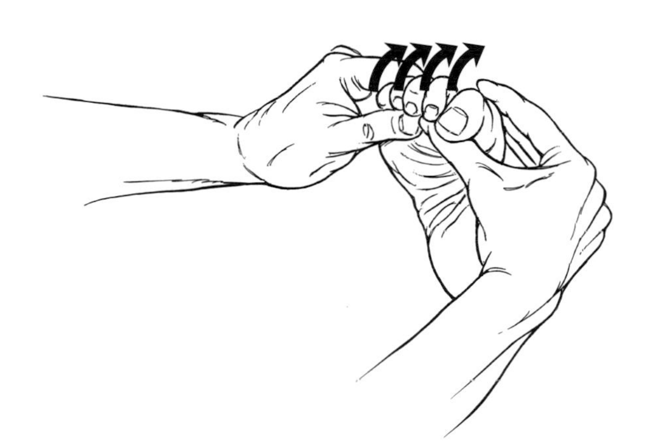

FIGURE 6-127

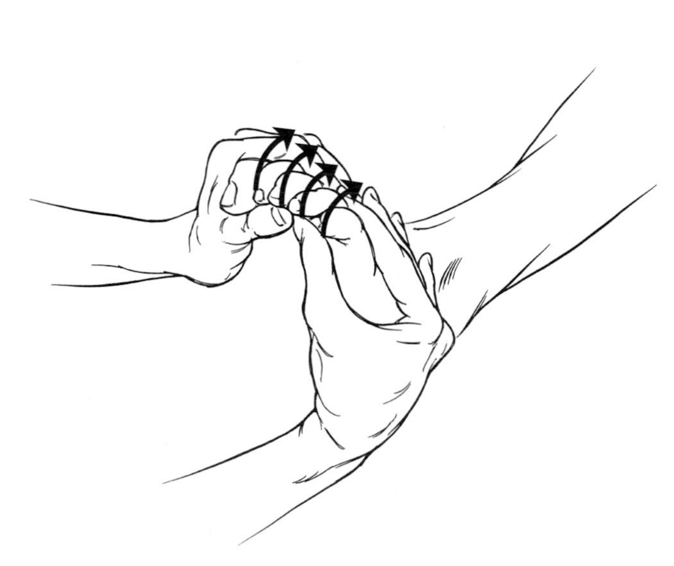

FIGURE 6-128

Test: Patient flexes the toes or hallux.

Instructions to Patient: "Curl your toes; hold it. Curl your big toe and hold it."

Grading

Grades 5 (Normal) and 4 (Good): Patient completes range of motion of toes and then hallux; resistance in both tests may be minimal.

Grades 3 (Fair) and 2 (Poor): Patient completes range of motion with no resistance (Grade 3) or completes only a partial range (Grade 2).

Grades 1 (Trace) and 0 (Zero): Minimal to no palpable contractile activity occurs. Tendon of the flexor hallucis longus may be palpated on the plantar surface of the proximal phalanx of the great toe.

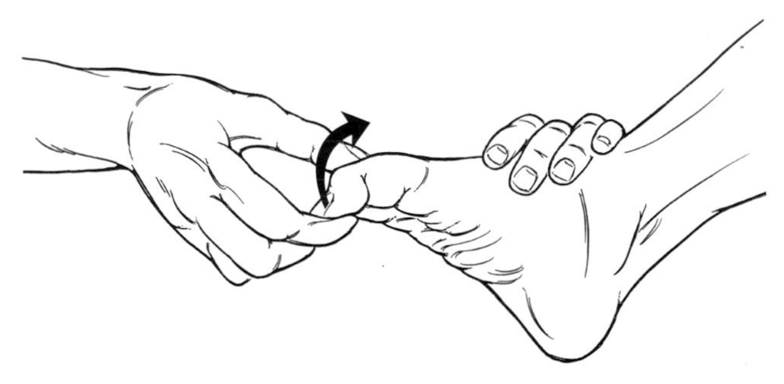

FIGURE 6-129

HALLUX AND TOE DIP AND PIP FLEXION

(Flexor digitorum longus, Flexor digitorum brevis, Flexor hallucis longus)

Helpful Hints

- As with all toe motions, the patient may not be able to move one toe separately from another or separate MP from IP activity among individual toes.
- Some people can separate hallux activity from toe motions, but fewer can separate MP from IP hallux activity.
- Many people can "pinch" with their great toe (adductor hallucis), but this is not a common clinical test.
- The abductor hallucis is not commonly tested because it is only rarely isolated. Its activity can be observed by resisting adduction of the forefoot, which will bring the great toe into abduction, but the lateral toes commonly extend at the same time.

(Extensor digitorum longus and brevis, Extensor hallucis longus)

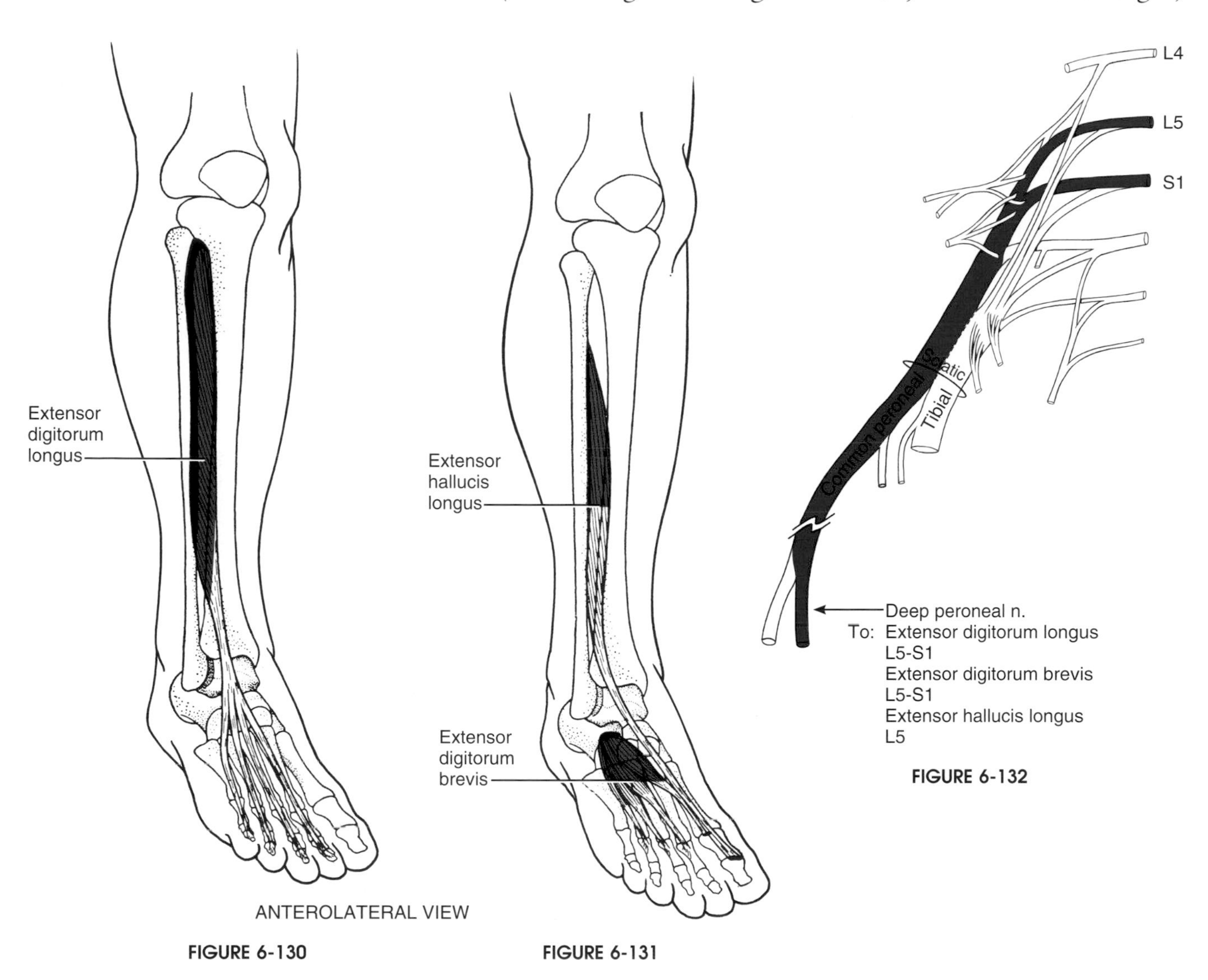

FIGURE 6-130

FIGURE 6-131

FIGURE 6-132

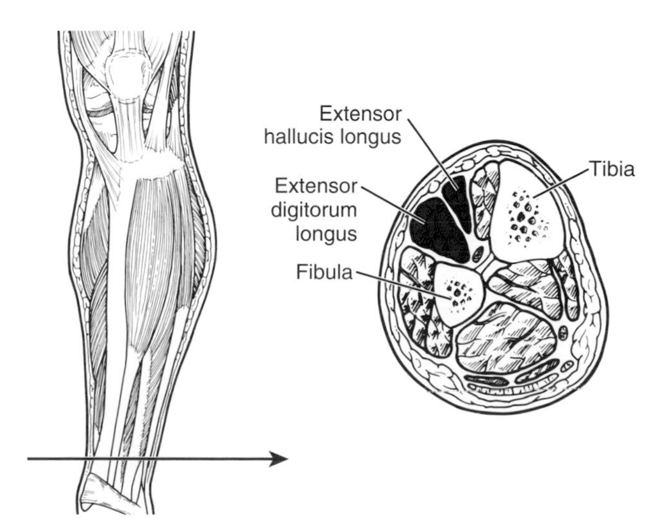

FIGURE 6-133 Arrow indicates level of cross section.

HALLUX AND TOE MP AND IP EXTENSION

(Extensor digitorum longus and brevis, Extensor hallucis longus)

Range of Motion
Hallux: 0° to 75°-80°
Digits 2-5: 0°-40°

Table 6-18 EXTENSION OF MP JOINTS OF TOES AND IP JOINT OF HALLUX

I.D.	Muscle	Origin	Insertion
211	Extensor digitorum longus	Tibia (lateral condyle) Fibula (shaft, proximal 3/4 of medial surface) Fascia cruris (deep) Interosseous membrane (anterior) Intermuscular septum	Toes 2-5 (to each middle and each distal phalanx, dorsal surface)
212	Extensor digitorum brevis	Calcaneus (anterior superolateral surface) Lateral talocalcaneal ligament Extensor retinaculum (inferior)	Ends in four tendons: Hallux (proximal phalanx, dorsal surface (may be named *extensor hallucis brevis*)) Toes 2-4: join tendons of extensor digitorum longus (lateral sides)
221	Extensor hallucis longus	Fibula (shaft, middle 1/2 of medial aspect) Interosseous membrane	Hallux (distal phalanx, dorsal aspect of base) Expansion to proximal phalanx

Grades 5 (Normal) to 0 (Zero)

Position of Patient: Sitting with foot on therapist's lap. Alternate position: supine. Ankle in neutral (midway between plantar flexion and dorsiflexion).

Position of Therapist: Sitting on low stool in front of patient, or standing beside table near the patient's foot.

Lateral Toes: One hand stabilizes the metatarsals with the fingers on the plantar surface and the thumb on the dorsum of the foot (Figure 6-134). The other hand is used to give resistance with the thumb placed over the dorsal surface of the proximal phalanges of the toes.

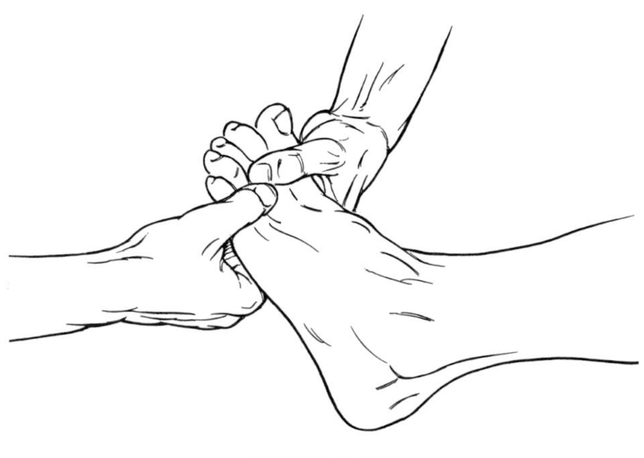

FIGURE 6-134

Grades 5 (Normal) to 0 (Zero) Continued

Hallux: Stabilize the metatarsal area by contouring the hand around the plantar surface of the foot with the thumb curving around to the base of the hallux (Figure 6-135). The other hand stabilizes the foot at the heel. For resistance, place thumb over the MP joint (see Figure 6-134) or over the IP joint (Figure 6-136).

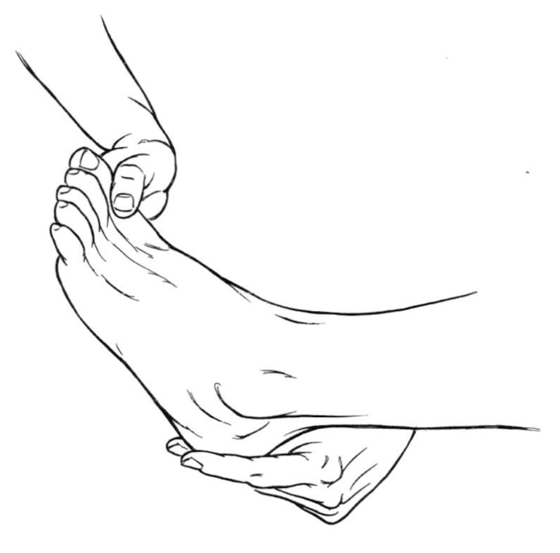

FIGURE 6-135

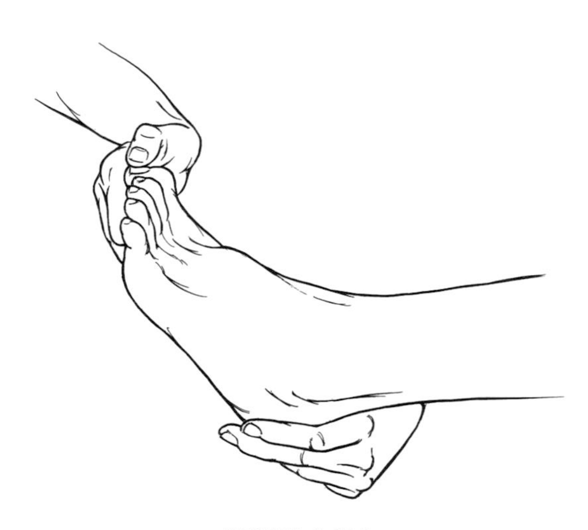

FIGURE 6-136

Test: Patient extends lateral four toes or extends hallux.

Instructions to Patient: "Straighten your big toe. Hold it." OR "Straighten your toes and hold it."

Grading

Grades 5 (Normal) and 4 (Good): Patient can extend the toes fully against variable resistance (which may be small).

Grades 3 (Fair) and 2 (Poor): Patient can complete range of motion with no resistance (Grade 3) or can complete a partial range of motion (Grade 2).

Grades 1 (Trace) and 0 (Zero): Tendons of the extensor digitorum longus can be palpated or observed over dorsum of metatarsals. Tendon of the extensor digitorum brevis often can be palpated on the lateral side of the dorsum of the foot just in front of the malleolus.

Palpable contractile activity is a Grade 1; no contractile activity is a Grade 0.

Helpful Hints

- Many (if not most) patients cannot separate great toe extension from extension of the four lateral toes. Nor can most separate MP from IP activity.
- The test is used not so much to ascertain strength as to determine whether the toe muscles are active.
- Normal strength in the ankle and foot muscles allows us to walk on uneven surfaces and supplies the major muscle forces needed for balance.

REFERENCES

Cited References

1. Sneath R. Insertion of the biceps femoris. J Anat. 1955;9:550-553.
2. Perry J, Weiss WB, Burnfield JM, et al. The supine hip extension manual muscle test: a reliability and validity study. Arch Phys Med Rehabil. 2004;85(8):1345-1350.
3. Bolgla LA, Uhl TL. Electromyographic analysis of hip rehabilitation exercises in a group of healthy subjects. J Orthop Sports Phys Ther. 2005;35:487-494.
4. Boudreau SN, Dwyer MK, Mattacola CG, et al. Hip-muscle activation during the lunge, single-leg squat, and step-up-and-over exercises. J Sport Rehabil. 2009;18:91-103.
5. Mirzabeigi E, Jordan C, Gronley JK, et al. Isolation of the vastus medialis oblique muscle during exercise. Am J Sports Med. 1999;27:50-53.
6. Bronikowski A, Kloda M, Lewandowska M, et al. Influence of various forms of physical exercise on bioelectric activity of quadriceps femoris muscle. Pilot study. Orthop Traumatol Rehabil. 2010;12:534-541.
7. Davlin CD, Holcomb WR, Guadagnoli MA. The effect of hip position and electromyographic biofeedback training on the vastus medialis oblique: vastus lateralis ratio. J Athl Train. 1999;34:342-346.
8. Eriksrud O, Bohannon RW. Relationship of knee extension force to independence in sit-to-stand performance in patients receiving acute rehabilitation. Phys Ther. 2003;83:544-551.
9. Davy DT, Kotzar GM, Brown RH, et al. Telemetric force measurements across the hip after total arthroplasty. J Bone Jt Surg. 1988;70:45-50.
10. Beaulieu FG, Pelland L, Robertson DG. Kinetic analysis of forwards and backwards stair descent. Gait Posture. 2008;27:564-571.
11. Mulroy S. Functions of the triceps surae during strength testing and gait. PhD dissertation, Department of Biokinesiology and Physical Therapy. University of Southern California: Los Angeles; 1994.
12. Lunsford BR, Perry J. The standing heel-rise test for ankle plantar flexion: criterion for normal. Phys Ther. 1995;75:694-698.
13. Jan MH, Chai HM, Lin YF, et al. Effects of age and sex on the results of an ankle plantar-flexor manual muscle test. Phys Ther. 2005;85:1078-1084.

Other Readings

Johnson CE, Basmajian JV, Dasher W. Electromyography of sartorius muscle. Anat Rec. 1972;173:127-130.

Jonsson B, Steen B. Function of the hip and thigh muscles in Romberg's test and "standing at ease." Acta Morphol Neerl Scand. 1962;5:267-276.

Joseph J, Williams PL. Electromyography of certain hip muscles. J Anat. 1957;91:286-294.

Keagy RD, Brumlik J, Bergen JL. Direct electromyography of the Psoas major muscle in man. J Bone Joint Surg. 1966;48(A):1377-1382.

Lee-Robinson A, Lee AT. Stepping up toe extension and flexion strength testing: a new method to record additional weakness. Am J Phys Med Rehabil. 2010;89:598-600.

Markee JE, Logue JT Jr, Williams M, et al. Two joint muscles of the thigh. J Bone Joint Surg. 1955;37A:125-142.

Mirzabeigi E, Jordan C, Gronley JK, et al. Isolation of the vastus medialis oblique muscle during exercise. Am J Sports Med. 1999;27:50-53.

Pare EB, Stern JT, Schwartz JM. Functional differentiation within the tensor fasciae latae. J Bone Joint Surg. 1981;63(A):1457-1471.

Perry J, Burnfield JM. Gait Analysis: Normal and Pathological Function, 2nd ed. Thorofare, NJ: Slack, Inc.; 2010.

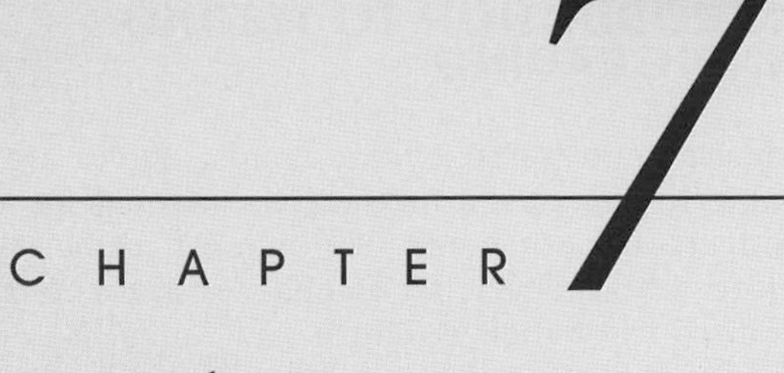

CHAPTER 7

Assessment of Muscles Innervated by Cranial Nerves

Jacqueline Montgomery

This chapter describes the muscles innervated by motor branches of the cranial nerves and describes test methods of assessing muscles of the eyelid, face, jaw, tongue, soft palate, posterior pharyngeal wall, and larynx. It also covers the extraocular muscles. The tests are appropriate for patients whose neurologic deficits are either central or peripheral. The only requirement for the patient to participate in the test is the ability to follow simple directions.

INTRODUCTION TO TESTING AND GRADING

Muscles innervated by the cranial nerves are not amenable to the classic methods of manual muscle testing and grading. In many, if not most, cases they do not move a bony lever, so manual resistance as a means of evaluation of their strength and function is not always the primary procedure.

The therapist needs to become familiar with cranial nerve innervated muscles in normal people. Their appearance, strength, excursion, and rate of motion are all variables that are unlike the other skeletal muscles. As for the infant and young child, the best way to assess the gross function of their muscles is to observe the child while crying or sucking, for example. In any event, experience with assessment requires considerable practice with both normal people and a wide variety of patients with suspected and known cranial nerve motor deficits emanating from both upper and lower motor neuron lesions.

The issue of symmetry is particularly important in testing the ocular, facial, tongue, jaw, pharyngeal, and palate muscles. The symmetry of these muscles, except for the laryngeal muscles, is visible to the therapist. Asymmetry is more readily detected merely by observation in these muscles (in contrast to the limb muscles) and should always be documented.

In all tests in this chapter, the movements or instructions may not be entirely familiar to the patient, so each test should be demonstrated and the patient should be allowed to practice. In the presence of unusual or unexpected test results, the therapist should inquire about prior facial reconstructive (e.g., cosmetic) surgery, and in this era, Botox injections.

General Grading Procedures

The distinction to be made in testing the muscles described in this chapter is to ascertain their relative functional level with respect to their intended activity. The scoring system, therefore, is a functional one, and motions or functions are graded as follows:

F: Functional; appears normal or only slight impairment.

WF: Weak functional; moderate impairment that affects the degree of active motion.

NF: Nonfunctional; severe impairment.

0: Absent.

Universal Precautions in Bulbar Testing

In testing the muscles of the head, oral cavity, and throat, the therapist frequently encounters body fluids such as saliva, tears, and bronchotracheopharyngeal secretions. The precaution of wearing gloves should always be followed. If the patient has any infectious disease or if there are copious secretions, the therapist should be masked and gowned as well as gloved.

The therapist should be cautious about standing directly in front of a patient who has been instructed to cough. This also is true in the case of the patient who has an open tracheostomy.

When a tongue blade is used, it should be sterile and care should be used about where it is placed between tests on a given patient.

Patient and Therapist Positions for All Tests

The short sitting position is preferred. The head and trunk should be supported as necessary to maintain normal alignment or to accommodate deformities. If the patient cannot sit for any reason, use the supine position, which will not influence testing of the head and eye muscles. When the muscles of the oral cavity and throat are tested, however, the head should be elevated as in sitting or using pillows if in the supine position. The therapist stands or sits in front of the patient but slightly to one side. A stool on casters is preferred so the therapist can move about the patient quickly and efficiently.

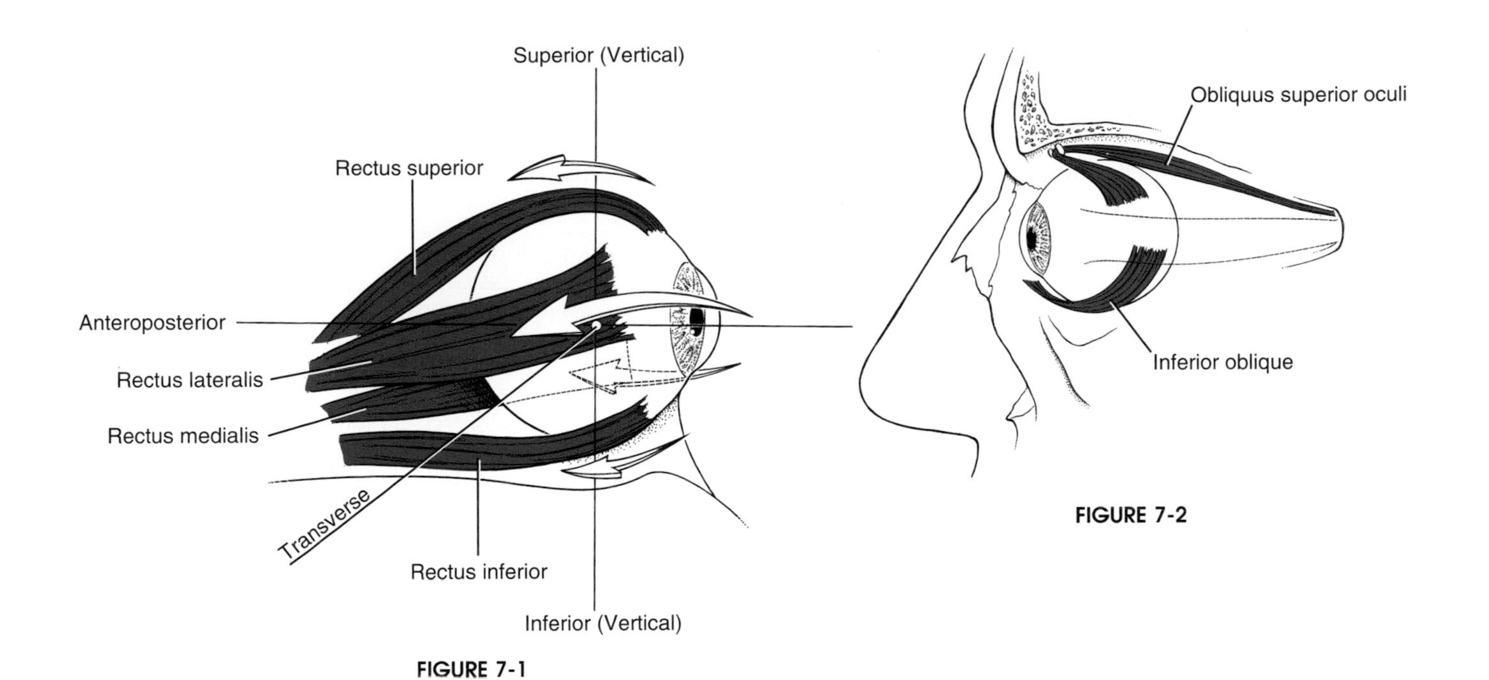

FIGURE 7-1

FIGURE 7-2

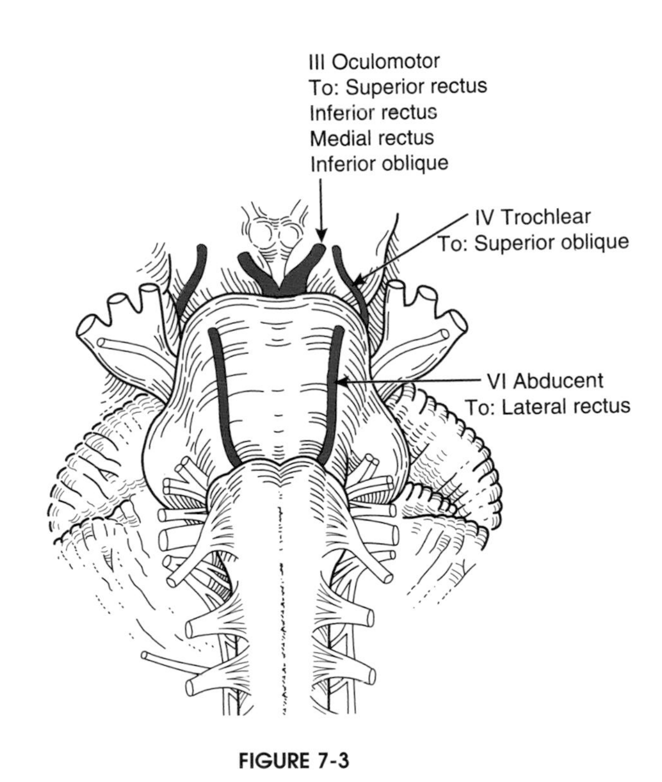

FIGURE 7-3

The six extraocular muscles of the eye (Figure 7-1 and Figure 7-2) move the eyeball in directions that depend on their attachments and on the influence of the movements themselves. It is usual that no muscle of the eye acts independently, and because these muscles cannot be observed, palpated, or tested individually, much of the knowledge of their function is derived from some variety of dysfunction. The extraocular muscles are innervated by cranial nerves III (oculomotor), IV (trochlear), and VI (abducent) (Figure 7-3).

Table 7-1 EXTRAOCULAR MUSCLES

I.D.	Muscle	Origin	Insertion
6	Rectus superior	Sphenoid bone (via common annular tendon)	Superior anterior sclera (via tendinous expansion)
7	Rectus inferior	Sphenoid bone (via common annular tendon)	Inferior sclera (via tendinous expansion)
8	Rectus medialis	Sphenoid bone (via common annular tendon)	Medial sclera (via tendinous expansion)
9	Rectus lateralis	Sphenoid bone (via common annular tendon)	Lateral sclera (via tendinous expansion)
10	Obliquus superior oculi (superior oblique)	Sphenoid bone (body) Tendon of rectus superior	Frontal bone (via a frontal bone pulley) Trochlea to the superolateral sclera behind the equator on the supralateral surface
11	Obliquus inferior oculi (inferior oblique)	Maxilla (orbital surface)	Lateral sclera behind the equator of the eyeball on lateral posterior quadrant

The Axes of Eye Motion

The eyeball rotates in the orbital socket around one or more of three primary axes (Figure 7-4), which intersect in the center of the eyeball.[1]

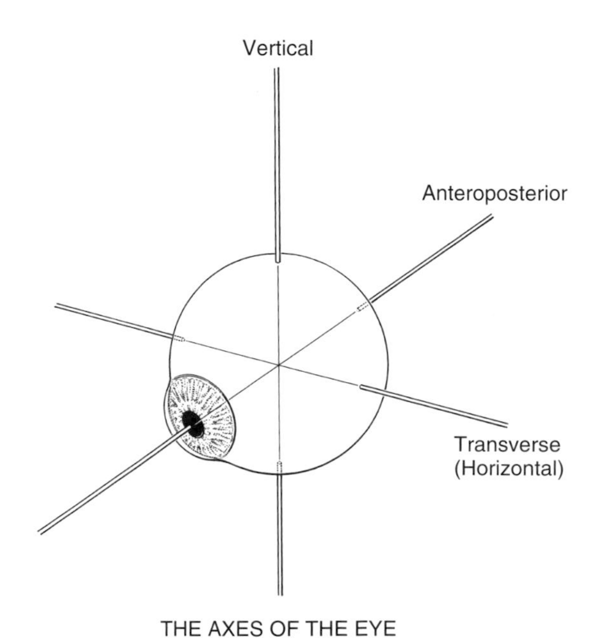

FIGURE 7-4 The three primary axes of the eye.

Vertical axis: Around this axis the lateral motions (abduction and adduction) take place in a horizontal plane.

Transverse axis: This is the axis of rotation for upward and downward motions.

Anteroposterior axis: Motions of rotation in the frontal plane occur around this axis.

The neutral position of the eyeball occurs when the gaze is straight ahead and far away. In this neutral position, the axes of the two eyes are parallel. Normally, the motions of the two eyes are conjugate, that is, coordinated, and the two eyes move together.

Eye Motions

The extraocular muscles seem to work as a continuum; as the length of one changes, the length and tension of the others are altered, giving rise to a wide repertoire of paired movements.[2,3] Despite this continuous commonality of activity, the function of the individual muscles can be simplified and understood in a manner that does not detract from accuracy but simplifies the test procedure.

Conventional clinical testing assigns the following motions to the various extraocular muscles (Figure 7-5).[1-3]

6. Rectus superior (III, Oculomotor)

Primary Movement: Elevation of the eyeball; movement is upward and inward.

Secondary Movements:
1. Rotation of the adducted eyeball so the upper end of the vertical axis is inward (see Figure 7-4).
2. Adduction of the eyeball to a limited extent.

7. Rectus inferior (III, Oculomotor)

Primary Movement: Depression of the eyeball; movement is downward and inward.

Secondary Movements:
1. Adduction of the eye.
2. Rotation of the adducted eyeball so the upper end of the vertical axis is outward.

8. Rectus medialis (III, Oculomotor)

Primary Movement: Adduction of the eyeball.

Secondary Movements: None.

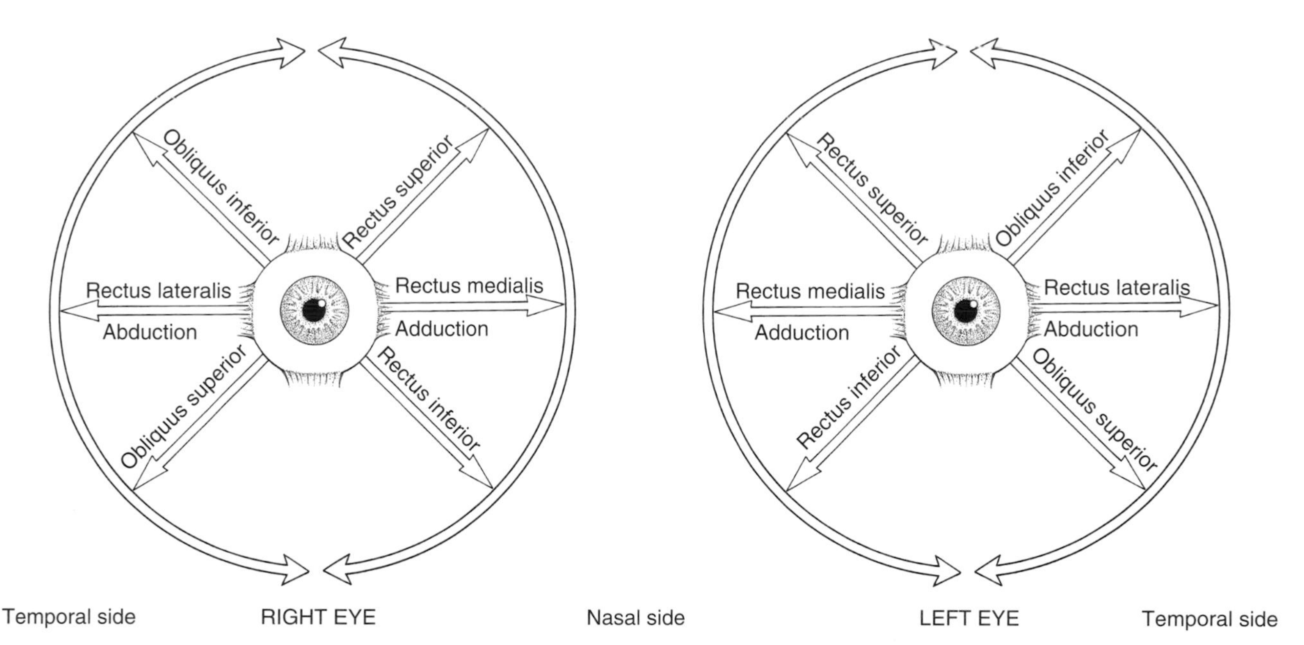

FIGURE 7-5 Extraocular muscles and their actions. The six extraocular muscles enable each eye to move in a circular arc, usually accompanied by head movements, though head position is static during testing. The traditional pairing of extraocular muscles is an oversimplification of their movement patterns. In any ocular rotation all six muscles change length. The reference point for description of the motions of the extraocular muscles is the center of the cornea.

Eye Motions Continued

9. Rectus lateralis (VI, Abducent)

Primary Movement: Abduction of the eyeball.

Secondary Movements: None. VI nerve lesions limit lateral movement. In paralysis the eyeball is turned medially and cannot be abducted.

10. Obliquus superior (IV, Trochlear)

Primary Movement: Depression of the eye.

Secondary Movements
1. Abduction of the eyeball.
2. IV nerve lesions limit depression, but abduction may be intact because abduction is the VI nerve.

11. Obliquus inferior (III, Oculomotor)

Primary Movement: Elevation of the eye, particularly from adduction; movement is upward and outward.

Secondary Movements:
1. Abduction of the eyeball.
2. Rotation of the eyeball so the vertical axis is outward.
3. Note: In paralysis, the eyeball is deviated downward and somewhat laterally; it cannot move upward when in abduction.
4. Note: In a III nerve lesion, the eye is outward and cannot be brought in. This lesion also results in ptosis, or drooping, of the upper eyelid.[2,3]

Eye Tracking

Eye movements are tested by having the patient look in the cardinal directions (numbers in parentheses refer to tracks shown in Figure 7-6).[2] All pairs in tracking are antagonists.

Laterally (1)	Upward and laterally (5)
Medially (2)	Upward and medially (7)
Upward (3)	Downward and medially (6)
Downward (4)	Downward and laterally (8)

Ask the patient to follow the therapist's slowly moving finger (or a pointer or flashlight) in each of the following tests. The object the patient is to follow should be at a comfortable reading distance. First, one eye is tested and then the other, covering the nontest eye. After single testing, both eyes are tested together for conjugate movements. Each test is started in the neutral position of the eye.

The range, speed, and smoothness of the motion should be observed, as well as the ability to sustain lateral and vertical gaze.[2-4] The therapist will not be able to use these observational methods to distinguish movement deviations accurately because accuracy requires the sophisticated instrumentation used in ophthalmology. The tracking movements will appear normal or abnormal, but little else will be possible.

Position of Patient: Head and eyeball in neutral alignment, looking straight ahead at therapist's finger to start. Head must remain static. If the patient turns the head while tracking the therapist's finger, the head will have to be held still with the therapist's other hand or by an assistant.

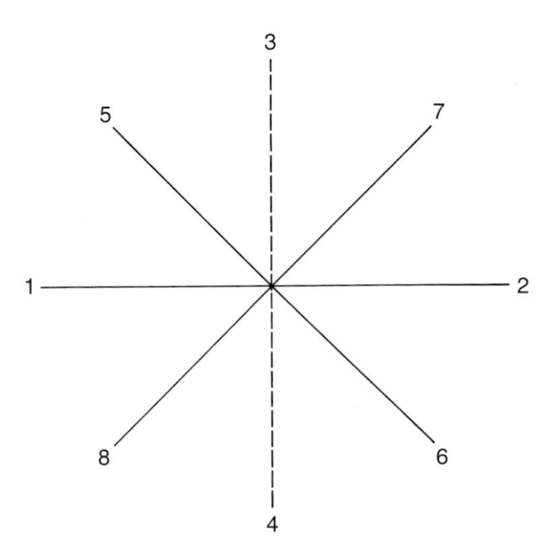

FIGURE 7-6

Eye Tracking Continued

Instructions to Patient: "Look at my finger. Follow it with your eyes" (Figure 7-7).

Test: Test each eye separately by covering first one eye and then the other. Then test both eyes together.

Examples of two bilateral tests show conjugate motion in the two eyes when tracking upward and to the right (Figure 7-8) and when tracking downward and to the left (Figure 7-9).

Criteria for Grading

F: Immediate tracking in a smooth motion over the full range. Completes full excursion of the test movement.

WF and NF: Not possible to distinguish accurately from Grade F or Grade 0 without detailed diplopia testing (by ophthalmologist).

0: Tracking motion in a given test is absent.

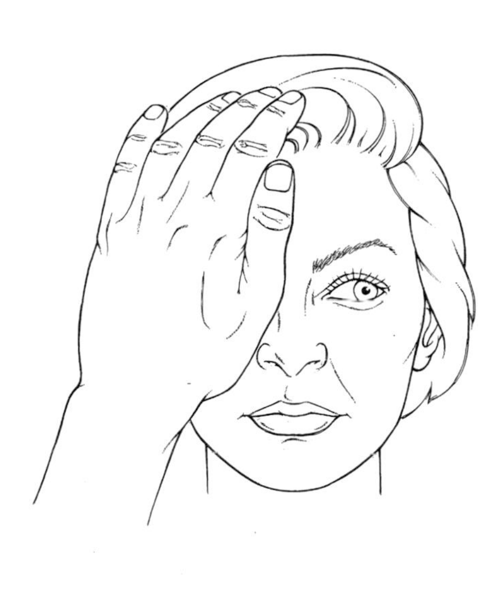

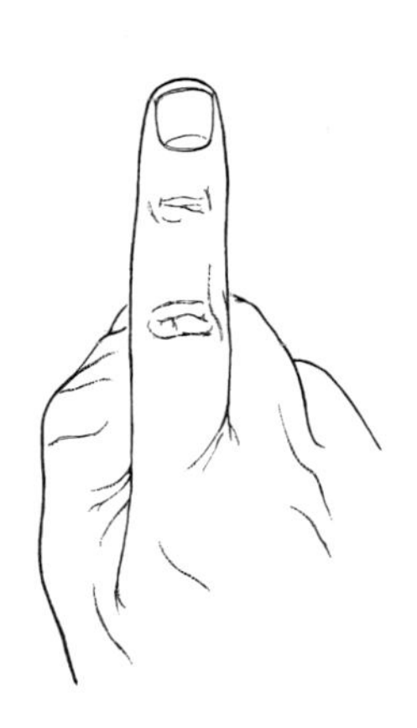

FIGURE 7-7

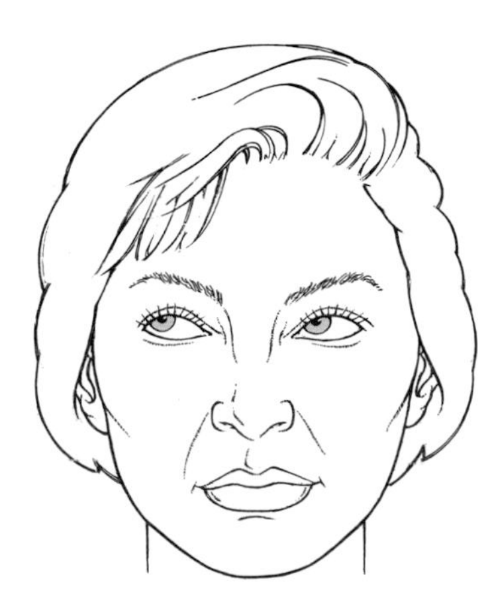

FIGURE 7-8 Patient tracks upward and to the right. The patient's right eye shows motion principally with the rectus superior; the left eye shows motion principally with the obliquus inferior.

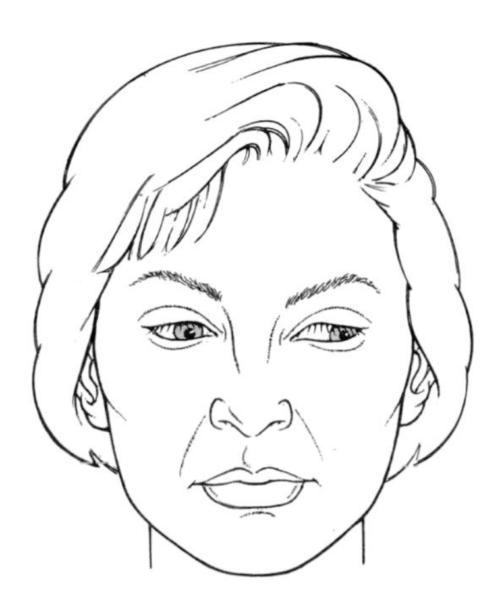

FIGURE 7-9 Patient tracks downward and to the left. The right eye movement reflects principally the obliquus superior; the left eye shows motion principally with the rectus inferior.

MUSCLES OF THE FACE AND EYELIDS

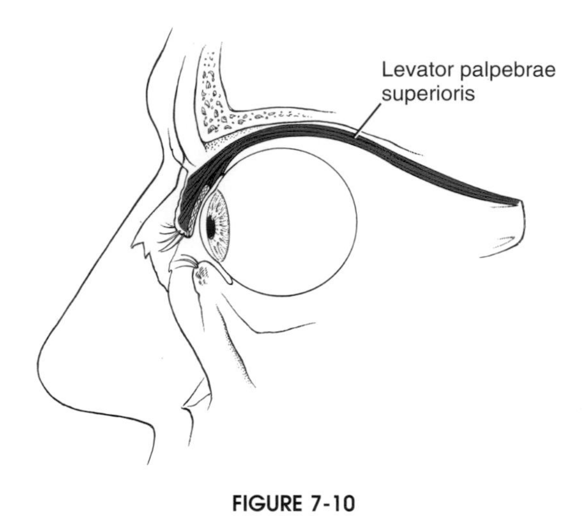

FIGURE 7-10

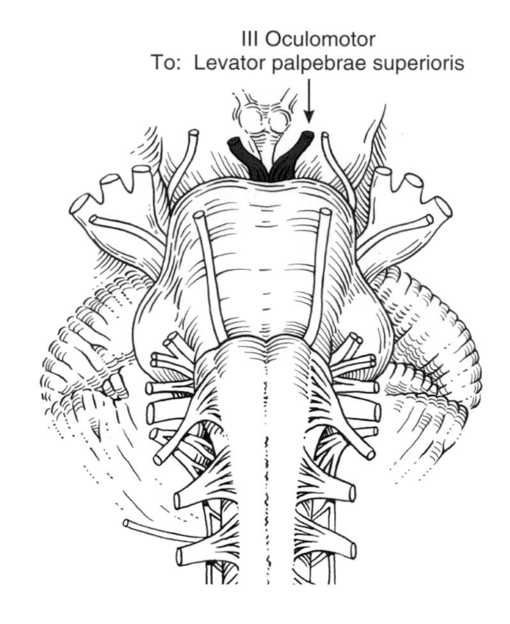

FIGURE 7-11

Table 7-2 MUSCLES OF THE EYELIDS AND EYEBROWS

I.D.	Muscle	Origin	Insertion
3	Levator palpebrae superioris	Sphenoid bone (lesser wing, inferior aspect) Roof of orbital cavity	Aponeurosis of orbital septum Superior tarsus of upper eyelid via aponeurosis Upper eyelid skin Sheath of rectus superior
4	Orbicularis oculi (has 3 parts)	***Orbital Part***	
		Frontal bone (nasal part) Maxilla (frontal process) Medial palpebral ligament	Blends with occipitofrontalis and corrugator supercilii Skin of the eyebrow
		Palpebral part	
		Medial palpebral ligament Frontal bone above and below ligament	Fibers form lateral palpebral raphe
		Lacrimal Part	
		Lacrimal fascia Lacrimal bone (crest)	Tarsi (superior and inferior) of eyelids
5	Corrugator supercilii	Frontal bone (superciliary arch)	Deep skin of eyebrow (above supraorbital margin)

The face should be observed for mobility of expression, and any asymmetry or inadequacy of muscles should be documented. A one-sided appearance when talking or smiling, a lack of tone (with or without atrophy), the presence of fasciculations, asymmetrical or frequent blinking, smoothness of the face, or excessive wrinkling are all clues to VII nerve involvement.

The facial muscles (except for motions of the jaw) convey all emotions via voluntary and involuntary movements.

Eye Opening (3. Levator palpebrae superioris)

Opening the eye by raising the upper eyelid is a function of the levator palpebrae superioris (see Figure 7-10). The muscle should be evaluated by having the patient open and close the eye with and without resistance. The function of this muscle is assessed by its strength in maintaining a fully opened eye against resistance.

The patient with an oculomotor (III) nerve lesion will lose the function of the levator muscle, and the eyelid will droop in a partial or complete ptosis. (A patient with cervical sympathetic pathology may have a ptosis but will be able to raise the eyelid voluntarily.) Ptosis is evaluated by observing the amount of the iris that is covered by the eyelid.

In the presence of a facial (VII) nerve lesion, the levator sign may be present.[2] In this case, the patient is asked to look downward and then slowly close the eyes. A positive levator sign is noted when the upper eyelid on the weak side moves upward because the action of the levator palpebrae superioris is unopposed by the orbicularis oculi.

Test: Patient attempts to keep the eyelids open against manual resistance (Figure 7-12). Both eyes are tested at the same time. **NEVER PRESS ON THE EYEBALL FOR ANY REASON!**

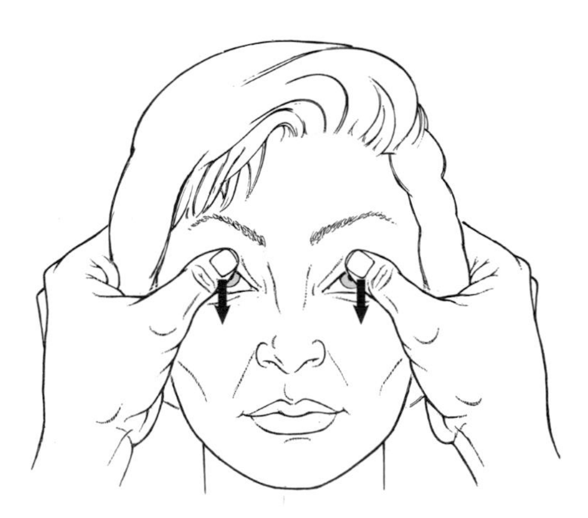

FIGURE 7-12

Manual Resistance: The thumb or index finger is placed lightly over the opened eyelid above the lashes, and resistance is given in a downward direction (to close the eye). The therapist is cautioned to avoid depressing the eyeball into the orbit while giving resistance.

Instructions to Patient: "Open your eyes wide. Hold them. Don't let me close them."

Criteria for Grading

F: Completes normal range of movement and holds against therapist's light manual resistance. Iris will be fully visible.

WF: Can open eye but only partially uncovers the iris and takes no resistance. Patient may alternately open and close the lids, but excursion is small. The frontalis muscle also may contract as the patient attempts to open the eye.

NF: Unable to open the eye and the iris is almost completely covered.

0: No eyelid opening.

Peripheral versus Central Lesions of the Facial (VII) Nerve

Involvement of the facial nerve may result from a lesion that affects the nerve or the nucleus (i.e., a peripheral lesion). Motor functions of the face also may be impaired after a central or supranuclear lesion. These two sites of interruption of the VII nerve lead to dissimilar clinical problems.[5]

The peripheral lesion results in a flaccid paralysis of all the muscles of the face *on the side of the lesion* (occipitofrontalis, corrugator, orbicularis oculi, nose and mouth muscles). The affected side of the face becomes smooth, the eye remains open, the lower lid sags, and blinking does not completely close the eye; the nose is depressed and may deviate to the opposite side. The cheek muscles are flaccid, so the cheek appears hollow and the mouth is drawn to one side. Eating and drinking are difficult because chewing and retention of fluids and saliva are impaired. Speech sounds, especially vowels or sounds that require pursing of the lips, are slurred.

When the VII nerve is affected central to the nucleus, there is paresis of the muscles of the lower face but sparing of the muscles of the upper face. This occurs because the nuclear center that controls the upper face has both contralateral and ipsilateral supranuclear connections, whereas that which controls the lower face has only contralateral supranuclear innervation. For this reason, a lesion in one cerebral hemisphere causes paresis of the lower part of the face *on the contralateral side* and there is sparing of the upper facial muscles. This may be called a "central VII syndrome."

One notable difference between peripheral and central disorders is that peripheral lesions often (but certainly not always) result in paralysis of all facial muscles; central lesions leave some function even of the involved muscles and are, therefore, notably weak but not paralytic.

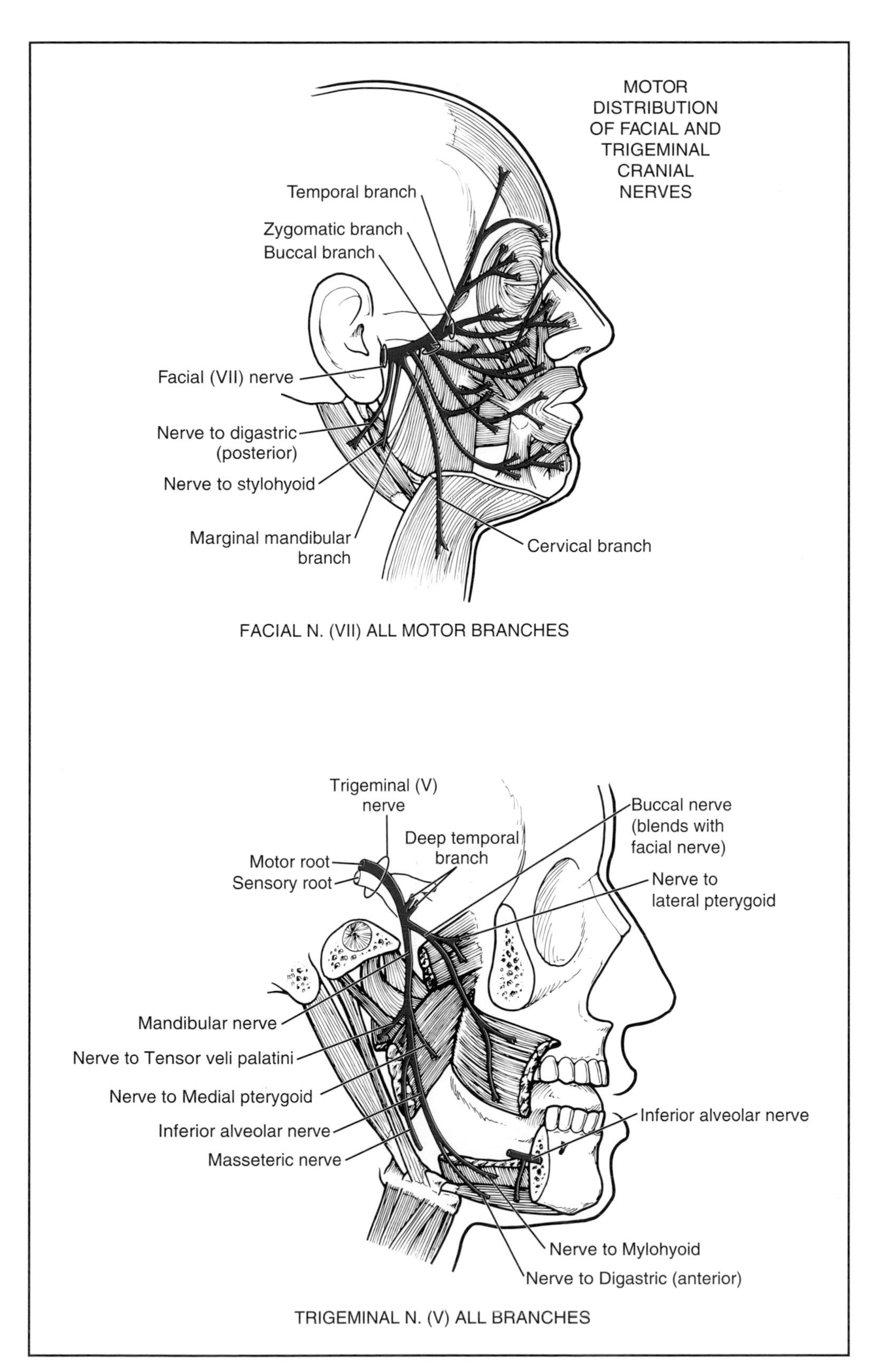
MOTOR DISTRIBUTION OF FACIAL AND TRIGEMINAL CRANIAL NERVES
Temporal branch
Zygomatic branch
Buccal branch
Facial (VII) nerve
Nerve to digastric (posterior)
Nerve to stylohyoid
Marginal mandibular branch
Cervical branch
FACIAL N. (VII) ALL MOTOR BRANCHES
Trigeminal (V) nerve
Motor root
Sensory root
Deep temporal branch
Buccal nerve (blends with facial nerve)
Nerve to lateral pterygoid
Mandibular nerve
Nerve to Tensor veli palatini
Nerve to Medial pterygoid
Inferior alveolar nerve
Masseteric nerve
Inferior alveolar nerve
Nerve to Mylohyoid
Nerve to Digastric (anterior)
TRIGEMINAL N. (V) ALL BRANCHES

PLATE 8

Closing the Eye (4. Orbicularis oculi)

The orbicularis oculi muscle is the sphincter of the eye (Figure 7-13).[1] Its lids are innervated by the facial (VII) nerve (temporal branch and zygomatic branch) (Figures 7-14 and 7-15). Its palpebral portion closes the eyelids gently, as in blinking and sleep. The orbital portion of the muscle closes the eyes with greater force, as in winking. The lacrimal portion draws the eyelids laterally and compresses them against the sclera to receive tears. All portions act to close the eyes tightly (Figure 7-16). Observation of the patient without specific testing will detect weakness of the orbicularis because the blink will be delayed on the involved side.

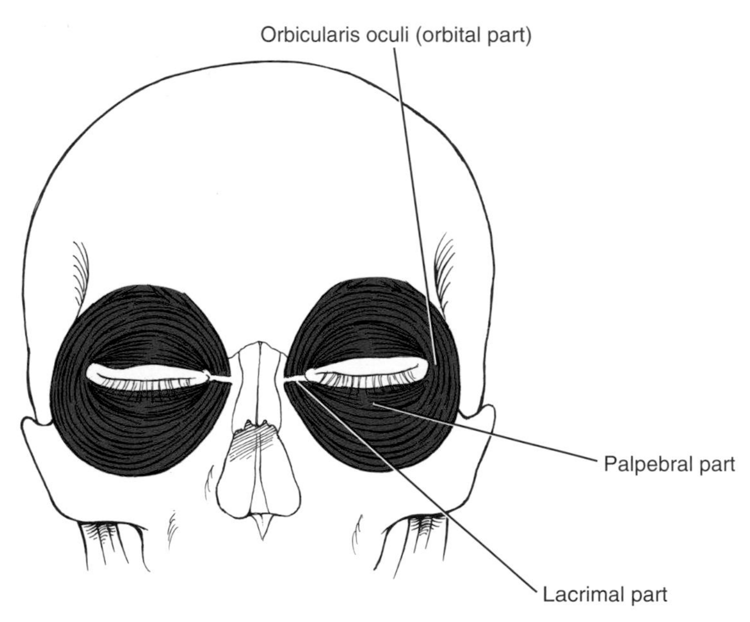

FIGURE 7-13

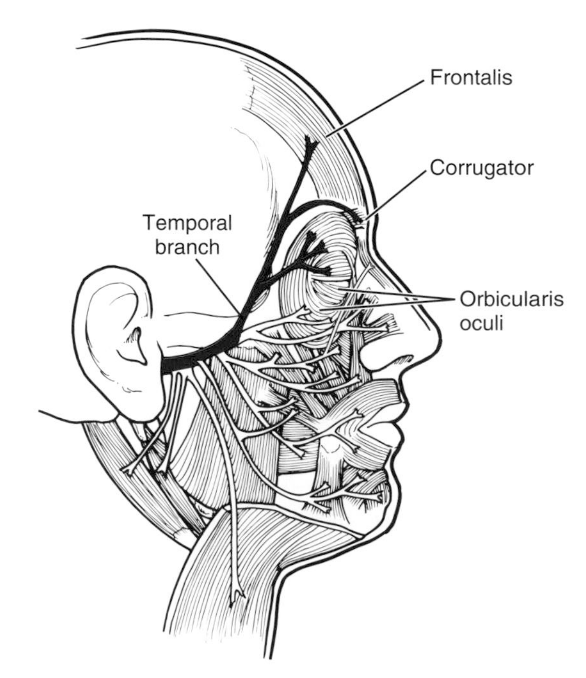

FACIAL N. (VII) TEMPORAL BRANCH

FIGURE 7-14

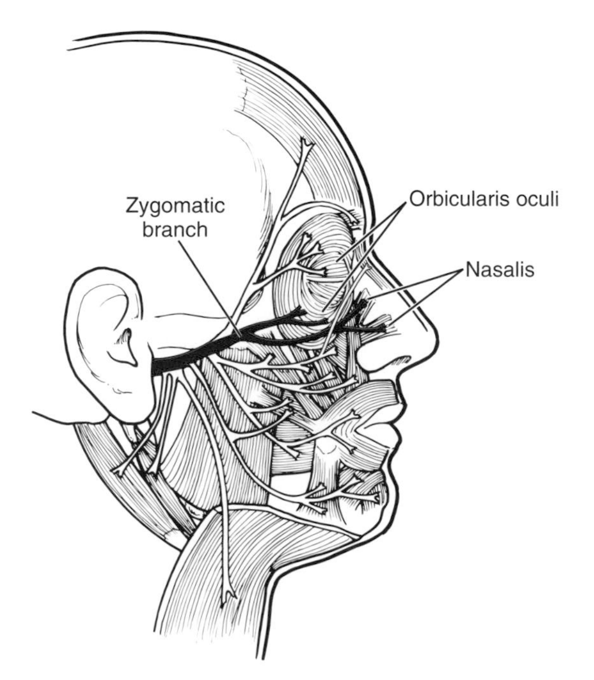

FACIAL N. (VII) ZYGOMATIC BRANCH

FIGURE 7-15

Closing the Eye (4. Orbicularis oculi) Continued

Test: Observe the patient opening and closing the eyes voluntarily, first together and then singly (Figure 7-16). (Single-eye closing is not a universal skill.) Patient closes eyes tightly, first together, then singly.

Rather than using resistance, the therapist may look at the depth to which the eyelashes are buried in the face when the eyes are closed tightly, noting whether the lashes are deeper on the uninvolved side.

Manual Resistance: Place the thumb and index finger below and above (respectively) each closed eye using a light touch (Figure 7-17). The therapist attempts to open the eyelids by spreading the thumb and index finger apart. **REMINDER: NEVER PRESS ON THE EYEBALL FOR ANY REASON.**

Instructions to Patient: "Close your eyes as tightly as you can. Hold them closed. Don't let me open them" OR "Close your eye against my finger."

Criteria for Grading

F: Closes eyes tightly and holds against therapist's resistance. Iris may not be visible.

WF: Takes no resistance to eye closure; closure may be incomplete, but only a small amount of the sclera and no iris should be visible. There may be closure of the eye, but the eyelid on the weaker side may be delayed in contrast to the quick closure on the normal side.

NF: Unable to close eyes so that the iris is completely covered. (These patients may need artificial eyedrops to prevent drying of the eye.)

0: No evidence of orbicularis oculi activity.

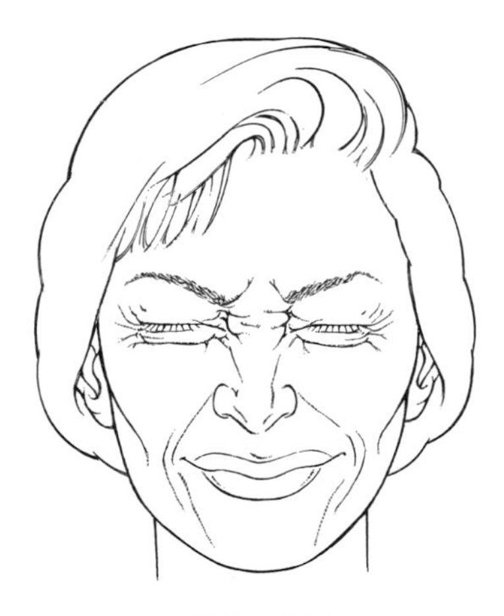

FIGURE 7-16

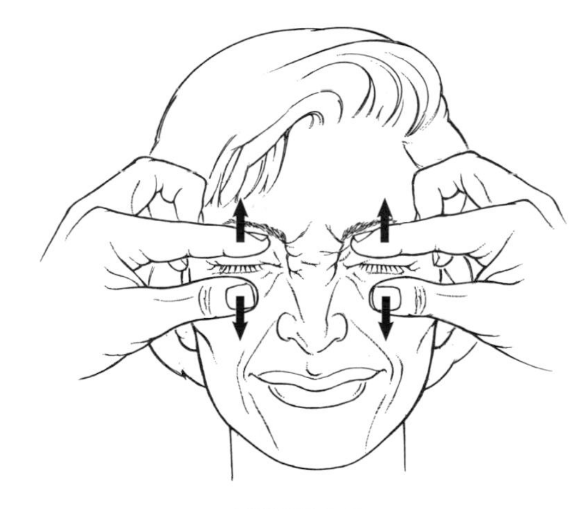

FIGURE 7-17

Helpful Hints

If the eyeball rotates upward when closing the eyes tightly, the patient is exerting effort to perform the test correctly. This upward rotation of the eyeball is called Bell's phenomenon. If the patient is not exerting effort, all protestations to the contrary, the eyeball will remain in the neutral position. This observation may give the therapist a clue to other testing done with this kind of patient.

Frowning (5. Corrugator supercilii)

To observe the action of the corrugator muscle (Figure 7-18; see also Figure 7-14), the patient is asked to frown. Frowning draws the eyebrows down and medially, producing vertical wrinkling of the forehead.

Test: Patient is asked to frown; the eyebrows are drawn down and together (Figure 7-19).

Manual Resistance: The therapist uses the thumb (or index finger) of each hand placed gently at the nasal end of each eyebrow and attempts to move the eyebrows apart (smooth away the frown) (Figure 7-20).

Instructions to Patient: "Frown. Don't let me erase it."

Criteria for Grading

F: Completes normal range (wrinkles are prominent) and holds against slight resistance.

WF: Frowns, but wrinkles are shallow and not too obvious; is unable to take resistance.

NF: Slight motion detected.

0: No frown.

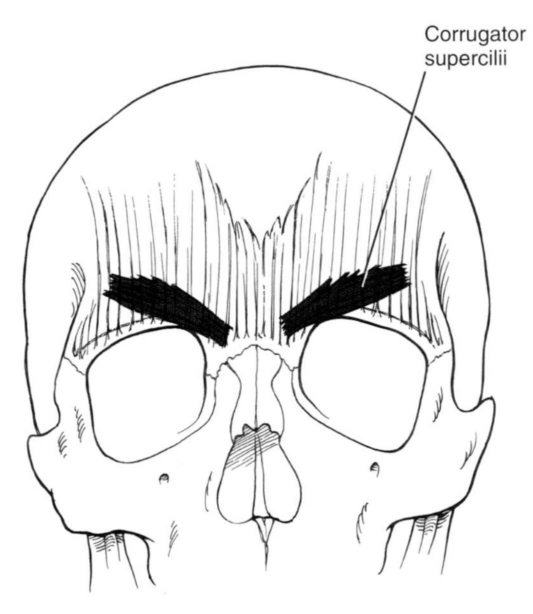

FIGURE 7-18

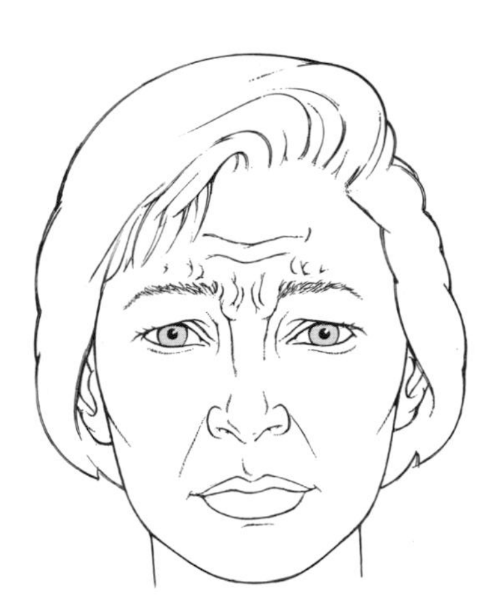

FIGURE 7-19

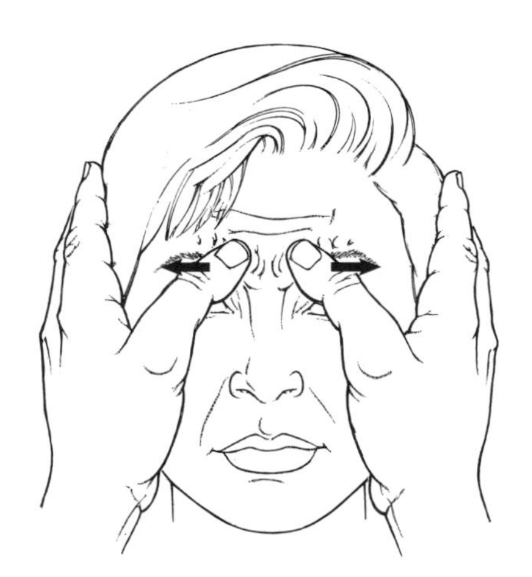

FIGURE 7-20

Raising the Eyebrows (1. Occipitofrontalis, frontalis part)

To examine the frontal belly of the occipitofrontalis muscle (Figure 7-21 and see Figure 7-14), the patient is asked to create an expression of surprise where the forehead skin wrinkles horizontally. The occipital belly of the muscle is not tested usually, but it draws the scalp backward.

Test: Patient raises the eyebrows so that horizontal forehead lines appear (Figure 7-22).

Manual Resistance: Therapist places the pad of a thumb above each eyebrow and applies resistance in a downward direction (smoothing the forehead) (Figure 7-23).

Instructions to Patient: "Raise your eyebrows as high as you can. Don't let me pull them down."

Criteria for Grading

F: Completes movement; horizontal wrinkles are prominent. Tolerates considerable resistance.

WF: Wrinkles are shallow and easily erased by gentle resistance.

NF: Only slight motion detected.

0: No eyebrow raising.

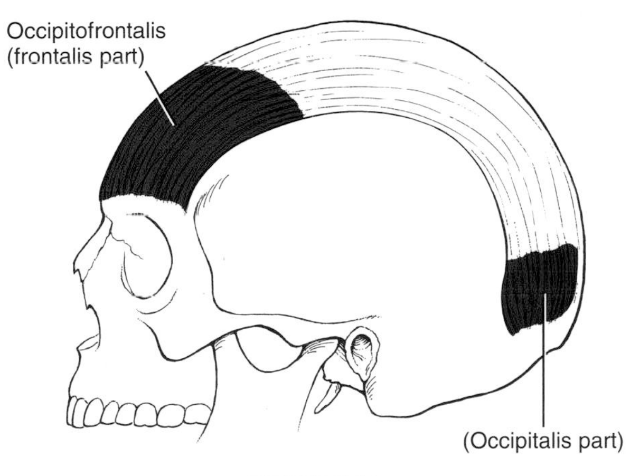

FIGURE 7-21

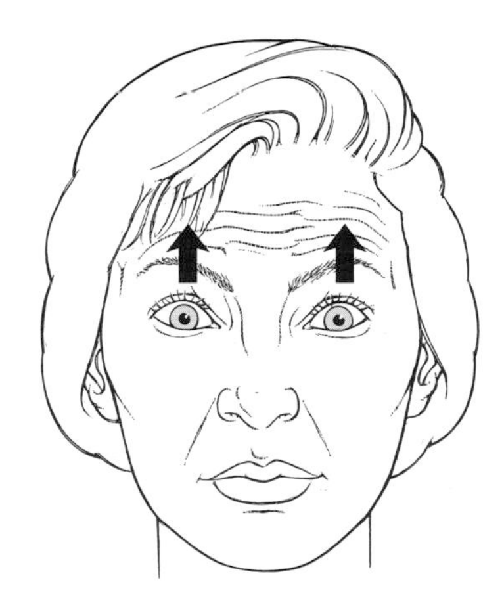

FIGURE 7-22

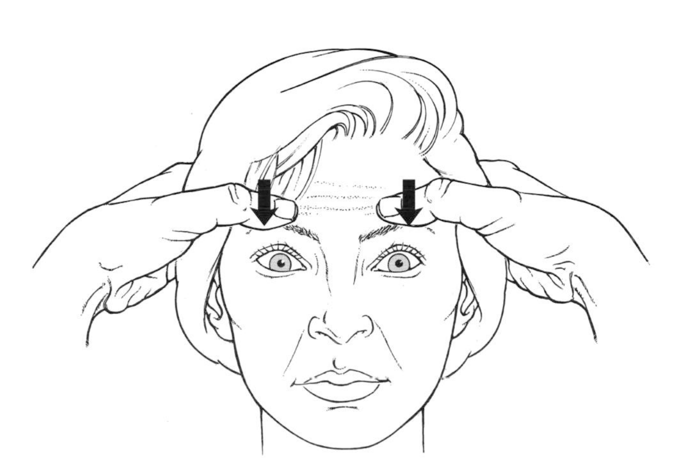

FIGURE 7-23

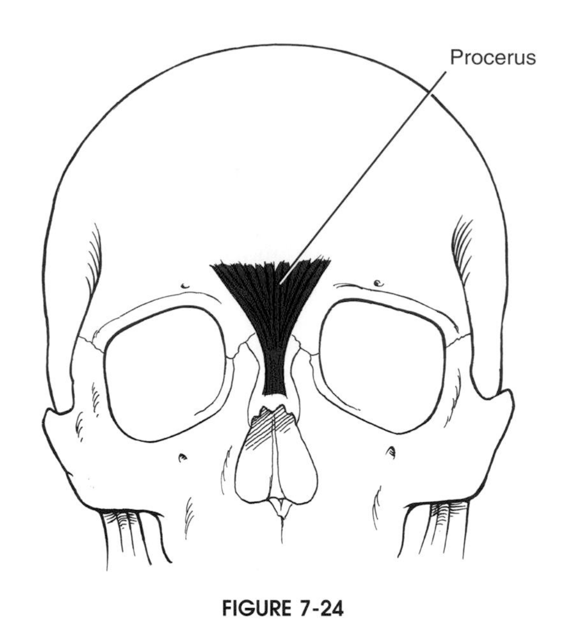

FIGURE 7-24

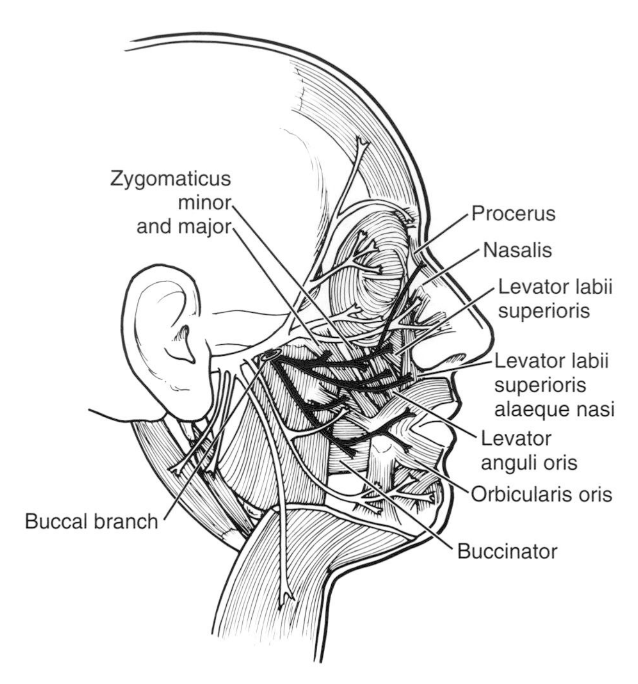

FACIAL N. (VII) BUCCAL BRANCH

FIGURE 7-25

Table 7-3 MUSCLES OF THE NOSE

I.D.	Muscle	Origin	Insertion
12	Procerus	Nasal bone aponeurosis Lateral nasal cartilage	Skin over lower forehead between eyebrows Joins occipitofrontalis
13	Nasalis		
	Transverse part (compressor nares)	Maxilla (above and lateral to incisive fossa)	Aponeurosis over bridge of nose
	Alar part (dilator nares)	Maxilla (above lateral incisor) Alar cartilage	Ala nasi cartilage Skin at tip of nose
14	Depressor septi*	Maxilla (above central incisor)	Nasal septum Alar cartilage

*The depressor septi often is considered part of the dilator nares.

The three muscles of the nose are all innervated by the facial (VII) nerve. The procerus (Figure 7-24) draws the medial angle of the eyebrows downward, causing transverse wrinkles across the bridge of the nose. The nasalis (compressor nares) depresses the cartilaginous portion of the nose and draws the ala down toward the septum (see Figure 7-15). The nasalis (dilator nares) dilates the nostrils. The depressor septi draws the alae downward, constricting the nostrils.

Of the three nose muscles only the procerus is tested clinically. The others are observed with respect to nostril flaring and narrowing in patients who have such talent.

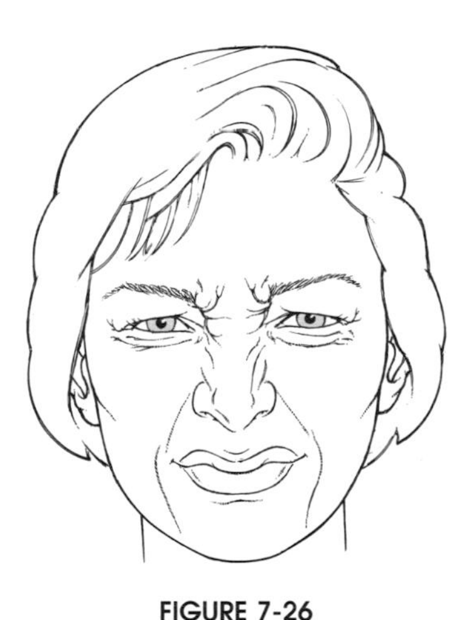

FIGURE 7-26

Wrinkling the Bridge of the Nose (12. Procerus)

Test: Patient wrinkles nose as if expressing distaste (Figure 7-26).

Manual Resistance: The pads of the thumbs are placed beside the bridge of the nose, and resistance is given laterally (smoothing the creases) (Figure 7-27).

Instructions to Patient: "Wrinkle your nose as if to say 'yuck.' "

Criteria for Grading

F: Prominent creases; patient tolerates some resistance.

WF: Shallow creases; patient yields to any resistance.

NF: Motion barely discernible.

0: No change of expression.

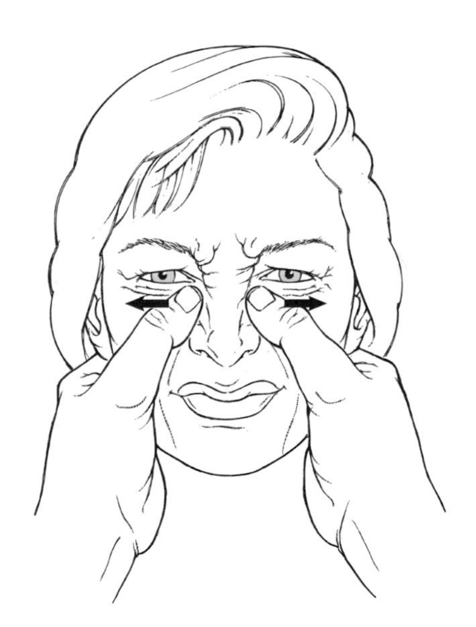

FIGURE 7-27

Helpful Hints

Isolated wrinkling of the nose is rare, and most patients use other facial muscles to perform this expressive movement.

MUSCLES OF THE MOUTH AND FACE

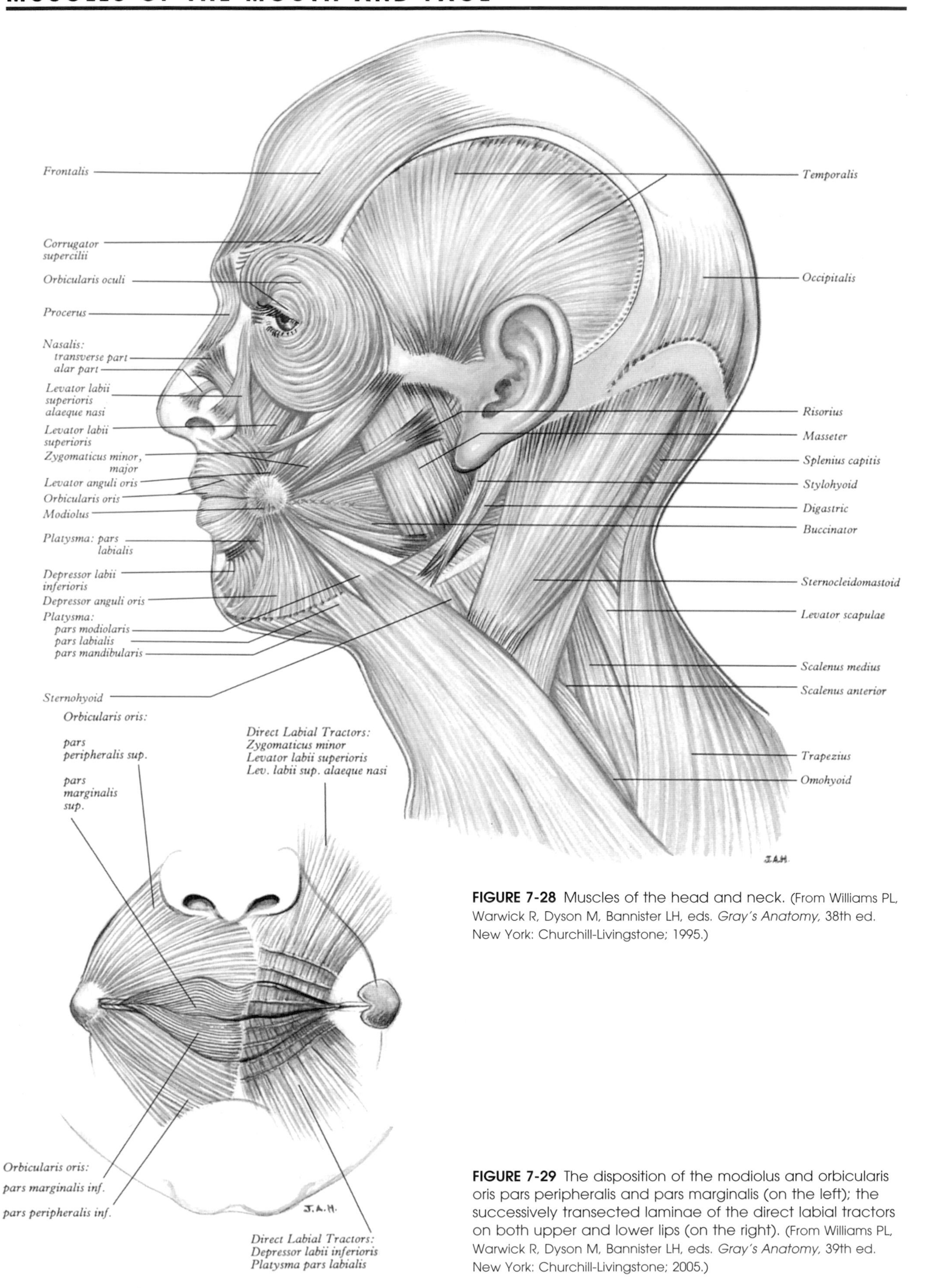

FIGURE 7-28 Muscles of the head and neck. (From Williams PL, Warwick R, Dyson M, Bannister LH, eds. *Gray's Anatomy,* 38th ed. New York: Churchill-Livingstone; 1995.)

FIGURE 7-29 The disposition of the modiolus and orbicularis oris pars peripheralis and pars marginalis (on the left); the successively transected laminae of the direct labial tractors on both upper and lower lips (on the right). (From Williams PL, Warwick R, Dyson M, Bannister LH, eds. *Gray's Anatomy,* 39th ed. New York: Churchill-Livingstone; 2005.)

Table 7-4 MUSCLES OF THE MOUTH

I.D.	Muscle	Origin	Insertion
15	Levator labii superioris	Orbit of eye (inferior) Maxilla Zygomatic bone	Upper lip (no bony attachment)
17	Levator anguli oris	Maxilla (canine fossa)	Modiolus
18	Zygomaticus major	Zygomatic bone	Modiolus
24	Depressor labii inferioris	Mandible (between symphysis and mental foramen)	Skin and mucosa of lower lip Modiolus Blends with its paired muscle from opposite side and with orbicularis oris
25	Orbicularis oris Accessory muscles: Incisivus labii superioris Incisivus labii inferioris	Modiolus No bony attachment	Modiolus Labial connective tissue Submucosa
26	Buccinator	Between maxilla and mandible (alveolar processes opposite molar teeth) Pterygomandibular raphe	Modiolus Submucosa of cheek and lips
21	Mentalis	Mandible (incisive fossa)	Skin over chin
23	Depressor anguli oris	Mandible (mental tubercle and oblique line)	Modiolus
Others			
16	Levator labii superioris alaeque nasi		
19	Zygomaticus minor		
20	Risorius		
22	Transversus menti		
88	Platysma		

The Modiolus

The arrangement of the facial musculature often causes confusion and misunderstanding. This is not surprising since there are 14 small bundles of muscles running in various directions, with long names and unsupported functional claims. Of all the muscles of the face, those about the mouth may be the most important because they have responsibility for both ingestion of food and for speech.

One major source of confusion is the relationship between the muscles around the mouth. The common description until recently was of uninterrupted circumoral muscles. In fact, the orbicularis oris muscle is not a complete ellipse but rather contains fibers from the major extrinsic muscles that converge on the buccal angle, as well as intrinsic fibers.[1,6,7] The authors and others do not describe complete ellipses, but most drawings illustrate such.[6]

The area on the face that has a large concentration of converging and diverging fibers from multiple directions lies immediately lateral and slightly above the corner of the mouth. Using the thumb and index finger on the outer skin and inside the mouth and compressing the tissue between them will quickly identify the knotlike structure known as the *modiolus*.[8-10]

The modiolus (from the Latin meaning nave of a wheel) is described as a muscular or tendinous node, a rather concentrated attachment of many muscles.[8,9] Its basic shape is conical (though this is oversimplified); it is about 1 cm thick and is found in most people about 1 cm lateral to the buccal angle. Its shape and size vary considerably with gender, race, and age. The muscular fibers enter and exit on different planes, superficial and deep, with some spiraling, but essentially they constitute a three-dimensional complexity.

Different classifications of modiolar muscles exist, but basically 9 or 10 facial muscles are associated with the structure:[9]

Levator anguli oris	Levator labii superioris
Orbicularis oris	Levator labii superioris alaeque nasi
Depressor anguli oris	Zygomaticus minor
Zygomaticus major	Mentalis
Buccinator	Depressor labii inferioris

Frequently associated are the special fibers of the orbicularis oris (incisive superior, incisive inferior), platysma, and risorius (the latter is not a constant feature in the facial musculature).

The orbicularis oris and the buccinator form an almost continuous muscular sheet, which can be fixed in a number of positions by the zygomaticus major, levator anguli oris, and depressor anguli oris (the latter three being the "stays" used to immobilize the modiolus in any position).

When the modiolus is firmly fixed, the buccinator can contract to apply force to the cheek teeth; the orbicularis oris can contract against the arch of the anterior teeth, thus sealing the lips together and closing the mouth tightly.[9] Similarly, control of the modiolar active and stay muscles enables accurate and fine control of lip movements and pressures in speech.

There are many muscles associated with the mouth, and all have some distinctive function, except perhaps the risorius. Rather than detail a test for each, only definitive tests will be presented for the buccinator and the orbicularis oris (the sphincter of the mouth). The function of the remaining muscles is illustrated, and individual testing is left to the therapist. All muscles of the mouth are innervated by the facial (VII) nerve.

Lip Closing (25. Orbicularis oris)

This circumoral muscle (Figures 7-28 and 7-29) serves many functions for the mouth. It closes the lips, protrudes the lips, and holds the lips tight against the teeth. Furthermore, it shapes the lips for such functional uses as kissing, whistling, sucking, drinking, and the infinite shaping for articulation in speech. (For innervation, see Figure 7-25.)

Test: Patient compresses and protrudes the lips (Figure 7-30).

Resistance: In deference to hygiene, a tongue blade rather than a finger is used to provide resistance. The flat side of the blade is placed diagonally across both the upper and lower lips, and resistance is applied inward toward the oral cavity (Figure 7-31).

Instructions to Patient: "Purse your lips. Hold it. Push against the tongue blade."

Criteria for Grading

F: Completely seals lips and holds against relatively strong resistance.

W: Closes lips but is unable to take resistance.

NF: Has some lip movement but is unable to bring lips together.

0: No closure of the lips.

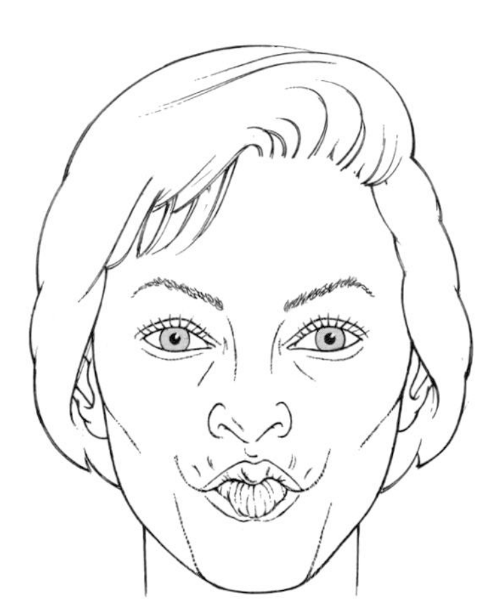

FIGURE 7-30

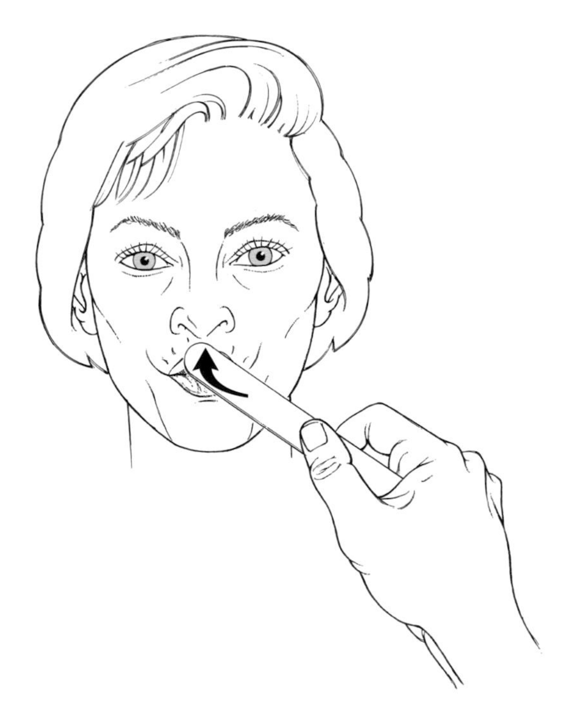

FIGURE 7-31

Cheek Compression (26. Buccinator)

The buccinator (see Figure 7-28) is a prime muscle used for positioning food for chewing and for controlling the passage of the bolus. It also compresses the cheek against the teeth and acts to expel air when the cheeks are distended (blowing). (For innervation, see Figure 7-25.)

Test: Patient compresses the cheeks (bilaterally) by drawing them into the mouth (Figure 7-32).

Resistance: A tongue blade is used for resistance. The blade is placed inside the mouth, its flat side lying against the cheek (Figure 7-33). Resistance is given by levering the blade inward against the cheek (at the angle of the mouth), which will cause the flat blade to push the test cheek outward.

Alternatively, the gloved index fingers of the therapist may be used to offer resistance. In this case, the index fingers are placed in the mouth (the left finger to the inside of the patient's left cheek and vice versa). The fingers are used simultaneously to try to push the cheeks outward. Use caution in this form of the test for patients with cognitive impairment (lest they bite!) or with those who have a bite reflex.

Instructions to Patient: "Suck in your cheeks. Hold. Don't let me push them out."

Criteria for Grading

F: Performs movement correctly and holds against strong resistance.

WF: Performs movement but is unable to hold against any resistance.

NF: Movement is detectable but not complete.

0: No motion of cheeks occurs.

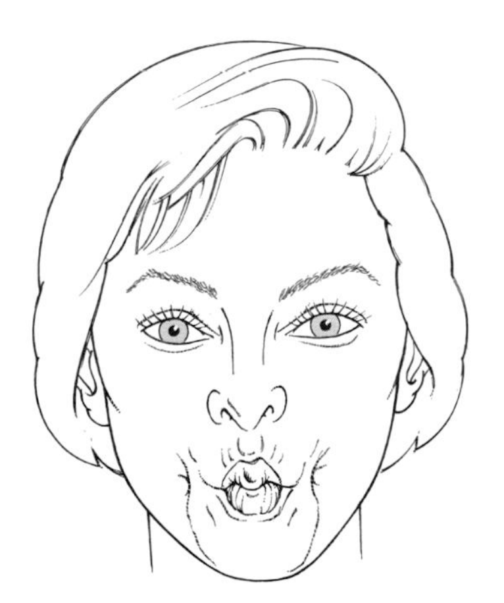

FIGURE 7-32

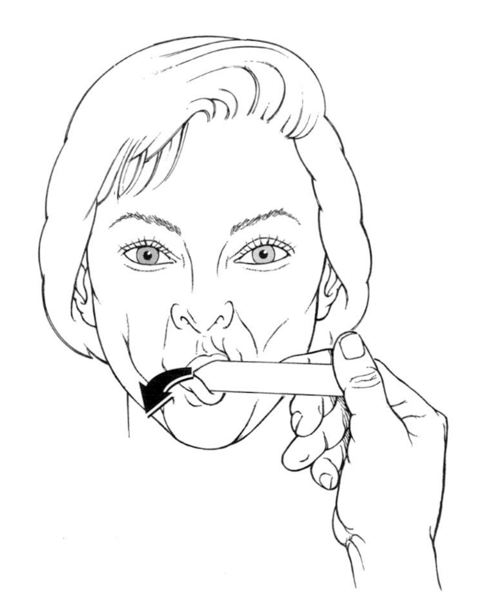

FIGURE 7-33

Other Oral Muscles

17. Levator anguli oris (for innervation see Figure 7-25)

This muscle elevates the angles of the mouth and reveals the teeth in smiling. When used unilaterally, it conveys the expression of sneering (Figure 7-34). The muscle creates the nasolabial furrow, which deepens in expressions of sadness and with aging.

15. Levator labii superioris (see Figures 7-25, 7-28, and 7-29)

This muscle raises and pushes out the upper lip and modifies the nasolabial fold (or furrow), which runs from the end of the nose to flatten out over the cheek. It is a prominent feature of the subnasal area in many people and deepens in sadness and sometimes anger.

16. Levator labii superioris alaeque nasi (see Figure 7-25)

These two levator labii muscles (15 and 16) elevate the upper lip (Figure 7-35). The labii superioris also protracts the upper lip, and the alaeque nasi dilates the nostrils.

18. Zygomaticus major (see Figure 7-28)

The major zygomaticus muscles draw the angles of the mouth upward and laterally as in laughing (Figure 7-36).

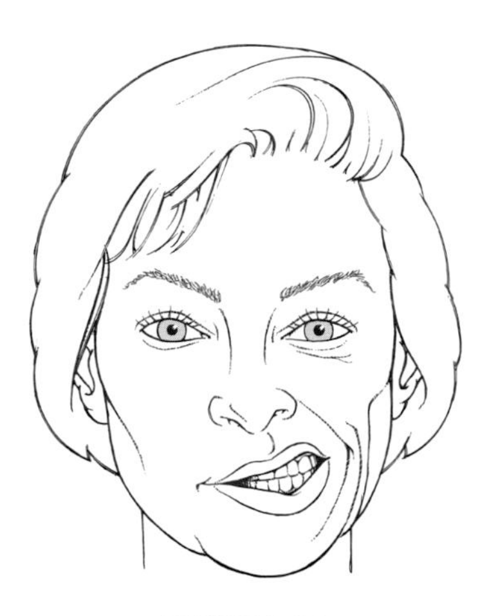

FIGURE 7-34

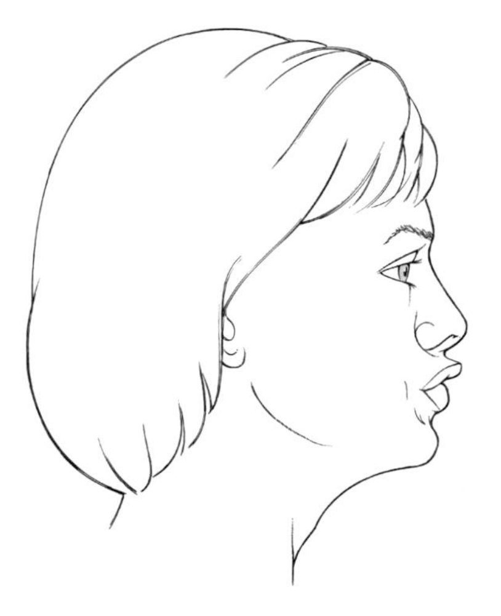

FIGURE 7-35

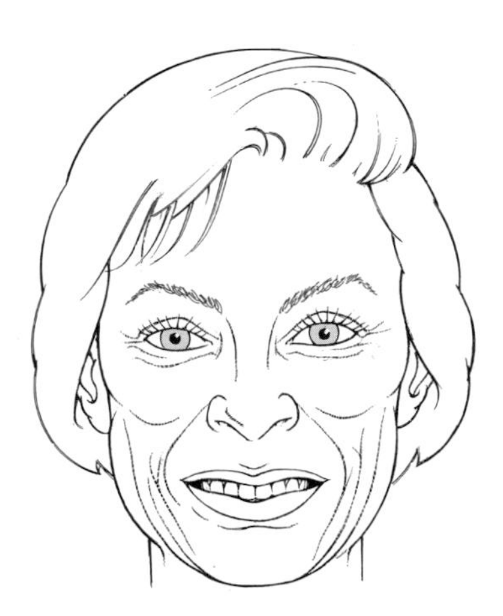

FIGURE 7-36

Other Oral Muscles Continued

21. Mentalis (Figure 7-37)

The mentalis protrudes the lower lip, as in pouting or sulking (Figure 7-38).

23. Depressor anguli oris (see Figure 7-37)

The depressor anguli oris crosses the midline to meet with its fellow muscles of the opposite side, forming the "mental sling." It draws down the angle of the mouth, giving an appearance of deep sadness (see Figure 7-38).

88. Platysma

These muscles depress the lower lip and the buccal angle of the mouth to give an expression of grief or sadness (Figure 7-39). The platysma draws the lower lip backward, producing an expression of horror, and it pulls up the skin of the neck from the clavicle (evoking the expression of "egad!"). This muscle may be tested by asking the patient to open the mouth against resistance or bite the teeth together tightly (Figure 7-40).

24. Depressor labii inferioris

This muscle draws the lower lip down and laterally, producing an expression of melancholy or irony (Figure 7-41).

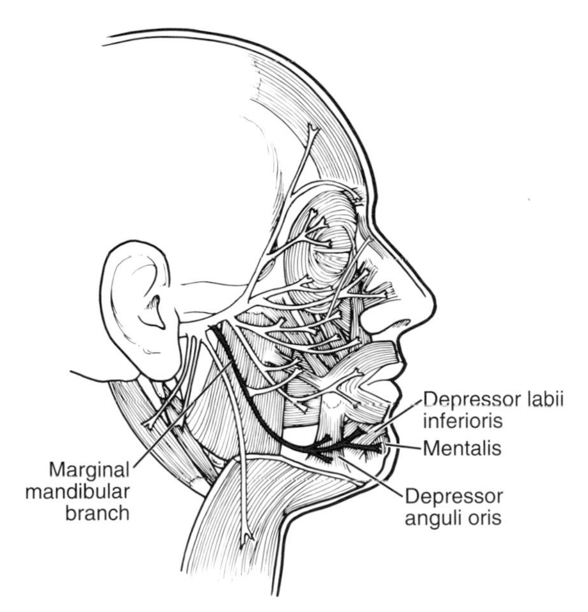

FIGURE 7-37

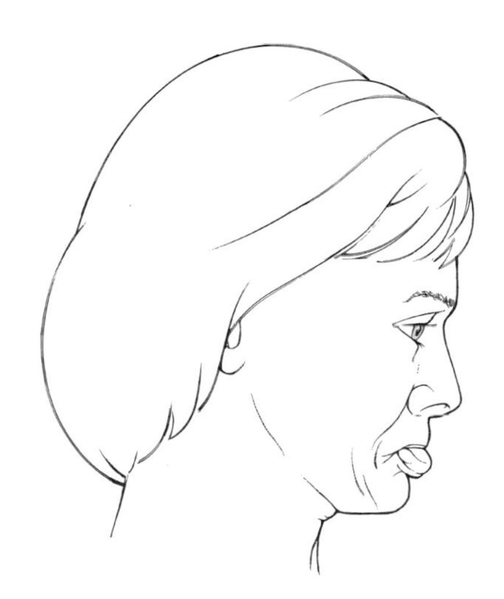

FIGURE 7-38

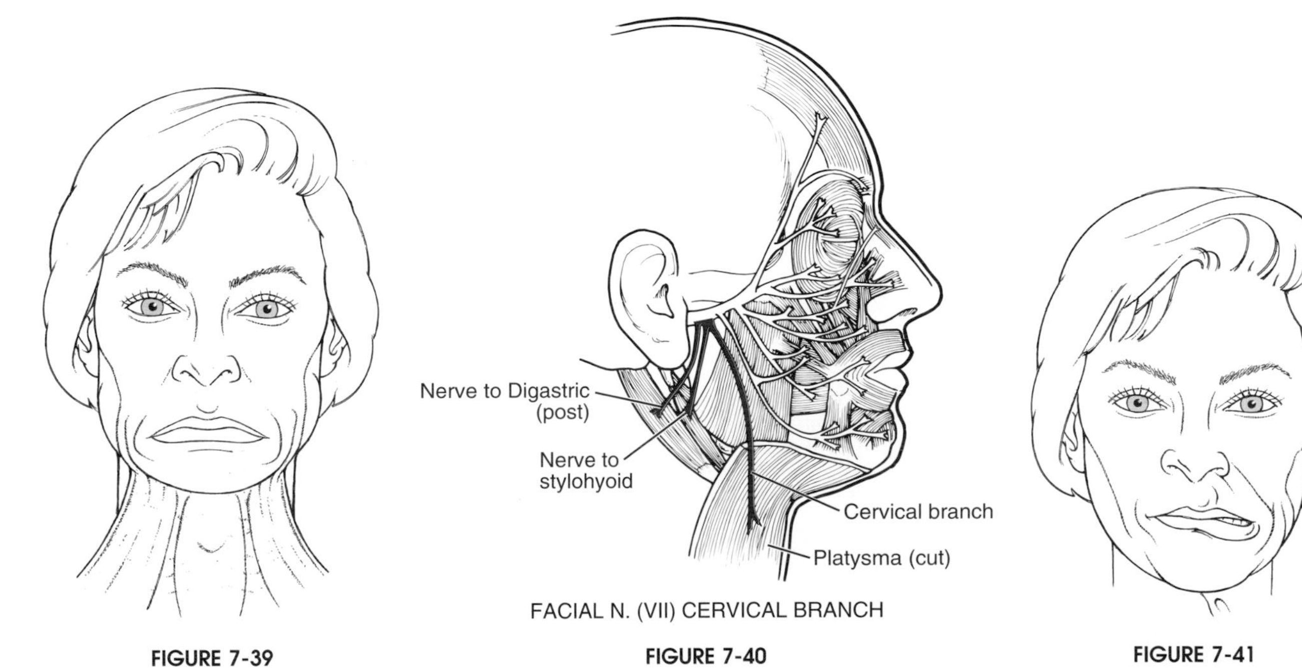

FIGURE 7-39

FIGURE 7-40

FIGURE 7-41

MUSCLES OF MASTICATION

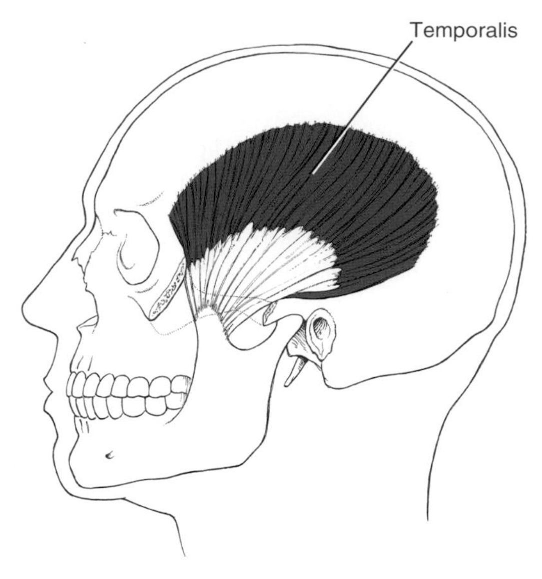

FIGURE 7-42

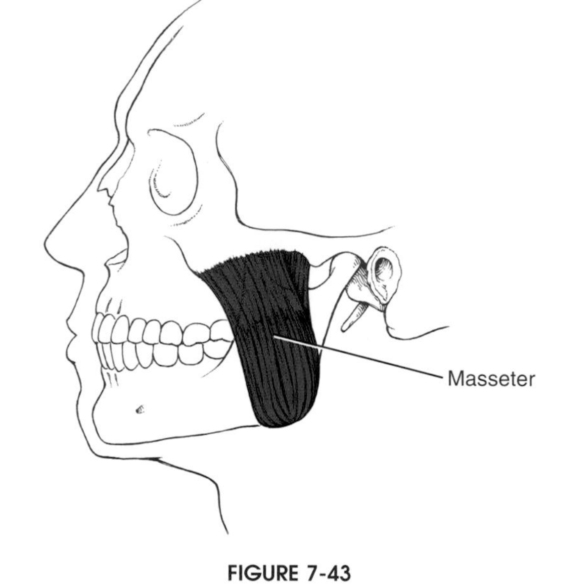

FIGURE 7-43

Table 7-5 MUSCLES OF MASTICATION

I.D.	Muscle	Origin	Insertion
28	Masseter (has 3 layers)		
	Superficial	Zygomatic bone (maxillary process) Maxilla zygomatic arch (inferior border)	Mandible (posterior and lateral ramus)
	Intermediate	Zygomatic arch (medial part of anterior 2/3)	Mandible (ramus)
	Deep	Zygomatic arch (posterior 1/3)	Mandible (ramus)
29	Temporalis	Temporal bone (whole fossa) Temporal fascia (deep surface)	Mandible (tendon to coronoid process; ramus near last molar)
30	Lateral pterygoid (has 2 heads)		*Both heads*
	Superior	Sphenoid bone (greater wing and its crest)	Mandible (condylar neck)
	Inferior	Sphenoid bone (lateral pterygoid plate)	Temporomandibular joint (articular capsule and disc)
31	Medial pterygoid	Sphenoid bone (lateral pterygoid plate, medial surface) Palatine bone (pyramidal process) Maxilla (tuberosity)	Mandible (ramus and angle)
75	Mylohyoid	Mandible (length of mylohyoid line)	Hyoid bone (front of body)
76	Stylohyoid	Temporal bone (styloid process)	Hyoid bone (body at junction with greater cornu)
77	Geniohyoid	Mandible (symphysis menti)	Hyoid bone (anterior aspect)
78	Digastric (has 2 bellies joined by tendon)		
	Posterior belly Anterior belly	Temporal bone (mastoid notch) Mandible (digastric fossa)	Hyoid bone and greater cornu (2 bellies meet in intermediate tendon that passes in a fibrous sling attached to hyoid bone)
Others			
Infrahyoids (2)			
84	Sternothyroid		
86	Sternohyoid		

Muscles of Mastication (28. Masseter, 29. Temporalis, 30. Lateral pterygoid, 31. Medial pterygoid)

The mandible is the only moving bone in the skull, and mandibular motion is largely related to chewing and speech. The muscles that control the jaw are all near the rear of the mandible (on the various surfaces and processes of the ramus), where they contribute considerable force for chewing and biting.[1] The muscles of mastication move the mandible forward (protraction) and backward (retraction) as well as shift it laterally. Excursion of the mandible is customarily limited somewhat, except in trained singers, who learn to open the mouth very wide to add to their vocal repertoire. The velocity of motions used for chewing is relatively slow, but for speech motions it is very rapid.

The muscles of mastication are all innervated by the motor division of cranial nerve V (trigeminal) (see Plate 8). The masseter elevates and protrudes the mandible. The temporalis elevates and retracts the mandible. The lateral pterygoids (Figure 7-44), acting in concert, protrude and depress the mandible; when one acts alone, it causes lateral movement to the opposite side. The medial pterygoids (see Figure 7-44) acting together elevate and protrude the mandible along with the lateral pterygoids, but acting alone they draw the mandible forward with deviation to the opposite side (as in chewing). The suprahyoid muscles (Figure 7-45 and Figure 7-46), acting via the hyoid bone, aid in jaw depression when the hyoid is fixed. The infrahyoids are weak accessories to jaw depression.

Lesions of the motor division result in weakness or paralysis of the motions of elevating, depressing, protruding, and rotating the mandible. In a unilateral lesion, the jaw deviates to the weak side; in a bilateral lesion, the jaw sags and is "paralyzed." The jaw should be examined for muscle tone, atrophy (jaw contour), and fasciculations.

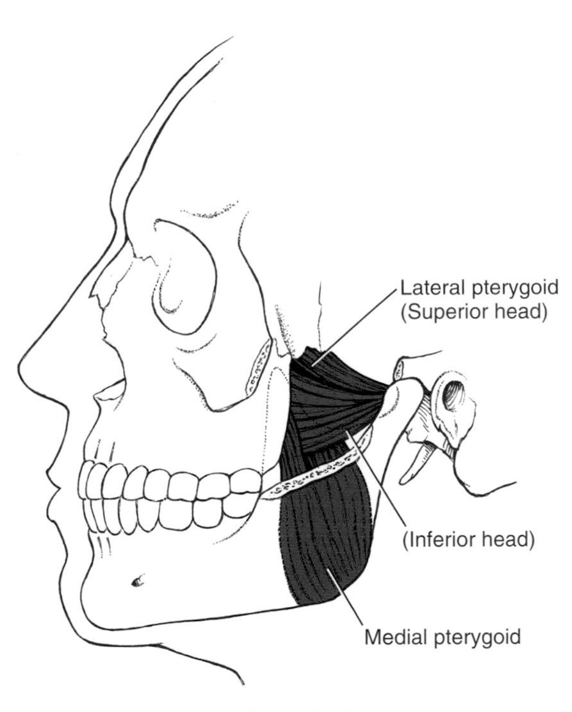

FIGURE 7-44

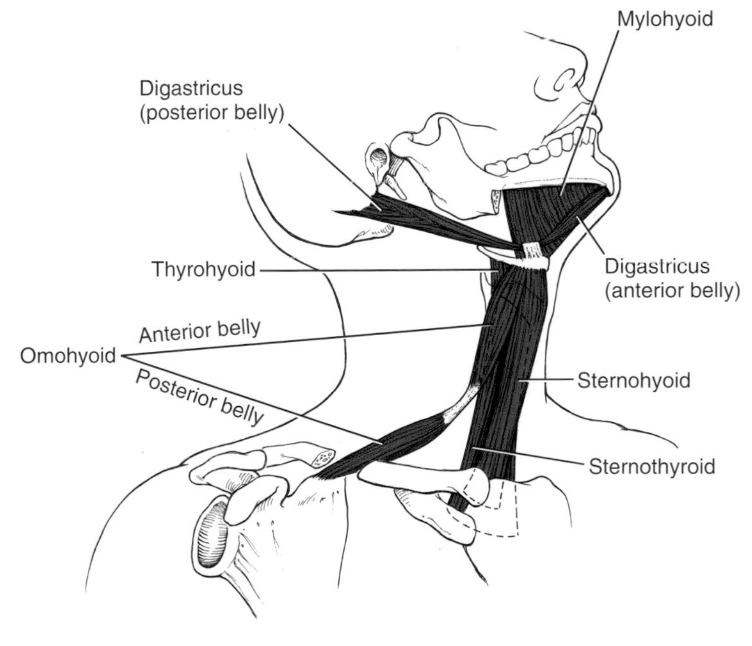

FIGURE 7-45

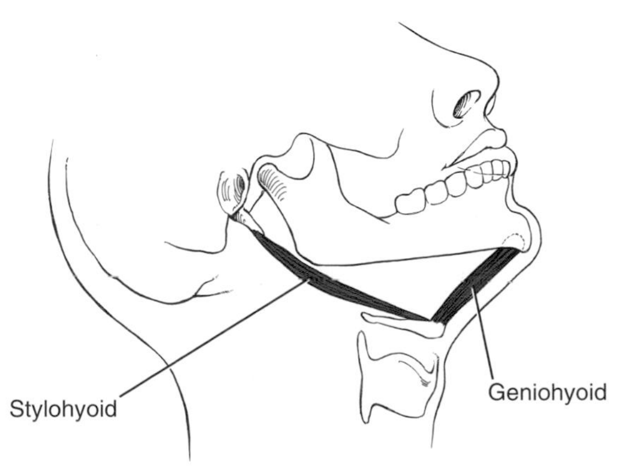

FIGURE 7-46

Jaw Opening (Mandibular Depression) (30. Lateral pterygoid, 75-78. Suprahyoid Muscles)

Note: Before testing the jaw muscles, the temporomandibular joint should be checked for tenderness and crepitus. If either is present, manual testing is avoided, and jaw opening and closing are simply observed.

Test: Patient opens the mouth as far as possible and holds against manual resistance.

Manual Resistance: One hand of the therapist is cupped under the chin; the other hand is placed on the crown of the head for stabilization (Figure 7-47). Resistance is given in a vertical upward direction in an attempt to close the jaw.

Instructions to Patient: "Open your mouth as wide as you can. Hold it. Don't let me close it."

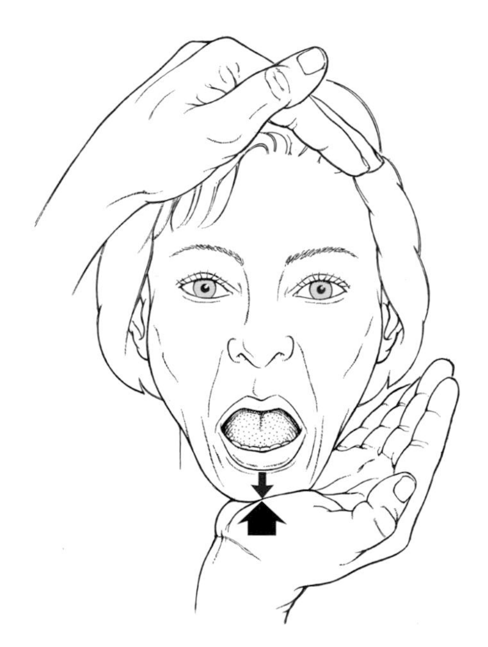

FIGURE 7-47

Criteria for Grading

F: Completes available range and holds against strong resistance. Indeed, this muscle is so powerful that in the normal person it can rarely be overcome with manual resistance. The mouth opening should accommodate three (sometimes four) stacked fingers (in an average-sized person), or 35 to 40 mm. There should be no deviation except downward.

WF: Can open mouth to accommodate two or fewer stacked fingers and can take some resistance.

NF: Minimal motion occurs. The lateral pterygoid can be palpated with a gloved finger inside the mouth, with the tip directed posteriorly past the last upper molar to the condyloid process of the ramus of the mandible. No resistance is tolerated.

0: No voluntary mandibular depression occurs.

Jaw Closure (Mandibular Elevation) (28. Masseter, 29. Temporalis, 31. Medial pterygoid)

Test: Patient clenches jaws tightly (for innervation, see Plate 8).

Manual Resistance: The chin of the patient is grasped between the thumb and index finger of the therapist and held firmly in the thumb web. The other hand is placed on top of the head for stability. Resistance is given vertically downward in an attempt to open the closed jaw (Figure 7-48).

Instructions to Patient: "Clench (or hold) your teeth together as tightly as you can, keeping your lips relaxed. Hold it. Don't let me open your mouth."

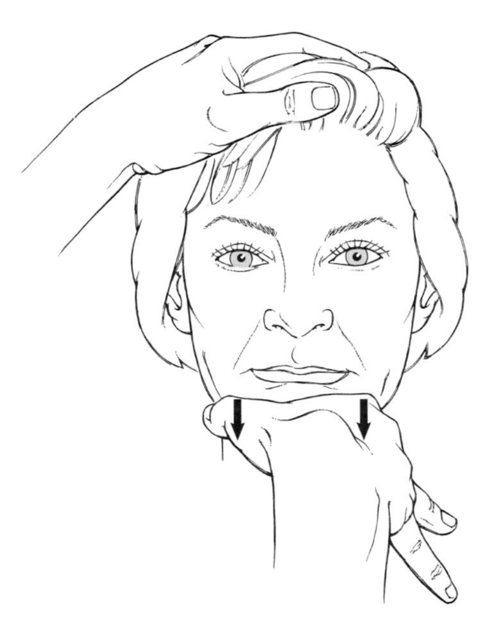

FIGURE 7-48

Criteria for Grading

F: Patient closes mouth (jaw) tightly. Therapist should not be able to open the mouth. This is a very strong muscle group. Consider circus performers who hang by their teeth!

WF: Patient closes jaw, but therapist can open the mouth with less than maximal resistance.

NF: Patient closes mouth but tolerates no resistance. The masseter and temporalis muscles are palpated on both sides. The masseter is palpated under the zygomatic process on the lateral cheek above the angle of the jaw. The temporalis muscle is palpated over the temple at the hairline, anterior to the ear and superior to the zygomatic bone.

0: Patient cannot completely close the mouth. This is more of a cosmetic problem (drooling, for example) than a significant clinical one.

In unilateral involvement, the jaw deviates to the strong side during attempts to close the mouth.

Alternate Test Procedure: The patient is asked to bite hard on a tongue blade with the molar teeth. Comparison of the depth of the bite marks from each side of the jaw is an indication of strength. If the therapist can pull out the tongue blade while the patient is biting, there is weakness of the masseter, temporalis, and lateral pterygoid muscles. (Note: This method of testing should never be used with a patient who has a bite reflex because the patient may break the blade and be injured by the splinters.)

Lateral Jaw Deviation (30. Lateral pterygoid, 31. Medial pterygoid)

When the patient deviates the jaw to the right, the acting muscles are the right lateral pterygoid and the left medial pterygoid. Deviation to the left is supported by the left lateral pterygoid and the right medial pterygoid.

With weakness of the pterygoids, when the patient opens the mouth there will be deviation to the side of the weakness.

The patient moves the jaw side to side against resistance. In V (trigeminal) nerve involvement, the patient can move the jaw to the paralyzed side but not to the unaffected side.

Test: Patient deviates jaw to the right and then to the left (for innervation, see Plate 8).

Manual Resistance: One hand of the therapist is used for resistance and is placed with the palmar side of the fingers against the jaw (Figure 7-49). The other hand is placed with the fingers and palm against the opposite temple to stabilize the head. Resistance is given in a lateral direction to move the jaw toward the midline.

Criteria for Grading

F: The range of motion for jaw lateral deviation is variable. Deviation is assessed by comparing the relationship between the upper and lower incisor teeth when the jaw is moved laterally from the midline. Do not assess deviation by the position of the lips. A pencil or ruler lined up vertically with the center of the nose may indicate mandibular deviation.

Most people can move the center point of the lower incisors laterally over three upper teeth (approximately 10 mm).[5] The patient tolerates strong resistance.

WF: Motion is decreased to lateral movement across one upper tooth, and resistance is minimal.

NF: Minimal deviation occurs, and no resistance is taken.

0: No motion occurs.

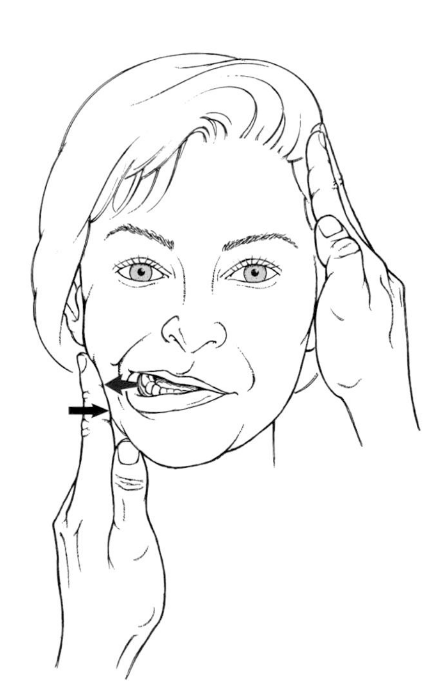

FIGURE 7-49

Jaw Protrusion (30. Lateral pterygoids, 31. Medial pterygoids)

The medial and lateral pterygoids act to protrude the jaw, which gives the face a pugnacious expression. The protrusion causes a malocclusion of the teeth, the lower teeth projecting beyond the upper teeth. With a unilateral lesion, the protruding jaw deviates to the weak side.

Test: Patient protrudes jaw so the lower teeth project beyond the upper teeth (for innervation, see Plate 8).

Manual Resistance: This is a powerful motion. The therapist stabilizes the head with one hand placed behind the head (Figure 7-50). The hand for resistance cups the chin in the thumb web with the thumb and index finger grasping the mandible. Resistance is given horizontally backward.

Instructions to Patient: "Push your jaw forward. Hold it. Don't let me push it back."

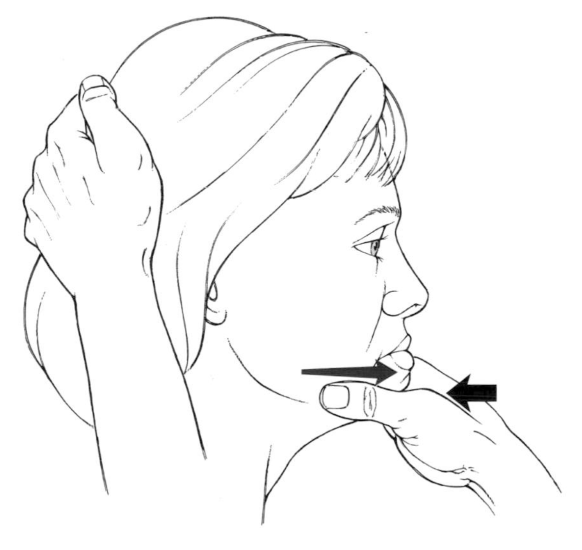

FIGURE 7-50

Criteria for Grading

F: Completes a range that moves the lower teeth in front of the upper teeth and can hold against strong resistance. There is sufficient space between the teeth in most people to see a gap between the upper and lower teeth.

WF: Moves jaw slightly forward but there is no discernible gap between the upper and lower teeth, and the patient tolerates only slight resistance.

NF: Minimal motion is detected, and the patient takes no resistance.

0: No motion and no resistance occur.

MUSCLES OF THE TONGUE

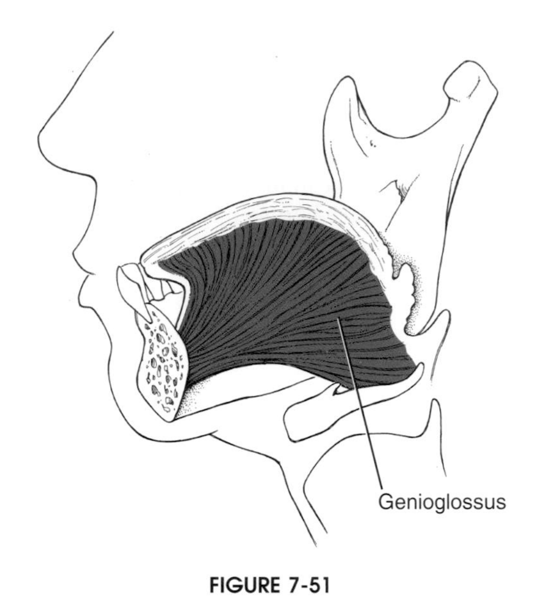

FIGURE 7-51

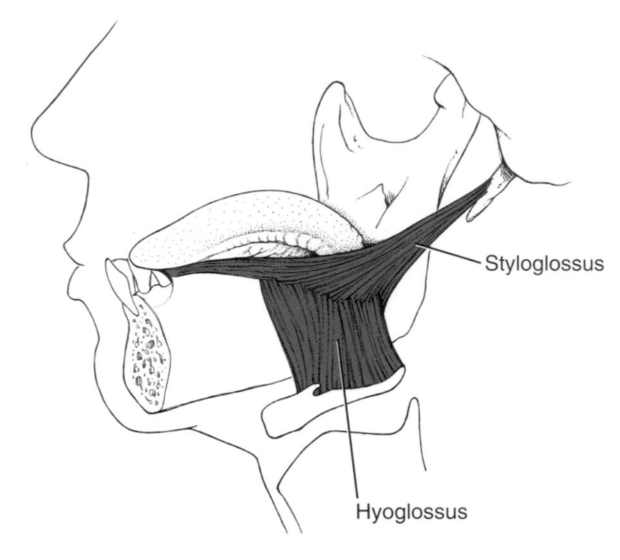

FIGURE 7-52

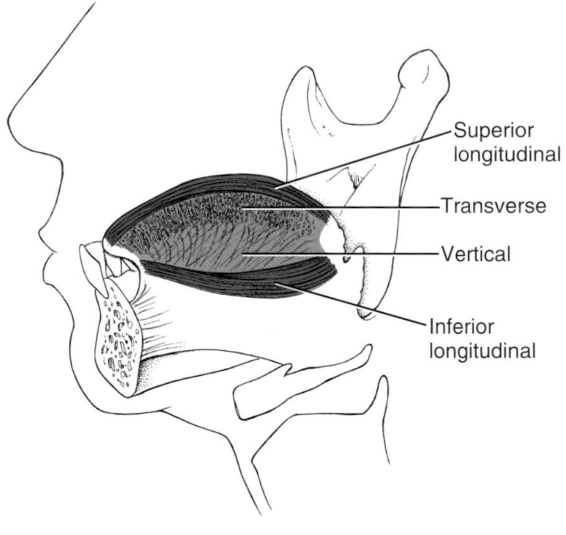

INTRINSIC TONGUE MUSCLES

FIGURE 7-53

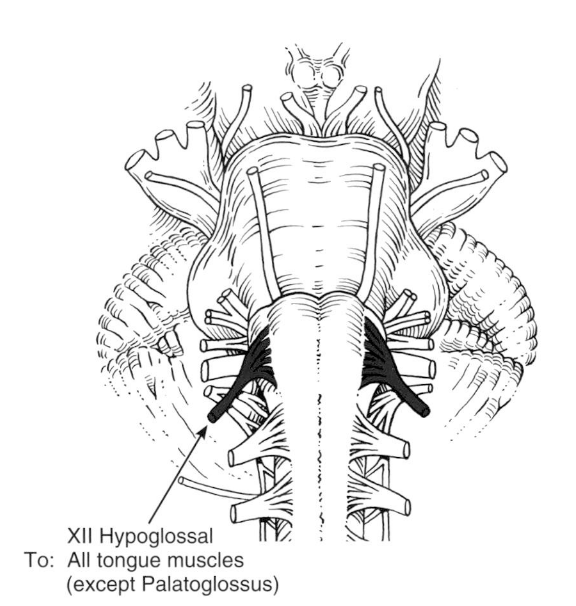

FIGURE 7-54

Table 7-6 MUSCLES OF THE TONGUE

I.D.	Muscle	Origin	Insertion
Extrinsic Muscles			
32	Genioglossus	Mandible (symphysis menti on inner surface of superior mental spine)	Hyoid bone (upper anterior side) Tongue (posterior and ventral surfaces) Blends with middle pharyngeal constrictor
33	Hyoglossus	Hyoid bone (greater cornu and side of body)	Tongue (merges on side with intrinsics)
34	Chondroglossus	Hyoid bone (lesser cornu and medial body)	Tongue (blends with intrinsic muscles on side)
35	Styloglossus	Temporal bone (styloid process, near apex) Stylomandibular ligament	Tongue (side then blends with intrinsics)
36	Palatoglossus	Soft palate (anterior)	Tongue (side to blend with transverse lingual)
Others			
Suprahyoid muscles			
75	Mylohyoid	Mandible (whole length of mylohyoid line from symphysis in front to last molar behind)	Hyoid bone (body, superior surface) Mylohyoid raphe (from symphysis menti of mandible to hyoid bone)
76	Stylohyoid	Temporal bone, styloid process (posterolateral surface)	Hyoid bone (body at junction with greater horn) Hyoid bone (body, anterior surface)
77	Geniohyoid	Mandible (symphysis menti, inferior mental spine)	Hyoid bone (body, anterior surface)
78	Digastric	Posterior belly: temporal bone (mastoid notch) Anterior belly: mandible (digastric fossa)	Intermediate tendon and from there to hyoid bone Atlas (tubercle on anterior arch) via a fibrous sling
Intrinsic Muscles			
37	Superior longitudinal	Tongue (oblique and longitudinal fibers on root and superior surface)	Tongue (to lingual margins)
38	Inferior longitudinal	Root of tongue (inferior surface)	Tongue (at tip) Hyoid bone (body) Blends with styloglossus
39	Transverse lingual	Median lingual septum	Tongue (dorsum and lateral margins) (Blends with palatopharyngeus)
40	Vertical lingual	Tongue (dorsum, anterolateral)	Tongue (ventral surface)

The extrinsic and intrinsic muscles of the tongue, except the palatoglossus, are innervated by the hypoglossal (XII) cranial nerve, a pure motor nerve. One XII nerve innervates half of the tongue (unilaterally). The hypoglossal nucleus, however, receives both crossed (mostly) and uncrossed (to a lesser extent) upper motor neuron fibers from the lowest part of the precentral gyrus via the internal capsule. Lesions of the XII nerve or its central connections may cause tongue paresis or paralysis.

Description of Tongue Muscles

The paired extrinsic muscles pass from the skull or the hyoid bone to the tongue. The intrinsic muscles rise and end within the tongue. The bulk of the tongue structure is muscle.

The principal muscle of the tongue is the genioglossus. It is a triangular muscle whose apex arises from the apex of the mandible, which is hard and immobile; its base inserts into the base of the tongue, which is soft and mobile. The genioglossus (Figure 7-51) is the principal tongue protractor, and it has crossed supranuclear innervation. The posterior fibers of the paired genioglossi draw the root of the tongue forward; a single genioglossus pushes the tongue toward the opposite side. The anterior fibers of the paired muscles draw the tongue back into the mouth after protrusion and depress it. The genioglossi acting together also depress the central part of the tongue, making it a tube.

The hyoglossi (paired) (Figure 7-52) and the chondroglossi retract and depress the sides of the tongue, making the superior surface convex. The two styloglossi (see Figure 7-52) draw the tongue upward and backward and elevate the sides, causing a dorsal transverse concavity.

The suprahyoid muscles influence the movements of the tongue via their action on the hyoid bone.

The intrinsic tongue muscles (Figure 7-53) are similarly innervated by the XII nerve (Figure 7-54). The superior longitudinal muscle shortens the tongue and curls its tip upward; the inferior longitudinal shortens the tongue and curls its tip downward. Their combined function is to alter the shape of the tongue in almost infinite variations to provide the tongue with the versatility required for speech and swallowing.

One test of a tongue motion used by therapists is called "channeling" in which the tongue is curled longitudinally; this motion may be considered to assist in sucking and directing the bolus of food into the pharynx. The difficulty presented with this motion, however, is that it is not a constant motion but rather a dominantly inherited trait that only 50% of the population can perform. Testing for channeling is acceptable as long as the inability to perform the motion is not considered a neurologic deficiency.

Examination of the Tongue

The tongue is a restless muscle, and when testing it, minor deviations are best ignored.[4] The test should start with observation of the tongue at rest on the floor of the mouth and then with the tongue protruded. The tongue is observed as it is curled up and down over the lip and then when the margins are elevated; both motions should be performed both slowly and rapidly. In all tests the ability to change the shape of the tongue is observed, but especially in tipping and channeling. One listens for difficulty in enunciation, especially of consonants.

The therapist must become familiar with the contour and mass of the normal tongue. The tongue should be examined for atrophy, which is evidenced by decreased mass, corrugations on the sides, and longitudinal furrowing. Unilateral atrophy is easy to detect and is usually accompanied by deviation to that side. When there is bilateral atrophy, the tongue will protrude weakly, if at all, and deviation also will be weak.

Fasciculations are easily visible in the tongue at rest (the surface of the tongue appears to be in constant

Examination of the Tongue Continued

motion) and can be separated from the normal tremulous motions that occur in the protruded tongue. The "tremors" that are a part of supranuclear lesions disappear when the tongue is at rest in the mouth, whereas the fasciculations of motor neuron disease such as amyotrophic lateral sclerosis continue. The hyperkinesias of parkinsonism are exaggerated when the tongue is protruded or during talking.

The therapist proceeds to examine protrusion and deviation of the tongue at slow and fast speeds. The normal tongue can move in and out (in the midline) with vigor and usually protrudes quite far beyond the lips.[11] The tongue deviates to the side of a weakness whether the cause of that weakness is a disturbance of the upper motor neuron (supranuclear disturbance) or the lower motor neuron (infranuclear disturbance).

Unilateral Weakness of the Tongue: At rest in the mouth, the tongue with a unilateral weakness may deviate slightly to the uninvolved side because of the unopposed action of the styloglossus.[11] The protruded tongue will deviate to the weak side and show weakness or inability to deviate to the normal side. Tipping may be normal because the intrinsic muscles are preserved. These functions may be impossible to evaluate if the clinical picture includes facial and jaw muscle weakness.

Early in the course of the disorder, before the onset of atrophy, the weak side of the tongue may appear enlarged and may ride higher in the mouth. After the onset of atrophy, the weak side becomes smaller, furrowed, and corrugated on the lateral edge. A unilateral weakness of the tongue may result in few functional problems, and speech and swallowing may be minimally disturbed, if at all.

Bilateral Paresis: In people with bilateral lesions, the tongue cannot be protruded or moved laterally. There will be indistinct speech, and swallowing may be difficult. Some patients experience interference with breathing when swallowing is impaired because the tongue may fall back into the throat. Total paralysis of the tongue muscles is rare (except in brain stem lesions or advanced motor neuron disease).

Supranuclear versus Infranuclear Lesions: In the presence of a supranuclear XII nerve lesion (central), the protruded tongue will deviate to the side of the weakness, which is the side opposite to the cerebral lesion. There is no atrophy of the tongue muscles. The tongue muscles also may evidence spasticity.[11]

In dyskinetic states (such as the athetosis of cerebral palsy, Huntington's chorea, or epileptic seizures), the tongue may protrude involuntarily as well as deviate to the opposite side. This is accompanied by other generally slow involuntary tongue movements that make speech thick and slow and difficult to understand.

Patients with hemiparesis after a vascular lesion (a unilateral corticobulbar lesion) may have a variety of bulbar symptoms, including tongue muscle dysfunction. In common with other bulbar manifestations, these symptoms generally are moderate and subside with time or are well compensated, so that little functional disability persists.[5] Only in patients with a second stroke or a bilateral stroke (because these muscles have bilateral cortical innervation) will the bulbar signs persist.

Inability to flick the tongue in and out of the mouth quickly (after some practice) may indicate a bilateral supranuclear lesion. In an infranuclear (peripheral) nerve lesion, the tongue will deviate to the side of the weakness, which also is the side of the lesion. There will be atrophy of the tongue muscles. Bilateral atrophy most commonly is caused by motor neuron disease. The tongue also may be weak in myasthenia gravis (fatiguing after a series of protrusions), but there will be no atrophy.

The distinction between a lower motor neuron lesion and an upper motor neuron lesion of the XII nerve depends on the presence of supporting evidence of other upper motor neuron signs and on the presence of classic lower motor neuron signs such as hemiatrophy, unilateral fasciculations, and obvious deviation to the side of the paralysis when the tongue is protruded.[4]

Tongue Protrusion, Deviation, Retraction, Posterior Elevation, Channeling, and Curling

Test for Protrusion (32. Genioglossus, Posterior Fibers)

Patient protrudes tongue so that the tip extends out beyond the lips.

Manual Resistance: Therapist uses a tongue blade against the tip of the tongue and provides resistance in a backward direction to the forward motion of the tongue (Figure 7-55).

Instructions to Patient: "Stick out your tongue. Hold it. Don't let me push it in."

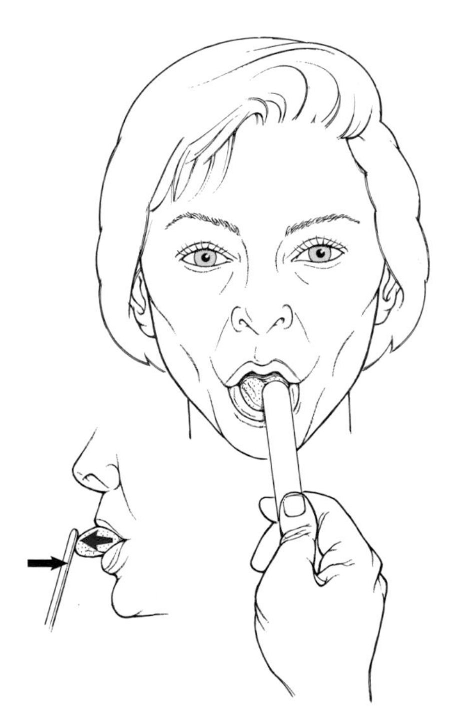

FIGURE 7-55

Test for Tongue Deviation (32. Genioglossus and Other Muscles)

Patient protrudes tongue and moves it to one side and then to the other.

Manual Resistance: Using a tongue blade, resist the lateral tongue motion along the side of the tongue near the tip (Figure 7-56). Resistance is given in the direction opposite to the attempted deviation.

Instructions to Patient: "Stick out your tongue and move it to the right." (Repeat for left side.)

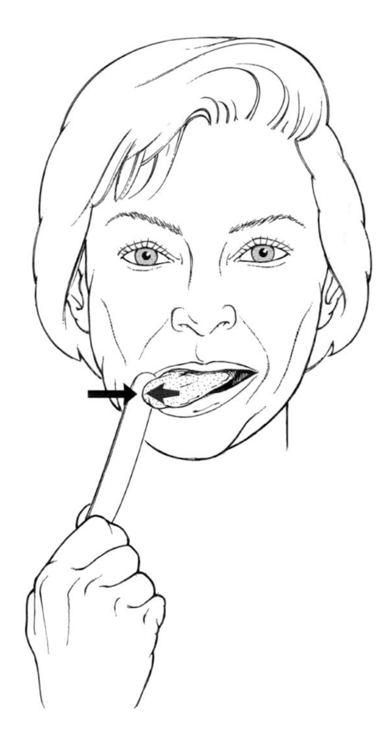

FIGURE 7-56

Tongue Protrusion, Deviation, Retraction, Posterior Elevation, Channeling, and Curling Continued

Test for Tongue Retraction (32. Genioglossus (anterior fibers), 35. Styloglossus)

Patient retracts tongue from a protruded position.

Manual Resistance: Holding a 3 × 4-inch gauze pad, securely grasp the anterior tongue by its upper and under sides (Figure 7-57). Resist retraction by holding the tongue firmly and gently pulling it forward. (The tongue is very slippery, but be careful not to pinch.)

Instructions to Patient: (Tell the patient you are going to grasp the tongue.) "Stick out your tongue. Now pull your tongue back. Don't let me keep it out."

Test for Posterior Elevation of the Tongue (36. Palatoglossus, 35. Styloglossus)

Patient elevates (i.e., "humps") the dorsum of the posterior tongue.

Manual Resistance: Therapist places tongue blade on the superior surface of the tongue over the anterior one-third. Placing the blade too far back will initiate an unwanted gag reflex (Figure 7-58). Resistance is applied in a down and backward direction, as in levering the tongue blade down, using the bottom teeth as a fulcrum (Figure 7-59).

Instructions to Patient: This is a difficult motion for the patient to understand. After directions are given, time is allowed for practice.

Begin the test by rocking the tongue blade back and forth so the patient experiences pressure on the middle to the back of the tongue.

"Push against this stick."

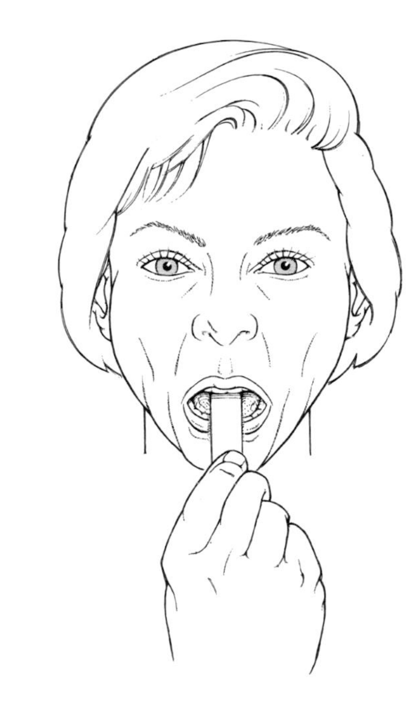

FIGURE 7-58

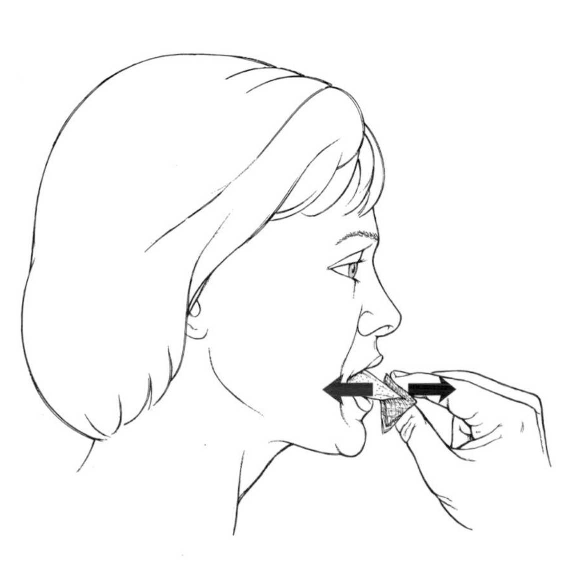

FIGURE 7-57

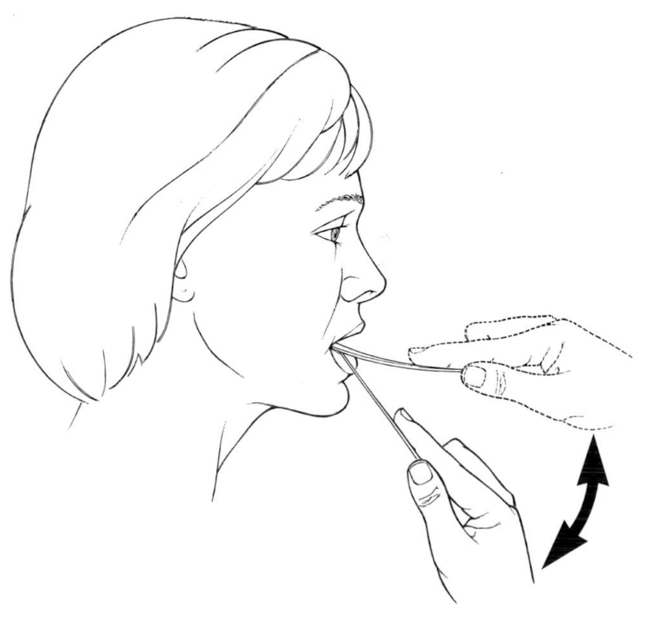

FIGURE 7-59

Tongue Protrusion, Deviation, Retraction, Posterior Elevation, Channeling, and Curling Continued

Test for Channeling the Tongue (32. Genioglossus, 37–40. Intrinsic tongue muscles)

The patient draws the tongue downward and rolls the sides up to make a longitudinal channel or tube, which is part of sucking and directing a bolus of food into the pharynx (Figure 7-60). Inability to perform this motion should not be recorded as a deficit because the motion is a dominantly inherited trait, and its presence or absence should be treated as such.

Manual Resistance: None.

Instructions to Patient: Demonstrate tongue motion to the patient. "Make a tube with your tongue."

Test for "Tipping" or Curling the Tongue (37, 38. Superior and Inferior longitudinals)

Patient protrudes tongue and curls it upward to touch the philtrum and then downward to the chin (Figure 7-61).

Manual Resistance: None.

Instructions to Patient: "Touch above your upper lip with your tongue."
"Touch your tongue to your chin."

Criteria for Grading Tongue Motions

F: Patient completes available range and holds against resistance.

Protrusion: Tongue extends considerably beyond lips.

Deviation: Tongue reaches some part of the cheek or the lateral sulcus (pocket between teeth and cheek).

Retraction: Tongue returns to rest position in mouth against resistance.

Elevation: Tongue rises so that the superior surface reaches the hard palate against considerable resistance; it blocks the oral cavity from the oropharynx.

Tipping: Tongue protrudes and touches area between upper lip and nasal septum (philtrum).

WF:

Protrusion: Tongue reaches margin of lips.

Deviation: Tongue reaches corner(s) of mouth.

Retraction: Tongue returns to rest posture but with slight resistance.

Elevation: Tongue reaches hard palate with slight resistance; oral cavity is blocked from oropharynx.

Tipping: Tongue protrudes and curls but does not reach philtrum.

NF:

Protrusion: Minimal protrusion and tongue does not clear mouth.

Deviation: Tongue protrudes and deviates slightly to side.

Retraction: Tongue tolerates no resistance and retracts haltingly.

Elevation: Tongue moves toward hard palate but does not occlude oropharynx from oral cavity.

0: All motions: None.

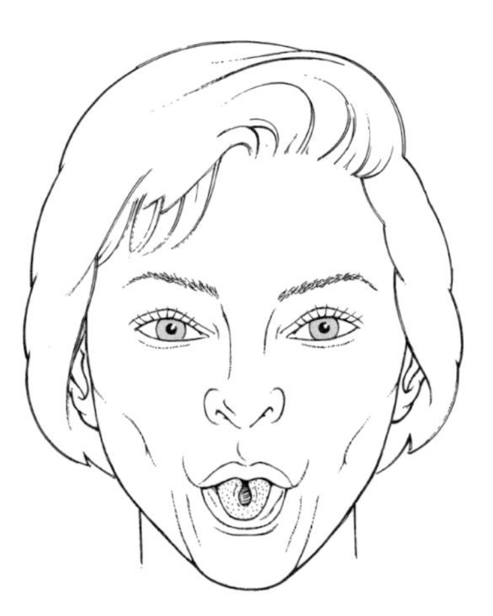

FIGURE 7-60

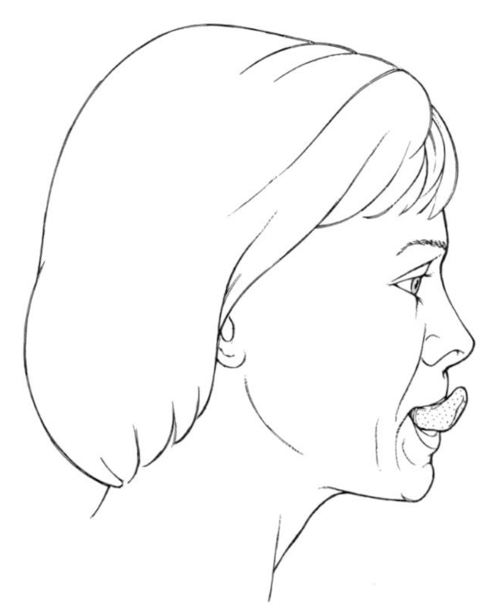

FIGURE 7-61

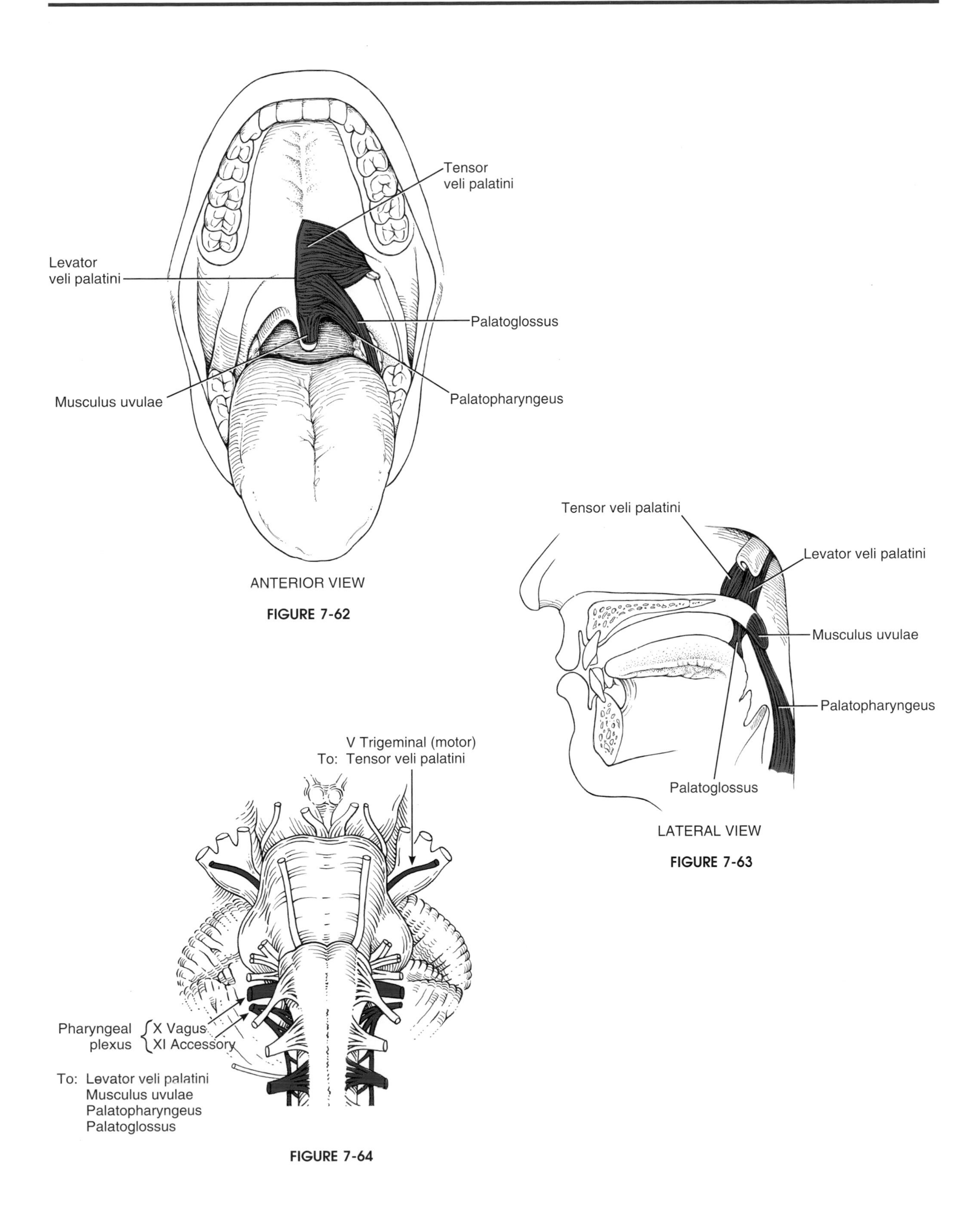

FIGURE 7-62

FIGURE 7-63

FIGURE 7-64

MUSCLES OF THE PALATE

Table 7-7 MUSCLES OF THE PALATE

I.D.	Muscle	Origin	Insertion
46	Levator veli palatini	Temporal bone Tympanic fascia Auditory (pharyngotympanic) tube (cartilage)	Palatine aponeurosis (Interlaces with its contralateral muscle to form a sling)
47	Tensor veli palatini	Auditory (pharyngotympanic) tube (cartilage, anterior) Sphenoid bone (spine and pterygoid process (scaphoid fossa))	Palatine aponeurosis Palatine bone (crest)
48	Musculus uvulae	Palatine bone (posterior nasal spine) Palatine aponeurosis (dorsal)	Uvula mucosa and connective tissue
49	Palatopharyngeus	Soft palate (pharyngeal aspect) Palatine aponeurosis Hard palate (posterior border)	Thyroid cartilage (posterior border) Pharynx (wall; crosses midline to join its contralateral muscle)

The muscles of the palate are innervated by the pharyngeal plexus (derived from the X [vagus] and XI [accessory] cranial nerves) (Figure 7-64), with the single exception of the tensor veli palatini, which derives its motor supply from the trigeminal (V) nerve (see Plate 8).

The tensor veli palatini elevates the soft palate, and paralysis of this muscle results in slight deviation of the uvula toward the unaffected side with its tip pointing toward the involved side. Weakness of the tensor as an elevator of the palate may be masked if the pharyngeal muscles innervated by the pharyngeal plexus are intact.[1,11-13] In any event, the levator veli palatini is a more important elevator of the palate than the tensor.[12,13]

The levator veli palatini also pulls the palate upward and backward to block off the nasal passages in swallowing. The musculus uvulae shortens and bends the uvula to aid in blocking the nasal passages for swallowing. The palatopharyngeus draws the pharynx upward and depresses the soft palate.

In the presence of a unilateral vagus (X) nerve lesion, the levator veli palatini (see Figure 7-64) and the musculus uvulae on the involved side are weak. There is a resultant lowering or flattening of the palatal arch, and the median raphe deviates toward the uninvolved side. With phonation, the uvula deviates to the uninvolved side.

With a bilateral vagus lesion, the palate cannot be elevated for phonation, but it does not sag because of the action of the tensor veli palatini (V nerve).[12] The nasal cavity is not blocked off from the oral cavity with the bilateral lesion, which may lead to nasal regurgitation of liquids. Also, during speaking, air escapes into the nasal cavity, and the change in resonance gives a peculiar nasal quality to the voice. Dysphagia may be severe.

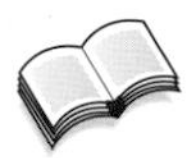

Description of the Palate

The palate, or roof, of the oral cavity is viewed with the mouth fully open and the tongue protruding (Figure 7-65). The palate has two parts: the hard palate is the vault over the front of the mouth, and the soft palate is the roof over the rear of the oral cavity.[1]

The hard palate is formed from the maxilla (palatine processes) and the horizontal plates of the palatine bones. It has the following boundaries: anterolaterally, the alveolar arch and gums of the teeth; posteriorly, the soft palate. The frontal mucosa is thick, pale, and corrugated; the posterior mucosa is darker, thinner, and not corrugated. The superior surface of the palate forms the nasal floor.

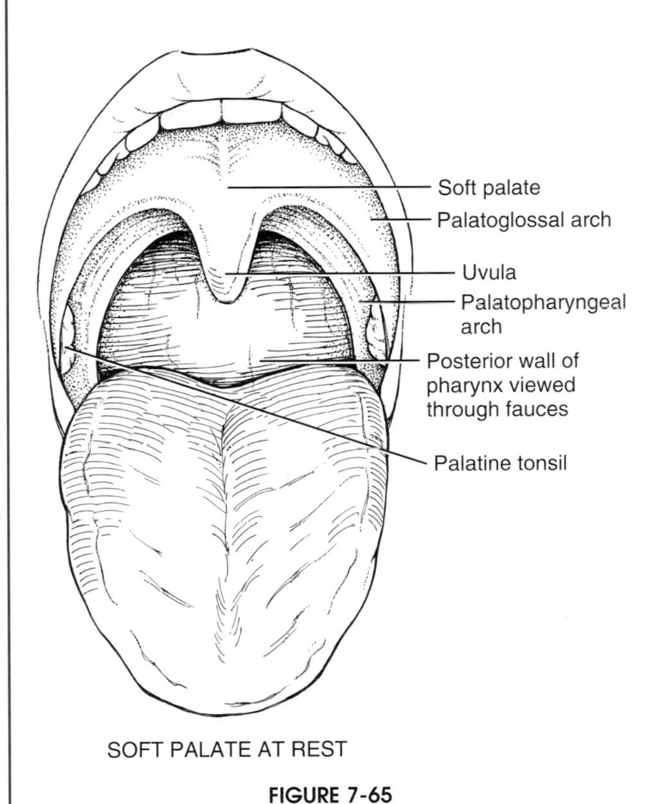

FIGURE 7-65

The soft palate is actually a rather mobile soft-tissue flap suspended from the hard palate, which slopes down and backward.[1] Its superior border is attached to (or continuous with) the posterior margin of the hard palate, and its sides blend with the pharyngeal wall. The inferior wall of the soft palate hangs free as a border between the mouth and the pharynx. The conical uvula drops from its posterior border.

The palatal arches are two curved folds of tissue containing muscles that descend laterally from the base of the uvula on either side. The anterior of these, the *palatoglossal arch,* holds the palatoglossus and descends to end in the lateral sides of the tongue. The posterior fold, the *palatopharyngeal arch,* contains the palatopharyngeus muscle and descends on the lateral wall of the oropharynx.[1,6] The palatine tonsils lie in a triangular notch between the diverging palatoglossal and palatopharyngeal arches.

The pharyngeal isthmus (or margin of the fauces) lies between the border of the soft palate and the posterior pharyngeal wall. The fauces forms the passageway between the mouth and the pharynx that includes the lumen as well as its boundary structures. The fauces closes during swallowing as a result of the elevation of the palate and contraction of the palatopharyngeal muscles (acting like a sphincter) and by elevation of the dorsum of the posterior tongue (palatoglossus).

In examining the soft palate, observe the position of the palate and uvula at rest and during quiet breathing and then during phonation. If the palatine arches elevate symmetrically, minor deviations of the uvula are insignificant (e.g., uvular changes often occur after tonsillectomy).[11] Check for the presence of dysarthria and dysphagia (both liquids and solids).

Normally the uvula hangs in the midline and elevates in the midline during phonation.

Elevation and Adduction of the Soft Palate (46. Levator veli palatini, 47. Tensor veli palatini, 36. Palatoglossus, 48. Musculus uvulae)

Test: Patient produces a high-pitched "Ah-h-h" to cause the soft palate to elevate and adduct (the arches come closer together, narrowing the fauces) (Figure 7-66).

To see the palate and fauces adequately, the therapist may need to place a tongue blade lightly on the tongue and use a flashlight to illuminate the interior of the mouth. Placing the tongue blade too far back or too heavily on the tongue may initiate a disagreeable gag reflex.

When this test does not give the desired information, the therapist may have to stimulate a gag reflex. Light touch stimulation, done slowly and gradually with an applicator (preferably) or tongue blade placed on the posterior tongue or soft palate, will evoke a reflex and produce the desired motion when phonation fails to do so.

Remember that the gag reflex is not a constant finding. Some normal people do not have one, and many people have an exaggerated reflex.

Resistance: None.

Instructions to Patient: "Use a high-pitched (soprano) tone to say 'Ah-a-a-a.'"

Criteria for Grading (Derived from Observation of Uvular and Arch Motion)

F: Uvula moves briskly and elevates while remaining in the midline. The palatoglossal and palatopharyngeal arches elevate and adduct to narrow the fauces.

WF: Uvula moves sluggishly and may deviate to one or the other side. Uvula deviation is toward the uninvolved side (Figure 7-67). The arches may elevate slightly and asymmetrically.

NF: Almost imperceptible motion of both the uvula and the arches occurs.

0: No motion occurs, and the uvula is flaccid and pendulous.

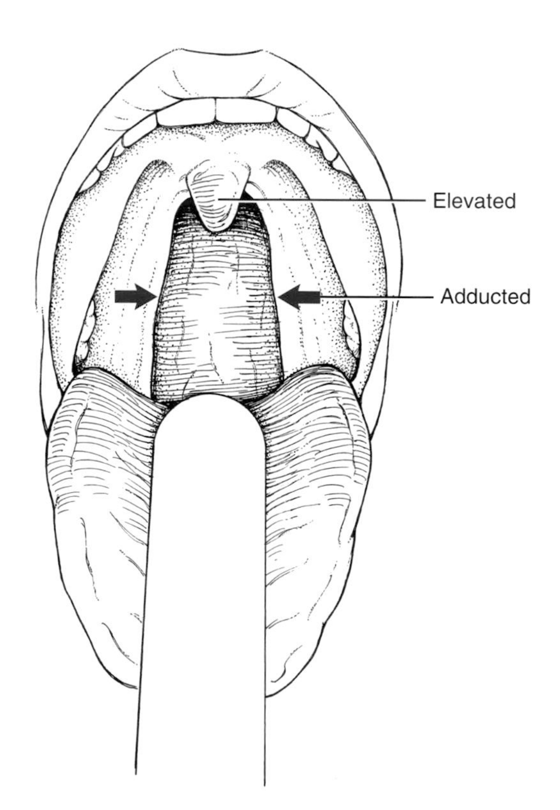

SOFT PALATE DURING TEST

FIGURE 7-66

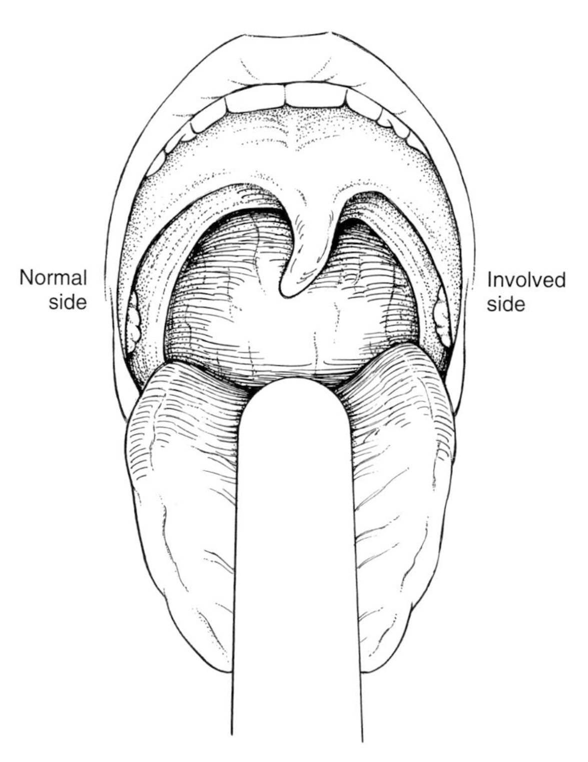

SOFT PALATE WEAKNESS

FIGURE 7-67

Occlusion of the Nasopharynx (49. Palatopharyngeus)

Test: Aiming at the therapist's finger, the patient blows through the mouth with pursed lips to occlude the nasopharynx via the palatopharyngeus. Place a slim mirror above the upper lip (horizontally blocking off the mouth) to check for air escape from the nostrils (the mirror clouds). Alternatively, place a small feather fixed to a small plastic platform right under the nose; the motion of the feather is used to detect air leakage.

Nasal speech is a sign of inability to close off the nasopharynx.

Resistance: None.

Instructions to Patient: "Blow on my finger."

Criteria for Grading

F: No leakage of air through the nose.

WF: Minimal leakage of air. Slight mirror clouding or feather ruffling.

NF to 0: Heavy mirror clouding or brisk feather ruffles.

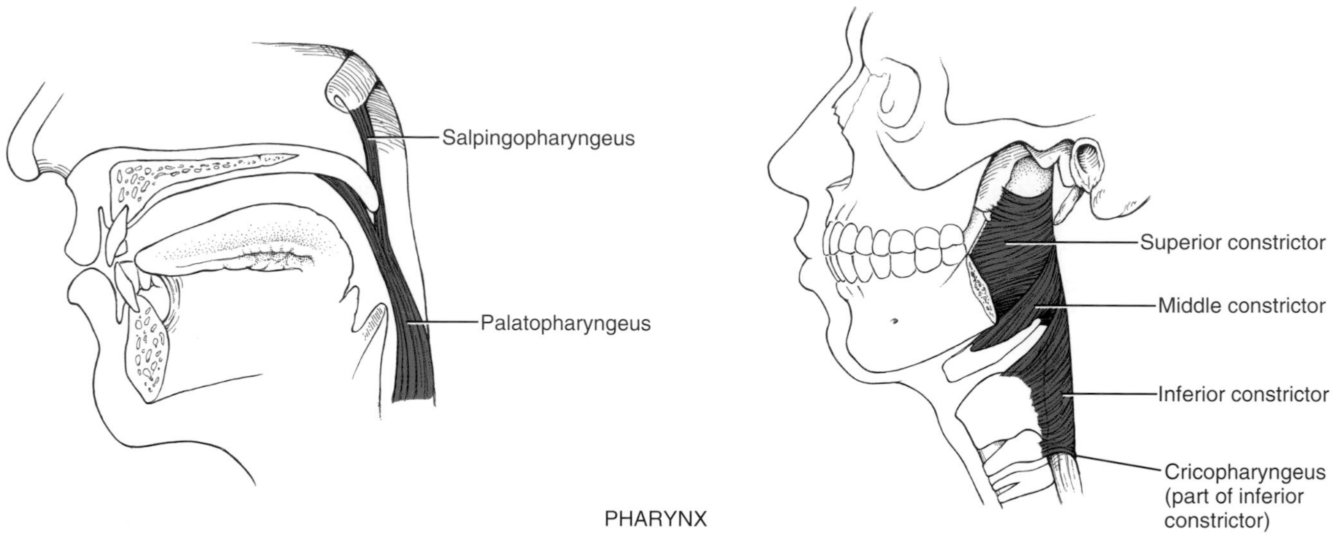

FIGURE 7-68

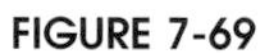
FIGURE 7-69

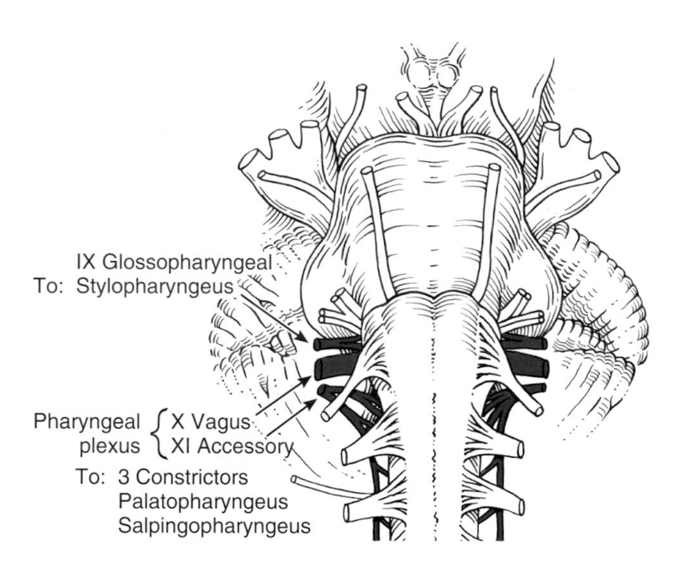

FIGURE 7-70

Table 7-8 MUSCLES OF THE PHARYNX

I.D.	Muscle	Origin	Insertion
41	Inferior pharyngeal constrictor	Cricoid cartilage Thyroid cartilage (oblique line) Hyoid bone (inferior cornu)	Pharynx (posterior median fibrous raphe)
42	Middle pharyngeal constrictor	Hyoid bone (lesser horn anterior; greater horn entire upper border) Stylohyoid ligament	Pharynx (posterior median fibrous raphe)
43	Superior pharyngeal constrictor	Sphenoid (medial pterygoid plate) Pterygoid hamulus Mandible (mylohyoid line) Tongue (side)	Pharynx (median fibrous raphe) Occipital bone (basilar part of pharyngeal tubercle)
44	Stylopharyngeus	Temporal bone (styloid process, medial base)	Thyroid cartilage (some fibers merge with constrictor muscles and palatopharyngeus)
45	Salpingopharyngeus	Auditory tube (inferior cartilage)	Blends with palatopharyngeus

The function of the pharyngeal muscles is tested by observing their contraction during phonation and their elevation of the larynx during swallowing. The pharyngeal reflex also should be invoked and the nature of the muscle contraction noted. The manner in which the patient handles solid and liquid foods, in addition to the quality and character of speech, should be described.

The motor parts of the glossopharyngeal (IX) cranial nerve (Figure 7-70) go to the pharynx but probably innervate only the stylopharyngeus muscle. The stylopharyngeus elevates the upper lateral and posterior walls of the pharynx in swallowing.[14]

The remaining pharyngeal muscles (inferior, middle, and superior constrictors, palatopharyngeus, and salpingopharyngeus) are innervated by the pharyngeal plexus composed of elements from the vagus (X) and accessory (XI) cranial nerves. The three constrictor muscles flatten and contract the pharynx in swallowing and are important participants in forcing the bolus of food into the esophagus, thereby initiating peristaltic activity in the gut. The salpingopharyngeus blends with the palatopharyngeus and elevates the upper portion of the pharynx.[1] Because the pharynx acts as a resonator box for sound, impairment of the pharyngeal muscles will alter the voice.

The inferior constrictor has two parts, which often are referred to as if they were separate muscles.[1] One, the cricopharyngeus, blends with the circular esophageal fibers to act as a distal pharyngeal sphincter in swallowing. These fibers prevent air from entering the esophagus during respiration and reflux of food from the esophagus back into the pharynx. It has been reported that when the system is at rest, the cricopharyngeus is actively contracted to prevent air from entering the esophagus.[15] When a swallow is initiated, some form of neural inhibition causes the cricopharyngeus to relax.[15,16] At the same time, the hyoid bone and the larynx elevate and move anteriorly, and the constrictor muscles act in a peristaltic manner, the sum of which permits passage of the bolus.[15]

The upper part of the inferior constrictor is the thyropharyngeus, which acts to propel the bolus of food downward.[1]

In unilateral lesions of the vagus (X) nerve, laryngeal elevation is decreased on one side, and in bilateral lesions it is decreased on both sides.

Constriction of the Posterior Pharyngeal Wall

Test: Patient opens mouth wide and says "Ah-h-h" with a high-pitched tone.

This sound causes the posterior pharyngeal wall to contract (the soft palate adducts and elevates as well).

Because it is difficult to observe the posterior wall of the pharynx, use a flashlight to illuminate the interior of the mouth. A tongue blade will probably be needed to keep the tongue from obstructing the view, but care must be taken not to initiate a gag reflex.

Patients with weakness may have an accumulation of saliva in the mouth. Ask the patient to swallow, or, if this does not work, use mouth suctioning. If the patient has a nasogastric tube, it will descend in front of the posterior wall and may partially obstruct a clear view.

If there is little or no motion of the pharyngeal wall, the therapist will have to stimulate the pharyngeal reflex to ascertain contractile integrity of the superior constrictor and other muscles of the pharyngeal wall. Patients do not like this reflex test.

The Pharyngeal Reflex Test: The pharyngeal reflex is tested by applying a stimulus with an applicator to the posterior pharyngeal wall or adjacent structures (Figure 7-71). The stimulus should be applied bilaterally. If positive, elevation and constriction of the pharyngeal muscles will occur along with retraction of the tongue.

Criteria for Grading

F: Brisk contraction of the posterior pharyngeal wall.

WF: Decreased movement or sluggish motion of the pharyngeal wall.

NF: Trace of motion (easily missed).

0: No contractility of the pharyngeal wall.

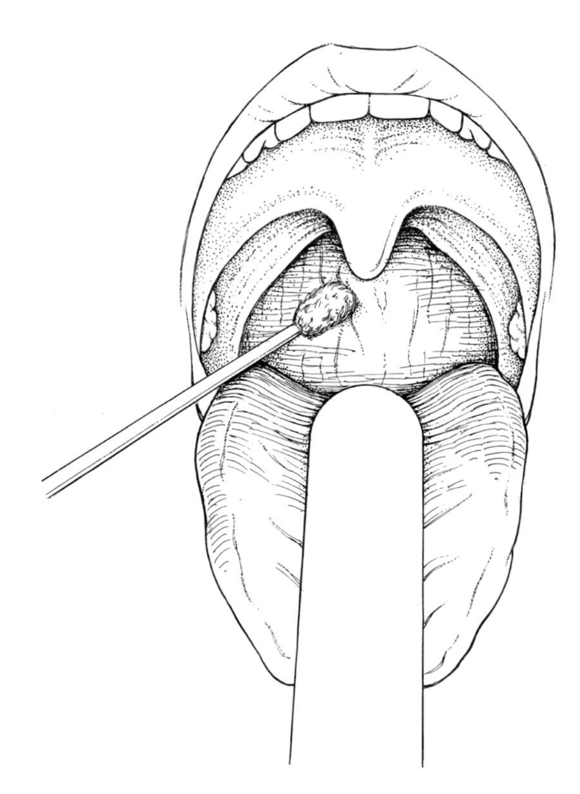

FIGURE 7-71 Soft palate just before touch.

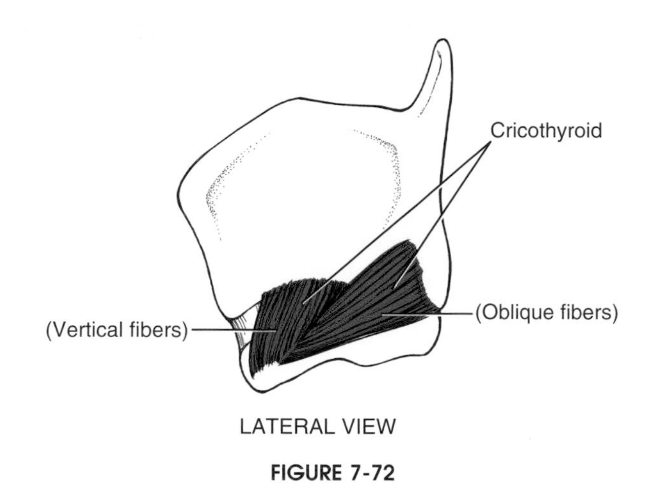

LATERAL VIEW

FIGURE 7-72

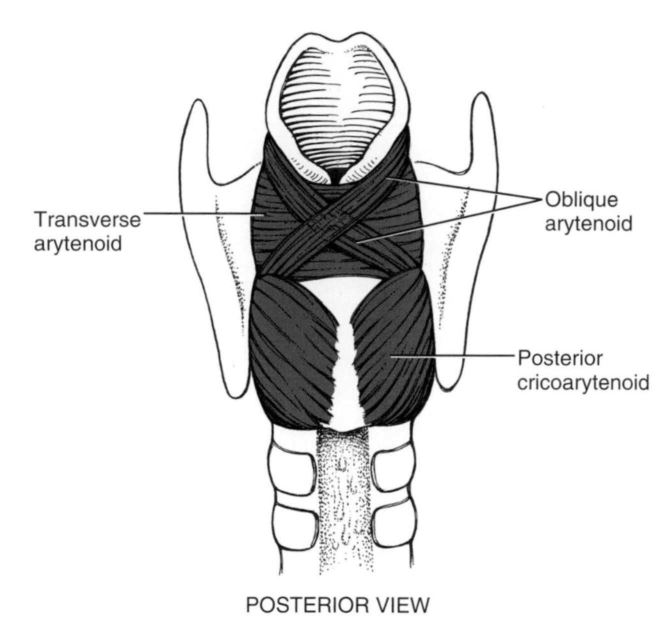

POSTERIOR VIEW

FIGURE 7-73

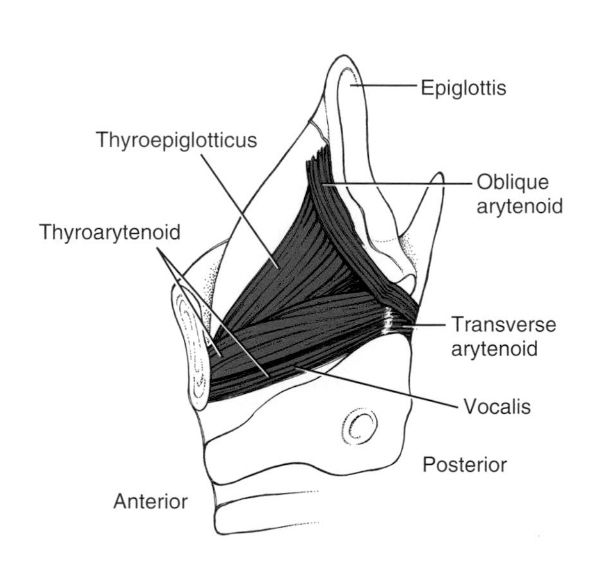

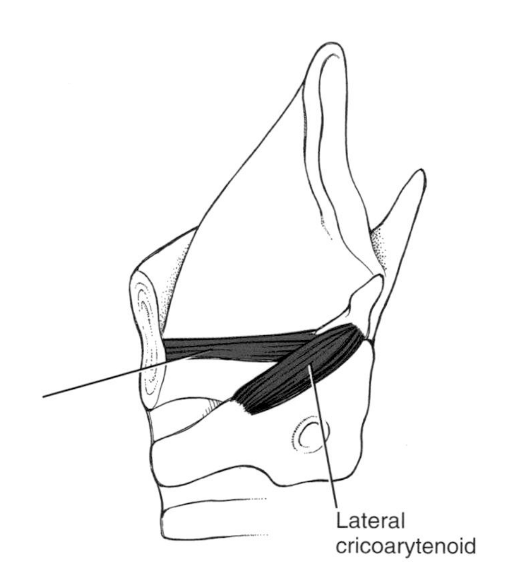

LATERAL VIEWS

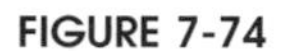

FIGURE 7-74

FIGURE 7-75

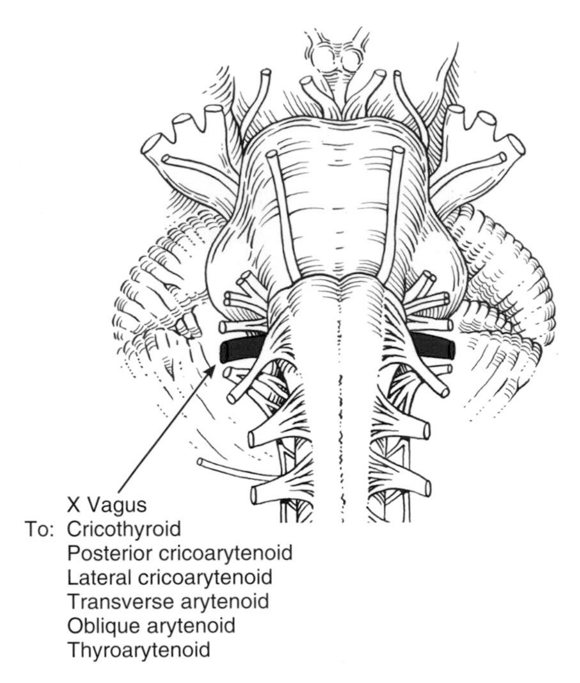

FIGURE 7-76

Table 7-9 MUSCLES OF THE LARYNX

I.D.	Muscle	Origin	Insertion
50	Cricothyroid	Cricoid cartilage (external aspect of arch)	Thyroid lamina Thyroid cartilage
51	Posterior cricoarytenoid	Cricoid cartilage (posterior surface)	Arytenoid cartilage (posterior on same side)
52	Lateral cricoarytenoid	Cricoid cartilage (arch)	Arytenoid cartilage (anterior on same side)
53	Transverse arytenoid (unpaired muscle)	Crosses transversely between the two arytenoid cartilages	Lateral border of both arytenoids Fills posterior concave surface between two arytenoids
54	Oblique arytenoid	Arytenoid cartilage (posterior) Cross back of larynx obliquely	Arytenoid cartilage (apex) on opposite side
55	Thyroarytenoid (vocalis muscle formed by band of fibers off lateral vocal process)	Thyroid cartilage (angle and lower half) Cricothyroid ligament	Arytenoid cartilage (anterior base) Vocal process (lateral)
Others			
Infrahyoid muscles			
84	Sternothyroid		
85	Thyrohyoid		
86	Sternohyoid		
87	Omohyoid		

Examination of the muscles of the larynx includes assessing the quality and nature of the voice, noting any abnormalities of phonation or articulation, impairment of coughing, and any problems with respiration. Also important is the rate of opening and closing of the glottis.

Some general definitions are in order. *Phonation* is the production of vocal sounds without the formation of words; phonation is a function of the larynx.[5] *Articulation,* or the formation of words, is a joint function of the larynx along with the pharynx, palate, tongue, teeth, and lips.

All the laryngeal muscles are innervated by the recurrent branches of the X (vagus) cranial nerve with the exception of the cricothyroid, which receives its motor innervation from the superior laryngeal nerve. The laryngeal muscles regulate the tension of the vocal cords and open and close the glottis by abducting and adducting the vocal cords. The vocal cords normally are open (abducted) during inspiration and adducted while speaking or during coughing.

The cricothyroids (paired) are the principal tensors owing to their action in lengthening the vocal cords.[1,5,11] The posterior cricoarytenoids (paired) are the main abductors and glottis openers; the lateral cricoarytenoids (paired) are the main adductors and glottis closers. The thyroarytenoids (paired) shorten and relax the vocal cords by drawing the arytenoid cartilages forward. The unpaired arytenoid (transverse and oblique heads) draws the arytenoid cartilages together; the oblique head acts as the sphincter of the upper larynx (called the aryepiglottic folds), and the transverse head acts as the sphincter of the lower larynx.

Paralysis of the laryngeal muscles on one side does not cause an appreciable change in the voice, in contrast to the difficulty resulting from bilateral weakness. Loss of the cricothyroids leads to loss of the high tones and the voice sounds deep and hoarse and fatigues readily, but respiration is normal. Loss of the thyroarytenoids bilaterally changes the shape of the glottis and results in a hoarse voice, but again, respiration is normal.

With bilateral paralysis of the posterior cricoarytenoids, both vocal cords will lie close to the midline and cannot be abducted, leading to severe dyspnea and difficult inspiratory effort (inspiratory stridor).[5] Expiration is normal.

In bilateral adductor paralysis (lateral cricoarytenoids), inspiration is normal because abduction is unimpaired. The voice, however, is lost or has a whisper quality.

With unilateral loss of both abduction and adduction, the involved vocal cords are motionless, and the voice is low and hoarse. In bilateral loss, all vocal cords are quiescent, and speech and coughing are lost. Marked inspiratory stress occurs, and the patient is dyspneic.

For a discussion of the functional anatomy of coughing, see Chapter 4, page 71.

Elevation of the Larynx in Swallowing

Test: The larynx elevates during swallowing. The therapist lightly grasps the larynx with the thumb and index finger on the anterior throat to determine the presence of elevation and its extent (Figure 7-77).

DO NOT PRESS DIRECTLY ON THE FRONT OF THE LARYNX, AND NEVER USE EXCESSIVE PRESSURE ON THE NECK.

Resistance: None.

Instructions to Patient: "Swallow."

Criteria for Grading

F: Larynx elevates at least 20 mm in most people.[14] The motion is quick and controlled.

WF: Laryngeal excursion may be normal or slightly limited. The motion is sluggish and may be irregular.

NF: Excursion is perceptible but less than normal. Aspiration may occur.

0: No laryngeal elevation occurs. (Aspiration will result in this event.)

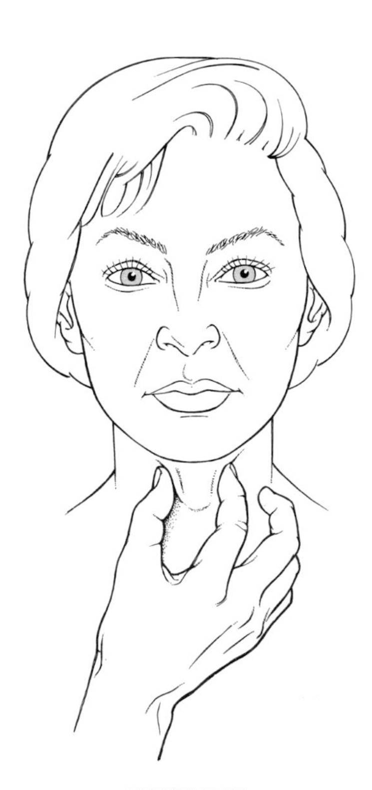

FIGURE 7-77

Vocal Cord Abduction and Adduction (51. Posterior cricoarytenoids, 52. Lateral cricoarytenoids)

In this test the therapist is looking for hoarseness, pitch and tone range, breathlessness, breathiness, nasal-quality speech, dysarthria, and articulation or phonation disturbances.

Test and Instructions to Patient: The patient is asked to respond to four different commands to determine the nature of airflow control during respiration, vocalization, and coughing.

1. "State your name." Patient should be able to say his or her name completely without running out of breath.
2. "Sing several notes in the musical scale," (do, re, mi, etc.) "first at a low pitch and then at a higher pitch." Patient should be able to sustain a tone (even if he or she "can't carry a tune") and vary the pitch.
3. "Repeat five times a hard staccato, interrupted sound: 'Akh, Akh, Akh.'" Therapist must demonstrate this sound to the patient. Patient should make and break sounds crisply with a definite halt between each sound in the series.
4. "Cough."

Evaluation of Cough in the Context of Laryngeal Function: Therapist determines whether the patient has a voluntary and effective cough. A voluntary cough is initiated on command. A reflex cough, because it cannot be initiated on command, must be evaluated when it occurs, which may be outside of the test session. The reflex cough occurs in response to irritation of the membranes of the postnasal air passages.

An effective or functional cough, voluntary or reflex, clears secretions from the lungs or airways. A functional cough is dependent on the coordination of the respiratory and laryngeal muscles.

Control of inspiration must be sufficient to fill the lungs with the necessary volume of air to produce a cough. Effective expiration of air during a cough is dependent on forceful contraction of the abdominal muscles. The vocal cords must adduct tightly to prevent air loss. Adduction of the vocal cords must be maintained before the expulsion of air.

A nonfunctional cough resulting from laryngeal deficiency sounds like clearing the throat or a low guttural sound, or there may be no cough sound at all.

For additional information, see "The Functional Anatomy of Coughing", in Chapter 4, page 71.

The kinesiology of swallowing is the subject of continued controversy. Many of the rapid actions described as sequential are close to simultaneous events. The means of studying swallowing are limited to a great extent by the limitations inherent in palpation and visualization of following ingested food. Videofluoroscopy, ultrasound, manometry, and acoustic measures improve assessment accuracy.

MUSCLE ACTIONS IN SWALLOWING

Ingestion of Food and Formation of Bolus (Oral Preparatory Phase)

- The food or liquid is placed in the oral cavity, and the orbicularis oris contracts to maintain a labial seal and to prevent drooling. The palatoglossus maintains a posterior seal by maintaining the tongue against the soft palate, which prevents leakage too early into the pharynx.[17]
- Foods are broken down mechanically by integrated action of the muscles of the tongue, jaw, and cheeks.
- Liquids: Intrinsic tongue muscles squirt fluids into the back of the mouth. The mylohyoid raises and bulges the back of the tongue into the oropharynx. Lips must be closed to retain fluids.
- Solids: Muscles of the tongue and cheek (buccinator) place the food between the teeth, which bite, crush, and grind it via action of the muscles of mastication (see Table 7-5). The food, when mixed with saliva (by the tongue intrinsics), forms a bolus behind the tip of the tongue.
- The tongue muscles (see Table 7-6) raise the anterior tongue and press it against the hard palate, which pushes the bolus back into the fauces.

The Oral Phase

- In this phase of swallowing, the bolus is squeezed against the hard palate by the tongue, the lip seal is maintained, and the buccinator continues to prevent pocketing or lodging of food in the lateral sulci.
- The tongue is drawn up and back by the styloglossus.
- The palate muscles (see Table 7-7) depress the soft palate down onto the tongue to "grip" the bolus.
- The hyoid bone and the larynx are elevated and moved forward by the suprahyoid muscles.
- The palatal arches are adducted by the paired palatoglossi.
- The bolus is driven back into the oropharynx.
- As a prelude to the act of swallowing, the hyoid bone is raised slightly, and this action is accompanied by a quiescence of all muscle action: chewing, talking, food movement in the mouth, capital and cervical motion, and facial movements. Even respiration is momentarily arrested.[16,17]
- The soft palate is raised (levator veli palatini) and tightened (tensor veli palatini) to be firmly fixed against the posterior pharyngeal wall. This leads to a tight closure of the pharyngeal isthmus (palatopharyngeus and superior constrictor), which prevents the bolus from rising into the nasopharynx.

The Engulfing Actions Through the Pharynx (Pharyngeal Phase)

- The epiglottis moves upward and forward, coming to a halt at the root of the tongue, and literally bends backward (possibly because of the weight of the bolus) to cover the laryngeal inlet. The bolus of food slides over its anterior surface. (The epiglottis in the human is not essential to swallowing, which is normal even in the absence of an epiglottis.[1])
- The fauces narrows (palatoglossi).

Note: The pharyngeal isthmus is at the border of the soft palate and the posterior pharyngeal wall and is the communication between the nasal and oral parts of the pharynx. Its closure is affected by the approximation of the two palatopharyngeus muscles and the superior constrictor, which form a palatopharyngeal sphincter.

- The larynx and pharynx are raised up behind the hyoid (salpingopharyngeus, stylopharyngeus, thyrohyoid, and palatopharyngeus).
- The arytenoid cartilages are drawn upward and forward (oblique arytenoids and thyroarytenoids), and the aryepiglottic folds approximate, which prevents movement of the bolus into the larynx.
- During swallowing, the thyroid cartilage and hyoid bone are approximated and there is a general elevation of the pharynx, larynx, and trachea. This causes the many laryngeal folds to bulge posteriorly into the laryngeal inlet, thus narrowing it during swallowing.[17,18]
- The bolus then slips further over the epiglottis, and partly by gravity and partly by the action of the constrictor muscles it passes into the lowest part of the pharynx. Passage is aided by contraction of the palatopharyngei, which elevate and shorten the pharynx, thus angling the posterior pharyngeal wall to allow the bolus to slide easily downward.[19]
- The laryngeal passage is narrowed by the aryepiglottic folds (posterior cricoarytenoids, oblique arytenoids, and transverse arytenoids), which close the laryngeal vestibule (glottis) and also form lateral channels to direct the bolus toward the esophagus.
- When the posterior cricoarytenoids are weak or paralyzed, the laryngeal inlet is not closed off in swallowing, the aryepiglottic folds move medially, and fluid or food enters the larynx (aspiration).

The Esophageal Phase

- At the beginning of this phase the compressed bolus is in the distal pharynx. The inferior constrictor pushes the bolus inferiorly (peristaltic action) to enter the esophagus. The distal fibers of the inferior constrictor, called the cricopharyngeus, are a distal sphincter and therefore must relax to allow the bolus to pass, but the mechanism of this action is in dispute.[19,20]
- After the passage of the bolus, the intrinsic tongue muscles move saliva around the mouth to cleanse away debris.

TESTING SWALLOWING

Swallowing is tested only when there is good cause to suspect that the swallowing mechanisms are faulty. Do not make an *a priori* assumption that the presence of a nasogastric tube, a gastrostomy, or a liquid diet precludes swallowing. The therapist also should review information from the patient's history and current chart to identify the site of the lesion, the presence of upper respiratory tract infections, and similar facts, which will assist the direction of the evaluation.

When a patient has a tracheostomy, a suctioning machine is essential and expertise with its use is required.

The therapist will have some prior information about patients from direct observation, such as how they handle saliva (swallowing it or drooling), whether and how they manage liquids and solids at mealtime, reports from nursing staff and family, and the nature of reported problems about swallowing. These all will suggest a starting point for testing.

In most swallowing tests, use a bib around the patient's neck to prevent soiling. Remember to protect yourself from sudden aspirates! Damp washcloths or tissues should be available for clean-up.

Position of Patient: Sitting preferred, supine if necessary, but head and trunk should be elevated to at least 30°. Maintain head and neck in neutral position.

Position of Therapist: Sitting in front of and slightly to one side of the patient.

Table 7-10 COMMON SWALLOWING PROBLEMS AND MUSCLE INVOLVEMENT

Problem	Possible Anatomical Cause
Drooling	Weakness of orbicularis oris
Pocketing in the lateral sulci	Weakness of the buccinator and intrinsic and extrinsic tongue muscles
Decreased ability to break down food mechanically during the oral preparatory phase	Weakness of the muscles of mastication
Decreased ability to form bolus	Weakness of the intrinsic and extrinsic tongue muscles Weakness of the buccinator
Decreased ability to maintain bolus in the oral cavity during the oral preparatory phase	Weakness of the palatoglossus or styloglossus or both
Nasal regurgitation	Weakness of the palatopharyngeus, levator veli palatini, or tensor veli palatini, individually or severally
Posterior pharyngeal wall residual after the swallow	Weakness of the pharyngeal constrictor(s) muscles
Coughing or choking prior to the swallow	Food may spill into an unprotected airway secondary to: Weakness of the intrinsic or extrinsic tongue muscles resulting in decreased ability to form a bolus (lack of bolus formation may result in spillage of the oral contents without initiation of a swallow) Weakness of the palatoglossus and styloglossus resulting in decreased ability to maintain the bolus in the oral cavity prior to initiation of a swallow
Coughing or choking during the swallow	Weakness of the muscles responsible for closing the true vocal folds, false vocal folds, and aryepiglottic folds
Coughing or choking after the swallow	Decreased strength of the genioglossus resulting in decreased tongue retraction with vallecular residual, which spills after the swallow into an unprotected airway Pharyngeal constrictor weakness with residual spillage from the pharyngeal walls after the swallow into an unprotected airway Decreased cricopharyngeal opening with overflow from the piriform sinus after the swallow into an unprotected airway

PRELIMINARY PROCEDURES TO DETERMINE CLINICALLY THE SAFETY OF INGESTION OF FOOD OR LIQUIDS

Test Sequence 1

Laryngeal Elevation: Therapist lightly grasps the larynx between the thumb and index finger on the anterior surface of the throat. Ask the patient to swallow. Ascertain if there is laryngeal elevation and its extent (see Figure 7-77).

Criteria for Grading

F: Larynx elevates at least 20 mm. Motion is quick and controlled.

WF: Laryngeal excursion may be normal or slightly limited. The motion may be sluggish or appear irregular.

NF: Elevation is perceptible but significantly less than normal.

0: No laryngeal elevation occurs.

Implications of Grade: If the patient is graded F (Functional) or WF (Weak functional), proceed with the swallowing assessment. If the patient is graded NF (Nonfunctional) or 0 and does not have a tracheostomy, discontinue the swallowing assessment. For patients with a tracheostomy, add a blue vegetable dye to the bolus to facilitate identification of any aspirated bolus during suctioning.

Test Sequence 2

Initial Ingestion of Water

Prerequisites: The patient has a grade of F or WF on Test Sequence 1.

There also must be at least a grade of WF or higher on the tests for posterior elevation of the tongue (see pages 313) and constriction of the posterior pharyngeal wall (see page 322).

Procedure: There are several ways to get water into the mouth to test swallowing. It does not matter which is used.

The first trial of swallowing begins with a small amount (1 to 3 mL) of water. The rationale is that should the patient not be able to swallow the water correctly and it is aspirated, the lungs can absorb this small quantity without penalty. There also is increasing evidence that differences in the pH of water can cause damage to the lungs, so the small amount of water is very important. Each procedure should be repeated at least three or four times.

1. If the patient is cognitively clear, offer a water impregnated cotton swab (large size) to the patient to suck. If the patient can extract the small amount of water from the swab and swallow it, a glass or cup containing a tiny amount of water is next offered for sipping. The test is successful if the water can be swallowed with one attempt, the swallow is inaudible, and the water is swallowed without any choking or coughing. If successful, proceed to Test Sequence 3.
2. If the patient cannot sip from a cup, offer a straw and ask the patient to suck a small amount. The shorter and wider the straw, the easier the task. If the swallowing attempt is successful as described in step 1, proceed to Test Sequence 3.
3. If the patient cannot sip or suck, trap water in a straw and place the straw in the side of the patient's mouth between the cheek and lower teeth. Tell the patient you are going to release the water and request a swallow. If successful, proceed to Test Sequence 3.
4. If the patient is not cognitively clear, control the amount of water available. This is most readily done by trapping water in a straw to give to the patient.
5. For the patient who cannot handle fluid, try thickening the water with gelatin to a consistency of thin gruel or thick pea soup.

Outcomes: If any of these trials are successful, proceed cautiously to a trial of pureed food. If none of these tests are successful and the patient does not have a tracheostomy, DO NOT give the patient food by mouth until further testing (e.g., fluoroscopy) can be conducted.

If the procedures with water are not successful and the patient has a tracheostomy (through which aspirated food can be suctioned), proceed cautiously to the use of pureed food, which usually is easier to swallow than water.

Test Sequence 3

Pureed Food

The most palatable commercial pureed foods are the pureed baby food fruits. The pureed meats and vegetables are totally unseasoned, which is unfamiliar and usually unpalatable to adults. Avoid milk products initially because they thicken the saliva. Ask about patient food preferences and try to use something enjoyable.

A suctioning machine is essential if the patient has a tracheostomy. It is recommended that the food be colored with vegetable dye (blue is readily seen and is not confused with body secretions or fluids) so that any aspiration can be readily detected as the color appears in tracheostomy secretions.

Criteria for Initiating Trials with Pureed Foods

1. Laryngeal elevation is Functional (F) or Weak functional (WF).
2. Posterior pharyngeal wall constriction is at least WF.
3. Patient has been successful in handling water in Test Sequence 2 or by observation.
4. Patient *must* have a functional cough (voluntary or reflex) or a tracheostomy. Some patients have a depressed gag reflex, but cough is the essential component in swallowing. The therapist cannot assume that a hyperactive gag reflex is synonymous with a functional cough.
5. The patient must have adequate cognition to attend to feeding.
6. There cannot be any respiratory problem present, such as aspiration pneumonia, that might be compromised by additional aspiration.

Procedures

1. Place a small amount (½ teaspoon) of food on the front of the tongue. Ask the patient to swallow, and observe ability to manipulate food in the mouth to position it for swallowing. Allow the patient to place the food in the mouth if possible because this will better coordinate feeding with the respiratory cycle.
2. If the patient cannot move the food in the mouth, push it back slightly with a tongue blade, being careful not to initiate a gag reflex. Ask the patient to swallow, while lightly palpating the larynx to check laryngeal elevation.
3. Ask the patient to open the mouth, and check to see that food has indeed been swallowed and that none of it has pooled in the pharyngeal isthmus or oral cavity.
4. To check for a clear airway, ask the patient to repeat three sequential crisp sounds: "Agh, Agh, Agh." Any gurgling indicates that food is in the airway; ask the patient to swallow again.

Repeat this procedure a number of times and check each response.

After four or five trials with pureed food, pause for about 10 minutes to ascertain that the patient does not have delayed coughing because of food collecting in the pharynx, larynx, or trachea. A blue aspirate from the tracheostomy tube may occur sometime after the actual ingestion of food.

Outcomes: If the patient has no immediate or delayed coughing, choking, or positive aspirate after swallowing and the airway is clear, the test is successful.

If the patient repeatedly coughs, chokes, or has a positive aspirate, this is solid evidence that there is inadequacy of swallowing, and the test should be terminated and no other food administered.

For patients who have been on a nasogastric tube and have demonstrated the ability to swallow water and pureed food without aspiration, proceed with feeding the pureed food until at least three fourths of the jar has been consumed. For the next meal, order a tray of pureed food. Observe the patient during eating; look for any problems and assess fatigue.

Use of a Mechanical Soft Diet: A mechanical soft diet (ground meat, ground vegetables if fibrous or hard) should be substituted for regular-consistency food for patients with any of the following: lack of teeth or dentures, poor intraoral control for chewing, fatigue during mastication (e.g., Guillain-Barré syndrome), limited jaw range of motion, limited attention span to complete the oral preparatory phase.

REFERENCES

Cited References

1. Strandring S. Gray's Anatomy. 40th ed. New York: Churchill Livingstone; 2008.
2. Biousse V. Walsh & Hoyt's Clinical Neuro-Ophthalmology: In Three Volumes. 6th ed. Baltimore: Lippincott, Williams & Wilkins; 2004.
3. Bender MB, Rudolph SH, Stacy CB. The neurology of the visual and oculomotor systems. In: Joynt RJ, ed. Clinical Neurology. Philadelphia: JB Lippincott; 1993.
4. Van Allen MW. Pictorial Manual of Neurologic Tests. Chicago: Year Book; 1969.
5. Haerer AF. DeJong's The Neurologic Examination. 5th ed. Philadelphia: JB Lippincott; 1992.
6. Clemente CD. Gray's Anatomy. 30th ed. Philadelphia: Lea & Febiger; 1991.
7. Jenkins DB. Hollingshead's Functional Anatomy of the Limbs and Back. 9th ed. Philadelphia: WB Saunders; 2008.
8. DuBrul EL. Sicher and DuBrul's Oral Anatomy. 8th ed. St. Louis: Ishiyaku EuroAmerica; 1988.
9. Nairn RI. The circumoral musculature: structure and function. Br Dent J. 1975;138:49-56.
10. Lightoller GH. Facial muscles: the modiolus and muscles surrounding the rima oris with remarks about the panniculus adiposus. J Anat. 1925;60:1-85.
11. Brodal A. Neurological Anatomy in Relation to Clinical Medicine. London: Oxford University Press; 1981.
12. Misuria VK. Functional anatomy of the tensor palatini and levator palatini muscles. Ann Otolaryngol. 1975;102:265.
13. Keller JT, Saunders MC, Van Loveren H, et al. Neuroanatomical considerations of palatal muscles: tensor and levator palatini. J Cleft Palate. 1984;21:70-75.
14. Jacob P, Kahrilas PJ, Logemann JA, et al. Upper esophageal sphincter opening and modulation during swallowing. Gastroenterology. 1989;97:1469-1478.
15. Miller AJ. Neurophysiological basis of swallowing. Dysphagia. 1986;1:91-100.
16. Doty R. Neural organization of deglutition. In: Handbook of Physiology, Section 6, Alimentary Canal. Washington, DC: American Physiologic Society; 1968.
17. Logemann JA. Evaluation and Treatment of Swallowing Disorders. San Diego: College-Hill Press; 1997.
18. Bosma J. Deglutition: pharyngeal stage. Physiol Rev. 1957;37:275-300.
19. Buthpitiya AG, Stroud D, Russell COH. Pharyngeal pump and esophageal transit. Dig Dis Sci. 1987;32:1244-1248.
20. Kilman WJ, Goyal RK. Disorders of pharyngeal and upper esophageal sphincter motor function. Arch Intern Med. 1976;136:592-601.

Other Readings

Cunningham DP, Basmajian JV. Electromyography of genioglossus and geniohyoid muscles during deglutition. Anat Rec. 1969;165:401-409.

Gates J, Hartnell GG, Gramigna GD. Videofluoroscopy and swallowing studies for neurologic disease: a primer. Radiographics. 2006;26:22.

Hrycyshyn AW, Basmajian JV. Electromyography of the oral stage of swallowing in man. Am J Anat. 1972;133:333-340.

Isley CL, Basmajian JV. Electromyography of the human cheeks and lips. Anat Rec. 1973;176:143-147.

Miller AJ. The Neuroscientific Principles of Swallowing and Dysphagia. (Dysphagia Series.) San Diego: Singular Publishing Group; 1998.

Palmer JB, Drennan JC, Baba M. Evaluation and treatment of swallowing impairments. Am Fam Phys. 2000;61:2453-2462.

Palmer JB, Tanaka E, Ensrud E. Motion of the posterior pharyngeal wall in human swallowing: a quantitative videofluorographic study. Arch Phys Med Rehabil. 2000;11:1520-1526.

Sonies BC. Dysphagia and post-polio syndrome: past, present, and future. Semin Neurol. 1996;16:365-370.

Vitti M, Basmajian JV. Electromyographic investigation of procerus and frontalis muscles. Electromyogr Clin Neurophysiol. 1976;16:227-236.

Vitti M, Basmajian JV, Ouelette PL, et al. Electromyographic investigation of the tongue and circumoral muscular sling with fine-wire electrodes. J Dent Res. 1975;54:844-849.

Wolf C, Meiners TH. Dysphagia in patients with acute cervical spinal cord injury. Spinal Cord. 2003;41:347-353.

Zablotny CM. Evaluation and management of swallowing dysfunction. In: Montgomery J, ed. Physical Therapy for Traumatic Brain Injury. New York: Churchill-Livingstone; 1995.

Zafar H. Integrated jaw and neck function in man. Studies of mandibular and head-neck movements during jaw opening-closing tasks. Swed Dent J Suppl. 2000;143:1-41.

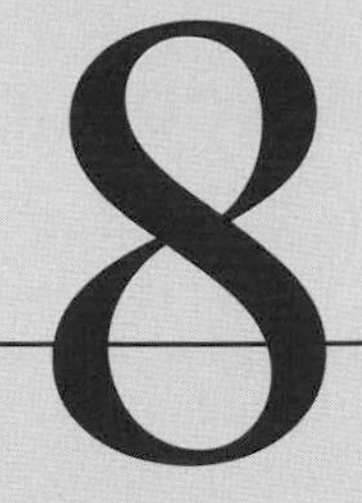

CHAPTER 8

Alternatives to Manual Muscle Testing

INTRODUCTION

Manual muscle testing is a foundational measure of strength that is widely used across the health professions for both diagnosis and rehabilitation. Yet manual muscle testing has specific limitations, as discussed in Chapter 2. Consequently, alternative strength measures are needed in certain cases such as when strength exceeds a functional threshold, when strength of the patient is greater than that of the therapist, when subtle differences exist between sides or between the agonist and antagonist, or when power or endurance need to be measured. The most commonly used alternatives to manual muscle testing are equipment-based tests.

There are many options for equipment-based testing, and each has its advantages and disadvantages. Choosing the best option depends on clinic space constraints, available budget, the type of patient, the goals of treatment, and how comprehensive the evaluation needs to be. For example, in a small outpatient clinic where most of the patients have low back or neck pain, the approach to equipment-based testing will differ substantially from that required in most acute care settings. Strength-testing instruments that can be used effectively for children and older adults will differ from those used for a sports team. The equipment-based tests presented in this chapter represent the more popular approaches, are appropriate for older adults, and also have demonstrated reliability and validity.

General Testing Considerations

It is presumed that any therapist conducting a strength testing session, particularly one requiring maximal effort from a large muscle group, will perform a prescreening exam for red-flag conditions. Maximal strength testing for the back extensors in a patient with severe osteoporosis, for example, may not be appropriate. Likewise, a patient with unstable blood pressure may have an adverse reaction while exerting maximum effort on a leg press, particularly if the patient—incorrectly—holds his or her breath. It is also presumed that muscular strength will be assessed after the patient has warmed up the muscle before testing. The typical warm-up includes completing three to five sub-maximal contractions at 40% to 50% of maximum using the muscle or muscle group that is being tested.[1] Active range of motion should be assessed to determine if adequate joint range and muscle length will allow maximum effort in the correct test position.

One-repetition Maximum Test

The one-repetition maximum (1-RM) test is regarded as the "gold standard" of standardized muscle strength testing. The 1-RM refers to the amount of load the patient can move one time (and one time only) through full range in a controlled manner with good form.[1] It is a safe technique, perhaps safer than a sub-maximum strength test, even though muscle soreness may occur and blood pressure may spike during a maximum exertion test.[2] 1-RM tests are highly reliable when specific procedures are followed, more so than any other type of strength assessment.[3] Additionally, the fundamental method for establishing 1-RM is the same for each muscle group and thus the 1-RM test is more precise than most.

Several factors are important in optimizing 1-RM performance. Obtaining a patient's maximum strength may serve to establish the amount of resistance needed for an exercise prescription; it may help determine the progress of a progressive, resistive exercise program; or it may be used to compare the patient to established norms. Many normative values for men and women of all ages exist for movements such as bench press, latissimus dorsi pull-down, leg press, and knee extension and are listed throughout this chapter.

Technique

The basic steps for performing a 1-RM are as follows:

1. Warm up by completing three to five sub-maximum repetitions. This warm-up also allows the patient to become familiar with the movement and to correct the form, if needed.
2. Select an initial weight that is within the patient's perceived capacity equivalent to 75% of capacity.
3. Determine the 1-RM within four repetitions with rest periods of 3 to 5 minutes between tests.
4. Increments of weight should be increased by 5 to 10 pounds until the patient cannot complete a repetition.
5. All repetitions should be performed at a constant and consistent rate of speed.
6. All repetitions should be performed through full range of motion (or the same range of motion if full range is not possible).

The final weight that the patient can move successfully is recorded as the definitive 1-RM.

One-repetition Maximum Test Continued

Selecting the Starting Weight

Selecting the amount of the starting weight is crucial because no more than four repetitions to reach 1-RM should be performed to avoid muscular fatigue and to prevent an underestimation of the true 1-RM. It is helpful for the tester to have knowledge of norms. For example, standing from a chair requires quadriceps strength of nearly half a person's body weight, no matter what the age. Therefore, when performing a 1-RM using a leg press to test the quadriceps of a person having difficulty standing from a chair, a starting weight might be 75% of the patient's body weight. Alternatively, norms exist for the leg press based on age. These norms might present a starting point for establishing a 1-RM. Other variables that can be factored into the clinical decision of the initial load are body size (muscular versus thin), fitness level, and the patient's self-perception of ability.

Other considerations that should also be attended to during 1-RM testing include breathing, form, and pain. First and foremost, patients should *not* hold their breath during the test. Thus, breath control should be practiced during the warm-ups. Second, the patient should maintain correct form throughout the test. For example, the patient should not be permitted to pitch the trunk forward during the knee extension test so as to avoid muscle substitution or the use of momentum. Joint movements during the test should be executed smoothly and consistently throughout the entire concentric and eccentric phase, in a controlled manner without jerking the bar or weight. If the test causes pain, an alternative to the 1-RM test should be selected, such as a multiple repetition maximum test.

Multiple-repetition Maximum Test

A multiple-RM test is based on the principles of a 1-RM test. The multiple-RM test is the number of repetitions performed using good form and proper breath technique at the point of muscle failure. Although not as exact as a 1-RM, a multiple-RM test may be desirable for certain situations. For example, some older adults are not comfortable exerting the kind of effort necessary for a true 1-RM. When joint or soft tissues are compromised (e.g., connective tissue disease, rotator cuff tear, ligamentous injury, post-surgery) a safer approach than a 1-RM may be preferred. The multiple-RM test, such as an 8- or 10-RM test is safer than the 1-RM test particularly for those with no exercise history and for patients who cannot tolerate high joint compression forces, such as those with osteo- and rheumatoid arthritis, or with systemic weakness.

A 1-RM test can be estimated from a multiple-RM test (Table 8-1), although this estimation has been shown to be quite variable (Table 8-2).[4] As the percent of 1-RM increases, the number of repetitions decreases (Table 8-3). Large muscle group exercises allow the completion of more repetitions than small muscle groups at the same relative intensity.[5] Because the volume of work is greater with a 10-RM than a 1-RM, fatigue will be a factor. The 1-RM and multiple-RM tests can be performed using the same equipment.

The number of repetitions performed at a given percent of 1-RM is influenced by the amount of muscle mass used because more repetitions can be performed during the back squat than either the bench press or arm curl.[5] The 4- to 6-RM is more accurate than the 10-RM. Variability increases with decreased loads.[6]

Table 8-1 ESTIMATING 1-RM FROM A MULTIPLE-RM TEST

Given a 1-RM of 100 pounds:	1-RM	2-RM	3-RM	4-RM	5-RM	6-RM	7-RM	8-RM	9-RM	10-RM
Multiple-RM loads are:	100	95	93	90	87	85	83	80	77	75

Table 8-2 NUMBER OF REPETITIONS PERFORMED AT 80% OF THE 1-RM[4]

	TRAINED		UNTRAINED	
Exercise	Men	Women	Men	Women
Leg press	19	22	15	12
Lat pull down	12	10	10	10
Bench press	12	14	10	10
Leg extension	12	10	9	8
Sit up	12	12	8	7
Arm curl	11	7	8	6
Leg curl	7	5	6	6

Table 8-3 MAXIMUM WEIGHT THAT CAN BE LIFTED DECREASES WITH THE NUMBER OF REPETITIONS

Given:	1-RM	2-RM	3-RM	4-RM	5-RM	6-RM	7-RM	8-RM	9-RM	10-RM
The load would be: (in pounds)	100	95	93	90	87	85	83	80	77	75
Number of repetitions	1	2	3	4	5	6	7	8	9	10

EQUIPMENT-BASED TESTING

Because practice patterns have changed so extensively since the advent of manual muscle testing, methods to identify muscle weakness have also evolved. The days of polio are behind us and the need to identify deficiencies from sports-related injuries, trauma, aging, and a host of other clinical conditions has resulted in the development of new and better testing techniques for the characterization of muscle weakness. This chapter segment will present an overview of some of the more popular approaches.

Equipment-based tests offer many advantages. The main advantage of using equipment (such as a strength-testing device) for repetition maximum testing is that the stability afforded by the device allows for highly controlled single plane movements, thus increasing the patient's safety. In addition, normative data for many movements are available with equipment-based testing. The disadvantages of using devices for testing are that 1) they take up space, 2) they can test only one plane of movement, and 3) they can test only a finite number of muscle groups.

Unilateral Knee Extension Test

Purpose: The unilateral knee extension test is used primarily to determine quadriceps strength when the strength of the patient exceeds the strength of the therapist. If manual muscle testing reveals Grade 4 or better strength, the therapist is incapable of discerning whether strength is greater than Grade 4 or actually "normal" (Grade 5). The unilateral knee extension test with weight is also superb for distinguishing side-to-side differences in quadriceps force output.

Testing Procedure: Select an initial weight based on the screening exam and have patient completely extend the knee through full range of motion. After a 30- to 60-second rest, another repetition with a higher weight is performed through full range of motion. After the load cannot be moved through full range or the patient loses form, the patient is asked to perform another repetition at that weight to verify muscle failure and confirm that the patient cannot complete another repetition.

Position of Patient: Seated comfortably on a knee extension machine that has been adjusted for leg length. A seat belt may be placed around patient's pelvis, if needed, to provide stability (Figure 8-1; seat belt not shown in figure). If necessary, padding may be placed beneath the thigh being tested for patient's comfort.

Position of Therapist: Standing adjacent to the patient.

Instructions to Patient: "Push against the bar and completely straighten your leg"

Scoring

Record the highest weight the patient could lift to reach full knee extension. The multiple-RM is recorded as the pounds at last repetition and the number of repetitions it took to achieve muscle failure. (Note: Extension through full range of motion, particularly the last 15° to 0°, must be achieved for a successful test.)

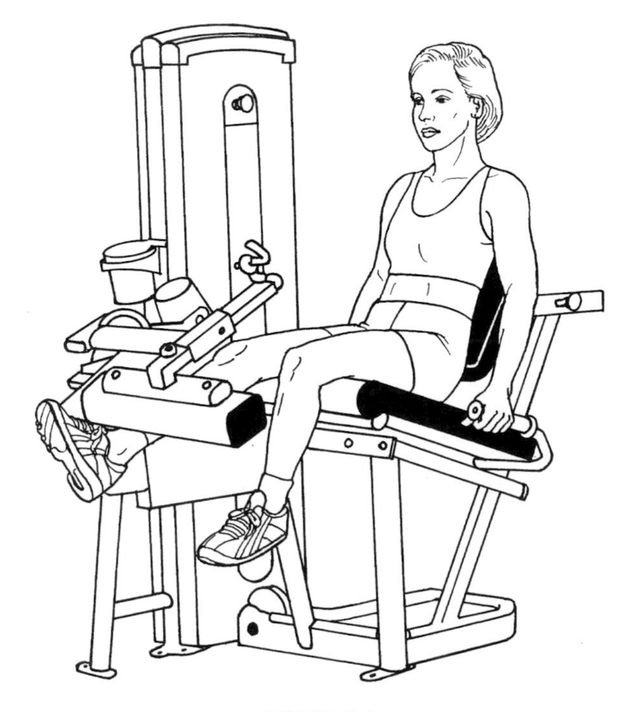

FIGURE 8-1

Helpful Hints

- If the patient can get up from a chair without use of the arms, a weight equivalent to 50% of the patient's body weight should be the initial starting weight on the knee extension device. Thus, if the patient weighs 150 pounds, 75 pounds would be a reasonable weight with which to start. If 75 pounds is successfully achieved through full range, with good form, in a controlled manner, another 10 pounds may be added.
- A patient will move less weight on a single-joint machine, such as a unilateral knee extension machine, than on a multiple-joint machine, such as a unilateral leg press, because of the amount of muscle mass involved (for example, quadriceps only versus quadriceps, gastrocnemius/soleus and gluteals combined).

Leg Press Test

The leg press machine is one of the most useful devices in a clinic. The force output generated by a patient will tell the therapist whether the patient has enough strength to be functional in activities of daily living or with sport activities requiring a huge amount of strength such as soccer.

Purpose: The leg press assesses the force output of all extensor muscles in both lower extremities: hip and knee extensors and plantar-flexors.

Testing Procedure: After the patient is comfortably seated on the machine, have him or her place both feet on the footplate, approximately 12 inches apart, directly under the hips. Adjust the seat distance so that the knees are bent to approximately 110°. Have the patient put his or her hands on the grab bars (Figure 8-2). Select the desired weight on the weight stack, put in the pin to keep weights in place and have the patient fully extend the footplate against the chosen resistance. The knees should be fully extended at the end of the push. Note: some leg press machines require the therapist to place weights on either side of the footplate bar (e.g., two 25-pound weights) and lock the weights in place.

Position of Patient: Seated comfortably on leg press machine with both feet on the foot plate, approximately 12 inches apart, directly under the hips, and hands on grab bars. Feet on the footplate in either the low position (Figure 8-3) or the high foot position (see Figure 8-2).

Position of Therapist: Standing adjacent to the patient.

Instructions to Patient: "Push the plate until your legs are straight. Don't hold your breath during the test."

Scoring

Record the highest weight the patient can push while fully extending the knees.

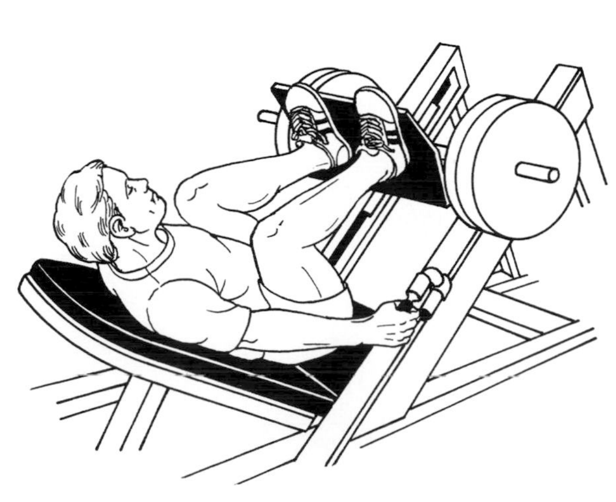

FIGURE 8-2

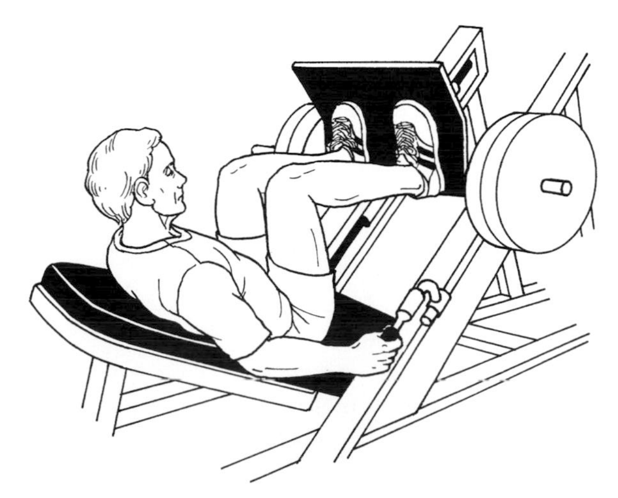

FIGURE 8-3

Helpful Hints

- The leg press is the only machine that uses the closed chain approach (distal end of the kinetic chain is fixed).
- Foot position low on the plate (see Figure 8-3) elicits greater muscle activity from the quadriceps and gastrocnemius than high foot position (see Figure 8-2), suggesting that the feet should routinely be positioned low on the plate.[7] Not all patients, however, can comfortably assume a low-foot position; in terms of importance, comfort should outweigh muscle activation. But be aware that if a patient cannot assume the low foot position, then maximal muscle activation is not likely to occur.
- There are established norms for leg press for men and women ages 20 through early 60s, which is hardly comprehensive of all age groups. Nonetheless, it is important to have an understanding of what should be expected in terms of "normal" strength. Norms are expressed as a ratio of force output to body weight. Thus, a typical ratio for a young woman in her 20s is 2.05, meaning that she should be able to generate force equivalent to twice her body weight. Normative data for the leg press and bench press on hundreds of men and women that have been tested by the Cooper Institute are presented in Table 8-4.

Table 8-4 LEG PRESS NORMS FOR MEN AND WOMEN IN VARIOUS AGE GROUPS VALUES REFLECT 1-RM/BODY WEIGHT

	20-29 YEARS		30-39 YEARS		40-49 YEARS		50-59 YEARS		60+ YEARS	
Percentile	Men	Women	Men	Women	Men	Women	Men	Women	Men	Women
90th	2.27	2.05	2.07	1.73	1.82	1.63	1.71	1.51	1.62	1.40
70th	2.05	1.66	1.85	1.50	1.74	1.46	1.64	1.30	1.56	1.25
60th	1.97	1.42	1.71	1.47	1.62	1.35	1.52	1.24	1.43	1.18
40th	1.83	1.36	1.65	1.32	1.57	1.26	1.46	1.18	1.38	1.15
30th	1.74	1.32	1.59	1.26	1.51	1.19	1.39	1.09	1.30	1.08
20th	1.63	1.25	1.52	1.21	1.44	1.12	1.32	1.03	1.25	1.04
10th	1.51	1.23	1.43	1.16	1.35	1.03	1.22	0.95	1.16	0.98

Descriptors for percentile rankings: 90, well above average; 70, above average; 50, average; 30, below average; 10, well below average.
Data for men provided by The Cooper Institute for Aerobics Research, The Physical Fitness Specialist Manual. Dallas, TX, 2005. http://hk.humankinetics.com/AdvancedFitnessAssessmentandExercisePrescription/IG/269618.indd.pdf
Data for women provided by the Women's Exercise Research Center, The George Washington University Medical Center, Washington, D.C., 1998.

Latissimus Dorsi Pull-down Test

The latissimus dorsi pull-down test (lat pull-down test) is a general measure of bilateral shoulder adduction and scapular downward rotation. The lat pull-down is available in most clinics and in all wellness centers and workout facilities. The test is one of the safest and easiest to perform of all upper extremity exercises.

Purpose: To measure the collective force of the latissimus dorsi muscles, rhomboids, and middle and lower trapezius.

Testing Procedure: Place the pull-down seat in a position so that the patient's feet are on the floor during the test. The patient is then seated astride a bench, typically facing the weight stack, with the back unsupported (Figure 8-4). Based on the initial physical therapy screening (e.g., can the patient pull against manual resistance easily?), select a weight stack that is relatively easy, such as 20 pounds for a woman and 40 pounds for a man. Have the patient reach overhead and grab a horizontal bar to which the weight stack is attached. The bar is grasped so that the arms are wide apart and the forearms are in pronation (more difficult) or supination (easier). Hands on the bar should be slightly further apart than the shoulders. After the patient has pulled the bar down to shoulder height in front of the body, the test is considered successful. The position of pulling down in front of the head provides the greatest activation of the latissimus dorsi.[8]

After a 30- to 60-second rest, the patient is asked to pull the bar down once again, this time with another 5 to 10 pounds added, depending on how easy or difficult the first repetition was. Additional weights are added in 5- to 10-pound increments until the patient reaches failure. Norms for the latissimus pull-down activity are typically 66% of body weight for young men and 50% of body weight for young women.[9] Norms for men and women who are middle-aged and older have not been established. This test is feasible for patients of nearly all ages.

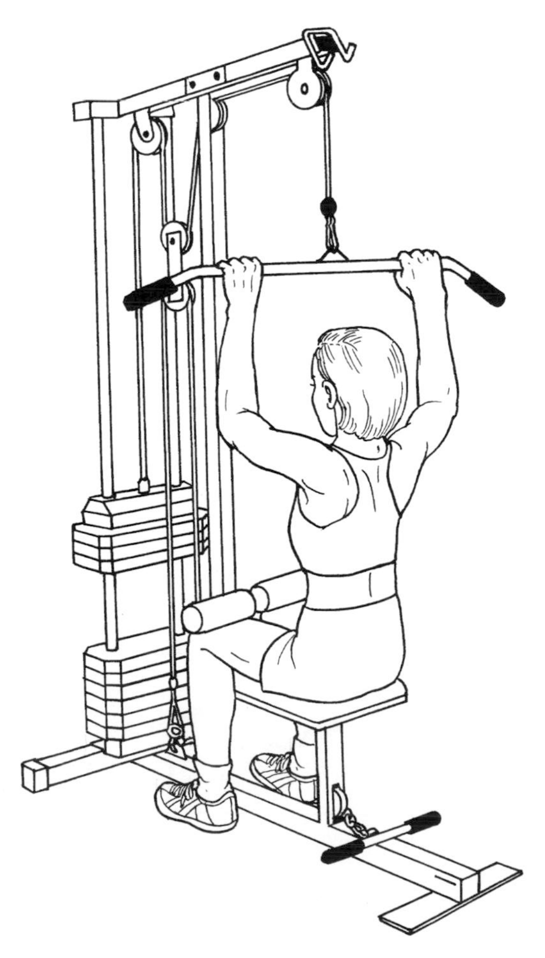

FIGURE 8-4

Position of Patient: Seated, facing the weight stack, feet flat on floor.

Position of Therapist: Standing behind the patient in case of test failure.

Instructions to Patient: "Pull the bar down in front of you level with your shoulders. Don't hold your breath."

Scoring

Record the highest weight the patient could pull down without losing form.

Note: If the first repetition is extremely easy, it may be reasonable to add 20 pounds for the second repetition. Using this method, four repetitions should be all that is required to reach failure.[9]

Free Weights Testing

Free weights are the "gold standard" for reliability and validity of the 1-RM method because of their ease of application. They offer a number of important advantages for muscle testing: 1) they permit the therapist to assess strength in both the concentric and eccentric modes, 2) they are readily available in any clinical setting and are readily accessible in the home where household items can easily be substituted for weights, and 3) they can be used through full range and through multiple planes.

Moreover, free-weight exercises require greater motor coordination and better balance, resulting in greater muscle recruitment. They employ important stabilizing muscles to complete a lift, compared with machines, which do not emphasize the stabilizing musculature because movements occur in only one plane of motion. And they allow the therapist the freedom to test different exercise variations compared to resistance machines.

Free Weights Testing Continued

Some disadvantages of using free weights are that: 1) greater control is required through all planes of movement; 2) testing can be unwieldy and proper positioning is critical for safety and test reliability; 3) free weights can be dropped, potentially causing injury; and 4) free weights can challenge the entire kinetic chain, thus stressing the "weakest link" rather than the targeted muscle, unless proper stabilization is provided. Probably the biggest disadvantage of using free weights is that maximum muscle loading only occurs at the weakest point in the range of motion.

Definition of Terms

Concentric activity refers to the shortening of a muscle as it contracts, as in the bending portion of a biceps curl or extension of the elbow when lifting an object overhead.

Eccentric activity refers to the lowering phase of an exercise, when the muscle lengthens, as in lowering the weight to the chest during the bench press or lowering oneself into a chair. Eccentric muscle activity is seen in many mobility-related functional tasks.

The *kinetic chain* refers to all the muscles and joints that are involved in producing a given movement. For example, in the movement of arising from a chair, the kinetic chain consists of the trunk, hip, knee, and ankle. Most exercises involve more than one muscle group and joint, which work simultaneously to produce the movement. Exercises in the kinetic chain can be performed two ways, open and closed, referred to as open chain and closed chain.

Open chain exercises are performed such that the distal end of the kinetic chain is free to move. An example of an open chain activity is quadriceps knee extension sitting on a plinth where the leg moves from 90° of flexion to full extension.

Closed chain exercises are performed with the distal end of the kinetic chain fixed. An example of a closed chain exercise for the quadriceps is squatting. The knee is again moving through 90° of movement but the leg is fixed in place and the thigh is moving over the fixed leg.

Elbow Flexion Test

The elbow flexion test is an example of how to use free weights to determine maximal muscle strength. In this instance the biceps, brachialis, and pronator teres are the muscles that will be challenged, particularly the biceps and brachialis. This test can easily discern side-to-side differences and whether strength is adequate for lifting during work.

Purpose: To determine maximum force capability of the biceps brachii and brachialis as well as the brachioradialis and pronator teres muscles.

Testing Procedure: Based on the patient's answers to prescreening questions (such as, can you lift a gallon of milk?), the therapist should pick a weight that is reasonably challenging. Normative strength is approximately 25% of body weight for women and 33% of body weight for men.[6] Another way to determine a starting point for less fit individuals is to ask the patient if he can easily carry a large bag of groceries (approximately 10 pounds). If the patient responds affirmatively, begin the test with 15 pounds of weight. The patient's elbow should be straight, with arm at the side. Put the 15-pound weight in the patient's hand and have the patient flex the elbow through full range of motion (Figure 8-5). If this movement is easy, select a 20-pound weight for the next repetition. After 20 pounds have been successfully lifted through full range of motion, select a 25-pound weight

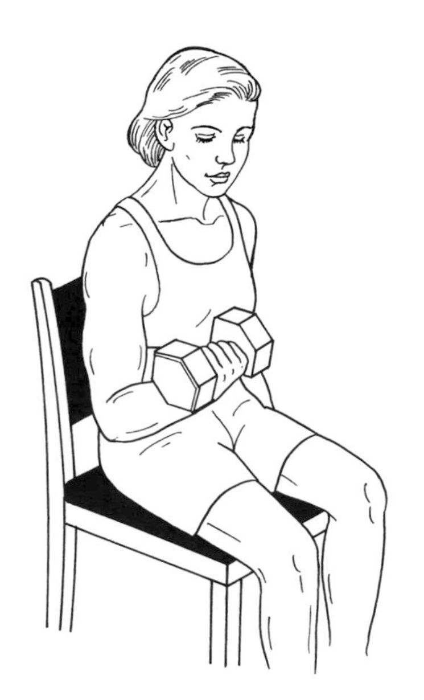

FIGURE 8-5

Free Weights Testing Continued

for the next repetition. If this movement is successful but difficult, increase the weight by 2.5 pounds. When the weight cannot be lifted through full range in a controlled manner, or if muscle failure occurs, the test is terminated and the last weight that was successfully lifted is the patient's 1-RM. Recall that 30 to 60 seconds of rest should be provided between repetitions.

If this movement is easy, increase weight for the next repetition by 5 to 10 pounds. If this movement is successful but difficult, increase the weight by 2.5 pounds.

When the weight cannot be lifted through full range in a controlled manner or if muscle failure occurs, the test is terminated 30 to 60 seconds of rest should be provided between repetitions.

Position of Patient: Seated comfortably in a standard chair with no arms. Provide seat belt if needed.

Position of Therapist: Standing adjacent to the patient.

Instructions to Patient: "Bend your elbow completely until the weight touches your arm."

Scoring

The last weight that was successfully lifted is the patient's 1-RM.

Note: The incremental increase in weight lifted is far less for the upper extremity compared to the lower extremity because of the difference in muscle mass.

Bench Press Test

The bench press is one of the most popular tests of upper extremity strength because it provides a composite value for a large number of muscles, similar to the leg press.

Purpose: To maximally challenge the larger anterior scapulohumeral muscles: pectoralis major, pectoralis minor, anterior deltoid, infraspinatus, serratus anterior, and upper and lower trapezius. In addition, the triceps brachii is critical to extend the elbow.

Testing Procedure: The patient is positioned supine on a low testing bench with a testing bar overhead. The patient's nipple line should be below the weight bar. Based on prescreening, two free weights are selected and one weight is placed at each end of the bench press bar and locked in place.

Hand placement should be gripping the bar with both hands placed slightly wider than shoulder width and the forearms in pronation (Figure 8-6). The bench press bar is lifted until the elbows are fully extended and the shoulders are at 90° of flexion. After the patient successfully completes the test, additional weight in 5- to 10-pound increments is added. Provide the patient 30 to 60 seconds of rest between lifts. Test failure is observed when the patient is unable to complete full range of motion.

Position of Patient: Supine on the testing bench with the knees at 90° of flexion and feet flat on the floor.

Position of Therapist: The therapist should be positioned above the patient's head to "spot" the patient throughout the movement (therapist not shown in figure).

Instructions to Patient: "Lift the weight straight up overhead until your arms are completely straight. Do not hold your breath."

Scoring

Record the highest weight that could successfully be lifted. The norms for men and women are listed in Table 8-5.

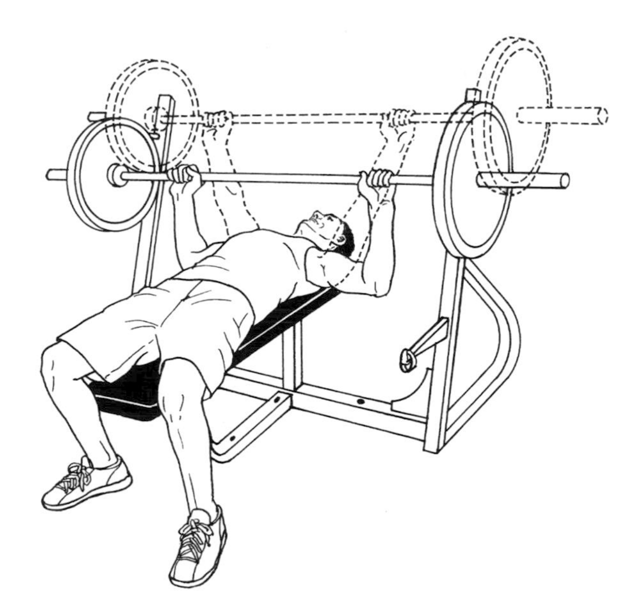

FIGURE 8-6

Helpful Hints

- Many bench press bars themselves weigh 20 pounds, which must be taken into consideration when determining ultimate load.
- It may be necessary for the therapist to take the weight bar away from the patient at test failure so the therapist should be sure (in advance) that he or she is physically capable of handling the weight bar being lifted.
- If there is no weight bench and the patient is lying on a plinth, the therapist must place the fully loaded lifting bar into position above the patient, again approximately 6 inches above the chest at nipple level. Help may be needed if the therapist is unable to handle the loaded weight bar. "Spotting" the patient is even more important in this adaptation of the bench press.

Table 8-5 BENCH PRESS NORMS BY GENDER AND AGE VALUES REFLECT 1-RM/BODY WEIGHT (IN POUNDS)

	20-29 YEARS		30-39 YEARS		40-49 YEARS		50-59 YEARS		60+ YEARS	
Percentile	Men	Women	Men	Women	Men	Women	Men	Women	Men	Women
90th	1.48	0.54	1.24	0.49	1.10	0.46	0.97	0.40	0.89	0.41
70th	1.32	0.49	1.12	0.45	1.00	0.40	0.90	0.37	0.82	0.38
60th	1.22	0.42	1.04	0.42	0.93	0.38	0.84	0.35	0.72	0.36
40th	1.14	0.41	0.98	0.41	0.88	0.37	0.79	0.33	0.72	0.32
30th	1.06	0.40	0.93	0.38	0.84	0.34	0.75	0.31	0.68	0.30
20th	0.99	0.37	0.88	0.37	0.80	0.32	0.71	0.28	0.66	0.29
10th	0.94	0.35	0.83	0.34	0.76	0.30	0.68	0.26	0.63	0.28

Descriptors for percentile rankings: 90, well above average; 50, average; 30, below average; and 10, well below average.
Data for women are derived from the Women's Exercise Research Center, The George Washington University Medical Center, Washington, D.C., 1998. Data for men were provided by the Cooper Institute for Aerobics Research, The Physical Fitness Specialist Manual, Dallas, TX, 2005.

Isokinetic Testing

Isokinetic testing was developed in the 1960s and has gained in popularity over the years for a variety of reasons. The advantages of isokinetic testing for evaluating muscles and muscle groups are notable and include testing through a spectrum of movement speeds (e.g., 0° to 400° per second), providing highly reliable data and providing safety in testing because movement control is assured. Most importantly, isokinetic machines (e.g., Biodex, KinCom) allow maximal resistance throughout the entire range of motion, something that no other testing methods can provide. It is also possible to assess eccentric strength.

The disadvantages of isokinetic testing include the cost and size (space occupying) of the equipment, the time it takes to set up the tests, the fact that only single planes can be tested, and from a biological perspective, the fact that isokinetic contractions are non-physiologic. Muscles simply do not contract isokinetically. Typically, muscle demand (percentage of force required) is highly variable throughout the range of motion. Normal physiologic contractions are concentric, eccentric, and isometric and the amount of force required differs by contraction type and the range employed. To use the knee extensors as an example, under physiologic conditions quadriceps strength demand is greatest at the end of the range where length-tension and the patella lever-arm are poorest.

The setup for isokinetics is straightforward, but the actual test execution requires skill, computer interaction, and know-how that is beyond the scope of this book. For complete instruction in isokinetic testing, the reader is referred to the remarkable amount of material on the internet and the instruction booklets from the makers of the Kin-Com and Biodex.[10]

Hand-held Muscle Dynamometry

Hand-held dynamometry has grown in popularity in the past decade as methods have become more reliable and tests can be conducted quickly. Other advantages include the objectivity of the dynamometer's numerical value, instant identification of side-to-side differences, and the portability of the device. Hand-held dynamometry can be performed anywhere, including the home health environment and at fitness centers. Disadvantages include the fact that one must properly isolate the desired joint and muscle group through careful positioning, as in manual muscle testing. Additionally, a considerable degree of skill is required to perform dynamometry consistently and thus it may be challenging for the new practitioner

Hand-held Muscle Dynamometry Continued

to achieve reliable results. Another disadvantage is that the numbers obtained may not provide relevant information about function and there are few norms available that translate into meaningful data. Probably the biggest disadvantage (as in manual muscle testing) is that the patient's strength may be greater than the therapist's. It is uncommon for example, for a woman to adequately test elbow flexion in a man, whether done manually or with a hand-held dynamometer. Thus, to distinguish between Grades 4 and 5, another form of testing may be necessary.

One hand-held muscle dynamometer that has grown in popularity is the microFET2, which fits easily in the palm of the hand and can replicate almost every manual muscle test. Instead of a manual grade, a number is provided, which, as noted, can identify subtle differences between sides. Other hand held dynamometers are available but most (including other versions of the microFET) require the practitioner to hold the device with the fingers, and thus the force output is limited by the finger strength of the therapist, which typically is not very high.

Several examples of specific hand-held muscle dynamometry testing follow.

Shoulder Abduction Test

Shoulder abduction is easily tested using the microFET2. Side-to-side differences are immediately identified using this device and the test is straightforward to execute.

Purpose: To determine maximum strength of the deltoid and rotator cuff muscles (infraspinatus, supraspinatus, teres minor, subscapularis). In addition, the serratus anterior and upper/lower trapezius must position the scapula for the deltoid to function properly. Thus the shoulder abduction test indirectly determines whether the muscles of scapular upper rotation are functioning properly.

Testing Procedure: For testing, the patient is seated with the shoulder in 90° of abduction. The therapist places the mircoFET on the distal humerus, and resistance is applied by the therapist in the same position and manner as for a manual muscle test (Figure 8-7). The test is repeated and the higher of the two values is recorded.

Position of Patient: Seated comfortably in a straight-backed chair.

Position of Therapist: Standing to the side of the patient.

Instructions to Patient: "Hold your arm in this position and don't let me push it down." (See Figure 8-7.)

Scoring

Record the highest of two repetitions or average the two trials.

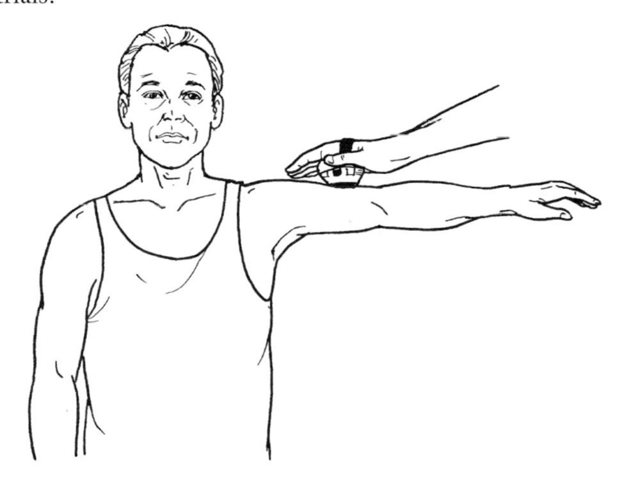

FIGURE 8-7

Hand-held Muscle Dynamometry Continued

Knee Extension Test

The primary reason to use a dynamometer for knee extension is to determine if one leg is weaker than the other. As with manual testing the knee extension test is only valid if the therapist is stronger than the patient.

Purpose: To determine maximum force output of the quadriceps.

Testing Procedure: The patient is seated on a plinth or low mat table with the thigh supported. The patient is then asked to extend the knee nearly to 0° (do not let the patient "lock" the knee in extension) and then hold the leg in this position as the therapist gradually applies maximal resistance through the dynamometer that is placed on the distal leg. A rolled towel may be placed under the distal thigh, if needed, for the patient's comfort. It may also be necessary to use padding under the dynamometer if the leg is bony (Figure 8-8; rolled towel and padding not shown). Because the quadriceps muscle group is so strong it is not uncommon for the patient to have more strength than the therapist and an alternate form of testing (e.g., such as a leg extension device or free weight) may be required.

Elastic Band Testing

Elastic band testing is a common form of strength testing that uses elastic bands of different resistances that are color coded according to level of resistance. These are available in nearly all clinics and for home use. Resistance of the band is based on the amount of material used in the band. Thicker bands provide more resistance. The force of elastic resistance depends on percentage of elongation, regardless of initial length. Force elongation in pounds for Thera-band elastic bands is listed in Table 8-6.

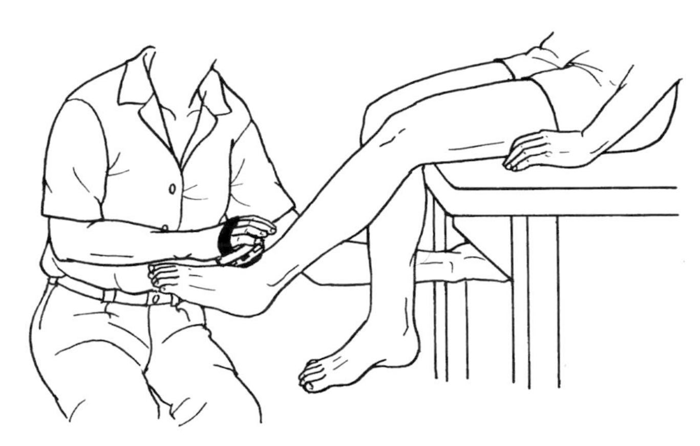

FIGURE 8-8

Table 8-6 FORCE-ELONGATION FOR THERA-BAND ELASTIC BANDS (VALUE = FORCE IN POUNDS)[10a]

Elongation (%)	Yellow	Red	Green	Blue	Black	Silver	Gold
25	1.1	1.5	2	2.8	3.6	5	7.9
50	1.8	2.6	3.2	4.6	6.3	8.5	13.9
75	2.4	3.3	4.2	5.9	8.1	11.1	18.1
100	2.9	3.9	5	7.1	9.7	13.2	21.6
125	3.4	4.4	5.7	8.1	11	15.2	24.6
150	3.9	4.9	6.5	9.1	12.3	17.1	27.5
175	4.3	5.4	7.2	10.1	13.5	18.9	30.3
200	4.8	5.9	7.9	11.1	14.8	21	33.4
225	5.3	6.4	8.8	12.1	16.2	23	36.6
250	5.8	7	9.6	13.3	17.6	25.3	40.1

The percentage of elongation (change in length) is calculated with the following formula: Percentage of elongation = (final length) − (resting length) / (resting length) × 100.

Elastic Band Testing Continued

There are a number of advantages to elastic band testing. First, it is the safest approach to strength testing. For those with soft-tissue compromise such as rotator cuff tear or fibromyalgia, elastic band testing will provoke the least amount of discomfort. Elastic band testing has an appeal to patients because the bands' resistance is color-coded, providing ready feedback about patients' progress. Disadvantages of elastic band testing include the difficulty of standardizing 1) distance of the pull, 2) positioning the patients and/or extremity, and 3) interpreting the tests. For example, if you have two patients and one patient abducts the hip only 10° against a gray elastic band (high strength demand) while another goes 20° against a green elastic band (low strength demand), which patient has better strength? Strength indexes help standardize this issue; however they are widely known only for Thera-band elastic bands.[11] Different manufacturers use different color codes and are not interchangeable with published strength indexes.

Most of the major muscle groups can be assessed using the standard method of elastic band testing. The elastic band should be the same length as the lever arm being tested to ensure elongation remains below 200%.[12] For example, if the length of the patient's leg, from hip to heel, is 50 inches, then a band of 50 inches should be used. For safety, test positions can be adapted. For example, testing of the elbow flexors can be done with the patient sitting or standing. See Figure 8-9 for an illustration of elastic band testing used to test shoulder abduction strength.

Shoulder Abduction Test

Purpose: To maximally challenge the shoulder abductors (deltoid and rotator cuff). Also required are the serratus anterior and upper/lower trapezius to upwardly rotate the scapula to support the humerus.

Testing Procedure: Before patient testing, a reasonably easy, moderate, or difficult color elastic band based on prescreening is selected for use. The patient is safely positioned in a standing position with something sturdy to hold onto if needed. One end of the elastic band is secured to an immovable object such as parallel bars and slack is removed from the band so that resistance of the band is zero at the beginning of the test. Place the band cuff around the wrist or attach a handle to the band to simplify the test for the patient (Figure 8-9). Have the patient move the shoulder into 90° of abduction, making sure the patient demonstrates proper form. With elastic band testing, resistance increases through the arc of motion and reaches its maximum at the end of the range. If the patient has a full 90° of active movement available but cannot abduct the shoulder 90° against resistance, the test is repeated with a lighter band. If the desired movement was completed through full range of motion against a specific color band, the therapist must consult a chart (provided by manufacturer) to determine how much force the patient exerted.

Position of Patient: Standing. If the patient cannot stand, the test can be performed in sitting.

Position of Therapist: Standing adjacent to the patient to monitor the pull.

Instructions to Patient: "Lift your arm out and away from the side of your body until it is horizontal with the floor. Don't hold your breath during the test."

Scoring

Record the color of the band used to complete a full 90° of abduction.

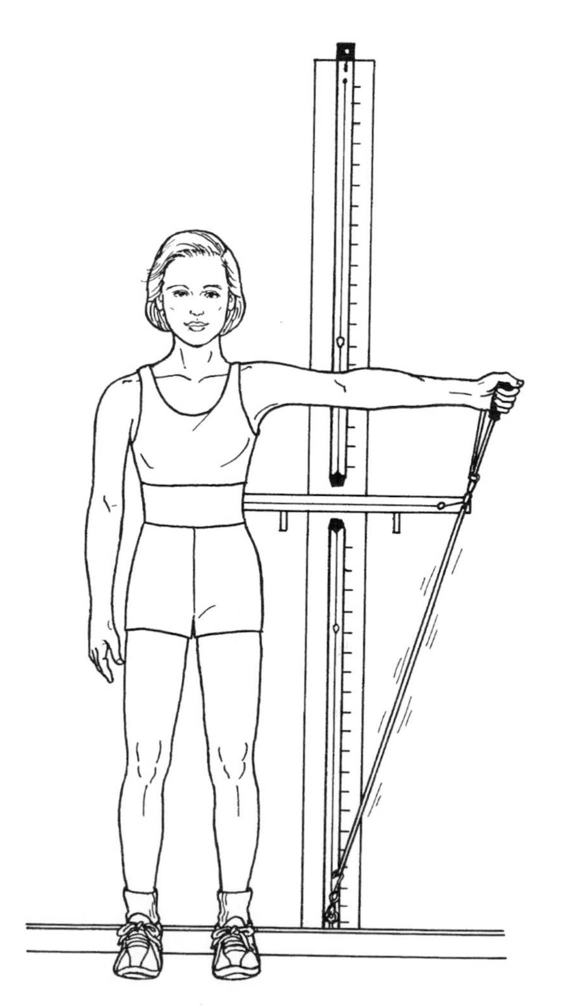

FIGURE 8-9

Helpful Hints

- With repeated use, elastic bands lose their elasticity and should be replaced. Bands should always be inspected for small tears or holes that may weaken the band and cause it to break during elongation. Periodic calibration will determine if it is time to discard the original band.
- In spite of the limitations of muscle testing with elastic bands, they are very practical to determine exercise intensity.

Cable Tensiometry Testing

As with all equipment-based tests, an advantage of cable tensiometry is that the patient's efforts produce numerical data. Repeat tests are highly reproducible. Tests are isometric, which makes this type of instrumentation safer than most. A disadvantage of cable tensiometry is that tensiometers test only one muscle group in one plane. Consequently, only a limited number of muscle groups can be tested using this method. Finally, it is difficult to perform tests specific to a particular pathology (e.g., scapular pain). An example of how to use cable tensiometry is provided in the next section.

Hip Adduction Test

Purpose: To obtain maximal force output of the hip abductors (adductors magnus, longus, brevis, and gracilis).

Testing Procedure: To test the hip adductors the patient stands adjacent to a tensiometer. The cuff of the tensiometer is then wrapped around the patient's ankle (Figure 8-10). The patient then adducts the thigh slowly to remove slack on the cable, and then over 1 to 2 seconds, attempts to push the thigh into further adduction. Typically, for the hip adductors, the cable placement permits force to be determined at approximately 10° to 15° of abduction, or at optimal length. Reset the needle on the tensiometer dial back to zero and repeat the test a second time.

Position of Patient: Standing adjacent to the tensiometer, with a fixed grab bar or railing to hold onto for stability.

Position of Therapist: Standing adjacent to the patient.

Instructions to Patient: "Slowly pull your leg in toward your body as hard as you can. Now pull a little further."

Scoring

Average the two trials or record the highest value.

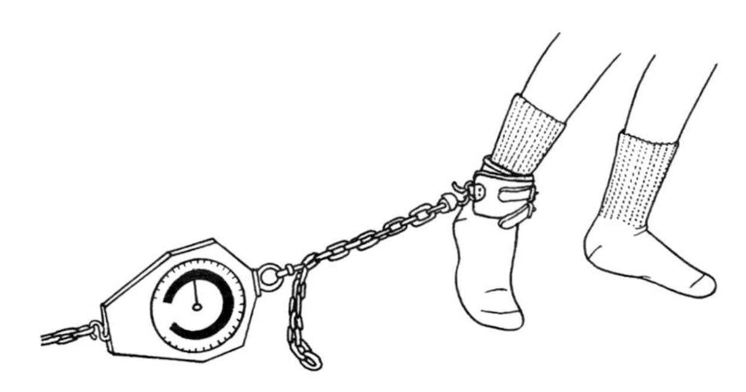

FIGURE 8-10

SPECIALIZED MUSCLE TESTING

The Perineometer Test

Purpose: Many women experience incontinence and/or sexual dysfunction, both of which may be a consequence of pelvic floor weakness. The perineometer is a device that was specifically developed to determine the amount of contractile force a woman can generate with the pelvic floor musculature (Figure 8-11). To perform the test, the perineometer is inserted into the vagina; typically, the inserted portion of the device is about 28 mm in diameter with an active measurement length of about 55 mm. Many types of perineometer devices are available and each works on the same principle as a blood pressure monitor.

Testing Procedure: The perineometer is first covered with a sterile sheath before being inserted into the vagina. A sterile hypoallergenic gel may be used on the sheath. After the probe is in place, the patient is asked to perform a Kegel exercise, exerting as much force against the probe as possible (squeezing it). The therapist must make sure the patient is not holding her breath while performing the pelvic contraction. The patient performs three contractions with a 10-second rest between each contraction.

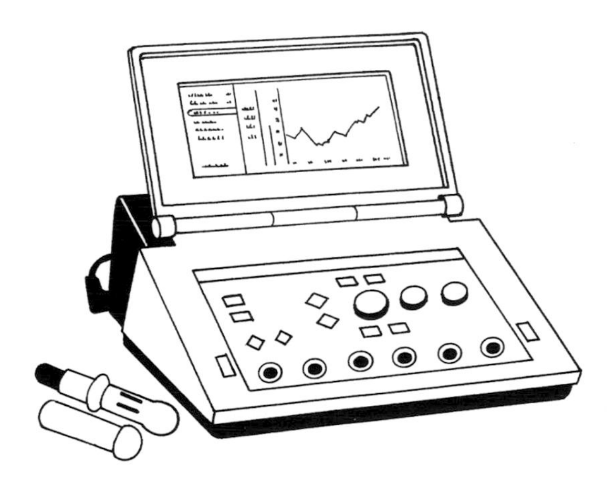

FIGURE 8-11 An example of a perineometer.

Position of Patient: Supine on a plinth with the knees flexed and the hips in some abduction.

Position of Therapist: Standing or sitting adjacent to the patient.

Instructions to Patient: "Squeeze as hard as you can against the probe and hold it."

Scoring

Record the highest force output or the average of the three contractions.

Helpful Hints

- One advantage of the perineometer over a manual muscle test is that the duration of the contraction hold can be determined. The reliability of the perineometer is comparable to that of manual muscle testing. Inter- and intra-rater reliability have been established.[13]
- The Kegel (pronounced KAY-gull) exercise is named after Dr. Arnold Kegel, who designed the exercise to strengthen the pelvic floor muscles, especially the pubococcygeal muscles. The exercise consists of tightening the pelvic floor muscles so as to stop a stream of urine. Strengthening the pelvic floor muscles increases vaginal tone, thus improving sexual response and limiting involuntary urine secondary to stress incontinence. Kegel exercises are often prescribed following childbirth or during or after menopause.

Grip Strength Test

There is a curvilinear relationship between grip strength and age. Grip strength peaks at 20 to 40 years and declines thereafter with advancing age.[14,15] In the older adult, grip strength has been shown to be a reliable predictor of mortality.[16] In many clinics, grip strength is used as a general indicator of total body strength.[17,18]

Purpose: To test the strength of the hand to determine any limitations that may affect functional activities. The extrinsic and intrinsic finger flexors, flexor pollicis longus and brevis, opponens pollicis, and thumb abductor are all involved in performing a hand-grip. The wrist extensors are also important to position the hand at optimal length.

Testing Procedure: Both hands are tested, one at a time. The therapist places the dynamometer in the patient's hand with the dial of the hand dynamometer facing away from the patient (Figure 8-12,*A*). The position of the dynamometer handle grip (e.g., Jamar dynamometer) is adjusted so that the fingers can comfortably grasp and squeeze the handle. Most often this is in the 2nd position (Figure 8-12,*B*). No visual or auditory feedback is provided. Scores are compared with the appropriate age and sex categories for accurate interpretation.[17]

Position of Patient: Seated with shoulders level, adducted and neutrally rotated. The elbow is flexed to 90°, forearm in neutral and wrist between 0° and 30° of extension (see Figure 8-12,*A*).[14]

Position of Therapist: Standing or sitting in front of the patient so as to see the dial.

Instructions to Patient: "I will be testing your grip strength. When I say go, give your maximum effort in a smooth manner. Do not jerk the tool while you are gripping. Stop immediately if you experience any unusual pain or discomfort. Are you ready? Go!" (See Figure 8-12,*B*.)

Scoring

Three trials are given for each hand, averaging the three for the final score.

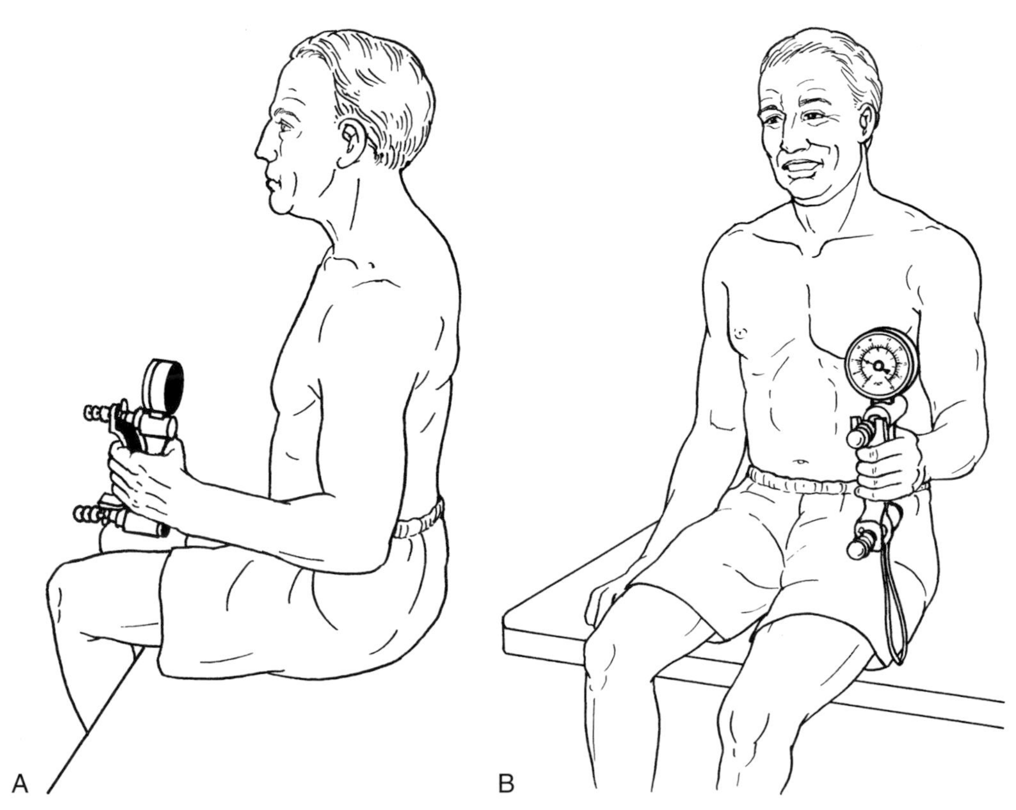

FIGURE 8-12

Table 8-7 MEAN NORMATIVE HAND GRIP STRENGTH (KG)[22a]

	MEN			WOMEN		
Age	Right	Left	BMI	Right	Left	BMI
20-29	47(9.5)	45(8.8)	26.4(5.1)	30(7)	28(6.1)	25.1(5.8)
30-39	47(9.7)	47(9.8)	28.3(5.2)	31(6.4)	29(6)	27.3(6.8)
40-49	47(9.5)	45(9.3)	28.4(4.6)	29(5.7)	28(5.7)	27.7(7.7)
50-59	45(8.4)	43(8.3)	28.7(4.3)	28(6.3)	26(5.7)	29.1(6.4)
60-69	40(8.3)	38(8)	28.6(4.4)	24(5.3)	23(5)	28.1(5.1)
70+	33(7.8)	32(7.5)	27.2(3.9)	20(5.8)	19(5.5)	27(4.7)

BMI, body mass index. Date collected using the position described in Figure 8-12,*A* and *B*.

Helpful Hints

- Grip strength of 9 kg (20 pounds) is commonly considered functional and is necessary to perform most daily activities.[15] A maximal grip strength of 5 kg (11 pounds) was found to be associated with a high risk of death in elderly women admitted to geriatric wards after acute illness.[16,17]
- A possible explanation for the relationship between weak grip strength and mortality is the fact that grip strength seems to be an indicator of nutritional status.[18] Protein deficiency may result in generalized muscle weakness and decreased cell-mediated immunity. Thus, weakness of grip may identify older patients at risk for dying as a result of protein malnutrition.[18]
- Grip strength also is correlated significantly with upper limb function in older adults and in people with certain disorders, but not in young, healthy patients.[19,20]
- Grip strength is affected by certain disorders that impair results, such as carpal tunnel syndrome, lateral epicondylitis, dementia, arthritis, and stroke.

Interpretation of Equipment-based Testing Data

Equipment-based testing data are informative only if used in context with other clinical findings. For example, if the therapist observes side-to-side strength differences for shoulder flexion, in conjunction with difficulty lifting or pain on the weaker side, the therapist's clinical decision-making is enhanced and treatment can be confidently and competently applied. If gait speed is slow and there is evidence of gait deviation, equipment-based testing will help inform the therapist about the reasons for the deviation and thus enhance treatment planning. Equipment-based testing, as with manual muscle testing, is only as good as the therapist and is useful only in conjunction with other important functional findings. Clinical competence develops with practice, practice, and more practice, which includes all testing procedures, particularly those that provide information about strength deficits. Investing the time to learn correct testing procedures results in improved treatment planning, more targeted goal setting, better documentation of the patient's status and rate of improvement, and greater success in receiving reimbursements from health care providers.

Summary

Except for the leg press, the procedures presented in this chapter are either isometric or concentric and patients are tested using the open chain approach. Day-to-day function requires performance of activities using a closed chain approach—for example, sitting down or climbing stairs. Activities that include multiple joints are often multiplanar, require some degree of balance, and are speed dependent. There are few instrumented options available for specifically and accurately assessing strength using the closed chain functional approach, but change is likely on the horizon. Currently, power and functional tests are the best options for use in the greatest number of clinical settings.

POWER TESTING

Power testing, also known as maximal anaerobic power testing, was initially developed to assess explosive strength in a sports setting. Since the early 1960s, numerous adaptations of the original Margaria stair run test[21] have been made as the relevance and importance of power testing has become evident. Maximal power is defined as force per unit of time and thus a power measure includes not just muscular force production but the rate of force development. The specific formula for power is:

Power = work/seconds

Powerful athletes are able to accelerate rapidly with explosive force output (for example, the 100-m Olympic dash). Rate of force development may be the critical determinant of a person's safety, especially in unexpected or emergency situations. For example, can a patient go from gas pedal to brake quickly enough to prevent a crash? One of the most important reasons for rapid force development is to prevent a fall. Once a person loses balance, only rapid limb movement can rescue the individual; rapid limb movement requires power. Recently, power has been identified as a major determinant of functional impairment in the older adult and is now considered even more important than strength (e.g., in the chair rise).[22] Thus, power is an important aspect of muscle performance.

Power testing is in its infancy. Although the concept of power determination has been around for half a century, actual tests for its measurement are limited. It is expected that more tests for power will be developed in the future or adaptations of existing tests will be made to include patients with muscular weakness and poor muscular endurance.

A few power tests are presented in the next section. None of these require extensive preparation and no special equipment is needed to execute the tests. Since maximal muscular activity is involved in performing power tests, they are anaerobic and are of short duration.

Original Margaria Test[21]

Purpose: To measure maximal anaerobic power of the lower extremities.

Testing Procedure: In this test, the patient runs up a flight of nine stairs, two steps at a time (each step 17.5 cm in height), at maximal speed.[21] Units of measure: vertical height achieved within 5 seconds (kg-m/kg sec). The formula given below takes into consideration the patient's body weight as well as the height (number of steps accomplished) and the time it took. Most patients achieve very little distance in the 5 seconds given, but a few people actually achieve an entire flight of stairs in less than 5 seconds.

The formula for calculating power is as follows:

Power (in kg-m) = Weight (body weight in kg) × Vertical height of stairs (or 9 stairs)/Time (seconds)

The advantage of the test is its ability to measure maximal anaerobic power quickly because it is a very rapid test (5 seconds) and it is highly reproducible. A disadvantage of the test is that only the young and healthy can perform it.

Other power tests that are easier to perform with lower impact are as follows.

Medicine Ball Throw Test

Purpose: To determine the power of important scapulothoracic and glenohumeral muscles, particularly the pectoralis major and minor, anterior deltoid, supra- and infraspinatus. Scapular upward rotation and abduction provide optimal positioning of the humerus, and prime movers are the serratus anterior and upper and lower trapezius. At the elbow, the prime movers are the triceps surae.

Medicine Ball Throw Test Continued

Testing Procedure: The ball (4 kg) is held close to the chest (like a basketball) and is subsequently thrust away from the body as rapidly as possible (Figure 8-13,*A*). The test is repeated three times. The maximum or average distance from the end of the chair to where the medicine ball lands is recorded. An alternate method is depicted in Figure 8-13,*B*. In this instance, the patient has to throw the ball using an overhead technique. Either technique is acceptable.

Position of Patient: Seated in a standard chair with no arms, with a seat belt around the pelvis if needed for stability (seat belt not shown in figure).

Position of Therapist: Standing to the side but in front of the patient to measure distance of throw.

Instructions to Patient: "Push the ball away from your chest as fast as you can and throw it as far as you can." (Alternative test: "Throw the ball as far away from you as you can.")

Scoring

The test is repeated three times. The maximum or average distance from the end of the chair to where the medicine ball lands is recorded.

Shot Put Test

Purpose: The primary muscles being tested are similar to those used for the medicine ball throw: the pectoralis major and minor, anterior deltoid, supra- and infraspinatus, serratus anterior, and upper and lower trapezius. At the elbow, the triceps surae is being tested.

As with the medicine ball throw, this test challenges the musculature of the glenohumeral and scapulothoracic muscles. The test is unilateral however, which permits side-to-side comparisons. Because the test is done standing, it also challenges balance.

Testing Procedure: Select a "shot" that is appropriate for the patient (4, 5, or 7 kg). The therapist then places the shot in the patient's hand. The patient brings the shot to the shoulder and balances it on the shoulder and chin (Figure 8-14). With a rapid thrust, the shot is cast away as far as possible. The trial is repeated three times and the furthest distance recorded.

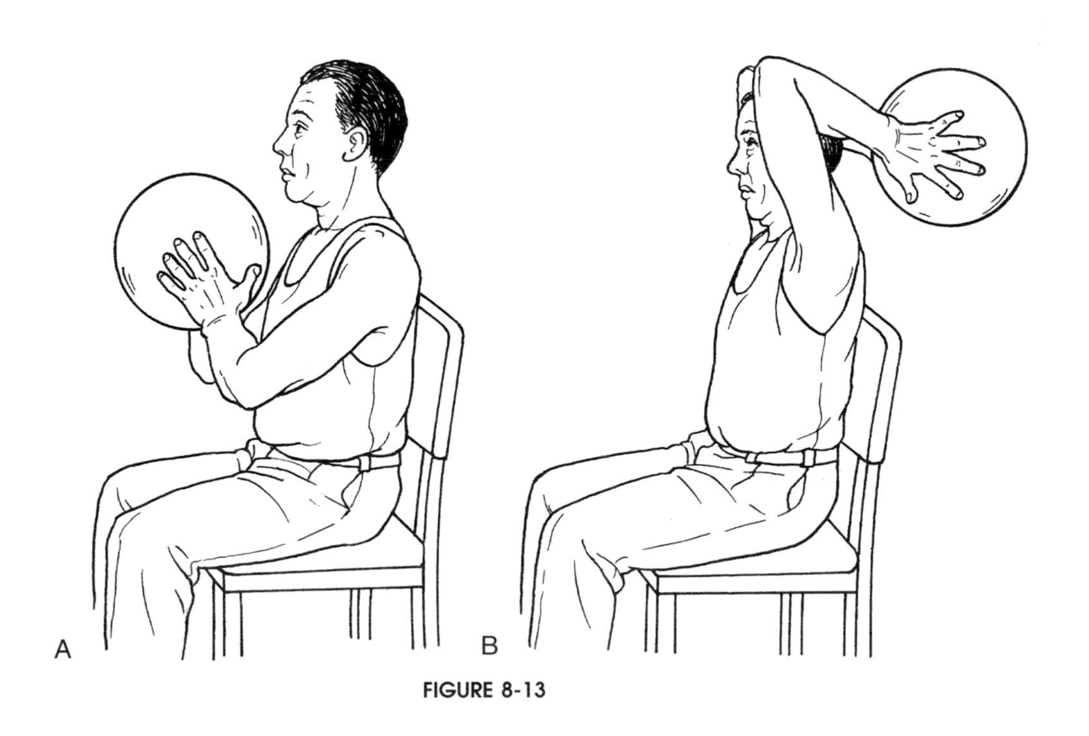

FIGURE 8-13

Shot Put Test Continued

Position of Patient: The patient is standing with one leg in front and the other behind, but using a reasonable stance width for support.

Position of Therapist: Standing adjacent but in front of the patient to record throw distance.

Instructions to Patient: "Thrust the shot away from you as far as you can. I will record the distance. Don't hold your breath."

Scoring

The trial is repeated three times and the furthest distance recorded.

Alternative Shot Put Test: Standing and using two hands, the patient leans forward, brings the shot down between the legs, and throws the shot forward as far as possible. The throw is underhand instead of overhand and involves both arms instead of just one. This test is safer and easier for the patient to perform. To score, record the distances once again.

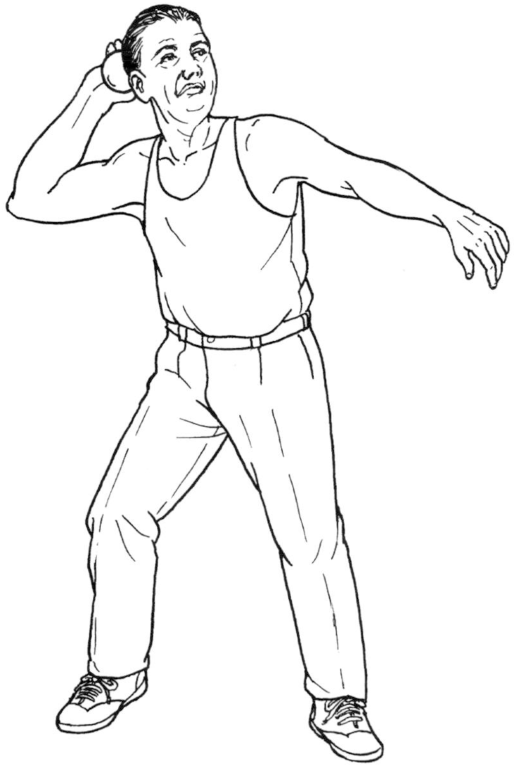

FIGURE 8-14

Vertical Jump Test

Purpose: This test of power challenges the extensors of the lower extremity, particularly the gluteus maximus and minimus, the hamstrings, quadriceps, gastrocnemius, and soleus. Only those with adequate balance can perform the test.

Testing Procedure: Tape a yardstick or piece of paper with height markings onto the wall. With the arm extended as far as possible, measure the height of the patient (distance between extended fingers and floor). Standing flat-footed the patient will jump as high as possible, touching the yardstick or paper at the end of the jump test (Figure 8-15). Chalk the fingers first before performing the test or have the patient hold onto a piece of chalk. Crouching to gain a better mechanical advantage is permitted. The patient jumps, marks the paper or wall once maximal height is reached, and distance jumped is recorded; the subject's height is subtracted from the final height to derive the jump distance.

Position of Patient: Standing.

Position of Therapist: Standing adjacent to the patient.

Instructions to Patient: "With your feet flat on the floor, crouch down and jump upwards as high as you can. Mark the paper with your fingers (or the chalk) at the highest point of your jump."

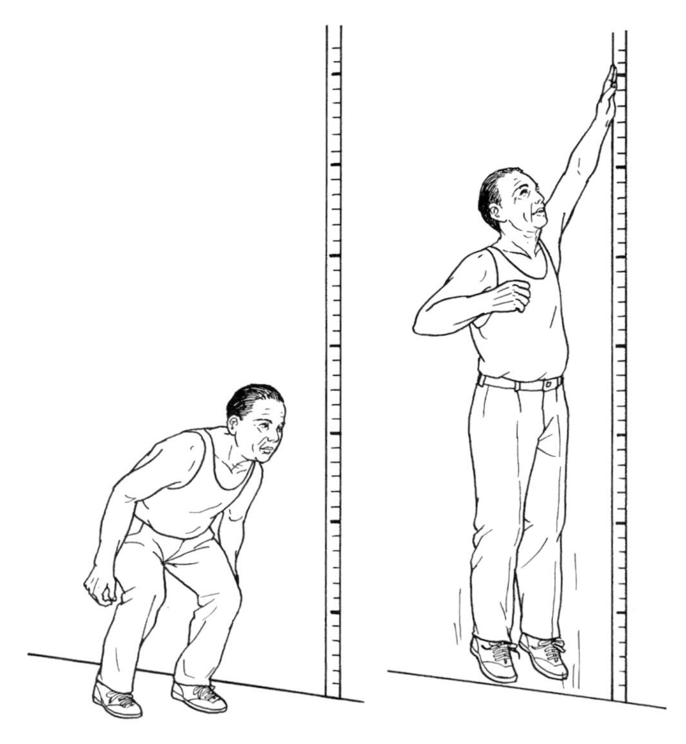

FIGURE 8-15

Vertical Jump Test Continued

Scoring

The total distance jumped is recorded; the subject's height is subtracted from the final height to derive the jump distance.

Hop Test

There are a number of variations on this particular power test. As depicted in Figure 8-16, the test can be done on one leg, alternating from side to side. It is also common to conduct a two-legged test where a patient will perform three jumps consecutively (Figure 8-17). For a more challenging examination (done frequently in athletic training centers), the patient is required to clear an obstacle with each jump, with some as high as 18 or more inches.

Purpose: To test the lower extremity extensors and pelvic stabilizers, particularly the gluteals, quadriceps, and plantar flexors. Patients cannot complete the tests without adequate abdominals and balance control.

Testing Procedure:

Single hop test: The patient stands on a line and when instructed, leaps forward and upward, completing three consecutive single leg hops (see Figure 8-16). The total distance achieved in the three hops is recorded.

Double hop test (standing broad jump): With both legs on the starting line, the patient is instructed to jump three times, as far forward as possible with each hop, without stopping (see Figure 8-17). The total three-hop distance is recorded.

Position of Patient: Standing.

Position of Therapist: Standing adjacent to the patient. Therapist follows trajectory of patient to facilitate recording of distance.

Instructions to Patient: "Hop three times in succession (on one leg or both legs). Hop as far as you can with each repetition."

Scoring

The cumulative total distance achieved in the three hops is recorded.

More difficult power tests are available but it is rare in physical therapy to use tests that are at the higher end of physical performance capacity. For more definitive work on this aspect of testing, the reader is referred to other sources.[23,24] Most power tests were developed for the young athlete. As a consequence, few of the existing power tests are appropriate for the older adult, those with significant weakness (Grade 3 or lower), or patients with painful conditions.

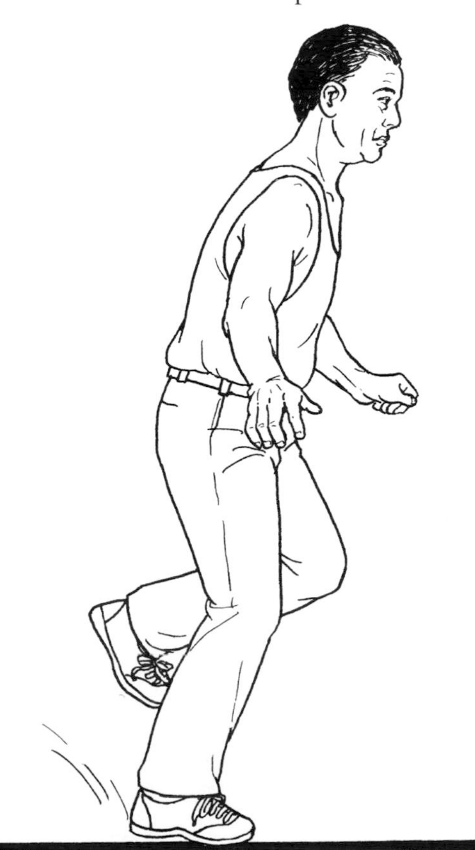

FIGURE 8-16

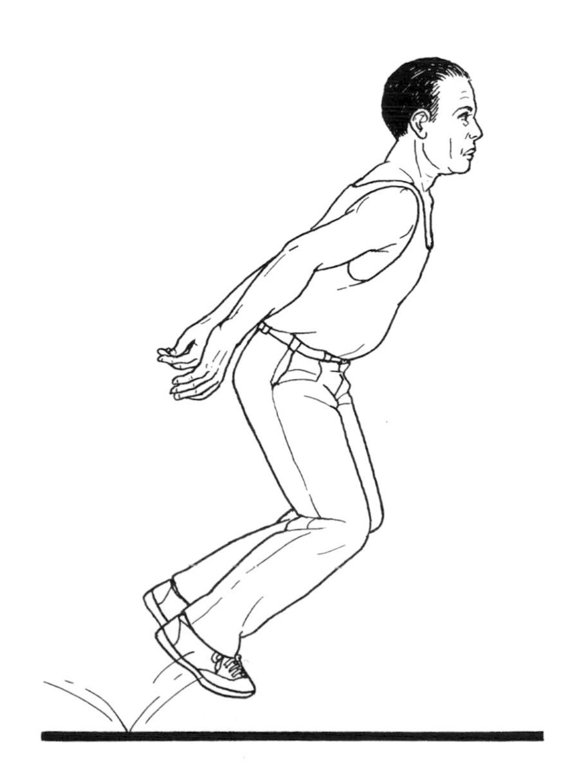

FIGURE 8-17

BODY-WEIGHT TESTING

Using body weight as resistance provides important information about the ability of patients to use the strength they possess to move their bodies in space. These tests are also effective exercises for strengthening the core as well as specified muscle groups. A number of the functional tests presented in Chapter 9 employ body-weight resistance. Presented below are several other tests that use body mass as resistance. All of these tests are high demand and should not be used for patients with undue weakness.

The Plank Test

Purpose: The plank is a superb challenge to the abdominals and muscles of the shoulder girdle, particularly the pectoralis major and minor, serratus anterior, anterior deltoid, and supra- and infraspinatus.

Testing Procedure: To perform this alternative test for the abdominals, the patient should assume the prone position and then push up so that body weight is born on the forearms. Some individuals prefer to clasp the hands for additional stability. If able, the patient should then raise his or her body so that the body is supported only by the forearms and the balls of the feet (Figure 8-18). If strength is adequate, the patient should maintain the trunk in a straight ramrod position, without arching the back or sticking the hips into the air. This position should be held for 60 seconds to be considered a "normal" test.[24]

Position of Patient: Prone on floor.

Position of Therapist: Standing adjacent to the patient.

Instructions to Patient: "Raise your bottom up into the air so that you are bearing weight only on your forearms and toes. Keep your body completely straight." (See Figure 8-18.)

Scoring

Hold times of less than 45 seconds are graded as 4 or less. Inability to assume the test position results in a grade of 3 or less.

Alternate Forms of Plank Testing

- An alternate form of baseline testing for patients not able to do a full plank is to time the distance the patient is able to hold a straight back while on knees and elbows only.
- An alternate position for the full plank is straight arms (elbows in extension) and toes with a straight back.

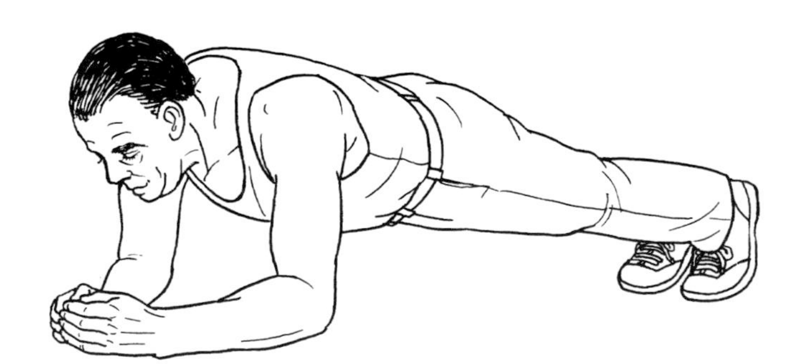

FIGURE 8-18

Pull-ups (Chin-ups) Test

Another rigorous test of strength for the shoulder (and scapular stabilizers), elbow, and wrist is the pull-up or chin-up.

Purpose: This test uses the patient's body weight to challenge the shoulder extensors (latissimus dorsi, teres major, triceps brachii, and posterior deltoid). The middle and lower trapezius, pectoralis minor, and rhomboids pull the scapula down. To pull the body up to the chin-up bar, the biceps brachii, brachialis and brachioradialis are contracting vigorously at the elbow. The wrist and finger flexors must also contract to hold the body on the bar.

Testing Procedure: To perform the test, the patient hangs from a chin-up bar with the forearms in supination and the elbows fully extended. Next, the patient lifts the entire body multiple times to exhaustion. For each repetition to count, the body must be raised so that the chin is brought above the bar. Subsequently, the body is lowered to the original starting position with the arms straight and another pull-up is performed. The number of pull-ups that can be performed successfully is recorded. There are norms that have been established for men and women by a number of sources such as the one presented in Table 8-8.

Position of Patient: Standing, arms up on the chin-up bar.

Position of Therapist: Standing adjacent to patient to record repetitions and determine when failure occurs.

Instructions to Patient: Pull yourself up to the bar to the level of your chin. Repeat the pull-up as many times as you can."

Scoring

The number of pull-ups that can be performed successfully is recorded. There are norms that have been established for men and women by a number of sources such as those presented in Table 8-8.

Helpful Hints

- Excess body weight may preclude performing the pull-up (chin-up) even if strength is adequate.
- If the patient has complaints of epicondylitis, test strength differently.
- Norms for boys and girls can be found at http://www.exrx.net/Testing/YouthNorms.html#anchor581034
- Norms used by the Marine Corps can be found at http://www.military.com/military-fitness/marine-corps-fitness-requirements/usmc-physical-fitness-test

Push-ups Test

Purpose: A test of strength, in this instance for the shoulder flexors, scapular stabilizers (especially serratus anterior), and triceps brachii. Push-ups are used not only as a test of strength but as a test of endurance, particularly in the U.S. Armed Forces.

Testing Procedure: The procedure for a correct push-up for males is to start with the "up" position with the hands a shoulder width apart, back straight, head up, and using the toes as the pivotal point. Females start in the bent knee position. The patient should lower the body until the chin touches the mat. The stomach should not touch the mat. For both men and women, the back should be straight at all times and the patient must push up to a straight arm position.[1]

Position of Patient: Lying prone on floor.

Position of Therapist: Standing adjacent to the patient to record number of repetitions.

Instructions to Patient: "Do as many push-ups as you can."

Table 8-8 NORMS FOR ADULTS FOR THE PULL-UP BY GENDER AND AGE

Gender	Excellent	Above Average	Average	Below Average	Poor
Male	>13	9-13	6-8	3-5	<3
Female	>6	5-6	3-4	1-2	0

From: McArdle WD, Katch FI, Katch CVL: Essentials of exercise physiology, 3 ed, Philadelphia, 2006, Lippincott, Williams & Wilkins.

Push-ups Test Continued

Scoring

The maximal number of push-ups performed consecutively without rest is counted as the score. Norms for young men and women from ages 20 to 60+ years are listed in Table 8-9.[2,25]

(Note: Norms for men and women over the age of 70 and for children below the age of 20 years have not been established. Most older adults cannot perform a push-up.)

Table 8-9 ADULT PUSH-UP FITNESS TEST RESULTS

Men	Age: 20-29	Age: 30-39	Age: 40-49	Age: 50-59	Age: 60+
Excellent	54 or more	44 or more	39 or more	34 or more	29 or more
Good	45-54	35-44	30-39	25-34	20-29
Average	35-44	24-34	20-29	15-24	10-19
Poor	20-34	15-24	12-19	8-14	5-9
Very poor	20 or fewer	15 or fewer	12 or fewer	8 or fewer	5 or fewer
Women	**Age: 20-29**	**Age: 30-39**	**Age: 40-49**	**Age: 50-59**	**Age: 60+**
Excellent	48 or more	39 or more	34 or more	29 or more	19 or more
Good	34-48	25-39	20-34	15-29	5-19
Average	17-33	12-24	8-19	6-14	3-4
Poor	6-16	4-11	3-7	2-5	1-2
Very poor	6 or fewer	4 or fewer	3 or fewer	2 or fewer	1 or fewer

Source: McArdle WD, Katch FI, Katch CVL: Essentials of exercise physiology, 3 ed, Philadelphia, 2006, Lippincott, Williams & Wilkins.

CYRIAX MODEL OF TESTING CONTRACTILE LESIONS

A common reason for strength testing in orthopedics is to diagnose the tissues contributing to musculoskeletal pain lesions. Since manual muscle testing typically requires completion of full range of motion to assign a grade, an alternative system is needed. James Cyriax developed a system to differentiate between painful contractile and non-contractile (inert) soft tissues.[26] Contractile tissues are parts of the muscle (belly, tendon, and their bony insertions). Inert lesions are those without the capacity to contract or relax such as joint capsule, ligaments, nerve roots and the dura mater. The therapist selects passive or active resisted movements to specifically stress inert (passive movement) or contractile tissue (resisted movement), respectively. If insert tissues are painful, both active and passive movement will be painful. If only contractile tissue is provoking pain, then only active movement will elicit pain. As an example, if a patient has a biceps tendonitis (long head), then resisted flexion (isometric, mid-range) will provoke pain. Passive movement through the flexion range of motion should not provoke pain. Once the biceps tendon lesion is identified, the therapist can provide the treatment needed for biceps tendonitis.

To test a muscle and its components (i.e., a contractile tissue, the therapist provides enough resistance to a limb segment so that the joint does not move [isometric]). The joint is held in mid-range so as to relax the inert tissue. No joint movement should occur so as to focus the tension on the muscle itself. If a contractile lesion is present, the resisted movement may provoke pain or demonstrate weakness, occasionally both. Normal contractions are strong and painless.

Because of the inherent strength of a nondiseased muscle, the therapist should stand in a position of maximum advantage with proper hand placement to exert the strongest possible force as appropriate. Additionally, the following rules, similar to manual muscle testing, should be followed:

- Muscles must be tested in such a way that the therapist's and the patient's strength are fairly evenly matched.
- The therapist must stand in the right place and use one hand for resistance, the other hand for counterpressure.
- Muscles other than those being tested must not be included. Proper hand placement should help isolate the muscle(s), for example, preventing supination when isolating the brachialis muscle.
- The joint that the muscles control must not move and should be held at near mid-range.
- The patient must be encouraged to try as hard as possible.

Only one study was found that has examined the reliability of the Cyriax selective tissue tension method.[27] In this small study of otherwise healthy individuals between the ages of 20 and 40 with either unilateral shoulder or knee pain of undiagnosed origin, for the knee, intra-rater reliability ranged from 0.74 to 0.82 and inter-rater reliability ranged from 0.42 to 0.46. Both intra-rater and inter-rater reliability were highest for knee flexion. For the shoulder, intra-rater reliability ranged from 0.44 to 0.67 and inter-rater reliability ranged from 0.00 to 0.45 with the highest values for shoulder abduction.[27] Nearly all the disagreements between therapists came from whether a contraction was painful or not. The authors concluded that intra-rater reliability for the knee was acceptable, but for the shoulder it was not. Inter-rater reliability was not acceptable for either joint.

Tips for Achieving Optimal Results in Alternative Muscle Testing

Before starting any of the alternative muscle tests described in this chapter, have all your tools and data collection materials ready so recording proceeds smoothly. Efficiency in testing will grow with clinical experience.

1. First and foremost, educate the patient. Explain and demonstrate each test and if feasible, allow the individual to perform the test with less weight or force. Patient cooperation is critical for achieving accurate results.
2. Provide a warm-up of some sort. Some clinics will have their patients walk on a treadmill or pedal a stationary cycle for 5 minutes before muscles are tested. It is also feasible to warm up cold muscles by performing the test with much less weight or resistance than what will be used during the testing session.
3. If there is suspected asymmetry in muscle performance, test the uninvolved side first. Side-to-side comparisons are critical and testing the uninvolved side also permits the patient to 'feel' what the test is going to entail on their weaker limb.
4. Stabilize the body part and patient. Depending on the test, each patient may need a seat belt, a stabilizing belt across the pelvis, or towels to position the arm or leg. After a part or extremity is stable, the test can be performed easily and accurately.
5. Standardize your commands to ensure that the test is performed exactly the same way each time.
6. Calibrate the device (if appropriate). Any device that records force or torque will drift away from accuracy over time. All testing devices should be routinely calibrated at least once a month, sometimes each session if deviations are suspected.
7. Allow the patient to rest between efforts. No one can duplicate a maximum effort without at least 30 seconds of rest before the next repetition can be performed to peak.
8. Provide a conducive test environment. The more diversions there are (such as radio noise or crowding), the more unlikely it is that an optimal effort will be made.
9. Provide feedback on the test. It is part of human nature to desire knowing if side-to-side differences exist, if test 1 is different from test 2, and so forth. Including the patient in the testing procedure optimizes their participation.

1. ACSM's Guidelines for Exercise Testing and Prescription. 8th ed. Baltimore, MD: Lippincott, Williams and Wilkins; 2010.
2. Lovell DI, Cuneo R, Gass GC. The blood pressure response of older men to maximum and submaximum strength testing. J Sci Med Sport. 2011;14:254-258.
3. LeBrasseur NK, Bhasin S, Miciek R, et al. Tests of muscle strength and physical function: reliability and discrimination of performance in younger and older men and older men with mobility limitations. J Am Ger Soc. 2008;56: 2118-2123.
4. Hoger WW, Hopkins DR, Barette SL, et al. Relationship between repetitions and selected percentages of one repetition maximum: a comparison between untrained males and females. J Strength & Cond Res. 1990;4:47-54.
5. Shimano T, Kraemer WJ, Spiering BA, et al. Relationship between the number of repetitions and selected percentages of one repetition maximum in free weight exercises in trained and untrained men. J Strength Cond Res. 2006;20:819-823.
6. Dohoney P, Chromiak JA, Lemire K, et al. Prediction of one repetition maximum (1-RM) strength from a 4-6 RM and a 7-10 RM submaximal strength test in healthy young adult males. JEP online. J Exercise Physiol. 2002;5(3). http://faculty.css.edu/tboone2/asep/Dohoney.pdf
7. Da Silva EM, Brentano MA, Cadore AL, et al. Analysis of muscle activation during different leg press exercises at submaximum effort levels. J Strength Cond Res. 2008; 22:1059-1065.
8. Signorile JF, Zink AJ, Szwed SP. A comparative electromyographical investigation of muscle utilization patterns using various hand positions during the lat pull-down. J Strength Cond Res. 2002;16:539-546.
9. Heyward VH. Advanced Fitness Assessment & Exercise Prescription. 2nd ed. Champaign, IL: Human Kinetics; 1991.
10. Brown L, ed. Isokinetics in Human Performance. Champaign, IL: Human Kinetics; 2000.
10a. Page P, Labbe A, Topp R. Clinical force production of Thera-band elastic bands. J Orthop Phys Ther 2000;30: A47-A48.
11. Page P, Ellenbecker TS, eds. The Scientific and Clinical Application of Elastic Resistance. Champaign IL: Human Kinetics; 2003.
12. Arborelius UF, Ekholm J. Mechanics of shoulder locomotion system using exercises resisted by weight-and-pulley circuit. Scand J Rehabil Med. 1978;10:171-177.
13. Hundley AF, Wu JM, Visco AG. A comparison of perineometer to brink score for assessment of pelvic floor muscle strength. Am J Obstet Gynecol. 2005;192: 1583-1585.
14. Fess EE. Grip Strength. 2nd ed. Chicago: American Society of Hand Therapists; 1992.
15. Bohannon RW, Bear-Lehman J, Desrosiers J, et al. Average grip strength: a meta-analysis of data obtained with a Jamar dynamometer from individuals 75 years or more of age. J Geriatr Phys Ther. 2007;30;28-30.
16. Shechtman O, Mann WC, Justiss MD, et al. Grip strength in the frail elderly. Am J Phys Med Rehabil. 2004;83: 819-826.
17. Desrosiers J, Bravo G, Hebert R, et al. Normative data for grip strength of elderly men and women. Am J Occup Ther. 1995;49:637-644.
18. Phillips P. Grip strength, mental performance and nutritional status as indicators of mortality risk among female geriatric patients. Age Ageing. 1986;15:53-56.
19. Kallman DA, Plato CC, Tobin JD. The role of muscle loss in the age-related decline of grip strength: Cross-sectional and longitudinal perspectives. J Gerontol. 1990; 45:M82-M88.
20. Hinson M, Gench BE. The curvilinear relationship of grip strength to age. Occup Ther J Res. 1989;9:53-60.
21. Margaria R, Aghemo P, Rovelli E. Measurement of muscular power (anaerobic) in man. J Appl Physiol. 1966;5: 1662-1664.
22. Bean JF, Kiely DK, LaRose S, et al. Are changes in leg power associated with clinically meaningful improvements in mobility in older adults? J Am Soc Geriatr. 2010;58: 2363-2368.
22a. Massey-Westropp NM, Gill TK, Taylor AW, et al. Hand grip strength; age and gender stratified normative data in population-based study. BMC Research Notes 2011; 4:127. http://www.biomedcentral.com/1756-0500/4/127
23. Wasserman B, Hansen J, Sue D, et al, eds. Principles of Exercise Testing and Interpretation. Philadelphia, PA: Lea and Febiger; 1987.
24. Hopkins WG, Schabort EJ, Hawley JA. Reliability of power in physical performance tests. Sports Med. 2001;31:211-234.
25. McArdle WD, Katch FI, Katch FL, et al. Exercise Physiology. 7th ed. Baltimore: Lippincott, Williams & Wilkins; 2010:518.
26. Cyriax J. Textbook of Orthopedic Medicine, volume 1. London: Bailliere Tindall; 1982.
27. Hayes KW, Petersen CM. Reliability of classifications derived from Cyriax's resisted testing in subjects with painful shoulders and knees. J Orthop Sports Phys Ther. 2003;33:235-246.

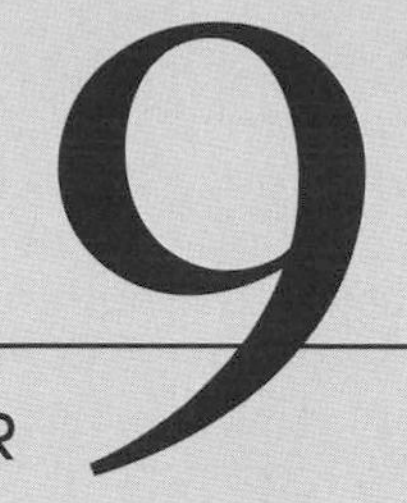

CHAPTER 9

Testing Functional Performance

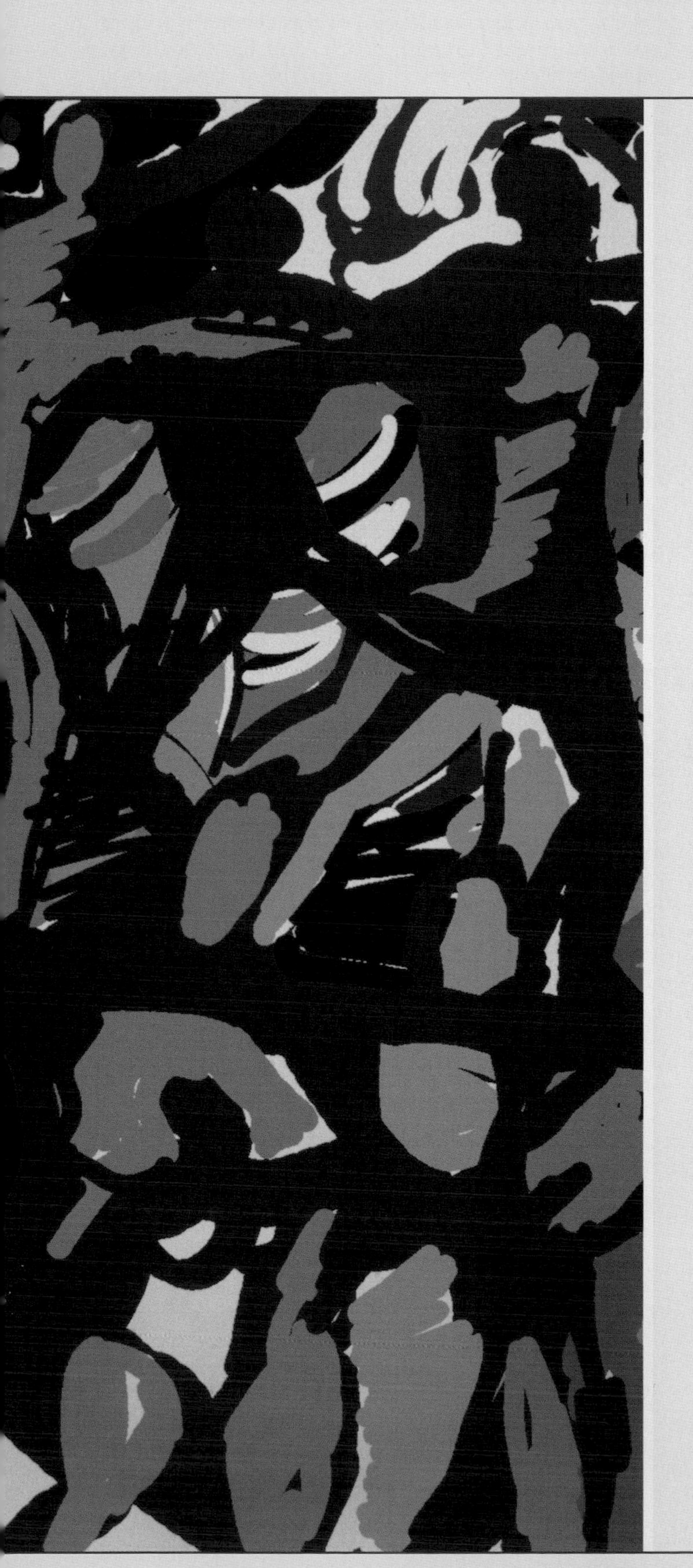

In current clinical practice, there is a growing need to emphasize the relationship between strength and functional movement, especially in older adults. Each person has a threshold of strength that is minimal for the performance of activities of daily living (ADLs). The larger or taller the person is, for example, the more strength will be needed. Third-party payers are requiring that therapists show a relationship between strength and function in their patients and if their assessments fail to show this relationship, payment is often denied. It has always been important for therapists to show that patients have strength deficits, but it is now critical for them to show that strength deficits are tied to the patient's ability, or lack thereof, to independently complete ADLs, perform a job task (such as bricklaying), or play with their children or grandchildren. This chapter presents a series of functional tasks, particularly relevant to older individuals, that can only be completed if strength is at a minimum threshold. Once an impairment is pinpointed, a strengthening program can be designed to help patients achieve their functional goals.

The functional assessment tests described in this chapter have been correlated to specific strength measures, and normative values are provided when available. The essential muscles involved in each movement are also identified. The list of muscles for each task is not comprehensive, but it provides a starting point for the beginning therapist to use in the design of exercises to improve task performance. In some cases, patients may be able to accomplish a task by compensating for a muscle weakness, but this weakness must be identified and corrected in order for the task to be performed successfully.

INTRODUCTION

Functional abilities represent a broad range of movements that require muscles to act in highly specific ways to achieve a desired purpose. These include ADLs such as dressing, eating, bathing, transferring, and walking, as well as other tasks of mobility such as rising from a chair, climbing stairs, lifting, writing, and rising from the floor. These functional activities are basic tasks of mobility that are required for all individuals to be independent in the home and community. Functional activity performance is especially important for older adults who may be at risk for institutionalization because of an inability to independently perform specific functional tasks. Higher level functional abilities such as those required for sports and work will not be discussed in this chapter.

The Nagi Model of Disablement[1] as well as the newer International Classification of Functioning (ICF) disablement model[2] describe the impact of disease and pathology within the context of both function and societal roles and provide a conceptual model to guide clinical practice. In these models, diminished muscle strength is seen as an impairment that affects a person's ability to perform functional tasks or to fulfill societal roles. Muscle strength testing takes place at the impairment level whereas testing performance of a functional task occurs at the function level. One goal of this chapter is to integrate impairment (strength deficit) and functional loss.

It is generally accepted that in the normal person, performance of basic functional tasks requires a relatively small amount of muscle strength in relation to the total amount of strength that existed before the injury, before a lifestyle of inactivity, or before the passage of years. The minimum amount of strength required is referred to as a "strength threshold." If patients have strength above the required threshold amount, they are unlikely to show deficits in performance. The relationship of strength to function up to a specific threshold is illustrated in Figure 9-1. According to the principle illustrated in this graph, if we strengthen a patient sufficiently and bring his or her strength value to the point at which the curve flattens out, a patient should be strong enough to perform the task. For example, about 45% of one's body weight is required to rise from a chair without using the arms.[3] If a person is unable to rise from a chair unassisted because of weakness in the lower extremities, strengthening will help to improve that function. Further strengthening will allow the person to rise more quickly and efficiently and will create a strength reserve to help preserve the ability to perform the task in the future.

Functional Testing

An analysis of any functional task shows that movements are multiplanar and asymmetrical, incorporate rotation, and are speed and balance dependent. Therefore, simply testing a muscle's maximum ability to generate force will not accurately represent its functional ability. Observation of the individual performing the functional task is the only way to accurately test functional ability. Such observation provides information about the quality of the performance, which in turn informs the therapist's clinical decision making. Inferring that a specific muscle is functional without direct observation of the functional task is incorrect and should be avoided. Table 9-1 shows the key muscles required for some basic functional tasks.

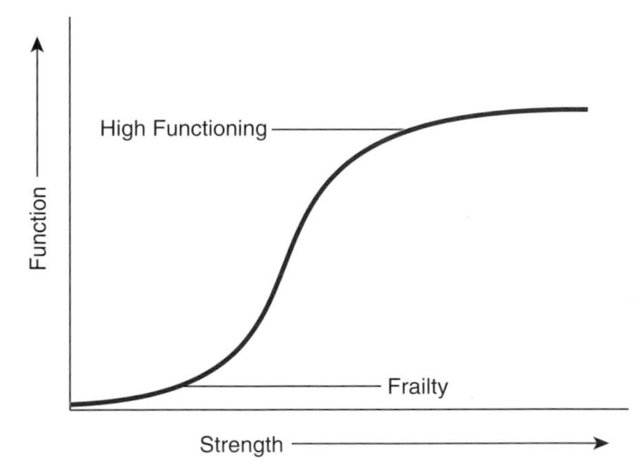

FIGURE 9-1 Conceptual diagram of curvilinear relationship between strength and function.

Table 9-1 KEY MUSCLES ESSENTIAL FOR FUNCTIONAL MOVEMENTS

Functional Movement	Key Muscles
Bed mobility	Abdominals, erector spinae, gluteus maximus
Transfers and squats	Gluteus maximus, medius, and obturator externus, piriformis, quadriceps
Ambulation and stair climbing	Abdominals, erector spinae, gluteus maximus and medius, obturator externus, piriformis, quadriceps, and anterior tibialis and gastrocsoleus
Floor transfers	Abdominals, erector spinae, gluteus maximus and medius, obturator externus, piriformis, quadriceps and gastrocsoleus
Fast gait and jumping	Gastrocsoleus, gluteus maximus and medius, quadriceps

Measurement

Functional task performance is measured in several ways. Ordinal scales showing hierarchical levels of performance are commonly used in both manual muscle testing and in some functional tests. In ordinal scales, numbers are sequentially and hierarchically assigned in accordance with the difficulty of the task. However, ordinal scales are limited by their susceptibility to subjectivity and their lack of responsiveness to small changes in performance. Therefore, measuring individual patient performance using ratio scales, such as time, is the preferred method. Timing task performance provides a strong measure of reliability and responsiveness. However, when a functional task is timed, such as when a patient is instructed to rise from a chair as quickly as possible, it should be noted that power is an additional component to strength. Ratio measures such as time and distance allow the therapist to compare an individual patient's performance against available normative data of similar individuals. This comparison aids in clinical decision-making.

Purpose: The chair stand test is a test of mobility specifically targeting the force production of the leg muscles.

Essential Muscle Movements for Task Performance: Hip extension, hip abduction from a flexed position, hip external rotation, knee extension, ankle plantar flexion, ankle dorsiflexion and inversion,[4] and trunk extension and flexion.

Reliability: Test-retest reliability for all versions of the Chair Stand Test ($r = 0.89$).[5]

Validity: Correlates with measures of lower extremity strength, walking speed, stair-climbing ability, and balance.[6,7] Correlates with one-repetition maximum (1-RM) leg press ($r = 0.78$ for men, 0.71 for women).[5]

Equipment: A standard, armless chair, 17 inches (42 cm) high, and a stopwatch.

Testing Procedure:

30-second Version: The test is *always* done without the use of the patient's arms. The patient rises from a sitting position and stands to a fully erect position as many times as possible in 30 seconds. The therapist starts timing when the patient begins to move (rather than on "Go!"). The last repetition is counted if the patient is standing, even if the patient hasn't returned to a sitting position when 30 seconds have elapsed. If indicated, the therapist should demonstrate the sit-to-stand movement before testing.

Timed Five-repetition Version: The test is *always* done without the use of the patient's arms. The patient comes to a full standing position five times as quickly as possible. The therapist begins timing on the command "Go!" The therapist times the effort from the command "Go!" until the patient returns to a seated position after five repetitions.

Position of Patient: Sitting with arms crossed over the chest. Feet are planted on the floor in the position chosen by the patient (Figure 9-2).

Position of Therapist: Standing to fully view the patient's quality of movement (Figure 9-3).

Instructions to Patient:

30-second Version: "When you're ready, stand up as many times as you can in 30 seconds without using your arms. I'll keep count. Make sure you stand all the way up."

Timed Five-repetition Version: "When you are ready, stand up 5 times, as quickly as you can without using your arms. I will be timing you. Make sure you stand all the way up."

Scoring

30-second Version: The number of repetitions is the patient's score. Count the repetition if the patient is more than halfway standing. If the patient cannot complete one repetition without the use of the arms, the score for the 30-second version is zero.

Timed Five-repetition Version: The time taken to complete five repetitions is the score. If 60 seconds elapse before five repetitions are accomplished, the test is terminated and the score of 60 seconds is recorded with a notation.

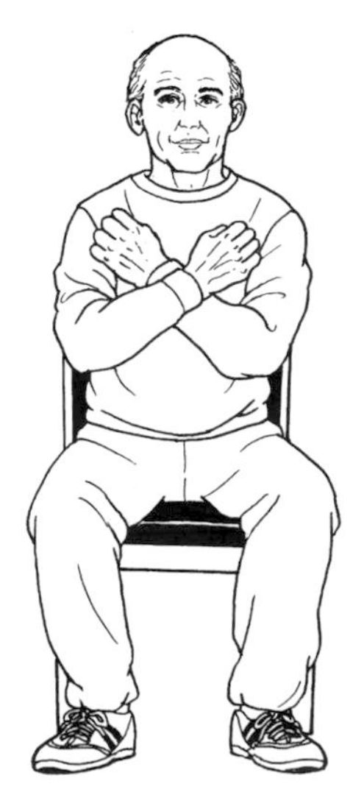

FIGURE 9-2

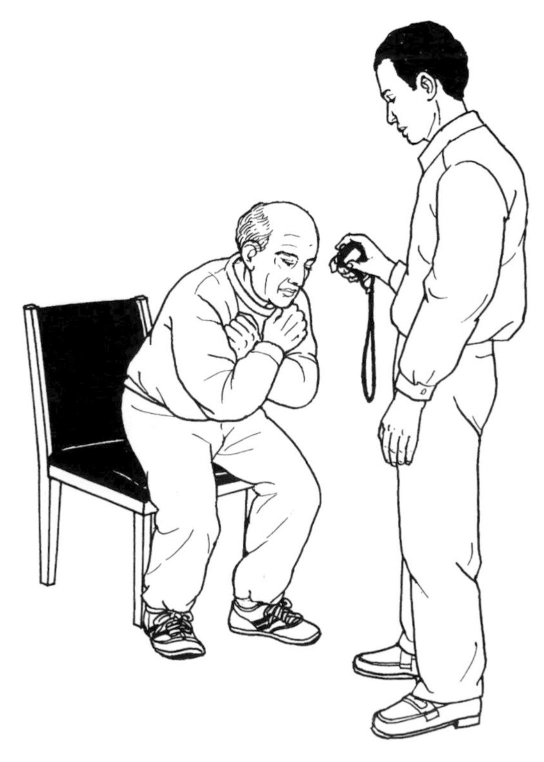

FIGURE 9-3

Helpful Hints

- Do not use a folding chair, a very soft chair, a deep chair, or a chair on wheels for the chair stand test. The chair should be placed against the wall for safety purposes.
- Allow the patient to perform the sit-to-stand movement first, without coaching. If the patient has difficulty rising, then offer tips such as scooting to the edge of the chair, leaning forward, etc.
- It is useful to observe the position of the hips while the patient is attempting to stand and sit. If the hips are adducted and/or internally rotated, this may indicate that the patient is primarily using the quadriceps to stand, rather than the gluteal muscles, and specific muscle testing is indicated, especially of the gluteus medius (Figure 9-4).
- Excessive bending forward of the trunk in order to stand may indicate that the patient has weak quadriceps (Figure 9-5).
- Although it is preferable to have the patient cross the arms over the chest, some patients may need to extend their arms forward to help them stand. If this occurs, it could indicate that the patient's legs are weak and that the trunk is being used to aid in standing (Figure 9-6).
- For every 1-second increase in the timed 5-repetition chair stand test, the odds of being disabled increases 1.4 times; inability to rise five times increases the odds ratio 2.5 times for severe mobility difficulty within 12 months.[8]
- If you suspect the patient will not be able to complete five repetitions, the 30-second chair stand is the preferred test because the patient is required to only complete a minimum of one repetition for a successful test.

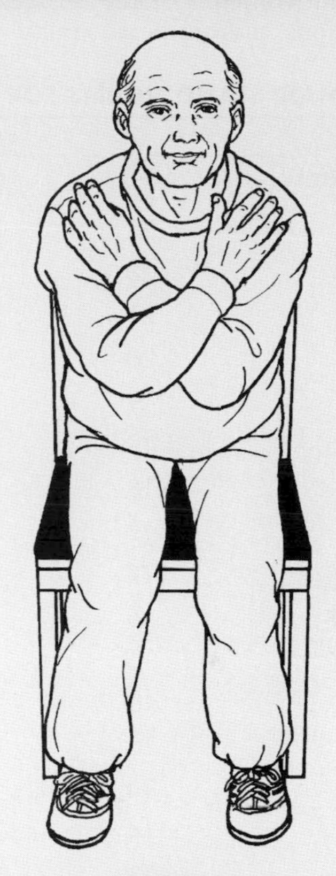

FIGURE 9-4

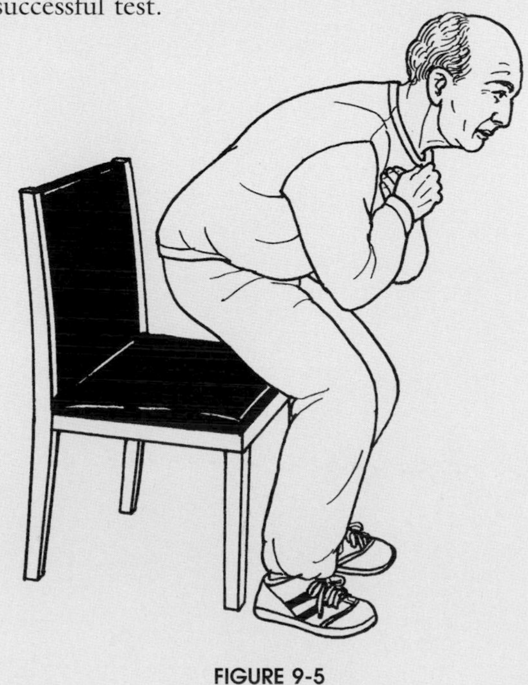

FIGURE 9-5

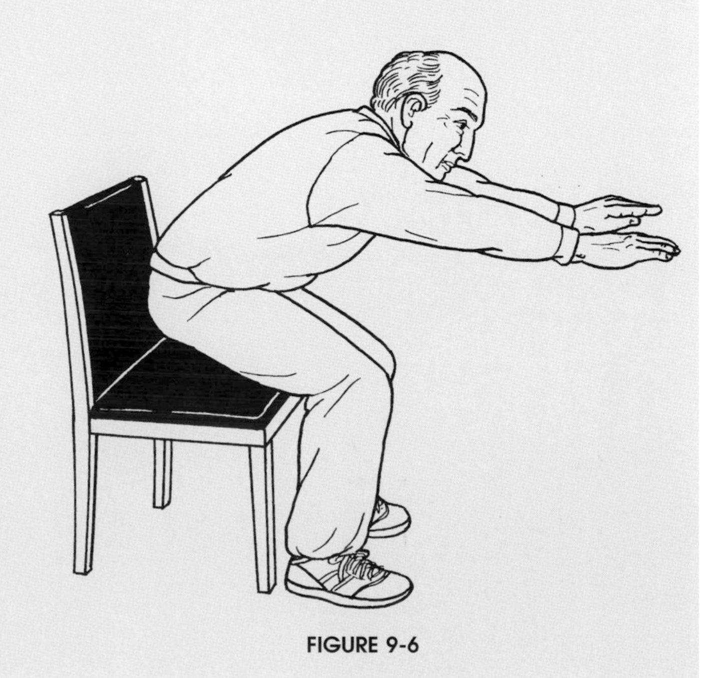

FIGURE 9-6

Table 9-2 shows normative ranges for physically active older men and women. For the 30-second chair stand, seven repetitions may indicate frailty in people with coronary artery disease.[9] Likewise, eight repetitions may be the threshold for physical disability.[5]

Table 9-2 CHAIR STAND NORMS FOR PHYSICALLY ACTIVE OLDER ADULTS

	CHAIR STAND TEST BY AGE (MEN)[5]						
Percentile Rank	60-64	65-69	70-74	75-79	80-84	85-89	90-94
95	23	23	21	21	19	19	16
90	22	21	20	20	17	17	15
85	21	20	19	18	16	16	14
80	20	19	18	18	16	15	13
75	19	19	17	17	15	14	12
70	19	18	17	16	14	13	12
65	18	17	16	16	14	13	11
60	17	16	16	15	13	12	11
55	17	16	15	15	13	12	10
50	16	15	14	14	12	11	10
45	16	15	14	13	12	11	9
40	15	14	13	13	11	10	9
35	15	13	13	12	11	9	8
30	14	13	12	12	10	9	8
25	14	12	12	11	10	8	7
20	13	11	11	10	9	7	7
15	12	11	10	10	8	6	6
10	11	9	9	9	7	5	5
5	9	8	8	8	6	4	3

Table 9-2 CHAIR STAND NORMS FOR PHYSICALLY ACTIVE OLDER ADULTS—cont'd

	CHAIR STAND TEST BY AGE (WOMEN)						
Percentile Rank	**60-64**	**65-69**	**70-74**	**75-79**	**80-84**	**85-89**	**90-94**
95	21	19	19	19	18	17	16
90	20	18	18	17	17	15	15
85	19	17	17	16	16	14	13
80	18	16	16	16	15	14	12
75	17	16	15	15	14	13	11
70	17	15	15	14	13	12	11
65	16	15	14	14	13	12	10
60	13	13	14	13	12	11	9
55	15	14	13	13	12	11	9
50	15	14	13	12	11	10	8
45	14	13	12	12	11	10	7
40	14	13	12	12	10	9	7
35	13	12	11	11	10	9	6
30	12	12	11	11	9	8	5
25	12	11	10	10	9	8	4
20	11	11	10	9	8	7	4
15	10	10	9	9	7	6	3
10	9	9	8	8	6	5	1
5	8	8	7	6	4	4	0

Source of data for women: Rikli RE, Jones CJ. Senior Fitness Test Manual. Champaign, IL: Human Kinetics; 2001.

Table 9-3 shows normative ranges for moderately disabled women—that is, those who have difficulty performing two ADL tasks. The Women's Health and Aging Study (of moderately to severely disabled women) found a mean time for ages 65 to 85 and older of 15.3 seconds.[10] The more time required, the more likely it is that the individual is frail.[11]

Table 9-3 CHAIR STAND PERFORMANCE FOR MODERATELY DISABLED WOMEN

5-Repetition Chair Stand	Total N = 1002	65-74 Y N = 388	75-84 Years N = 311	85+ Y N = 303
Unable to do (%)	25.2	17.8	25.9	44.9
Mean Time to rise 5 × (seconds)	15.3	14.7	15.7	16.3
5th percentile	24.5	21.9	25.5	24.1
25th percentile	17.4	16.7	17.5	18.5
50th percentile	14.2	13.9	14.4	15.0
75th percentile	12.3	12.1	12.4	12.7
95th percentile	10.0	9.6	10.3	10.0

Adapted from Ferrucci L, Guralnik JM, Bandeen-Roche KL, et al. Performance measures from the Women's Health and Aging Study. http://www.grc.nia.nih.gov/branches/ledb/whasbook/chap4/chap4.htm. Accessed January 8, 2012.
Y, age in years.
Moderately disabled women were those with difficulty in two or more activities of daily living tasks.

Purpose: Gait speed is a functional test of one's ability to walk at a comfortable (usual) speed. A fast-paced walk can demonstrate available reserve and the ability to accelerate rapidly, such as in the need to get across a street. Possible gait speed times range from the fastest sprinters to the slowest possible gait, often seen in individuals residing in nursing homes. Gait speed has been called the sixth vital sign because of its validity in predicting functional ability, frailty, nursing home placement, and the ability to walk in the community.[15] It can be measured in any person who can walk, even those using assistive devices.

Essential Muscle Movements for Task Performance: Hip extension and abduction, knee extension, ankle plantar flexion, and ankle dorsiflexion with inversion.[12] Hip flexion also contributes to walking velocity.[13] The reader is referred to the gait section of this chapter for a more specific list of muscles that are imperative for smooth and normal gait.

Reliability: $r = 0.90$[14]

Validity: Gait speed is related to age (Figure 9-7).[15] Gait speed at "usual pace" was found to be a consistent predictor of disability, cognitive impairment, institutionalizations, falls, and/or mortality.[16] A speed of less than 0.8 meters per second (m/s) is a predictor of 8-year mortality in predisabled women 75 years or older[17] and is considered pathologic.[18] A speed of less than 1.0 m/s identifies well-functioning people at high risk of health-related outcomes[19] and impaired function.[20] In one study, the mean gait speed used by 139 pedestrians was 1.32 (SD, 0.31) m/s.[21] A cutoff score of 0.57 m/s can indicate that the person is in need of physical therapy.[22]

Equipment: A 4- to 8-meter-long walkway and a stopwatch. It is helpful to have 2 meters or so before and after the 4-meter test course to allow for acceleration and deceleration. However, although this extra distance is desirable, it is not necessary to perform the test.

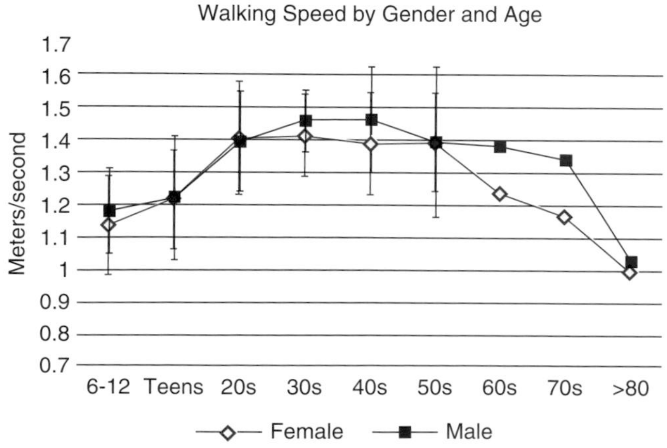

FIGURE 9-7 Self-selected walking speed categorized by gender and age.

Testing Procedure: First, describe the test clearly to the individual. Demonstrate the test if needed, taking care not to walk too fast. Then, have the patient perform two trials with adequate rest in between, scoring the faster one. Test both comfortable (usual) and fast gait speeds. Begin timing the individual when the first foot crosses the line at the beginning of the course (Figure 9-8,*A*) and stop timing when the first foot crosses the end line (Figure 9-8,*B*). Any part of the foot will do; it is just important to be consistent.

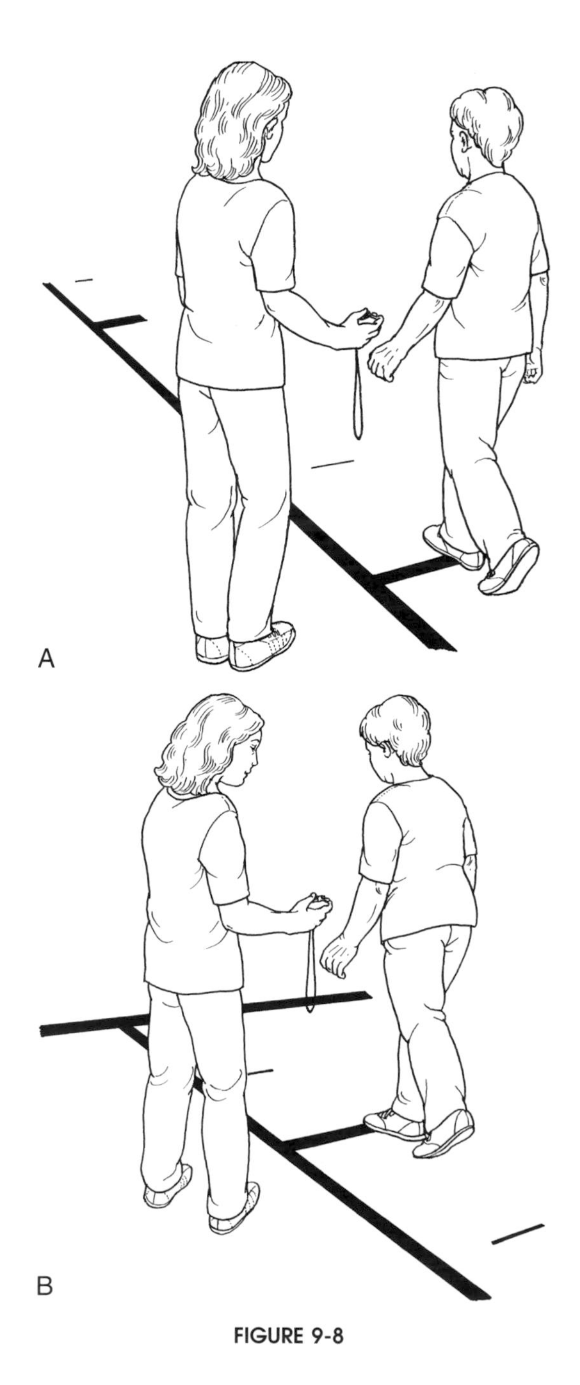

FIGURE 9-8

Position of Patient: Standing, facing a marked-off walkway. Patient may use an assistive device if needed.

Position of Therapist: Standing, holding the stop-watch perpendicular to the starting line. Therapist will walk with the patient to obtain an accurate view of when the first foot crosses the finish line. The therapist will begin timing when the first foot (or part of the first foot) crosses the start line of the 4-meter walkway (see Figure 9-8,*A*).

Instructions to Patient: "First, walk at your usual and comfortable speed from this line to the other line on the floor (indicate which line). I will be timing you. The first trial is the practice trial and then we'll test you twice. OK? Ready, Go!" (The same directions are given for the fast-paced walk, with the patient instructed to walk as quickly, but as safely, as possible.)

Scoring

The time taken to walk 4 meters is divided into 4 for a result in meters per second (m/s). There are many gait speed standards. Gait speeds of 1.75 m/s to 2.25 m/s are normal in high-functioning older adults, whereas gait speeds slower than 0.5 m/s are common in nursing home residents. Table 9-4 indicates some conversions from meters/second to feet/second and miles/hour. Tables 9-5, 9-6 and 9-7 list normative values for gait speed by age.

Helpful Hints

- Gait speed can be measured in patients who use an assistive device. When retesting performance in the same patient, retest using the same assistive device.
- Studies have shown that additional distance for acceleration and deceleration is not necessary; however, we recommend using a further end-point target to prevent patients from slowing down as they approach the finish line (see Figure 9-8,*B*).
- If walking with the individual, be careful not to set the pace but walk slightly behind the individual. This will allow you to get a more realistic view of the patient's actual performance. While always maintaining a safe test situation, do not inhibit the individual by standing too close or providing too many instructions. Certainly, use a gait belt if it is warranted.
- Knowing when to start and stop timing requires skill and practice. It is recommended to use a specific "event," such as when the first foot crosses the line, as the moment to begin and end timing but any such event will do; just be consistent!

Table 9-4 CONVERSIONS FOR GAIT SPEED

Meters/ Second	Feet/ Second	Minutes/ Mile	Miles/ Hour
0.25	0.82	106.7	0.6
0.30	0.98	88.9	0.7
0.35	1.15	76.2	0.8
0.40	1.31	66.7	0.9
0.45	1.48	59.3	1.0
0.50	1.64	53.3	1.1
0.55	1.80	48.5	1.2
0.60	1.97	44.4	1.4
0.65	2.13	41.0	1.5
0.70	2.30	38.1	1.6
0.75	2.46	35.6	1.7
0.80	2.62	33.3	1.8
0.85	2.79	31.4	1.9
0.90	2.95	29.6	2.0
0.95	3.12	28.1	2.1
1.00	3.28	26.7	2.3
1.10	3.61	24.2	2.5
1.20	3.94	22.2	2.7
1.30	4.26	20.5	2.9
1.40	4.59	19.0	3.2
1.50	4.92	17.8	3.4
1.60	5.25	16.7	3.6
1.70	5.58	15.7	3.8
1.80	5.90	14.8	4.1
1.90	6.23	14.0	4.3
2.00	6.56	13.3	4.5

Table 9-5 MEAN USUAL GAIT SPEED TIME FOR MEN AND WOMEN AGE 20 YEARS AND OLDER

Sex/ age	COMFORTABLE GAIT SPEED (M/S)		MAXIMUM GAIT SPEED (M/S)	
	$\bar{x}$	SD	$\bar{x}$	SD
Men				
20s	1.39	0.15	2.53	0.29
30s	1.46	0.09	2.46	0.32
40s	1.46	0.16	2.46	0.36
50s	1.39	0.23	2.07	0.45
60s	1.36	0.21	1.93	0.36
70s	1.33	0.20	2.08	0.36
Women				
20s	1.41	0.18	2.47	0.25
30 s	1.42	0.13	2.34	0.34
40s	1.39	0.16	2.12	0.28
50s	1.40	0.15	2.01	0.26
60s	1.27	0.21	1.77	0.25
70s	1.27	0.21	1.75	0.28

Data from Bohannon RW. Comfortable and maximum walking speed of adults aged 20-79 years: reference values and determinants. Age Ageing. 1997;26(1):15-19.
SD, standard deviation; x, mean.

Table 9-6 NORMS FOR USUAL GAIT SPEED TIME (M/S) FOR MODERATELY DISABLED WOMEN AGE 65 AND OLDER

	Total n = 1002	65-74	75-84	85+
Mean	0.6	0.7	0.6	0.4
5th percentile	0.2	0.3	0.2	0.1
25th percentile	0.4	0.5	0.4	0.3
50th percentile	0.6	0.6	0.6	0.6
75th percentile	0.7	0.7	0.8	0.6
95th percentile	1.1	1.1	1.1	0.8

Adapted from: Ferrucci L, Guralnik JM, Bandeen-Roche KL, et al. Performance measures from the women's health and aging study. http://www.grc.nia.nih.gov/branches/ledb/whasbook/chap4/chap4.htm. Accessed January 8, 2012.
M/s, meters per second; n, number of subjects.
Moderately disabled women were those with difficulty in two or more activities of daily living tasks.
Subjects were asked to walk at their usual and customary pace for 4 m.

Table 9-7 NORMS FOR FAST GAIT SPEED TIME (M/S) FOR MODERATELY DISABLED WOMEN AGE 65 AND OLDER

	Total n = 1002	65-74	75-84	85+
Mean	0.9	1	0.9	0.7
5th percentile	0.2	0.4	0.3	0.2
25th percentile	0.6	0.8	0.6	0.4
50th percentile	0.9	1	0.9	0.7
75th percentile	1.1	1.3	1.1	0.9
95th percentile	1.7	1.7	1.7	1.3

Adapted from: Ferrucci L, Guralnik JM, Bandeen-Roche KL, et al. Performance measures from the women's health and aging study. http://www.grc.nia.nih.gov/branches/ledb/whasbook/chap4/chap4.htm. Accessed January 8, 2012.
M/s, meters per second; n, number of subjects.
Moderately disabled women were those with difficulty in two or more activities of daily living tasks.

Purpose: The short physical performance battery (SPPB) can be used to assess how well older adults perform mobility-related tasks and tasks that are important to the performance of daily activities. This test battery can predict future disability, hospitalization, and death even in patients who report no disability at initial testing.[23] Early identification of these people, who are presumably in a preclinical stage of disability, can provide an opportunity for early intervention that may prevent further progression of disability. Most of the tasks in the battery are timed, providing some norms to compare specific patient performance.

The SPPB was developed by the National Institute on Aging for the Established Populations for Epidemiologic Studies of the Elderly and has been used in many research studies. A free download of the instructions (with script) and DVD are available at http://www.grc.nia.nih.gov/branches/ledb/sppb/index.htm.

Essential Muscle Movements for Task Performance:

Balance Tasks: Ankle dorsiflexion with inversion, plantar flexion, foot inversion, foot eversion with plantar flexion, knee extension, and hip abduction and extension.

Gait Speed Task: Hip extension and abduction, knee extension, ankle plantar flexion, and ankle dorsiflexion with inversion.[12] Hip flexion also contributes to walking velocity.[13] The reader is referred to the gait section of this chapter for a more specific list of muscles that are imperative for smooth and normal gait.

Chair Stand Task: Hip extension, hip abduction from a flexed position, hip external rotation, knee extension, ankle plantar flexion,[4] ankle dorsiflexion and inversion, and trunk extension and flexion.

Reliability: Reliability ranges from 0.97 to 0.79, depending on the task.[24,25]

Validity: Poorer scores were predictive of nursing home admission,[26] with lower scores (0-4) predicting longer hospital stays.[27] A 1-point increase was associated with a 0.5-day reduction in hospital stay.[27] Walking speed was the most powerful predictor of impending disability of any task in the SPPB.[28]

Equipment: Stopwatch, a 4-meter path for gait speed, a 17-inch-high armless chair with a hard seat for the chair stand task and a scoring form.

Testing Procedure: The tasks for the three physical performance areas of the SPPB must be performed in order: balance tasks, usual gait speed, and chair stand. Demonstrate each portion of the test, especially the balance tasks, as you are explaining the test to the patient. Generally, two trials are given, with the poorest performance scored. However, in the gait speed task, the faster of the two trials is scored. (Note: It is recommended that the lowest score be used because of the need to accurately record the patient's performance in the clinical setting. While performance may improve with repeated trials, the most genuine performance, reflective of the real world, may be the lowest timed or poorest performance.)

Position of Therapist *(All SPPB Tests)*: The therapist should stand as close to the patient as necessary to ensure the patient's safety but not so close as to impede the patient's performance. The therapist may assist the patient in achieving the balance positions, but then must not have physical contact with the patient during timing (safety not withstanding). During the gait speed portion of the test, the therapist should walk with the patient, but slightly behind, to assure accurate timing when the first foot crosses the starting and finish line but not so as to pace the patient. The therapist records the time for each task on the scoring form.

Balance Tasks

The tasks of balance provide an assessment of the patient's ability to hold three balance positions independently with the eyes open. These positions are side-by-side stance (Figure 9-9), semi-tandem (Figure 9-10), and full tandem stance (or heel-to-toe) (Figure 9-11) and are performed in this order. Patients performing these tasks must be able to stand unassisted without using a cane or a walker.

Testing Procedure: The patient assumes the correct foot position for each position and initially may be supported by the therapist if necessary. Once the patient appears to be steady, the therapist asks if the patient is ready. When the patient says yes, the therapist says, "Ready, begin," then starts timing, relinquishing support if support was given. The timing is continued until the patient moves his or her feet, grasps the therapist for support, or 10 seconds have elapsed. Record any time less than 10 seconds to the nearest hundredth of a second on the scoring form.

Side-by-side Stance: The first balance position tested is the side-by-side stance. In this balance task, the patient is requested to stand with the feet together in a side-by-side position for 10 seconds (see Figure 9-9).

Semi-tandem Stance: The second balance task is the semi-tandem stance. The patient starts with the heel of one foot placed to the side of and against the big toe of the other foot. Either foot can be placed in the forward position (see Figure 9-10). Only one foot forward is tested.

Full Tandem Stance: The third and final position is the tandem stance. To assume the tandem stance position, the heel of one foot is placed directly in front of the toes of the other foot. Either foot can be placed in the forward position (see Figure 9-11). Only one foot-forward is tested.

Position of Patient:

Side-by-side Stance: Standing with feet together.

Semi-tandem Stance: Standing with heel of one foot placed to the side of and against the big toe of the other foot.

Full Tandem Stance: Standing with heel of one foot placed directly in front of the toes of the other foot.

Instructions to Patient:

Side-by Side Stance: "I want you to try to stand with your feet together for 10 seconds. You may use your arms, bend your knees, or move your body in order to maintain your balance, but try not to move your feet and you cannot hold on. Try to hold this position until I tell you to stop."

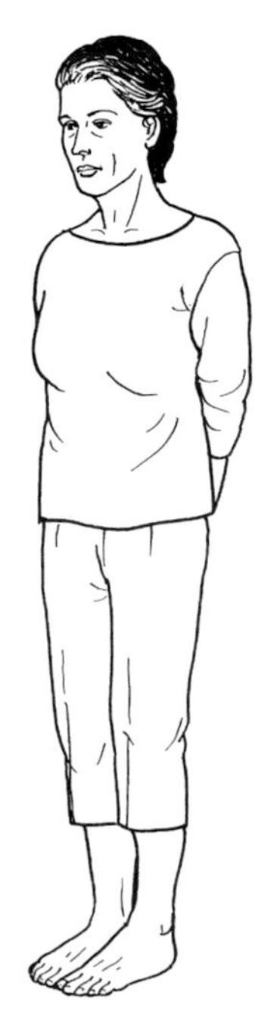

FIGURE 9-9

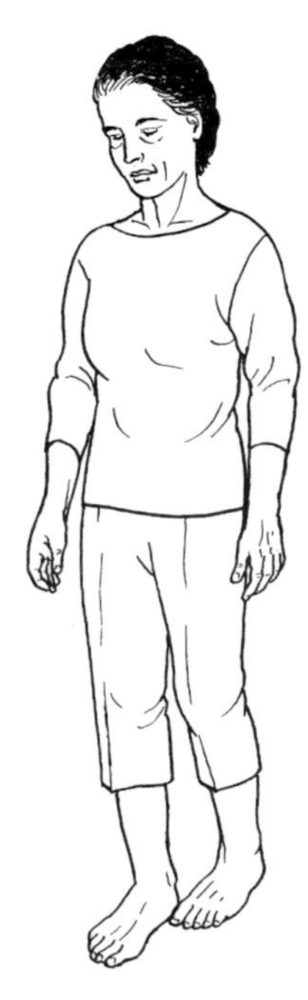

FIGURE 9-10

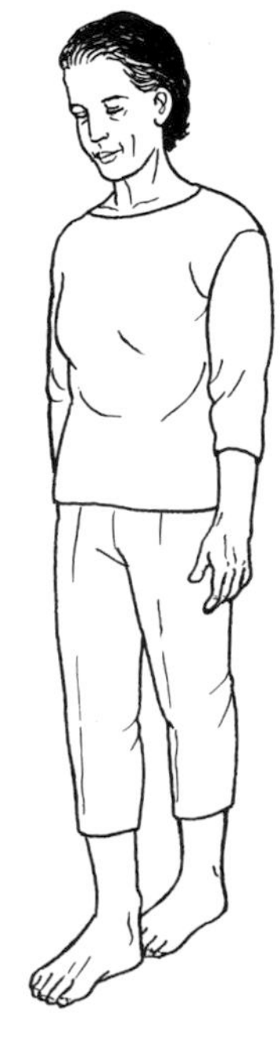

FIGURE 9-11

Balance Tasks Continued

Semi-tandem Stance: "I want you to try to stand with the side of the heel of one foot touching the big toe of the other foot for 10 seconds. You may put either foot in front, whichever is more comfortable for you. You may use your arms, bend your knees, or move your body to maintain your balance, but try not to move your feet or use your hands to maintain your balance. Try to hold this position until I tell you to stop."

Full Tandem Stance: "I want you to try to stand with the heel of one foot in front of and touching the toes of the other foot for 10 seconds. You may put either foot in front, whichever is more comfortable for you. You may use your arms, bend your knees, or move your body to maintain your balance, but try not to move your feet. Try to hold this position until I tell you to stop."

Scoring

Successful completion of each balance task for the full 10 seconds earns 1 point for the side-by-side and semi-tandem stance positions and 2 points for the full tandem stance position. If the patient was able to hold the tandem stance position, but not for the full 10 seconds, only 1 point is awarded. A total of 4 points for the balance portion of the SPPB is possible. If the patient was unable to hold any of three positions independently for 10 seconds, no points are assigned for that balance position.

Gait Speed Task

Testing Procedure: Patients are instructed to walk at their comfortable (usual) speed over an unobstructed 4-meter course. Timing commences when the first foot crosses the starting line and is stopped when the first foot completely crosses the 4-meter mark. The faster of two timed walks is used for scoring purposes.

Position of Patient: Standing at the starting line of a 4-meter walkway (Figure 9-12). Patient should be wearing comfortable, low-heeled shoes.

Instructions to Patient: "I am going to observe how you normally walk. If you use a cane or other walking aid and you feel you need it to walk this distance, then you may use it. I want you to walk to the other end of the course at your comfortable and usual speed, just as if you were walking down the street to go to the store. Walk all the way past the other end of the tape before you stop. I will walk with you. Ready? Begin." After an appropriate rest (only if necessary), begin second trial. "Now I'd like for you to repeat the walk. Remember to walk at your comfortable and usual pace and go all the way past the other end of the tape."

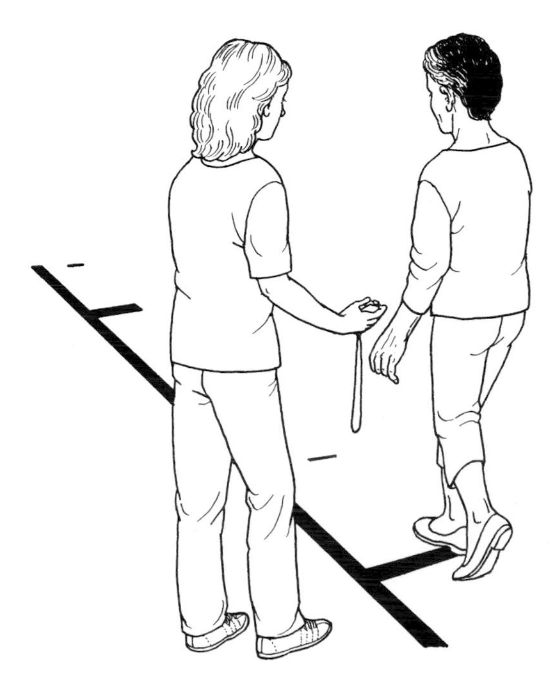

FIGURE 9-12

Gait Speed Task Continued

Scoring

Scoring of the 4-meter gait speed test is based on established categories of completion times.

- More than 8.70 seconds to complete the 4-meter walk receives 1 point.
- 6.21-8.70 seconds receives 2 points.
- 4.82-6.20 seconds receives 3 points.
- Less than 4.82 seconds receives the full 4 points.
- Inability to complete the walk in less than 60 seconds results in a score of 0.

Chair Stand Task

Testing Procedure: The chair stand task is a test of leg strength. The patient is first asked to stand from the chair with arms folded across the chest one time while the therapist observes. If the patient is successful at rising from the chair once without the use of his or her arms, the patient is then asked to stand up and sit down five times as quickly as possible. Timing begins as soon as the command to stand is given and continues until the patient is fully upright at the end of the fifth stand.

Position of Patient: Seated, with arms crossed over the chest. Feet are planted on the floor in any position desired by the patient (Figure 9-13). It is not necessary to have the patient's back against the back of the chair. The patient may chose to sit close to the front of the chair for maximum advantage.

Instructions to Patient: "This test measures the strength of your legs. First, fold your arms across your chest and sit so that your feet are on the floor. Then, stand up, keeping your arms folded across your chest" (Figure 9-14). (After observing that the patient can safely stand independently, proceed to the timed five-repetition part of the chair stand test.)

"Please stand up straight, as quickly as you can. Do this five times without stopping in between. After standing up each time, sit down and then stand up again. Keep your arms folded across your chest. I'll be timing you."

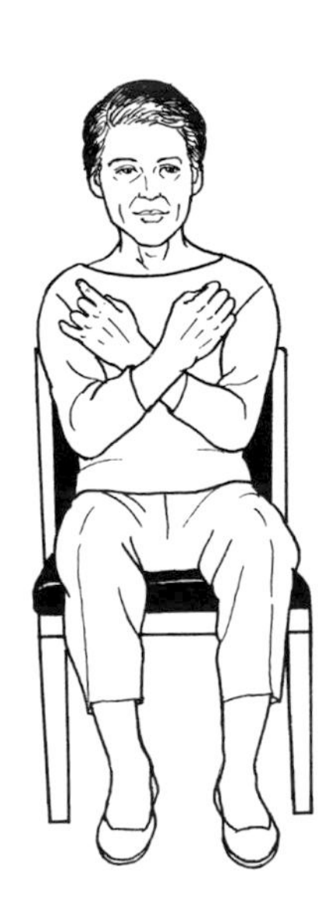

FIGURE 9-13

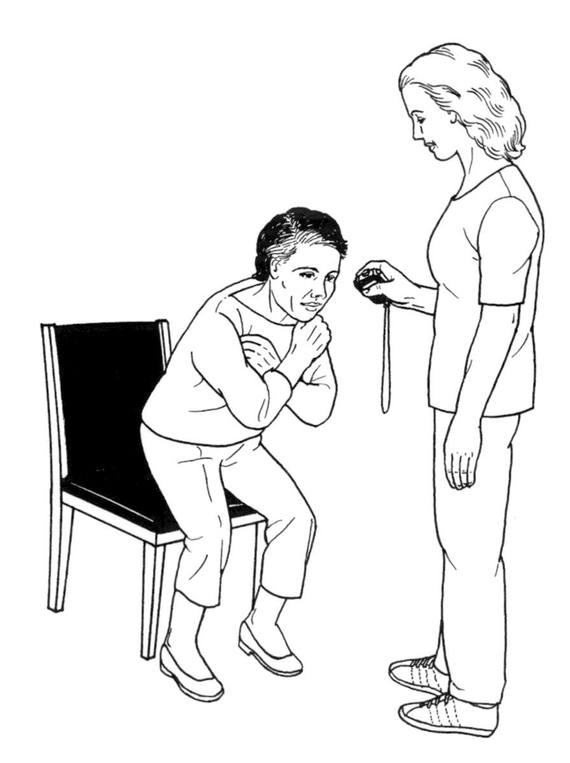

FIGURE 9-14

Chair Stand Task Continued

Scoring

The patient must be able to complete five repetitions to achieve a score. Mark the form if the patient was able to stand independently. If the patient was unable to stand without using the arms, the score is zero. Scoring of the chair stand task is based on established categories of times for completion of five repetitions:

- More than 16.70 but less than 60 seconds receives 1 point.
- Between 13.70 and 16.69 seconds receives 2 points.
- Between 11.20 and 13.69 seconds receives 3 points.
- Less than 11.20 seconds receives 4 points.

Scoring the Full SPPB

Recording Inability or Refusal to Complete the Test: For purposes of correct scoring of the SPPB, it is important to distinguish between the patient who is unwilling to perform a task and one who is physically unable. Differentiating between these two alternatives is a responsibility of the therapist and can be a difficult decision. If someone refuses to participate in any of the tasks, the therapist would generally mark on the scoring form that the patient has refused, unless it is quite clear that the patient is refusing because the patient cannot do the task or is afraid to attempt it (Figure 9-15).

Final Score

The composite score for the whole battery is simply the sum of the scores of the three individual components. The maximum score that a patient can receive is 12 points (see Figure 9-15).

Helpful Hints

- Ensure the patient's safety. Although it is ideal for the patient to perform the tasks independently, you may need to use a gait belt and/or have another person supervise the patient while you provide the directions and observe the patient's performance. If the patient does not wish to perform a task, do not force it, but score the test appropriately.
- A cane or walker may be used during the gait speed portion of the test, but if people with such devices can walk short distances without them, they should be encouraged to do so. Many people with assistive devices use them only when they walk outdoors or for long distances indoors. Doing the test without the device provides a much more accurate assessment of the functional limitations of the patient. Ask the patient if she ever walks at home without the device. Then ask the patient if she thinks that she can walk a short distance for the test. Patients who normally use assistive devices and opt to walk without it should be watched particularly closely during the test to prevent falling.
- The position of the therapist is critical for the gait speed task. If you stand too close to the patient, you may inadvertently set the pace or impede the patient's performance. If you are too far behind, you will not be in a good position if the patient starts to fall or to observe the foot crossing the finish line. The best position to maintain during the gait speed task is to the side and slightly behind the patient, outside of the patient's visual field.
- The gait speed task can also serve as an independent gait speed test. A score is obtained by dividing the time taken to walk 4 meters into 4 to obtain a score in meters/second.
- Do not use a folding chair, a very soft chair, a deep chair, or a chair on wheels for the chair stand test. The chair should be placed against the wall for safety purposes.
- Score the poorest performance, as long as your directions were clear and the patient understood them.
- Each task is performed twice. Subsequent trials often improve performance but may not provide a realistic view of the patient's performance on a novel task.
- Watch the patient and be prepared to stop timing if the patient steps out of position or grabs your arm. Do not watch the stopwatch continuously during the test so as to miss observing the quality of the performance or safety issues.

Short Physical Performance Battery (SPPB) Scoring Form

Web address for free download of the instructions (with script):
http://www.grc.nia.nih.gov/branches/ledb/sppb/index.htm

Balance Tests

The subject must be able to stand unassisted without the aid of a cane or walker.

A. Side-by-side Stance

____(1) Held for 10 seconds
____(0) Not held for 10 seconds
____(0) Not attempted ____

Number of seconds held
if less than 10 seconds ______

If 0 points, end Balance Test

B. Semi-tandem Stance

____(1) Held for 10 seconds
____(0) Not held for 10 seconds
____(0) Not attempted ____

Number of seconds held
if less than 10 seconds ______

If 0 points, end Balance Test

C. Full Tandem Stance

____(2) Held for 10 seconds
____(1) Held for 3 to 9 seconds
____(0) Not held for at least 3 seconds
____(0) Not attempted ____

Number of seconds held
if less than 10 seconds ______

D. Total Balance Score ______ (sum points)

If any test was NOT performed,
please choose the reason that most closely represents why the subject did not perform the test. Write that number in the appropriate blank after the test NOT performed.

Tried but unable ...1

Subject could not stand unassisted ...2

Not attempted, you felt unsafe ...3

Not attempted, subject felt unsafe ...4

Subject unable to understand instructions ...5

Other (SPECIFY)________________________________...6

Subject refused ...7

Comments:

____

____

____

____

Page 1 of 3

FIGURE 9-15 Short Physical Performance Battery (SPPB) scoring form.

Gait Speed Tests

Subject may use an assistive device.
Measure 4 meters. Instruct the subject to walk at his/her usual and customary pace.

A. Time for First Usual Walk (in seconds)

1. Time for 4 meters ____ seconds
2. IF NOT ATTEMPTED/COMPLETED:
   Refer to boxed options on page 1. ____
   (GO TO CHAIR STAND TEST)
3. Aids for first walk:
   None__ Cane__ Other __

Comments:

____

____

____

____

B. Time for Second Usual Walk (in seconds)

1. Time for 4 meters ____ seconds
2. IF NOT ATTEMPTED/COMPLETED:
   Refer to boxed options on page 1. ____
   (GO TO CHAIR STAND TEST)
3. Aid for first walk:
   None__ Cane__ Other __

WHAT IS THE TIME FOR THE FASTER OF THE USUAL PACED 2 WALKS?
Record the shorter of the two times ____ seconds (if only 1 walk done, record that time)

For 4-Meter Walk:
____(0) If the subject was UNABLE to do the walk
____(1) If time is more than 8.70 seconds
____(2) If time is 6.21 to 8.70 seconds
____(3) If time is 4.82 to 6.20 seconds
____(4) If time is less than 4.82 seconds

Page 2 of 3

FIGURE 9-15, cont'd

Continued

Chair Stand Tests

30-second Chair Stand

A. Safe to stand without help — YES — NO

B. Results:

	YES	NO
Subject stood without arms	____	____ Go to FIVE-REPETITION CHAIR STANDS
Subject used arms to stand	____	____ Ends CHAIR STANDS
Test not completed	____	____ Ends CHAIR STANDS
		Refer to boxed options on page 1.____

(Go to end of TOTAL TEST SCORES.)

Five-repetition Chair Stands

Instruct the subject to stand up as quickly as he/she can five times without stopping. Keep arms folded across chest. Instruct the subject you will be timing the effort. Count repetitions.

A. Safe to stand five times (CIRCLE) YES NO

B. IF FIVE STANDS DONE SUCCESSFULLY, RECORD TIME IN SECONDS.
Time to complete five stands ____ seconds.

C. IF NOT COMPLETED/NOT ATTEMPTED:
Refer to boxed options on page 1. ____

Scoring Five-repetition Chair Stands

____(0) If the subject was unable to complete the 5 chair stands or completes stands in over 60 seconds
____(1) If chair stand time is 16.70 seconds or more
____(2) If chair stand time is 13.70 to 16.69 seconds
____(3) If chair stand time is 11.20 to 13.69 seconds
____(4) If chair stand time is 11.19 seconds or less

SCORING OF THE SPPB

TOTAL TEST SCORES

Balance Test score ___________ points

Gait Speed Test score _________ points

Chair Stands Test score _______ points

Total SCORE _______________ (sum points)

Page 3 of 3

FIGURE 9-15, cont'd

Purpose: The physical performance test (PPT) measures aspects of physical function and ADLs in older adults using nine items that emphasize mobility tasks. There are two versions of the test: one with seven items and one with nine; the nine-item version also includes stair-climbing tasks.

Essential Muscle Movements for Task Performance:

Writing Task: (If arm is supported, only hand and wrist muscles may be essential.) Wrist flexion and extension, finger metacarpophalangeal (MP), proximal phalanges (PIP), and distal phalanges (DIP) flexion.

Eating Task: Shoulder flexion, shoulder internal rotation, elbow flexion, forearm supination and pronation, wrist flexion and extension, and finger MP, PIP, and DIP flexion.

Lifting a Book: Scapular protraction and upward rotation, shoulder flexion, shoulder external rotation, elbow flexion and extension, forearm supination and pronation, wrist flexion and extension, and finger MP, PIP, and DIP flexion.

Putting On and Taking Off a Garment (Depending on Technique): Scapular protraction and upward rotation, shoulder flexion, shoulder external rotation, elbow flexion and extension, forearm supination and pronation, wrist flexion and extension, and finger MP, PIP, and DIP flexion. Core stability (for sitting or standing). If task is performed in standing: hip extension and abduction, knee extension, ankle plantar flexion, and ankle dorsiflexion with inversion.

Picking Up a Coin: Back extension, hip extension, knee extension, ankle plantar flexion, elbow flexion and extension, forearm supination and pronation, wrist flexion and extension, and finger MP, PIP, and DIP flexion.

360° Turn: Ankle dorsiflexion with inversion, plantar flexion, foot inversion, foot eversion with plantar flexion, knee extension, hip abduction and extension, and core stability.

Walking Task: Hip extension and abduction, knee extension, ankle plantar flexion, and ankle dorsiflexion with inversion.[12] Hip flexion also contributes to walking velocity.[13] The reader is referred to the gait section of this chapter for a more specific list of muscles that are imperative for smooth and normal gait.

Stair Climb Tasks: Ascent: hip flexion and extension, knee flexion, ankle plantar flexion, ankle dorsiflexion, spine extension, and core stability. Descent: eccentric knee extension, hip flexion, and core muscles. For a test that requires stability and balance however, any lower extremity muscle or group will be used at some point during the task.

Reliability: Seven-item version has a Cronbach alpha coefficient of 0.79 and correlation coefficient of 0.83 for inter-rater reliability.[29]

Validity: Predictive validity for classifying level of care as dependent or independent.[30] Construct validity based on self-reported ADL and instrumental ADL performance.[29] Predictive of major health outcomes such as death and nursing home placement.[31] Predictive of first time fall (within 12 months)[32] and recurrent falls.[33]

Equipment:

Scoring form
Stopwatch
Table and chair
Bowl
Spoon
Coffee can
5 dry (uncooked) kidney beans
5.5-pound book
2 adjustable shelves
Front-opening garment such as a jacket or lab coat
25-foot walkway
One flight of stairs (10-12 stairs)

Testing Procedure: The PPT takes about 10 minutes to complete. The test items can be done in any order; however, they will be described here in the order in which they appear on the scoring form. Each task is timed, except for task 6 (turning 360°) and task 9 (climbing four flights of stairs). Each task is scored on a 0-4 scale. Two trials of each task are performed, except for the stair climb task, with the lowest performance recorded as the score for that task. (It is recommended to use the lowest score because of the need to accurately record the patient's performance in the clinical setting. Although performance may improve with repeated trials, the most genuine real-life performance may be the lowest timed or poorest performance.) The seven-item version does not include the stair climbing tasks. A total possible score for the seven-item version is 28, whereas the nine-item version is a total possible score of 36.

An assistive device can be used for the walking and stair climbing tasks, but not for the other tasks. All tasks are to be completed unassisted and without support.

The nine tasks are:

1. Writing a sentence
2. Simulated eating
3. Lifting a book onto a shelf
4. Putting on and taking off a garment
5. Picking up a coin from the floor
6. 360° turn
7. 50-foot walk
8. Climbing one flight of stairs
9. Climbing four flights of stairs

1. Writing a Sentence

Testing Procedure: The patient is to write a sentence. Ideally, the sentence should be written on the back of the test form so there will be a record of the result. The therapist writes the sentence first: "Whales live in a blue ocean." A period is placed at the end of the sentence. Then, on the command of "Go!" the patient writes the same sentence. Timing begins on Go! and ends when the period is placed at the end of the sentence. The therapist records the time it took the patient to write the sentence legibly (Figure 9-16).

Instructions to Patient: "The first task is a writing task. I am going to write the sentence 'Whales live in a blue ocean.' Then I want you to write the same sentence while I time you."

2. Eating Task

Testing Procedure: The second task is a simulated eating task. Five kidney beans are placed in a bowl 5 inches from the edge of the table in front of the patient. An empty coffee can is placed on the table at the patient's nondominant side. A teaspoon is placed in the patient's dominant hand. The patient is asked on the command "Go!" to pick up the beans, one at a time with the spoon, and place them in the coffee can (Figure 9-17). Timing begins with the command "Go!" and ends when the last bean is heard hitting the bottom of the can. The patient can use the other hand to steady the bowl, but not to move it in any way. The other hand cannot help steady the can or complete the task except to help pick up a dropped bean. Sometimes, the use of a nonskid mat may be indicated. If the patient drops a bean, timing continues while the patient uses his or her dominant hand to pick up the bean.

Instructions to Patient: "This second task is an eating task. When I say 'Go!' I want you to use your spoon to move one bean at a time from this can to the bowl, like this. You cannot use your other hand except to steady the bowl. Are you ready? Go!"

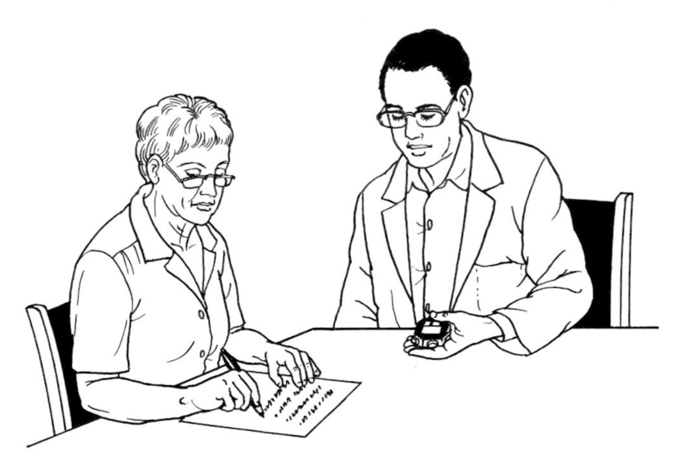

FIGURE 9-16

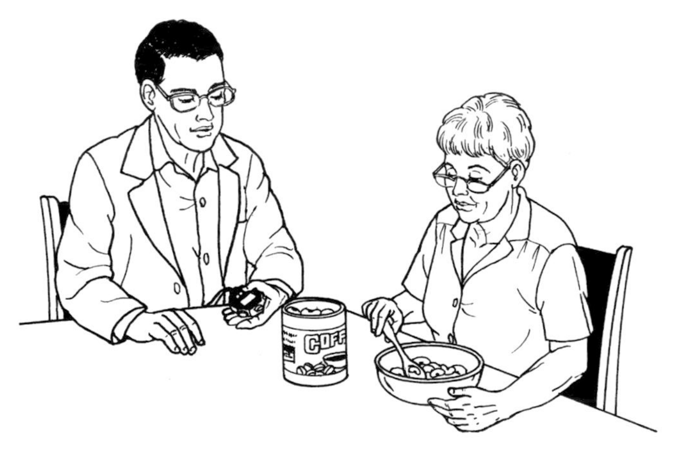

FIGURE 9-17

3. Lifting a Book onto a Shelf

Testing Procedure: The third task is done with the patient sitting on a chair (or other surface) (Figure 9-18), or standing (Figure 9-19), depending on whether you want to assess the patient's standing or sitting balance while lifting. It is handy to use an open cabinet with multiple and/or two adjustable shelves, usually available in a clinic. Having multiple or two adjustable shelves helps accommodate the patient's height. The countertop can serve as the starting position for the book placement.

Adjust the higher shelf so that it is 12 inches above the patient's shoulders. A 5.5-pound book, similar to a *Physicians' Desk Reference*, is placed on the edge of the counter, with the book hanging slightly off the edge of the counter to make it easy for the patient to grab. On "Go!" the patient lifts the book to the upper shelf with timing stopped when the patient removes his or her hand from the book after it is placed on the top shelf. In the original PPT test, the patient is seated during the task (see Figure 9-18). However, the task can be performed standing if desired (see Figure 9-19).

The therapist should demonstrate this task to assure understanding. The time is recorded on the scoring form.

Instructions to Patient: "For this task, I want you to lift this book to this shelf while I time you. Do you understand? Now, I'll demonstrate. OK, when I say 'Go!' you may begin."

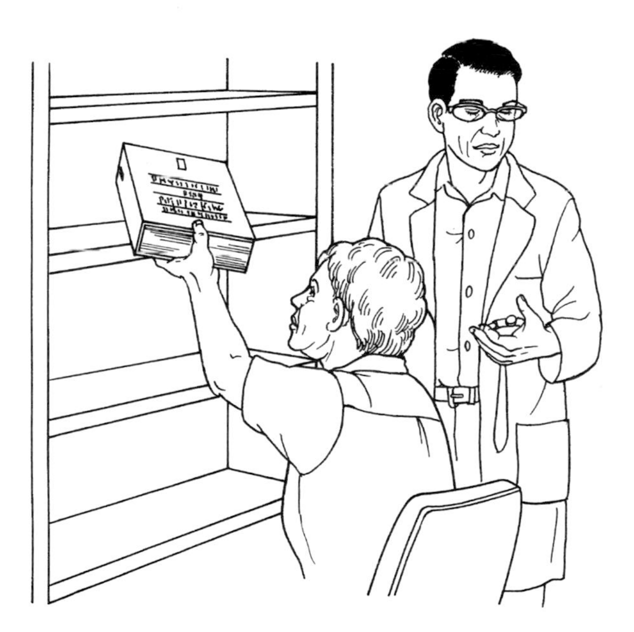

FIGURE 9-18

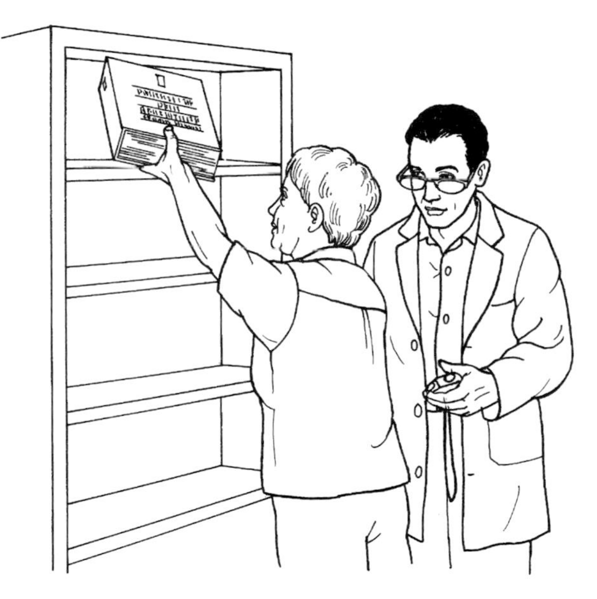

FIGURE 9-19

4. Putting On and Taking Off a Garment

Testing Procedure: The fourth task involves putting on and removing a garment in a standing position. An extra-large bathrobe, front-buttoned shirt, or hospital gown can be used and put on so that it opens in the front. If the patient has a jacket or sweater that opens in the front, use that. Make sure the garment is large enough to put on over any clothes the patient is wearing. To start, the garment is held so the label inside the garment is facing the patient (Figure 9-20).

The patient is instructed to start with arms at sides and on "Go!" to take the garment, put it on (Figure 9-21), square it on the shoulders, and then remove it completely, holding it out to the therapist. Timing begins on "Go!" and ends when the patient hands the jacket to the therapist.

Instructions to Patient: "This task involves putting on and taking off this jacket while I time you. When I say 'Go!' I want you to take the jacket from me, put it on so that it is square on your shoulders, and then take it off and hand it back to me. Now Go!"

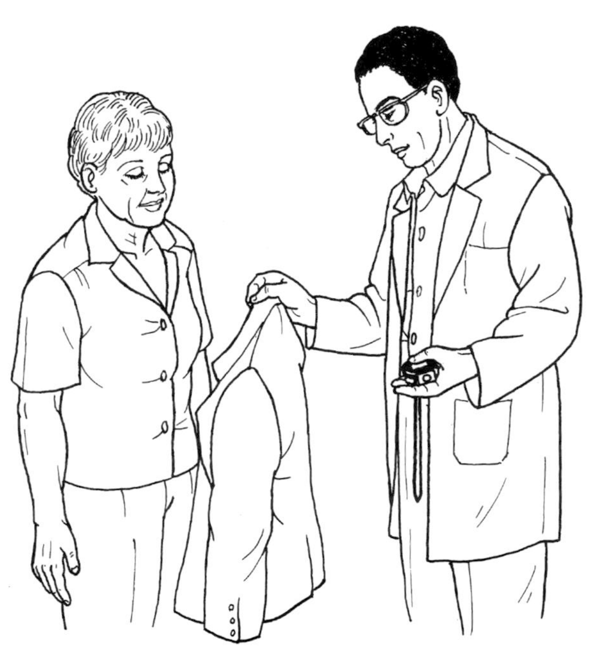

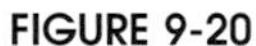

FIGURE 9-20

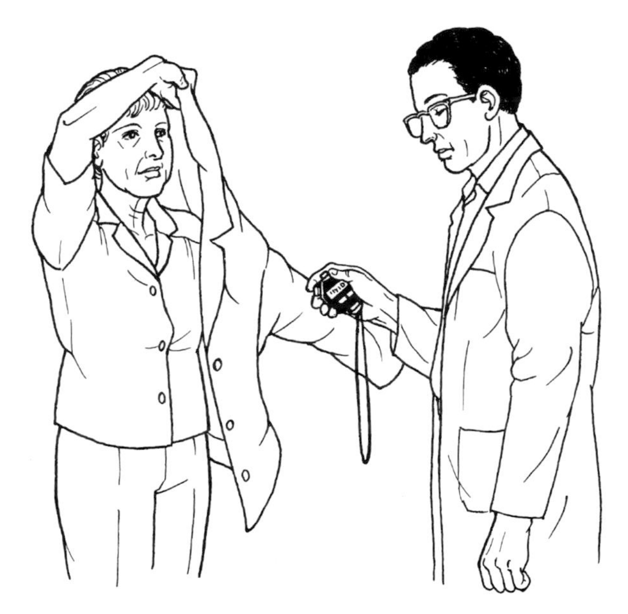

FIGURE 9-21

5. Picking Up a Coin From the Floor

Testing Procedure: This task involves picking up a coin from the floor. This task is also timed. A coin is placed approximately 12 inches from the patient's foot (usually the dominant side). On the command "Go!" the patient picks up the coin from the floor and returns to a fully upright position (Figure 9-22). The timing will begin with the command "Go!" and end when the patient is standing erect with coin in hand.

Instructions to Patient: "I'm going to put a coin on the floor and on 'Go!' I want you to pick it up, completely stand up, and hand it to me. OK. Are you ready? Good. Remember, I'm timing you."

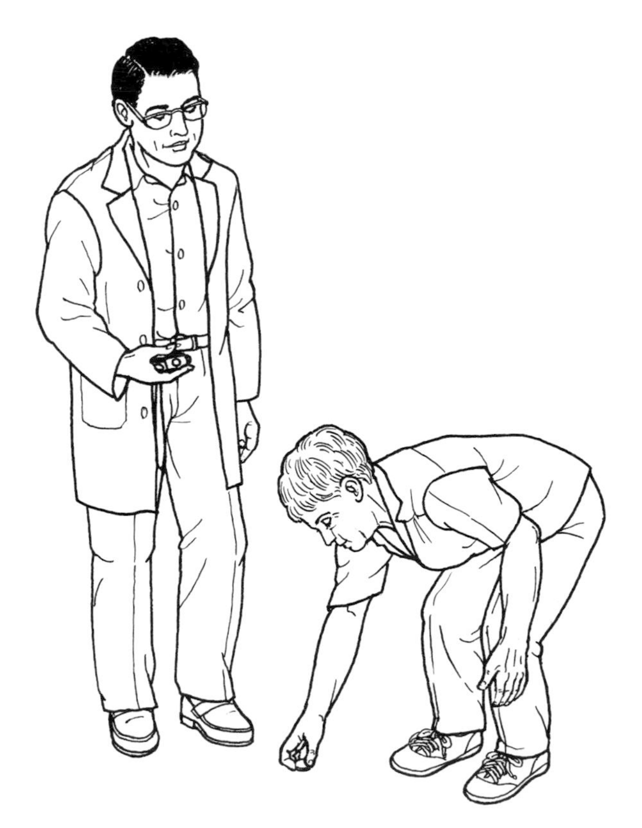

FIGURE 9-22

6. 360° Turn

Testing Procedure: This task involves making a complete 360° turn to test the patient's ability to turn around in a circle in both directions (Figure 9-23). This effort is not timed, but rather is scored in terms of the quality and safety of the effort.

The patient is instructed to turn 360° at a comfortable pace (in either direction) beginning with the toes pointed forward and ending when the toes are pointed forward again. This task should be demonstrated before testing. The demonstration speed of turning should not be so fast that it encourages the patient to mimic it, thus compromising the patient's safety. Both directions will be examined, so it does not matter which direction is performed first. Typically, the patient will choose his or her best direction to perform first. The performance is evaluated for continuity of movement and steadiness.

Instructions to Patient: "I want you to turn in a full circle so that your toes are back on this line. You can choose whichever direction you want to go toward first, since I will ask you to go in the other direction next. I will not be timing you."

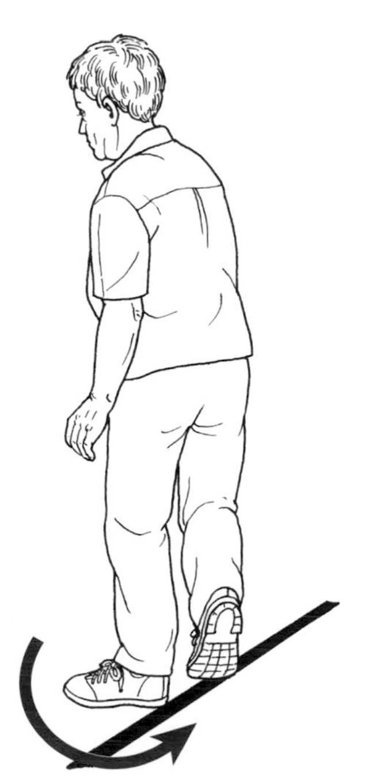

FIGURE 9-23

7. Timed 50-foot Walk

Testing Procedure: This is a timed 50-foot walk task designed to examine gait speed and observe the quality of the patient's gait. The patient is brought to the start of a 50-foot walk test course that consists of a walkway 25 feet out and 25 feet back. No acceleration or deceleration distance is needed because of the distance. The patient is asked, on the command "Go!" to walk to the 25-foot mark and back. Timing begins with the command "Go!" and ends when the starting line is crossed on the way back. The time is recorded on the scoring form. An assistive device may be used, and the type of device should be documented. Typically, demonstration is not needed on this task because walking is a familiar task.

Instructions to Patient: "This is a walking task over 50 feet. I'd like you to walk out and back as quickly but as safely as you can. You will turn around at the end of the walkway and return to this spot. I will be timing you." (Note: It is not as important to time according to foot placement as in the 4-meter gait speed test because the distance is much longer.)

Once the seventh task is performed, the seven-item version of the PPT is complete. If you do not intend to have the patient perform stair climbing, add up the scores for the seven items now.

The next two items involve the stair climbing tasks, which are included in the nine-item version.

8. Climbing One Flight of Stairs

Testing Procedure: Note that the stair climb tasks, (climbing one flight of stairs and climbing four flights of stairs) may be performed together, but they are scored separately. Before beginning these two tasks, the patient is alerted to the possibility of developing chest pain or shortness of breath and is told to inform the test administrator if any of these symptoms occur. Vital signs should be monitored as indicated. Indications to monitor vital signs include evidence of more than ordinary effort expended in any previous task such as complaints of fatigue and the need to rest between tasks.

For task 8, the timed stair climb, the patient is asked to climb one flight of stairs that has 9 to 12 steps. The timing starts with the command "Go!" and ends when the patient's first foot reaches the top of the top step. The patient may use a handrail and/or assistive device and this should be noted on the scoring form as well as the time taken to climb one flight of stairs.

Instructions to Patient: "This task involves climbing a flight of stairs as quickly but as safely as you can (Figure 9-24). You may use the handrail if you need to. For this task, you are only required to go up to the landing. Stair climbing may require more than usual effort, so please let me know if you experience any tightness or pain in your chest or if you are short of breath and need to stop. OK? Go!"

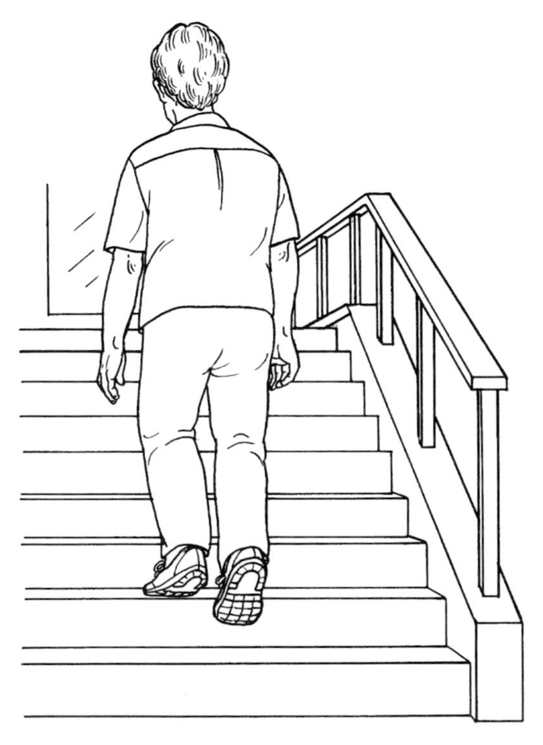

FIGURE 9-24

9. Climbing Four Flights of Stairs

Testing Procedure: In this task, the patient is asked to climb four flights of stairs. The scoring is based on how many flights, up and down, the patient was able to complete. The patient is asked on the command "Go!" to begin descending the first flight of stairs, counted as one, and to reclimb the same flight. This up and down climbing is to continue until the patient feels tired and wishes to stop, or until four flights, four ups and four downs total, have been climbed.

Record the number of flights (maximum of four) climbed (up and down is one flight). A handrail and/or an assistive device may be used.

Typically, a demonstration is not needed and only one trial is given. It is also wise to ask the patient how many flights he or she thinks can be completed to give some idea of the anticipated level of performance. Patients should be gently encouraged but not coerced or forced to do more than they feel they can safely and comfortably do.

Instructions to Patient: "Now, the next task is to climb, up and down, as many as four flights of stairs. You can determine how many flights you feel comfortable doing. You are scored based on the number of flights. Are you willing to try? How many flights do you think you can do?"

Position of Patient: Dependent on task. See specific task instructions.

Position of Therapist: Dependent on task. Safety should always be a concern, but the therapist's presence should not impede performance.

Scoring

Each task's performance is recorded on the PPT scoring form (Figure 9-25). Reuben and Siu established percentile norms based on the performance of a 79-year-old male who is independent in all activities of daily living.[29]

25th percentile ... 21 (9-item), 15 (7-item)
75th percentile ... 29 (9-item), 22 (7-item)
90th percentile ... 31 (9-item), 24 (7-item)

Helpful Hint

Timing a patient during task performance should be done with the utmost awareness of the influence of timing. Many patients may move faster than is safe, because of a competitive nature. In some cases, it may not be best practice to tell the patient the task is timed, especially in cases where balance is significantly impaired.

Physical Performance Test Scoring Sheet

			Physical Performance Test		
			Time	**Scoring**	**Score**
1	Writing task: (Write the sentence "Whales live in a blue ocean.")	Sec*		≤10 sec = 4 10.5–15 sec = 3 15.5–20 sec = 2 >20 sec = 1 unable = 0	
2	Eating task (simulated eating)	Sec		≤10 sec = 4 10.5–15 sec = 3 15.5–20 sec = 2 >20 sec = 1 unable = 0	
3	Lift a book and put it on a shelf Book: approximately 5.5 lbs Bed height: 23 in Shelf height: 46 in	Sec		≤2 sec = 4 2.5–4 sec = 3 4.5–6 sec = 2 >6 sec = 1 unable = 0	
4	Put on and remove a garment 1. Standing 2. Use of bathrobe, button-down shirt, or hospital gown	Sec		≤10 sec = 4 10.5–15 sec = 3 15.5–20 sec = 2 >20 sec = 1 unable = 0	
5	Pick up a coin from the floor	Sec		≤2 sec = 4 2.5–4 sec = 3 4.5–6 sec = 2 >6 sec = 1 unable = 0	
6	Turn 360°		Discontinuous steps = 0 Continuous steps = 2 Unsteady (grabs, staggers) = 0 Steady = 2		
7	50-foot walk test (15.24 meters) <15 sec = 3.33 feet/sec or 1.0 m/sec	Sec		≤15 sec = 4 15.5–20 sec = 3 20.5–25 sec = 2 >25 sec = 1 unable = 0	
8	Climb one flight of stairs	Sec		≤5 sec = 4 5.5–10 sec = 3 10.5–15 sec = 2 >15 sec = 1 unable = 0	
9	Climb four flights of stairs		Number of flights of stairs up and down (maximum of 4)		
	TOTAL SCORE (maxium 36 for nine-item; 28 for seven-item)				
	*For time measurements, round to nearest 0.5 seconds			Total score	

Data from: Reuben DB, Siu AL. An Objective Measure of Physical Function of Elderly Outpatients (the Physical Performance Test). *Journal of the American Geriatric Society* 1990; 38(10): 1105-1112.

FIGURE 9-25 Physical Performance Test (PPT) scoring form.

Purpose: The modified physical performance test (MPPT)[34] is similar to the nine-item PPT, except the two measures of hand function are replaced with tests of balance and leg strength from the SPPB. Thus, the MPPT, as with the PPT, measures aspects of physical function and activities of daily living in older adults using nine different items that emphasize mobility tasks.

Essential Muscle Movements for Task Performance:

Balance Tasks: Ankle dorsiflexion with inversion, plantar flexion, foot inversion, foot eversion with plantar flexion, knee extension, and hip abduction and extension.

Chair Stand: Hip extension, hip abduction from a flexed position, hip external rotation, knee extension, ankle plantar flexion, ankle dorsiflexion and inversion,[4] and trunk extension and flexion.

Lifting a Book onto a Shelf in Sitting or Standing: scapular upward rotation and protraction shoulder flexion, shoulder external rotation, elbow flexion and extension, forearm supination and pronation, wrist flexion and extension, and finger MP, PIP, and DIP flexion

Putting On and Taking Off Garment (Depending on Technique): Scapular protraction and upward rotation shoulder flexion, shoulder external rotation, elbow flexion and extension, forearm supination and pronation, wrist flexion and extension, and finger MP, PIP, and DIP flexion. Core stability (for sitting or standing). If task is performed in standing: hip extension and abduction, knee extension, ankle plantar flexion, and ankle dorsiflexion with inversion.

Picking Up a Coin: Back extension, hip extension, knee extension, ankle plantar flexion, elbow flexion and extension, forearm supination and pronation, wrist flexion and extension, and finger MP, PIP, and DIP flexion.

360° Turn: Ankle dorsiflexion with inversion, plantar flexion, foot inversion, foot eversion with plantar flexion, knee extension, hip abduction and extension, and core stability.

Walking Task: Hip extension and abduction, knee extension, ankle plantar flexion, ankle dorsiflexion with inversion.[12] Hip flexion also contributes to walking velocity.[13] The reader is referred to the gait section of this chapter for a more specific list of muscles that are imperative for smooth and normal gait.

Stair Climb Tasks: Ascent: hip extension, knee flexion, ankle plantar flexion, ankle dorsiflexion, spine extension, and core stability. Descent: eccentric knee extension, hip flexion, and core muscles. For a task that requires stability and balance however, any lower extremity muscle or group will be used at some point during the task.

Reliability: Not tested.

Validity: The MPPT can indicate whether an individual is frail.[34]

Equipment:

Scoring form
Stopwatch
Coin
Standard chair without arms
5.5-pound book
A bookshelf with two adjustable shelves
Patient's jacket or front-button sweater or extra-large lab coat, hospital gown, or other front-opening garment
25-foot walkway
One flight of stairs (9 to 12 stairs)

Testing Procedure: The MPPT will require approximately 10 minutes to complete. The nine tasks can be done in any order; however, here they are described in the order they appear on the scoring form. Each task is timed, except for task 9 (climbing four flights of stairs) and task 6 (turning 360°). A total of 36 points is possible. An assistive device can be used for the walking and stair climbing tasks, but not for the other tasks. Each task is performed twice, with the lowest performance used for scoring. (Note: It is recommended to use the lowest score because of the need to accurately record the patient's performance in the clinical setting. Although performance may improve with repeated trials, the most genuine real-life performance may be the lowest timed or poorest performance.)

As in all tests, the patient's safety should be assured. Although assistance from the therapist is not permitted during performance of the test, the therapist should be vigilant for balance problems. A gait belt is always recommended during test performance.

The nine tasks are:

1. Standing static balance
   a. Side-by-side stance
   b. Semi-tandem stance
   c. Full tandem stance
2. Chair stand (five-repetition)
3. Lifting a book onto a shelf
4. Putting on and taking off a garment
5. Picking up a coin from the floor
6. 360° turn
7. 50-foot walk
8. Climbing one flight of stairs
9. Climbing four flights of stairs

1. Standing Static Balance Tasks

Testing Procedure: These balance tasks examine the patient's ability to stand in three positions: side-by-side, semi-tandem, and full tandem. The three positions should be tested in order because they increase in difficulty. All three balance positions are timed. If the patient cannot perform one position, then the next position is not performed but rather is scored as "unable." These positions are designed to maximally challenge balance, so the therapist should be alert for balance difficulties and maintain the patient's safety at all times.

Each balance position is timed for a maximum of 10 seconds. The semi-tandem and tandem positions are tested with each foot forward (unlike the SPPB, where only one foot is tested) with the poorest performance scored. Foot positioning should be strictly observed. No out-toeing is permitted. If the patient cannot attain the proper position, the score is zero for that stance task. Only one trial is allowed for each position. (The original instructions, stated here, were for research purposes. In the clinical situation, patients may not be able to assume the ideal position because of severe valgus, for example. Therefore, the therapist should score the best attempt, with a notation of the position assumed.)

Each position is practiced before testing. If necessary, the patient is assisted to assume the positions because during testing the positioning is strictly observed; however, when timing starts, no support is given. Once the patient appears to be steady, the therapist asks if the patient is ready. When the patient says yes, the therapist says "Ready, begin," then starts the timing (relinquishing support if it was initially needed to assume the correct position). The timing is continued until the patient moves the feet, grasps the therapist for support, or 10 seconds have elapsed. Record any time less than 10 seconds to the nearest hundredth of a second on the test form.

a. Side-by-side Stance

Testing Procedure: The first balance task is the side-by-side stance. In this position, the patient is requested to stand for 10 seconds with the feet together in a side-by-side stance position (Figure 9-26).

Instructions to Patient: "The balancing tasks involve you standing in three different positions and holding each position for up to 10 seconds. First we'll start with the side-by-side stance position. You can use me to get into the position but then you have to stand by yourself. I will be timing you when you are steady enough to let go.

"First, I want you to place your feet completely together, like this. Then hold that position as long as you can. Ready? Begin."

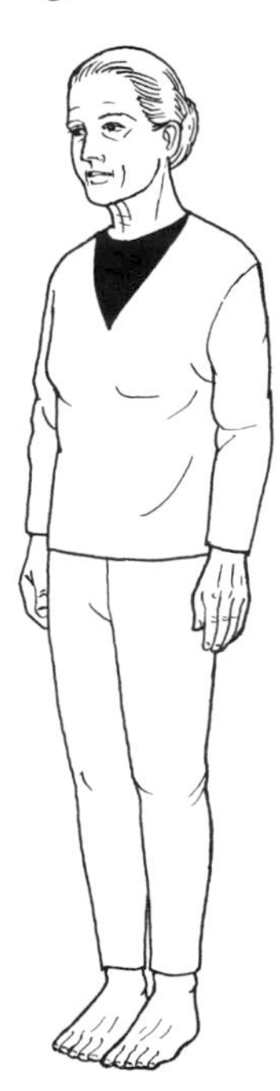

FIGURE 9-26

b. Semi-tandem Stance

Testing Procedure: The second balance task is the semi-tandem stance position. The patient starts with the heel of one foot placed to the side of and touching the big toe of the other foot. Each foot should be placed in the forward position and timed separately (Figure 9-27). (Note: This task should be performed only in patients who were able to perform the previous side-by-side task.)

Instructions to Patient: "Move one foot in front of the other so that the heel of the front foot is against the side of the big toe of the other foot, like this. Make sure you do not turn your foot out. You can choose which ever foot you like, because I will test you on both sides. Begin! Great! Now let's try the other side. Ready, begin!"

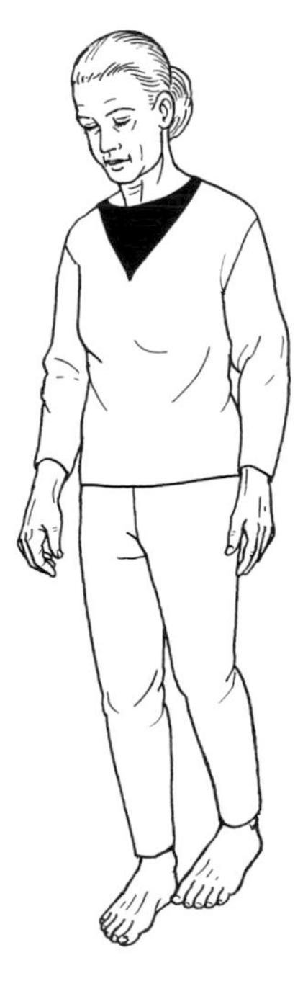

FIGURE 9-27

c. Full Tandem Stance

Testing Procedure: The third and final position is the tandem stance position. To assume the tandem stance position, the heel of one foot is placed directly in front of the toes of the other foot. Either foot can be placed in the forward position (Figure 9-28). (Note: This task should be performed only in patients who were able to perform the semi-tandem stance.)

Instructions to Patient: "Place the heel of one foot directly in front of the toes of the other foot, like this." (Demonstrate the correct position for the patient.) "Either foot can be placed in the forward position because we will be testing both of your feet. I will hold you, if necessary, until you are ready. Are you ready? Now begin."

Helpful Hint

Allowing the patient to choose which foot to place forward in the semi-tandem or full tandem stance may indicate which foot the patient feels is stronger.

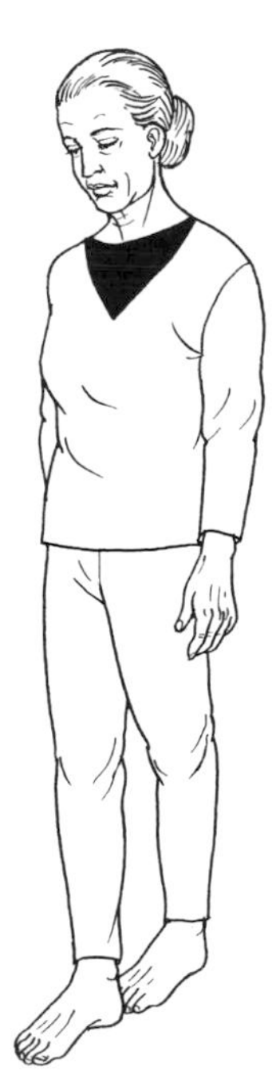

FIGURE 9-28

2. Chair Stand (Five-repetition)

Testing Procedure: The chair stand task is a test of leg strength. The patient is first asked to stand from the chair with the arms folded across the chest while the therapist observes. If the patient is able to rise from the chair once, the patient is then asked to stand up and sit down five times as quickly as possible. Timing begins as soon as the command to stand is given and continues until the patient is fully upright at the end of the fifth stand.

Position of Patient: Seated, with arms crossed over the chest. Feet are planted on the floor in a comfortable position (Figure 9-29).

Instructions to Patient: "This task measures the strength of your legs. First, fold your arms across your chest and sit so that your feet are on the floor. Then, stand up, keeping your arms folded across your chest." (After it is observed that the patient can safely stand independently without the use of the arms, proceed to the timed five-repetition part of the chair stand task.) "Now stand up straight, as quickly as you can, five times, without stopping in between. After standing up each time, sit down and then stand up again. Keep your arms folded across your chest. I'll be timing you with a stopwatch."

3. Lifting a Book onto a Shelf

Testing Procedure: For this task, the height of two shelves is adjusted—one at the patient's waist level and the other 12 inches above the patient's shoulders. A 5.5-pound book, similar in size to a *Physicians' Desk Reference*, is placed on the edge of the lower shelf, with the book hanging slightly off the shelf to make it easy for the patient to grab. The patient is then asked to lift the book from the lower shelf to the upper shelf while the effort is timed. The therapist should demonstrate this task to ensure understanding.

Position of Patient: Standing, facing the shelf. (Figure 9-30).

Instructions to Patient: "I want you to lift this book from this shelf to the higher shelf. I'll be timing you. Let me show you. Do you understand? Good. Ready, begin."

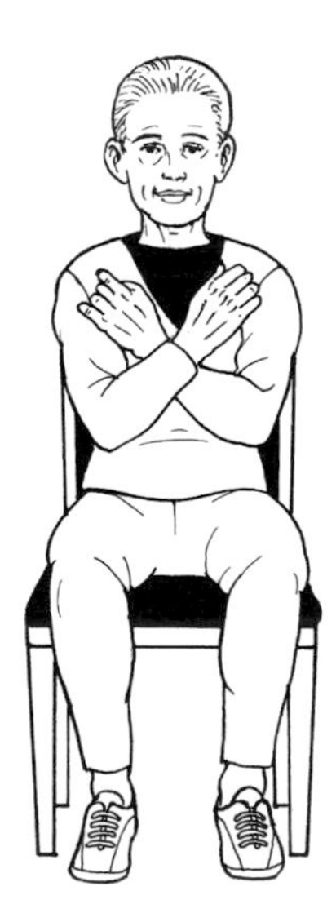

FIGURE 9-29

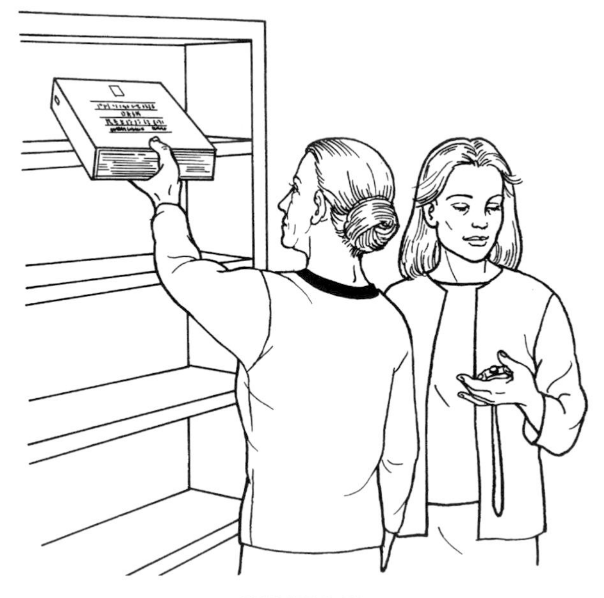

FIGURE 9-30

4. Putting On and Taking Off a Garment

Testing Procedure: This task involves putting on and removing a garment in a standing position. An extra-large bathrobe, front-buttoned shirt, lab coat, or hospital gown can be used, putting it on so that it opens in the front. If the patient has a jacket or front opening sweater, use that, or have a garment large enough to go over the patient's clothes.

Position of Patient: Patient standing, arms at sides.

Position of Therapist: The garment is held so the label inside the garment is facing the patient (Figure 9-31).

Instructions to Patient: When I say "Go!" I want you to take this jacket, put it on, square it on your shoulders, and then take it off and hand it to me. You can put the jacket on any way you like, but you must square the shoulders. I'll be timing you. Ready? Begin."

5. Picking Up a Coin from the Floor

Testing Procedure: This is a timed task of the patient's ability to pick up a coin from the floor. A coin is placed approximately 12 inches from the patient's foot on the dominant side. On the command "Go!" the patient is asked to pick up the coin from the floor and return to a fully upright position (Figure 9-32). The timing will begin with the command "Go!" and end when the patient is standing erect with coin in hand.

Position of Patient: Standing with coin in front of dominant foot.

Instructions to Patient: "I'm going to put this coin on the floor and on 'Go!' I want you to pick it up, completely stand up and hand it to me. You will have two tries. I'll demonstrate first. Are you ready? Go!"

Helpful Hint

- If working with a patient with low vision, someone who may not be able to visualize a coin on the floor, substitute a larger sized item such as a pencil or pen. Substituting a larger item obviates the need for a patient to spend excess time with their head down near the ground because they can't find the coin.

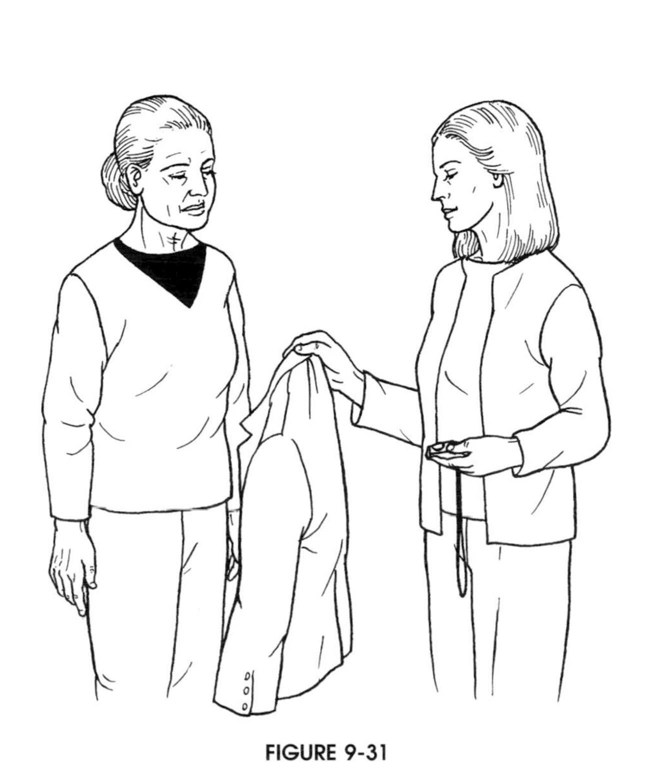

FIGURE 9-31

FIGURE 9-32

6. 360° Turn

Testing Procedure: The 360° turn task examines the patient's ability to turn in a complete circle in both directions. This effort is not timed, but rather scored for the quality and safety of the effort.

The patient is instructed to place his or her toes on a line, then turn 360° at a comfortable pace (in either direction) until the toes are back on the line (Figure 9-33).

This task should be demonstrated before testing. The demonstration speed of turning should not be so fast that it encourages the patient to mimic it, thus compromising his or her safety. Both directions will be examined, so it does not matter which direction is performed first. Typically, the patient will choose his or her best direction to perform first. The performance is evaluated for continuity of movement and steadiness.

Position of Patient: Standing, with toes pointed forward, toward the line.

Instructions to Patient: "I want you to turn in a full circle so that your toes are back in the starting position on this line. You can choose whichever direction you want to go towards first, because I will ask you to go in the other direction next. This effort is not timed, so take your time to be safe. Let me show you. Whenever you are ready, begin. Good. Now turn in the other direction."

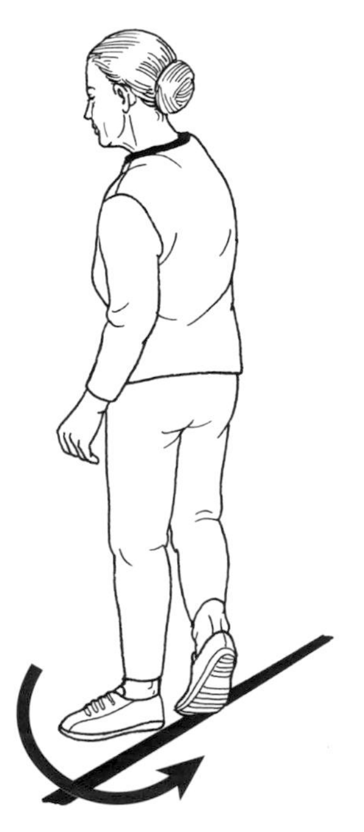

FIGURE 9-33

7. 50-foot Walk

Testing Procedure: This task is a measure of gait speed over 50 feet. The patient is brought to the start of a 50-foot walk test course that consists of a walkway 25 feet out and 25 feet back. No acceleration or deceleration distance is needed because of the distance. The patient is asked, on the command "Go!" to walk to the 25-foot mark and back. Timing is begun with the command "Go!" and ends when the starting line is crossed on the way back. The time is recorded on the scoring form. An assistive device may be used, and the type of device should be documented. Demonstration is not needed on this task because walking is a familiar task.

Instructions to Patient: "I want you to walk out and back as quickly but as safely as you can. You will turn around at the end of the walkway and return to this spot. I will be timing you, and you'll do this twice. Are you ready? Begin." When the patient is ready, retest again. (Note: It is not as important to time according to where the foot crosses the start and finish line as in the 4-meter gait speed test because the distance is much longer.)

8. Climbing One Flight of Stairs

Testing Procedure: The stair climb tasks (climbing one flight of stairs and climbing four flights of stairs) may be performed together, but they are scored separately. Generally, only one trial is given.

For the timed stair climb task, the patient is asked to climb one flight of stairs that has 9-12 steps. The timing starts with the command "Go!" and ends when the patient's first foot reaches the top of the top step. The patient may use a handrail and/or assistive device and this should be noted on the scoring sheet.

9. Climbing Four Flights of Stairs

Testing Procedure: In this task, the patient is asked to climb four flights of stairs. The scoring is based on how many flights, up and down, the patient was able to complete. This task is not timed. The patient is asked on the command "Go!" to begin descending the first flight of stairs, counted as one, and to reclimb the same flight. This up-and-down climbing is to continue until he or she feels tired and wishes to stop, or until four flights, four ups and four downs, have been completed (Figure 9-34). Record the number of flights (maximum of four) completed (up and down is one flight).

Before beginning the task, the patient is alerted to the possibility of developing chest pain or shortness of breath and is told to inform the test administrator if any of these symptoms occur. Vital signs should be monitored as indicated.

Typically, a demonstration is not needed and only one trial is given. It is also wise to ask the patient how many flights he or she thinks he or she can complete to give some idea of the anticipated level of performance. Patients should be gently encouraged but not coerced or forced to do more than they feel they are capable of.

A handrail and/or an assistive device may be used to ensure safety.

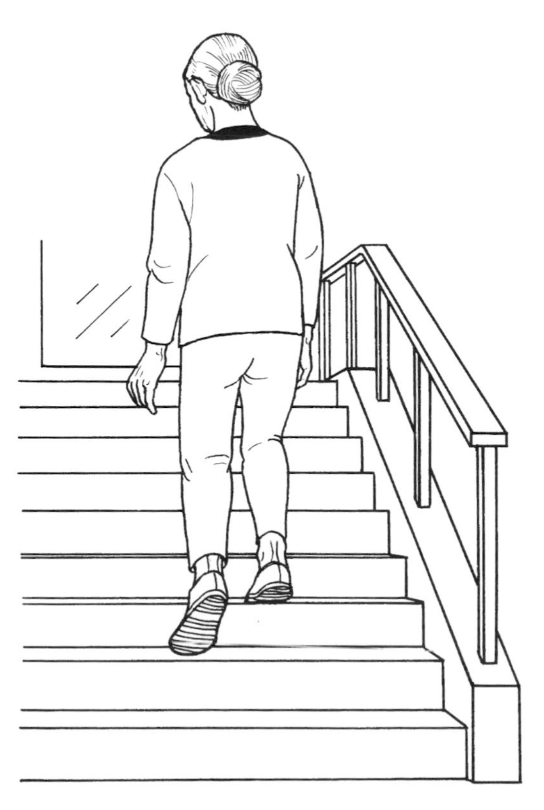

FIGURE 9-34

Instructions to Patient: "This task involves climbing this flight of stairs as quickly but as safely as you can. You may use the handrail. For the first part, you are only required to go up to the landing, then stop before beginning the next part.

"Stair climbing may require more than usual effort, so please let me know if you experience any tightness or pain in your chest or if you are short of breath and need to stop.

Are you ready? Go!"

"Now, the next task is to climb, up and down, as many as four flights of stairs. You can determine how many flights you feel comfortable doing. You are scored based on the number of flights. This part is NOT timed. You may turn around at the landing at any time you feel too tired or uncomfortable to continue. Are you ready? Begin."

Scoring

See scoring form in Figure 9-35. For any task that the patient is unable to perform, score a zero.

Helpful Hints

- Completing the 50 feet (15.24 meters) in 15 seconds is equal to a 1.0 m/s pace. You can calculate the patient's gait speed by dividing the distance walked by the time.
- Gait speeds of over 0.8 m/s are typically required for safe community ambulation.

Modified Physical Performance Test

1.	Standing Static Balance	Feet Together: ____sec	Semi-tandem: ____sec	Tandem: ____sec	Score
		❑ 10 sec	❑ 10 sec	❑ 10 sec	❑ 4
		❑ 10 sec	❑ 10 sec	❑ 3–9.9 sec	❑ 3
		❑ 10 sec	❑ 10 sec	❑ 0–2.9 sec	❑ 2
		❑ 10 sec	❑ 0–9 sec	Unable	❑ 1
		❑ 0–9 sec	Unable	Unable	❑ 0
			Time	**Scoring values**	Score
2.	Chair stand (5 × without arms)			≤11 sec = 4 11.1–14 sec = 3 14.1–17 sec = 2 >17 sec = 1 unable = 0	
3.	Lift a book and put it on a shelf			≤2 sec = 4 2.1–4 sec = 3 4.1–6 sec = 2 >6 sec = 1 unable = 0	
4.	Put on and remove a garment			≤10 sec = 4 10.1–15 sec = 3 15.1–20 sec = 2 >20 sec = 1 unable = 0	
5.	Pick up a coin from the floor			≤2 sec = 4 2.1–4 sec = 3 4.1–6 sec = 2 >6 sec = 1 unable = 0	
6.	Turn 360°		Discontinuous steps = 0 Continuous steps = 2		
			Unsteady (grabs, staggers) = 0 Steady = 2		
7.	50-foot walk			≤15 sec = 4 15.1–20 sec = 3 20.1–25 sec = 2 >25 sec = 1 unable = 0	
8.	Climb one flight of stairs			≤5 sec = 4 5.1–10 sec = 3 10.1–15 sec = 2 >15 sec = 1 unable = 0	
9.	Climb four flights of stairs		Number of flights of stairs up and down (maximum 4)		
TOTAL SCORE				9-item score	/36

FIGURE 9-35 Scoring form for Modified Physical Performance Test (MPPT).

Purpose: The timed up and go test (TUG) is a test of general mobility that involves standing from a standard-height chair, walking, turning and sitting down.[35] The test can be performed with an assistive device.[36] Typically, performance time increases with the use of an assistive device.

The TUG takes only seconds to perform and can be used in all health care settings because of the minimal equipment and space required. The test can be used to identify impairments related to mobility.

Essential Muscle Movements for Task Performance: Hip extension, hip abduction from a flexed position, hip external rotation, knee extension, ankle plantar flexion, ankle dorsiflexion and inversion,[4] and trunk extension and flexion. Hip flexion also contributes to walking velocity.[13] The reader is referred to the gait section of this chapter for a more specific list of muscles that are imperative for smooth and normal gait.

Reliability: Intra-class correlation coefficient (ICC) = 0.99; test-retest reliability ICC – 0.99.[37] In individuals with Alzheimer's disease, ICC = 0.97.[38]

Validity: The TUG is a valid test for determining fall risk, with 13.5 seconds or more as a cutoff with 0.80 sensitivity and 1.0 specificity.[37] Construct validity is for independence in mobility (the time taken is strongly correlated to the level of functional mobility).[37] Similar to gait speed, it can predict global health and new ADL difficulty.

Equipment: Standard 17-inch-high chair with arms, stopwatch, and 3 meters measured on floor.

Testing Procedure: The test involves the patient standing, walking at the patient's usual and comfortable speed 3 meters to a specified mark on the floor, turning around and walking back to the chair, and sitting all the way back down in the chair. A chair with arms is placed against a wall to prevent the chair from moving. Then a distance of 3 meters is measured from the patient's toes with the patient seated in the chair. A line or other object should indicate the 3-meter mark (Figure 9-36). Timing starts when the therapist says "Go!" rather than when the patient starts to rise. Be clear so that the patient knows you are about to start the test. You will want to make sure the patient can hear you and waits for your "Go!" Stop timing when the patient is fully seated with his or her back against the chair. A practice trial is given before the two test trials are performed.

Position of Patient: Initially seated in a chair with arms with his or her feet in contact with the floor and his or her back against the back of the chair.

Position of Therapist: Standing to the side of the patient. The therapist may choose to walk with the patient if safety is a concern (Figure 9-37).

Instructions to Patient: "On 'Go!' I want you to stand up and walk as quickly but as safely as you can to the mark on the floor, turn, and return to the chair, sitting down with your back against the back of the chair. I'll be timing you, OK?"

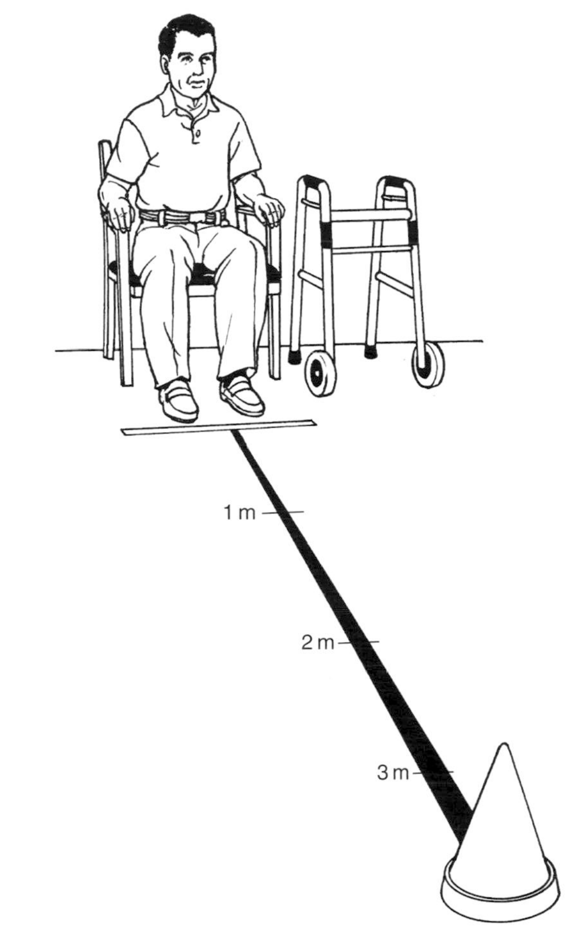

FIGURE 9-36

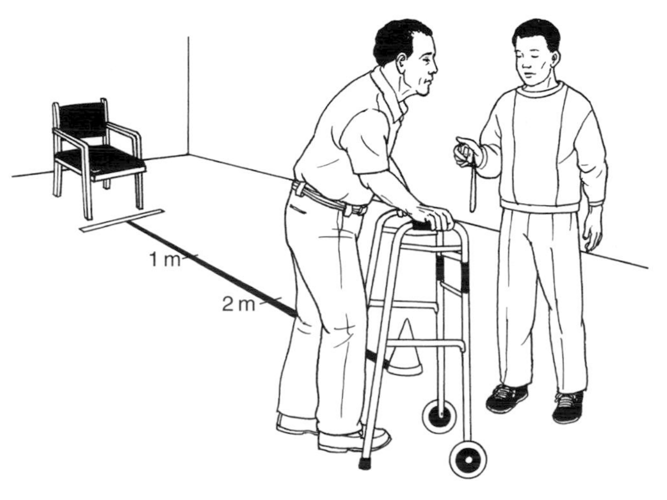

FIGURE 9-37

Scoring

The fastest time taken to perform the TUG is the score.

10 seconds or faster indicates the patient is freely mobile.

13.5 seconds or slower indicates a risk for falls.[37]

24 seconds or slower is predictive of falls within 6 months after hip fracture.[39]

30 seconds or slower indicates the patient is dependent in mobility.[40]

Norms

A total of 92% of community-dwelling older adults had TUG times of less than 12 seconds, whereas only 9% of institutionalized patients performed the TUG in that time. Community-dwelling women between 65 and 85 years of age should be able to perform the TUG in 12 seconds or less.[41]

TUG times are worse than average if they exceed 9.0 seconds for 60- to 69-year-olds, 10.2 seconds for 70- to 79-year-olds, and 12.7 seconds for 80- to 99-year-olds.[42] Table 9-8 lists normative values for the TUG test.

Table 9-8 NORMATIVE REFERENCE VALUES FOR THE TIMED UP AND GO TEST

Age Group	Time in Seconds (95% Confidence Interval)
60-69 y	8.1 (7.1-9.0)
70-79 y	9.2 (8.2-10.2)
80-89 y	11.3 (10.0-12.7)

Data from Bohannon RW. Reference values for the timed up and go test: a descriptive meta-analysis. J Geriatr Phys Ther. 2006;29(2):64-68.

Helpful Hints

- Measure the distance from the patient's toes.
- If using an object to mark the farthest point of the 3-meter distance, make sure it is moved forward of the 3-meter mark to avoid lengthening the course as the patient walks around the object (see Figure 9-37).
- Always retest using the same assistive device as used in the original test.
- Avoid overcoaching. Valuable information that will inform clinical decision-making can be obtained from observing how the patient chooses to perform the test.
- Using the general procedure for the TUG, a timed performance can be obtained from any surface, such as a couch or car seat, to assist in clinical decision-making and objective documentation.

Purpose: The stair climb test assesses the ability to climb a flight of stairs. Qualitative and quantitative assessment can be made to determine the amount of assistance a patient needs, identify impairments that may contribute to stair climbing, and indicate how quickly and/or safely the patient can accomplish the task. The stair climb test is also used as a functional test of power.[43,44]

Essential Muscle Movements for Task Performance: Ascent—hip extension, knee flexion, ankle plantar flexion, ankle dorsiflexion, spine extension, and core stability. Descent—eccentric knee extension, hip flexion, and core muscles. For a test that requires stability and balance, however, any lower extremity muscle or group will be used at some point during the task.

Reliability: ICC = 0.99[45]

Validity: Predictor of fall risk (descent); ascent (borderline predictor of fall risk).

Ascent: When 5 seconds or more are needed to climb eight stairs, the test indicates a risk for multiple falls with a positive likelihood ratio (LR) of 1.29 (sensitivity [Sn] = 0.54; specificity [Sp] = 0.58).[46]

Descent: When 5 seconds or more are needed to descend eight stairs, the test indicates a risk for multiple falls with a postitive LR of 1.40 (Sn = 0.63; Sp = 0.55).[46]

Equipment: Any flight of stairs with a railing can be used.

Testing Procedure: Timing starts when the patient's first foot is lifted from floor and is stopped when both feet are on the top stair. Because descent is typically more difficult, the therapist should score ascent and descent separately. The therapist should document the use of handrails, assistive devices, gait belts, and the number of stairs.

Position of Therapist: Safety of the patient should be the therapist's primary concern. Therefore, the therapist may need to closely guard the patient, ascending and descending the stairs with the patient (Figure 9-38). If safety is not a concern, the therapist can choose to remain at the bottom of the flight of stairs during the test.

Instructions to Patient: "I want to see how safely and how quickly you can climb this flight of stairs. Do you feel safe to climb these stairs? You may hold onto the railing if you want to. Please stop at the top of the stairs before coming down so I can time how long it takes you to descend. Ready? Go!"

Scoring

Scoring the time it takes the patient to ascend and descend stairs must include the number of stairs. In nondisabled individuals, 0.5 seconds/stair is typical. Stair ascent and descent decreases with age from 2.5 stairs/sec in 20- to 39-year-olds to 1.2 stairs/second in 90+ year olds.[47]

Helpful Hints

- Carefully observe the patient's use of the handrail. The patient may use the handrail for balance or may use the handrail for weight bearing to off-load a painful joint or compensate for weakness. Watch for the patient pulling him- or herself up by the handrail. This observation can inform clinical decision-making.
- Note the position of the feet during stair descent, which may indicate compensation for muscle weakness or pain.
- Stair climbing without a handrail typically increases ground reaction forces by 7 times the body weight.[48,49]
- If a patient with eyeglasses has difficulty descending stairs, don't encourage him or her to move faster. Glasses sometimes cause the patient to see a step where it isn't and increased speed may result in a fall.

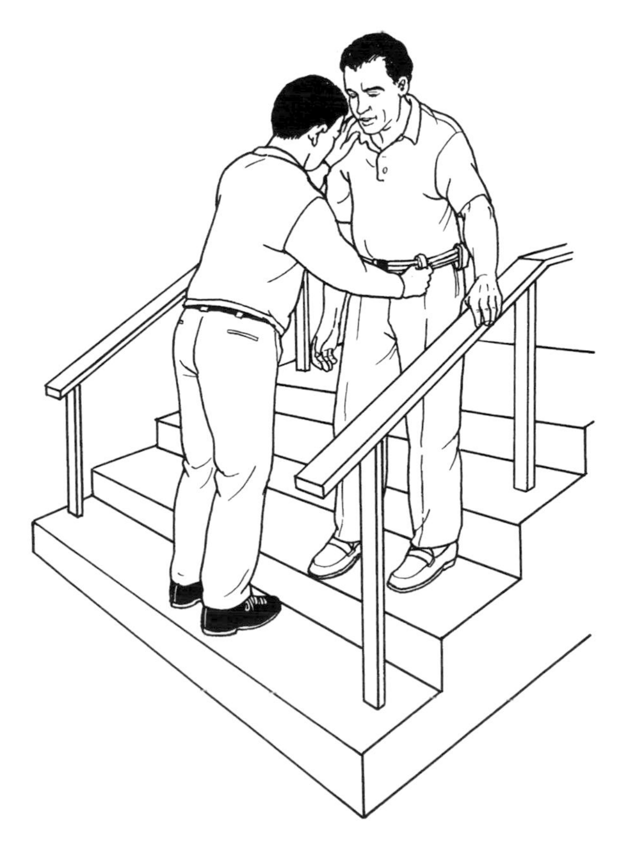

FIGURE 9-38

FLOOR RISE

Purpose: Floor rise ability is necessary for a patient's safety and confidence. Anyone who falls should be able to rescue themselves from the floor (unless they have become seriously injured). The floor rise test assesses the patient's ability to descend and rise from the floor, thereby identifying impairments, functional ability, and informing clinical decision-making.

Essential Muscle Movements for Task Performance: Knee extension, ankle plantar flexion, hip extension, core stability, and trunk rotation. If arms are needed to assist, scapular adduction and downward rotation, scapular depression and adduction, elbow extension, and shoulder horizontal adduction.

Reliability: Not known.

Validity: An inability to rise from the floor is associated with older age, increased mortality, and lower functional abilities and risk for serious injury.[50]

Equipment: Stopwatch, chair with arms, and an unobstructed floor surface that allows the patient to lie flat.

Testing Procedure: The therapist should demonstrate the lowering of the body to the floor, lying supine, and rising again. During the test, the patient should lie supine so that 75% of the body is in contact with the floor. The patient may choose to place the head and trunk flat on the floor, bending the knees or lying flat with only the head and shoulders raised (Figure 9-39). Either position is acceptable. A chair should be nearby to be used by the patient if needed. Timing begins on "Go!" and ends when the patient is fully standing again and steady. Document the type of assistance needed to rise, as appropriate.

Instructions to Patient: "I want you to get onto the floor, without assistance if possible, lying flat so that most of your body is flat on the floor, then get up again. You may get up in any way you choose and if you need to, you may use this chair. I can help you if you can't get up by yourself. I will demonstrate. I will be timing you and will stop timing when you are fully standing and steady. Are you ready? Good. Go!"

Scoring

The score is the time it takes to complete the floor transfer. There are no norms for this test, but in the author's experience, more than 10 seconds often involves the need for assistance with the transfer.

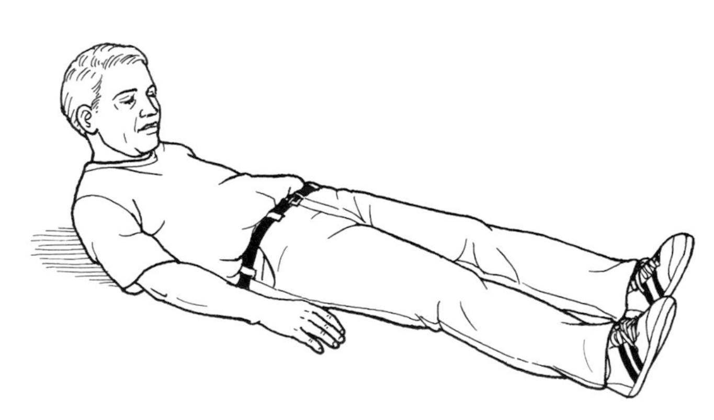

FIGURE 9-39

Helpful Hints

- When an individual has difficulty getting up from the floor, it often involves an inability to shift weight from the hips as in side-sitting to the knees.
- The therapist should note the "cause" of any difficulty in rising—such as pain, weakness, or an inability to motor plan. These causes may form the basis of a treatment plan.
- Because there are several ways to rise from the floor, the method used by the patient should be noted in the documentation. The position requiring the most strength is rising without assistance (Figure 9-40); using one knee to rise requires less strength (Figure 9-41); and using assistance such as a chair requires the least amount of strength. (Figure 9-42).

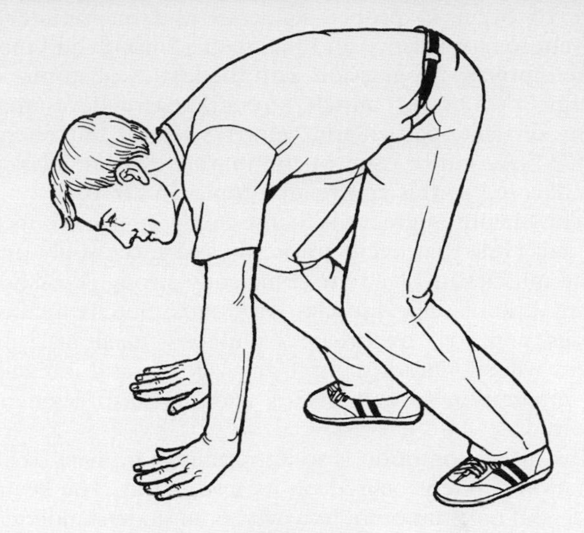

FIGURE 9-40

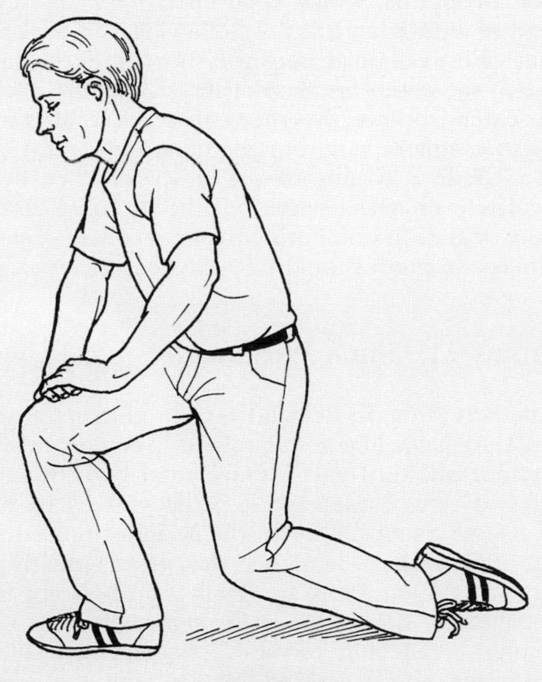

FIGURE 9-41

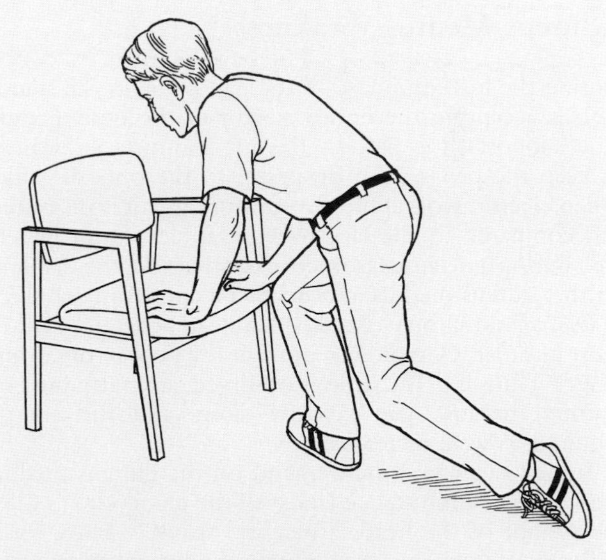

FIGURE 9-42

Human gait is a remarkable feat. Each step is a complex integration of muscular and neural events, all of which have to occur in proper sequence and magnitude to prevent loss of balance and maintain a smooth and integrated forward progression with the least expenditure of energy.[51,52] Loss of muscle strength has a devastating effect on gait, particularly velocity, safety, and energy cost.[53,54] An entire issue of the journal *Physical Therapy* was devoted to this and related topics in 2010.[55]

This chapter segment is focused only on five events in the gait cycle that occur smoothly and successfully only if the muscles involved are sufficiently strong. Weakness in any one of these muscles or groups gluteus medius, tibialis anterior, quadriceps, gluteous maximus, and soleus will significantly blunt gait velocity and interrupt the integration of gait events and the limb segments involved.

Because locomotion is so important to humans, rehabilitation is often focused on its restoration. The key to successful rehabilitation, however, is an understanding of which muscles or muscle groups are weak. What follows are some common deviations in the gait cycle that are directly linked to specific muscle weakness. These deviations are relatively easy to spot with the eye and once they are observed the therapist should immediately turn to specific muscle testing for confirmation.

Gluteus Medius Weakness

During the loading phase of the gait cycle, as the stance limb is accepting the entire weight of the body (single limb support), the gluteus medius contracts vigorously to keep the pelvis from dropping to the opposite side. When electromyographic output during gait is measured and compared to the electromyographic output generated during a maximal isometric contraction, the demand on the gluteus medius appears to be approximately 25% of its maximum force capacity. Thus, in general, strength must be at least Grade 3 to prevent the pelvis from dropping.[56] Thus, if pelvic drop is observed, strength must be restored because gait velocity slows and the energy required to walk increases.[53]

Inman calculated the demand on the gluteus medius during single limb stance (most of the gait cycle) as 2.5× the weight of the head, arms, and trunk.[57] Thus, for a 150-pound individual, the gluteus medius must generate approximately 100 pounds of torque with each step. If the therapist is strength testing with a hand-held dynamometer, a minimum of 100 pounds should be the expected value in a 150-pound person.

Tibialis Anterior Weakness

Immediately following heel strike, the tibialis anterior (TA) decelerates the foot to the floor.[56] This eccentric contraction is a rapid event that places high demand on the muscle, estimated at between 45% and 75% of its maximum strength.[56,58] A demand this high requires a manual muscle grade of at least 4. Weakness of the TA immediately eliminates the foot-lowering portion of the normal gait cycle. With moderate weakness (approximately Grade 3) the therapist will observe a foot flat approach.[56] Stride length is shortened to permit the foot flat landing. A shorter stride results in slower gait velocity. Thus, if the therapist observes a patient who fails to execute heel strike and approaches each step with a foot flat approach, test the TA to confirm its strength loss. If there is severe weakness the therapist will observe (and hear) a foot slap gait.

Quadriceps Weakness

Another key event in the stance phase of gait is shock absorption at the knee shortly after heel strike.[56] During this instant in the gait cycle, the knee (in a normal person) rapidly goes from full extension to 15° of flexion and the quadriceps absorb a high amount of force, estimated to be 75% of maximum.[56] With shock absorption, the quadriceps permit a smooth transition to mid-stance. If the quadriceps are weak the entire shock absorption process disappears, which is another observable event. Instead of a brisk knee flexion following heel strike, the patient with weak quadriceps will shorten the stride and approach the entire first half of the stance phase with a nearly extended knee. No shock absorption takes place. Strength estimates vary, but the quadriceps must be at least a Grade 3 to absorb the shock of knee flexion immediately after heel strike.[56] If the therapist observes a failure of knee flexion during the initial phase of stance, quadriceps strength should be evaluated.

Gluteus Maximus Weakness

The highest strength demand on the gluteus maximus occurs during loading response and is complete by the mid-stance phase of gait.[59] Once total body weight is transferred onto the stance leg, the gluteus maximus must assume responsibility for the upright trunk (muscle acting on its origin). If muscle weakness is present, the patient will exhibit a forward trunk lean. Forward trunk lean may occur during the entire stance phase or occur suddenly, a "pitching forward," suggesting a sudden failure of the muscles to hold the trunk upright. Gluteus maximus strength should be sufficient to hold the weight of the head, arms, and trunk, or about 60% of body mass.[56] If suspected gluteus maximus weakness exists, as evidenced by a forward trunk lean during stance, with subsequent slowing of gait, further muscle testing is indicated for confirmation.

Gastrocnemius-soleus Weakness

When the gastrocnemius and soleus act on their insertion, they produce plantar flexion and stabilize the ankle during roll-off.[58,60,61] The soleus is one of the

Gastrocnemius-soleus Weakness Continued

most important muscles of the leg because it works not just to control the foot and ankle complex but has a critical role in stabilizing the knee.[62] Equally important is the role of the soleus to prevent forward translation of the tibia toward the end of the stance phase. If the soleus is functioning adequately, the ankle is stable and heel rise occurs.[56] The demand on the gastrocnemius and soleus is extremely high, measured at 75% of maximum for the gastrocnemius and at more than 80% for the soleus. When gastrocnemius-soleus muscle strength is at least Grade 4, the ankle will lock and heel rise will occur, which is another key event in the gait cycle that markedly influences velocity.[63] If heel rise is noticeably diminished or nonexistent, further muscle testing is indicated.

Each of the five gait events described has been identified as one of the "critical determinants of gait."[62-64] Without these five critical determinants, gait velocity is markedly diminished, and as noted, if gait speed gets low enough, community ambulation is no longer feasible and/or independence may be lost. Indeed, loss of gait function is a major reason for nursing home placement in a person's later years.[65]

Hicks and colleagues reported the collective strength required to walk is 24% of normal.[66] By the time strength gets down to 24% of normal, profound changes in gait speed have already occurred, and a person with this much weakness is on the threshold of frailty and loss of independence. Physical therapists are in a position to recognize subtle but highly observable gait deviations long before strength losses become catastrophic. Muscle testing techniques as presented in this book permit identification of strength losses in the early phase of loss, when rehabilitation is more feasible and successful.

REFERENCES

Cited References

1. American Physical Therapy Association. Guide to physical therapist practice. Phys Ther. 1997;77:1163-1650.
2. Rauch A, Cieza A, Stucki G. How to apply the international classification of functioning, disability and health (ICF) for rehabilitation management in clinical practice. Eur J Phys Rehabil Med. 2008;44(3):329-342.
3. Eriksrud O, Bohannon RW. Relationship of knee extension force to independence in sit-to-stand performance in patients receiving acute rehabilitation. Phys Ther. 2003;83(6):544-551.
4. Gross MM, Stevenson PJ, Charette SL, et al. Effect of muscle strength and movement speed on the biomechanics of rising from a chair in healthy elderly and young women. Gait Posture. 1998;8(3):175-185.
5. Jones CJ, Rikli RE, Beam WC. A 30-s chair stand test as a measure of lower body strength in community-residing older adults. Res Q Exer Sport. 1999;70(2):113-119.
6. Bohannon RW. Sit to stand test for measuring performance of lower extremity muscles. Perceptual Motor Skills. 1995;80:163-166.
7. Csuka M, McCarty DJ. A simple method for measurement of lower extremity muscle strength. Am J Med. 1985;78:77-81.
8. Rivera JA, Fried LP, Weiss CO, et al. At the tipping point: predicting severe mobility difficulty in vulnerable older women. J Am Geriatr Soc. 2008;56(8):1417-1423.
9. Purser JL, Kuchibhatla MN, Fillenbaum GG, et al. Identifying frailty in hospitalized older adults with significant coronary artery disease. J Am Geriatr Soc. 2006;54(11):1674-1681.
10. Ferrucci L, Guralnik JM, Bandeen-Roche KL, et al. Performance measures from the women's health and aging study. http://www.grc.nia.nih.gov/branches/ledb/whasbook/chap4/chap4.htm. Accessed Jan. 8, 2012.
11. Brown M. Quick tests to aid in the diagnosis of physical frailty. GeriNotes. 1998;15(4):15.
12. Neptune RR, Sasaki K, Kautz SA. The effect of walking speed on muscle function and mechanical energetics. Gait Posture. 2008;28:135-143.
13. Chang RW, Dunlop D, Gibbs J, et al. The determinants of walking velocity in the elderly. An evaluation using regression trees. Arthritis Rheum. 1995;38(3):343-350.
14. Bohannon RW. Comfortable and maximum walking speed of adults aged 20-79 years: Reference values and determinants. Age Ageing. 1997;26(1):15-19.
15. Fritz S, Lusardi M. White paper: "Walking speed: The sixth vital sign." J Geriatr Phys Ther. 2009;32(2):2-5.
16. Abellan van Kan G, Rolland Y, Andrieu S, et al. Gait speed at usual pace as a predictor of adverse outcomes in community-dwelling older people: an International Academy on Nutrition and Aging (IANA) task force. J Nutr Health Aging. 2009;13(10):881-889.
17. Blain H, Carriere I, Sourial N, et al. Balance and walking speed predict subsequent 8-year mortality independently of current and intermediate events in well-functioning women aged 75 years and older. J Nutr Health Aging. 2010;14(7):595-600.
18. Montero-Odasso M, Schapira M, Varela C, et al. Gait velocity in senior people. An easy test for detecting mobility impairment in community elderly. J Nutr Health Aging. 2004;8(5):340-343.
19. Guralnik JM, Seeman TE, Tinetti ME, et al. Validation and use of performance measures of functioning in a non-disabled older population: MacArthur studies of successful aging. Aging (Milano). 1994;6(6):410-419.
20. Verghese J, Wang C, Holtzer R. Relationship of clinic-based gait speed measurement to limitations in community-based activities in older adults. Arch Phys Med Rehabil. 2011;92(5):844-846.
21. Andrews AW, Chinworth SA, Bourassa M, et al. Update on distance and velocity requirements for community ambulation. J Geriatr Phys Ther. 2010;33(3):128-134.

REFERENCES

22. Harada N, Chiu V, Damron-Rodriguez J, et al. Screening for balance and mobility impairment in elderly individuals living in residential care facilities. Phys Ther. 1995;75(6): 462-469.
23. Guralnik JM, Simonsick EM, Ferrucci L, et al. A short physical performance battery assessing LE function. J Gerontol. 1994:49(2):M85-M94.
24. Guralnik JM, Ferrucci L, Pieper CF, et al. Lower extremity function and subsequent disability: consistency across studies, predictive models, and value of gait speed alone compared with the short physical performance battery. J Gerontol Med Sci. 2000;55A:M221-M231.
25. Ostir GV, Volpato S, Fried LP, et al. Reliability and sensitivity to change assessed for a summary measure of lower body function: results from the Women's Health and Aging Study. J Clin Epidemiol. 2002;55: 916-921.
26. Guralnik JM, Simonsick EM, Ferrucci L, et al. A short physical performance battery assessing lower extremity function: association with self-reported disability and prediction of mortality and nursing home admission. J Gerontol. 1994;49:M85-M94.
27. Fogel JF, Hyman RB, Rock B, et al. Predictors of hospital length of stay and nursing home placement in an elderly medical population. J Am Med Dir Assoc. 2000;1(5): 202-210.
28. Volpato S, Cavalieri M, Sioulis F, et al. Predictive value of the short physical performance battery following hospitalization in older patients. J Gerontol A Biol Sci Med Sci. 2011;66(1):89-96.
29. Reuben DB, Siu Al. An objective measure of physical function of elderly outpatients: the Physical Performance Test. J Am Geriatr Soc. 1990;38(10):1105-1112.
30. Beissner KL, Collins JE, Holmes H. Muscle force and range of motion as predictors of function in older adults. Phys Ther. 2000;80:556-563.
31. Reuben DB, Siu Al, Kimpau S. The predictive validity of self-report and performance-based measures of function and health. J Gerontol. 1992;47:M106-M110.
32. Delbaere K, Van den Noortgate N, et al. The Physical Performance Test as a predictor of frequent fallers: a prospective community-based cohort study. Clin Rehabil. 2006;20(1):83-90.
33. VanSwearingen JM, Paschal KA, Bonino P, et al. Assessing recurrent fall risk of community-dwelling, frail older veterans using specific tests of mobility and the physical performance test of function. J Gerontol Med Sci. 1998;53A:M457-M464.
34. Brown M, Sinacore DR, Binder EF, et al. Physical and performance measures for the identification of mild to moderate frailty. J Gerontol Med Sci. 2000;55A(6): M350-M355.
35. Herman T, Giladi N, Hausdorff JM. Properties of the 'timed up and go' test: more than meets the eye. Gerontology. 2010;57(3):203-210.
36. Mathias S, Nayak US, Isaacs B. Balance in elderly patients: the "get-up and go" test. Arch Phys Med Rehabil. 1986;67(6):387-389.
37. Podsiadlo D, Richardson S. The timed "up and go": a test of basic functional mobility for frail elderly persons. J Am Geriatr Soc. 1991;39:142-148.
38. Ries JD, Echternach JL, Nof L, et al. Test-retest reliability and minimal detectable change scores for the timed "up & go" test, the six-minute walk test, and gait speed in people with Alzheimer disease. Phys Ther. 2009;89(6): 569-579.
39. Kristensen MT, Foss NB, Kehlet H. Timed "up & go" test as a predictor of falls within 6 months after hip fracture surgery. Phys Ther. 2007;87(1):24-30.
40. Steffen T, Seney M. Test-retest reliability and minimal detectable change on balance and ambulation tests, the 36-item short-form health survey, and the unified Parkinson disease rating scale in people with parkinsonism. Phys Ther. 2008;88(6):733-746.
41. Bischoff HA, Stahelin HB, Monsch AU, et al. Identifying a cut-off point for normal mobility: a comparison of the timed "up and go" test in community-dwelling and institutionalised elderly women. Age Ageing. 2003;32(3): 315-320.
42. Bohannon RW. Reference values for the timed up and go test: a descriptive meta-analysis. J Geriatr Phys Ther. 2006;29(2):64-68.
43. Zech A, Steib S, Sportwiss D, et al. Functional muscle power testing in young, middle-aged, and community-dwelling nonfrail and prefrail older adults. Arch Phys Med Rehabil. 2011;92(6):967-971.
44. Roig M, Eng JJ, MacIntyre DL, et al. Associations of the stair climb power test with muscle strength and functional performance in people with chronic obstructive pulmonary disease: a cross-sectional study. Phys Ther. 2010;90(12): 1774-1782.
45. LeBrasseur NK, Bhasin S, Miciek R, et al. Tests of muscle strength and physical function: reliability and discrimination of performance in younger and older men and older men with mobility limitations. JAGS. 2008;56: 2118-2123.
46. Tiedemann A, Shimada H, Sherrington C, et al. The comparative ability of eight functional mobility tests for predicting falls in community-dwelling older people. Age Ageing. 2008;37(4):430-435.
47. Butler AA, Menant JC, Tiedemann AC, et al. Age and gender differences in seven tests of functional mobility. J Neuroeng Rehabil. 2009;6:31.
48. Teh KC, Aziz AR. Heart rate, oxygen uptake, and energy cost of ascending and descending the stairs. Med Sci Sports Exerc. 2002;34:695-699.
49. Stolk J, Verdonschot N, Huiskes R. Stair climbing is more detrimental to the cement in hip replacement than walking. Clin Orthop Relat Res. 2002;405:294-305.
50. Bergland A, Laake K. Concurrent and predictive validity of "getting up from lying on the floor." Aging Clin Exp Res. 2005;17(3):181-185.
51. Kuo AD, Donelan JM. Dynamic principles of gait and their clinical implications. Phys Ther. 2010;90:157-176.
52. Borghese NA, Bianchi L, Lacquaniti F. Kinematic determinants of human locomotion. J Physiol. 1996;494: 863-879.
53. Waters RL. The energy expenditure of normal and pathological gait. Gait Posture. 1999;9:207-231.
54. Bianchi L, Angelini D, Orani GP, et al. Kinematic coordination in human gait: relation to mechanical energy cost. J Neurophysiol. 1998;79:2155-2170.
55. Jacquelin Perry special issue: stepping forward with gait rehabilitation. Phys Ther. 2010;90(2):142-305.
56. Perry J, Burnfield JM. Gait Analysis: Normal and Pathological Function. 2nd ed. Thorofare NJ: Slack Inc; 2010:3-260.
57. Inman V. Functional aspects of the abductor muscles of the hip. J Bone Joint Surg. 1947;29:607-619.
58. Dubo HIC, Peat M, Winter DA, et al. Electromyographic temporal analysis of gait: normal human locomotion. Arch Phys Med Rehabil. 1976;57:415-420.

59. Lyons K, Perry J, Gronley JK, et al. Timing and relative intensity of hip extensor and abductor muscle action during levels and stair ambulation. Phys Ther. 1983;63: 1597-1605.
60. Sutherland DH, Cooper L, Daniel D. The role of the ankle plantar flexors in normal walking. J Bone Joint Surg. 1980;62A:354-363.
61. Simon SR, Mann RA, Hagy JL, et al. Role of the posterior calf muscles in normal gait. J Bone Joint Surg. 1978;60A: 465-475.
62. Kerrigan DC, Della Croce U, Marciello M, et al. A refined view of the determinants of gait: significance of heel rise. Arch Phys Med Rehabil. 2000;81:1077-1080.
63. Saunders JB, Inman VT, Eberhardt HD. The major determinants in normal and pathological gait. J Bone Joint Surg. 1953;35A:543-548.
64. Pandy MG, Berme N. Quantitative assessment of gait determinants during single stance via a three-dimensional model-part 1. Normal gait. J Biomech. 1989;22: 717-724.
65. Studenski S, Perera S, Patel K, et al. Gait speed and survival in older adults. JAMA. 2011;305:70-78.
66. Hicks GE, Shardell M, Alley DE, et al. Absolute strength and loss of strength as predictors of mobility decline in older adults: the InCHIANTI study. J Gerontol A Biol Med Sci. 2012;67(1):66-73.

OTHER READINGS

Chair Stand

Cesari M, Onder G, Zamboni V, et al. Physical function and self-rated health status as predictors of mortality: results from longitudinal analysis in the ilSIRENTE study. BMC Geriatr. 2008;22(8):34.

Onder G, Penninx BW, Ferrucci L, et al. Measures of physical performance and risk for progressive and catastrophic disability: results from the Women's Health and Aging Study. J Gerontol A Biol Sci Med Sci. 2005;60(1):74-79.

Studenski S, Perera S, Wallace D, et al. Physical performance measures in the clinical setting. J Am Geriatr Soc. 2003;51(3):314-322.

Wang CY, Yeh CJ, Hu MH. Mobility-related performance tests to predict mobility disability at 2-year follow-up in community dwelling older adults. Arch Gerontol Geriatr. 2011;52(1):1-4. Epub 2009 Nov 27.

Jones CJ, Rikli RE. Measuring functional fitness. Active Aging 2002;1(2):24-27.

Gait Speed

Fiser WM, Hays NP, Rogers SC, et al. Energetics of walking in elderly people: factors related to gait speed. J Gerontol A Biol Sci Med Sci. 2010;65(12):1332-1337.

Guralnik JM, Seeman TE, Tinetti ME, et al. Validation and use of performance measures of functioning in a non-disabled older population: MacArthur studies of successful aging. Aging (Milano). 1994;6(6):410-419.

Hasselgren L, Olsson LL, Nyberg L. Is leg muscle strength correlated with functional balance and mobility among inpatients in geriatric rehabilitation? Arch Gerontol Geriatr. 2011;52(3):e220-e225. Epub 2010 Dec 14.

Mayson DJ, Kiely DK, Larose SI, et al. Leg strength or velocity of movement: which is more influential on the balance of mobility limited elders? Am J Phys Med Rehabil. 2008;87(12):969-976.

Studenski S, Perera S, Wallace D, et al. Physical performance measures in the clinical setting. J Am Geriatr Soc. 2003;51(3):314-322.

Viccaro LJ, Perera S, Studenski SA. Is timed up and go better than gait speed in predicting health, function, and falls in older adults? J Am Geriatr Soc. 2011;59(5):887-892.

SPPB

Puthoff ML, Nielsen DH. Relationships among impairments in lower-extremity strength and power, functional limitations, and disability in older adults. Phys Ther. 2007;87:1334-1347.

TUG

Schaubert KL, Bohannon RW. Reliability and validity of three strength measures obtained from community-dwelling elderly persons. J Strength Cond Res. 2005;19(3): 717-720.

Shumway-Cook A, Brauer S, Woollacott M. Predicting the probability for falls in community-dwelling older adults using the Timed Up & Go Test. Phys Ther. 2000;80(9): 896-903.

Steffen TM, Hacker TA, Mollinger L. Age- and gender-related test performance in community-dwelling elderly people: Six-minute walk test, Berg balance scale, timed up & go test, and gait speeds. Phys Ther. 2002;82(2):128-137.

van Iersel MB, Munneke M, Esselink RA, et al. Gait velocity and the timed-up-and-go test were sensitive to changes in mobility in frail elderly patients. J Clin Epidemiol. 2008; 61(2):186-191.

Yeung TS, Wessel J, Stratford PW, et al. The timed up and go test for use on an inpatient orthopaedic rehabilitation ward. J Orthop Sports Phys Ther. 2008;38(7):410-417.

Stair Climb

Panzer VP, Wakefield DB, Hall CB, et al. Mobility assessment: sensitivity and specificity of measurement sets in older adults. Arch Phys Med Rehabil. 2011;92(6):905-912.

Tiedemann AC, Sherrington C, Lord SR. Physical and psychological factors associated with stair negotiation performance in older people. J Gerontol A Biol Sci Med Sci. 2007;62(11):1259-1265.

Floor Rise

Bergland A, Wyller TB. Risk factors for serious fall related injury in elderly women living at home. Inj Prev. 2004;10(5):308-313.

Fleming J, Brayne C, Cambridge City over-75s Cohort (CC75C) Study Collaboration. Inability to get up after falling, subsequent time on floor, and summoning help: Prospective cohort study in people over 90. BMJ. 2008; 337:a2227.

Hofmeyer MR, Alexander NB, Nyquist LV, et al. Floor-rise strategy training in older adults. J Am Geriatr Soc. 2002;50(10):1702-1706.

Manckoundia P, Buatois S, Gueguen R, et al. Clinical determinants of failure in balance tests in elderly subjects. Arch Gerontol Geriatr. 2008;47(2):217-228.

Wang CY, Olson SL, Protas EJ. Physical-performance tests to evaluate mobility disability in community-dwelling elders. J Aging Phys Act. 2005;13(2):184-197.

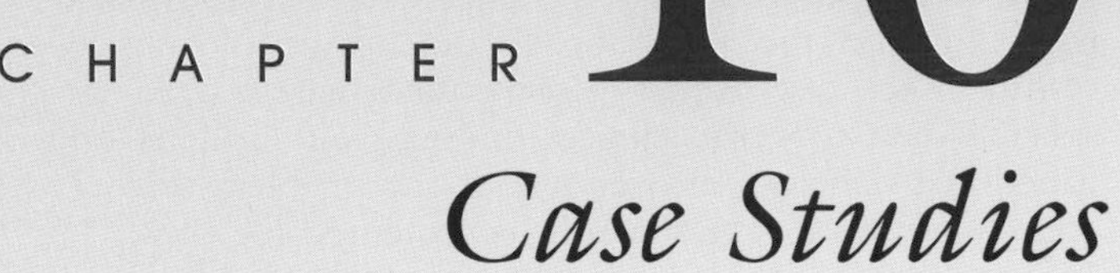

Case Studies

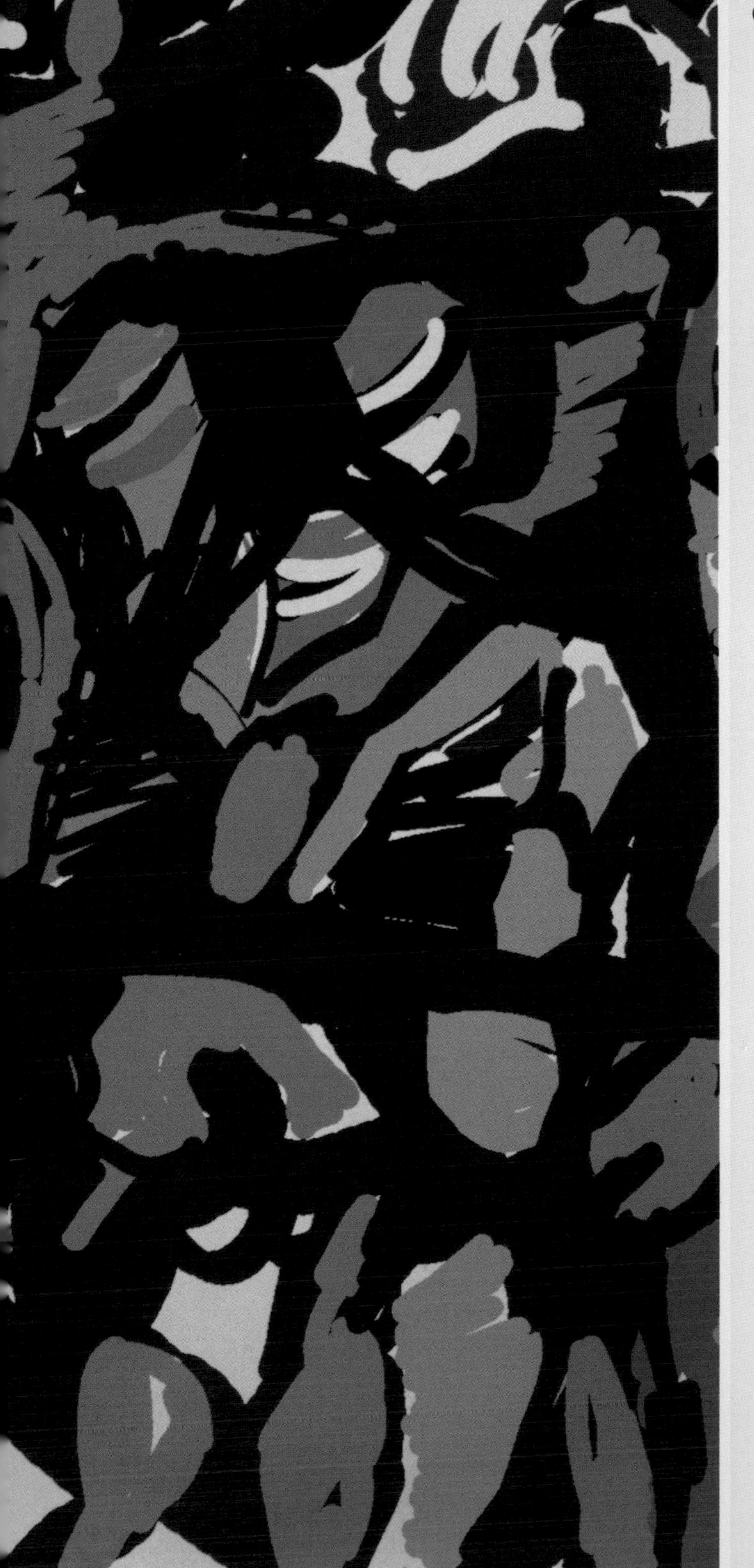

CASE STUDIES

INTRODUCTION

This chapter serves as a brief summary of the muscle testing performance concepts presented throughout this book. Concepts are amplified using a series of case studies that illustrate the need for various forms of muscle testing. Each case features a real patient with a need for specific data to verify clinical findings and understand functional deficits. An overview of the problem-solving approach used by the therapist is presented for each.

The variety of tests available to therapists is illustrated in these case studies. The diagnoses presented are common and each case is intended to highlight the rationale for specific muscle test selection. The cases are unique in both their presentation and the clinical data they require, thus providing a glimpse into the decision-making required to thoroughly evaluate the range of muscle performance deficits seen in various patients.

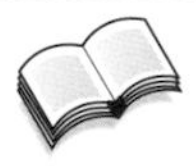

Case 1. Shoulder Pain

The patient was a 56-year-old male investment banker who developed right shoulder pain after a weekend of working with his arms extended over his head while painting and wallpapering his home. On examination, he presented with Grade 3 strength of the right external rotators (teres minor and infraspinatus). Abductor strength, when tested in 15° of abduction, was weak (Grade 4) and painful. Internal rotation, flexion, and extension strength were all Grade 5 and nonpainful. Given his pattern of pain and weakness, shoulder joint impingement with supraspinatus tendonitis was suspected.

Attention to scapular function became the focus of evaluation. Because glenohumeral joint movement is only possible if the scapula moves simultaneously, muscle testing of the scapular stabilizers was performed as a key element of his problems.

The scapular retractors (middle and lower trapezius, rhomboids); downward rotators (also middle and lower trapezius, rhomboids); and muscles that perform upward rotation (serratus anterior, pectoralis minor, upper and lower trapezius) were tested. In this patient example, the retractors and downward rotators were graded at the 4 level. The upward rotators were a Grade 3. Active and passive shoulder movement revealed tightness of the pectoralis minor (Grade 3).

Treating the muscles only at the glenohumeral joint will not resolve this patient's problem because a major cause of his pain is weakness of the scapulohumeral muscles, specifically the serratus anterior and lower trapezius, and tightness of the pectoralis minor. Strengthening of the serratus and lower trapezius and stretching of the pectoralis minor opens the sub-acromial space, allowing more freedom for the supraspinatus to slide beneath. This decreases the impingement and may ultimately resolve the patient's complaints and prevent a recurrence.

This case example reflects a typical patient who is referred to physical therapy. The original symptom was pain, but the patient's discomfort was the consequence of muscle weakness coupled with diminished muscle length. Knowledge of anatomy, kinesiology, and manual muscle testing enabled the therapist to isolate the root causes of the patient's painful condition.

Clinical Comments

- Pectoralis minor tightness is a common clinical finding that often is a significant contributor to impingement at the glenohumeral joint.[1,2] Tightness of the pectoralis minor and weakness of the serratus anterior and lower trapezius results in a downward and forward position of the acromion. The downward and forward position decreases the sub-acromial space and results in an impingement of the rotator cuff muscles that ordinarily slide freely under the acromion during overhead activities.[3] Repetitive impingement causes irritation of the supraspinatus portion of the rotator cuff, resulting in pain and decreased strength.[1,2]
- To confirm an inflamed supraspinatus tendon, alternate the position of the supraspinatus and the infraspinatus (posterior rotator cuff muscles for internal rotation with arm at the side) to test only the contractile tissue. If these muscles are strong and testing does not cause pain, progress to the manual muscle positions of external rotation and shoulder flexion. If pain results from the alternate position, do not use the traditional test position (which involves more torque).
- If supraspinatus tendonitis exists, shoulder abduction and flexion muscle tests will often cause pain and reveal weakness. If the scapula downwardly rotates during shoulder abduction and flexion, it will cause compression of the humeral head into the acromion process and impinge the supraspinatus tendon (painful). Downward rotation of the scapula per se is not usually painful or weak. If the scapula moves into downward rather than upward rotation, it is not properly positioning the humerus, and the supraspinatus becomes compressed. This condition is often seen in patients who have kyphotic posture and in men and women of all ages who stand with rounded shoulders.

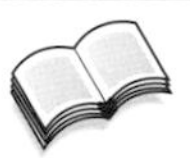

Case 2. Compromised Gait and Function Secondary to Muscle Weakness

The patient is a 68-year-old retired man. One weekend he went to the movies with his wife and after 2 hours of sitting found he could not get up from the chair without a great amount of effort. This embarrassing incident prompted him to seek help and he referred himself to an older adult wellness clinic.

Evaluation revealed a pleasant appearing gentleman with flexed hips (~20°) and knees (~15°) when standing upright. He was of average height (68 in.) but was overweight, stating that he weighed about 240 pounds at the time of initial evaluation (body mass index = 36, which is obese). He clearly had difficulty rising from the standard 17-in. chair in the treatment area, as evidenced by using his arms and rocking back and forth several times. Gait evaluation revealed the following: slow gait speed (2 mph or 0.9 m/s), forward trunk lean during the entire gait cycle, slight pelvic drop bilaterally during the stance phase (exhibited by a "waddling" gait), no flexion at the knee (exhibited by failure to flex the knee at loading), and no heel rise at the end of the stance phase as exhibited by a flat foot and shortened stride. These observations suggested possible weakness of the following muscle groups: back extensors, hip extensors, hip abductors, knee extensors, and plantar flexors. Thus, additional muscle testing was done.

Because this man was large, it became immediately apparent to the therapist that manual muscle testing was not feasible given the therapist's size in relation to the patient's. Therefore alternative testing using the leg press and the one repetition maximum (1-RM) method was chosen. The patient was also tested using the standard 25× heel rise test for plantar flexors (described in Chapter 6, page 254).

Total Lower Extremity Extension

The leg press provides a composite value for total lower extremity extension (ankle plantar flexion, knee extension and hip extension). If it is suspected that there is weakness in the entire kinetic chain, wider testing to get a general idea of patient capability is useful as an index of general lower body strength. The leg press is ideal because norms are available for men and women of all ages (see Chapter 8). The patient was seated on a leg-press device that was adjusted to a position of comfort that was compatible with the patient's leg length. A 68-year-old man should be able to complete a leg press equivalent to approximately 1.4 times his body weight (see Chapter 8).

Because of this patient's difficulty rising from a chair, a functional task that requires a minimum of 50% of the body's weight, that is, a weight stack of 150 pounds was chosen (60% of body weight); however he could not move the weight stack. The amount of resistance was adjusted downward to 110 pounds (40% of body weight) based on his inability to move the stack or rise from a chair. The patient did complete a full leg extension with 110 pounds. Thus, another 10 pounds was added (120 pounds) and another full leg extension elicited, which he completed, but barely. To confirm the 120-pound maximum, a final 5 pounds was added to the weight stack and then he could not complete leg extension.

If one considers the fact that this 240-pound man could leg press only 120 pounds, it is no surprise he had difficulty getting out of a chair. To provide a different context, on a manual muscle test, if enough resistance could realistically be applied, he would have scored a maximum of Grade 4. It is unreasonable to believe that a therapist can apply sufficient resistance to discern the difference between Grade 4 and Grade 5 for total lower extremity extension, particularly when a leg is so large and heavy. Thus, manual testing is not appropriate to determine the leg strength required to rise from a seated position.

For a more thorough understanding of this patient's weakness, it is essential to determine the strength of specific muscle groups, particularly those that evidence weakness in the gait cycle. Thus, specific selective resistance tests were done in addition to the leg press (e.g., leg extension, knee extension, and plantar flexion).

Hip Extension

Initially, the patient was positioned prone on a plinth and a hip extension manual muscle test was performed on each leg, first as a Grade 3 (no resistance but to assess the patient's ability to move and complete range). The patient was able to raise each leg against gravity and was able to hold the position against some manual resistance; therefore, the hip extensors were graded a 4. To establish the appropriate amount of resistance for effective strengthening, 1-RM testing was chosen. Weight was added progressively around the ankle beginning at 5 pounds. The patient was able to lift 5 pounds, so another 5 pounds of weight was added. With 10 pounds of ankle weights, he could not extend his hip through full range of motion. Thus, 5 pounds was recorded as his maximum for the first leg tested. The test was repeated on the other leg.

Knee Extension

A 1-RM using the leg extension machine (open chain approach) was used to isolate the knee extensors. The patient was seated on the leg extension machine and initially 50 pounds was selected from the weight stack to test one leg at a time. Fifty pounds was chosen because it is slightly less than half of the bilateral leg press 1-RM. The patient was not able to complete the full range, so the weight was decreased by 10 pounds. He was then able to complete full range with utmost effort. To confirm the RM, the patient was asked to perform as many repetitions as possible. He was unable to do another repetition with full range; therefore, his 1-RM for the first leg was 40 pounds. The test was then repeated on the other side. (Note: Open chain movements generally produce less force than what is achieved on the leg press because of the isolation of the knee extensors.)

Hip Abduction

Given the patient's size, the only feasible option for accurate testing was a cable tensiometer affixed to an immovable object such as the wall. The patient was placed against the wall and instructed to hold onto a grab bar for stability. A cuff was placed around his ankle. The tension on the cable was set to zero while he was in the neutral stance position. He was then asked to abduct his leg as hard as possible while

Continued

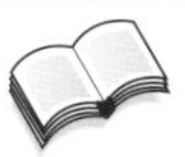

Case 2. Compromised Gait and Function Secondary to Muscle Weakness—cont'd

keeping his opposite heel against the wall. The tensiometer cable was set so that the contraction elicited was isometric in the nearly hip neutral position, which is consistent with muscle demand in gait. Three repetitions were requested and the top value of 92 pounds was recorded. The weight of this patient's head, arms, and trunk (i.e., the demand on his hip abductors) would be approximately 160 pounds. Thus, a 92-pound force output is not sufficient to keep his pelvis in the midline during gait. His force output would correspond to a manual muscle test Grade 4. Although not reported, the other hip was also tested and values were comparable.

Plantar Flexion

The traditional plantar flexion test (page 254) requires 25 repetitions of at least 2-inch clearance.[4] Norms for a male of 60+ years require completing from 4 to 27 heel raises of at least 2-inch clearance.[5] This test was ideal for the patient given its functionality and using his body weight as resistance. Given a lack of heel rise during gait, it was expected the patient would be in the lower part of the range of normal. Actual testing of both legs revealed an ability to accomplish a total of eight repetitions, which corresponds to a Grade 4 (barely).

In summary, this patient's knee extension strength was Grade 4 with a 1-RM of 40 pounds, hip extensors were Grade 4 with a 10-pound 1-RM, and hip abductors and plantar flexors were Grade 4. These grades indicate muscle weakness of a magnitude that compromises functional activity: a normal gait pattern and rising from a chair without using the arms. The instrumented tests provided specific numbers that could be used in context with the body weight demands of daily activities and help establish the appropriate amount of resistance for an effective exercise program.

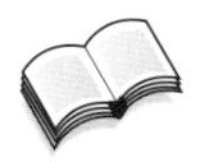

Case 3. Fatigue Secondary to Muscle Weakness

The patient was a physical therapy student participating in the muscle testing laboratory. During testing it was noticed that he could not walk on his toes symmetrically, and on questioning he admitted that he had calf muscle fatigue after walking across campus that seemed to affect his ability to walk quickly. On further questioning, he reported a history of multiple ankle sprains on the left side with the most recent being 6 months earlier while he was playing volleyball. Initially he treated the sprain with ice and compression, and had limited his weight-bearing until the swelling decreased. He never sought the consultation of a physician or physical therapist after any of his sprains. It took several months for the ankle stiffness to resolve and he reported there was some swelling after activity such as walking across campus. He was playing volleyball once again but did not feel he had regained his ability to jump, cut side to side, or go for a ball with confidence.

There was no ankle pain at examination but there was limited range of motion at the end range of dorsiflexion, eversion, and inversion. Strength was evaluated using manual muscle testing. Manual muscle testing was chosen for the following reasons: the therapist can compare strength values side to side, the forces produced by the evertors and invertors are small enough to resist manually, and body weight resistance is used to challenge the plantar flexors.

To test plantar flexion, the student was asked to remove his shoes and stand next to a wall where he could use a finger or two for balance. He was then asked to rise up onto the ball of the foot 25 times (traditional test), first on his unaffected side, and then the sprained side. On the unaffected ankle he could easily achieve 25 heel rises, clearing at least 2 inches with each repetition. On the sprained side, he completed (barely) seven repetitions before muscle fatigue occurred as evidenced by a lack of range.

Inversion and eversion were then tested using manual resistance. The unaffected side was again tested first and was evaluated as Grade 5 in both movements. Further testing revealed that strength on the affected side was Grade 5 for inversion but Grade 3+ for eversion. It took barely any resistance before the fibularis longus and brevis (aka peroneal muscles) failed to hold against resistance. There was no pain with muscle resistance.

This case reflects a common finding: residual muscle strength deficits following what appears to be a simple injury. His involved plantar flexors were Grade 4 and his evertors were Grade 3. Given his commonplace injury, he expected a complete return of strength and range and did not seek the services of a clinician. He could have gone through life unable to fully participate in sports at his level of inherent skill and strength. It was the serendipity of being a student in a clinical program that resulted in evaluation and subsequent treatment. How many other men and women are "getting by" with diminished strength following a simple injury?

Case 4. Muscle Weakness Following Nerve Injury

The patient is a 34-year-old male who was referred to the clinic because of weakness in his forearm, wrist, and hand. History taking revealed the patient was caught in the 2010 earthquake in Haiti and suffered a crush injury of the arm when a portion of a wall collapsed on it. He had open reduction internal fixation surgery to repair the crush damage to the radius and ulna and his arm and forearm were in a cast for 3 to 4 months (patient unclear of duration). After cast removal, he was placed in a cast brace that permitted some movement at the elbow, wrist, and fingers. The patient wore the cast brace for approximately 4 more months. Now, on his first clinical visit he is many months after removal of the cast brace (lack of insurance hampered access to further care), his fractures are healed, and he is cleared for all resistance activities for the upper extremity including wrist and hand.

Initial screening revealed a profoundly weak grip with inability to hold onto an empty water glass. The patient's fingers were stiff as well but movement was observable toward finger closure, finger opening, and spreading the fingers a small distance (abduction). Thumb movement was minimal in all directions. Gross sensory testing revealed diminished sensation along the forearm over the muscle bellies of the wrist extensors and over the dorsum of the thumb. Sensation was also diminished on the thumb pad and over the skin of the thumb web.

The initial major findings were severe muscle weakness following 6 months of immobility, generalized hand/finger stiffness, reduced range of motion throughout the forearm, wrist, and hand, and diminished sensation at multiple sites. The therapist strongly suspected nerve injury over and above the inactivity-related atrophy and chose to do a manual muscle test to confirm nerve injury and identify which muscles(s) were affected by more than immobility.

If this were your patient, what muscle tests would you perform? It is not uncommon for physical therapists to diagnose unsuspected findings, and in this instance, it was radial and median nerve damage. Nerve damage was not complete in either nerve and there were signs of recovery beginning to occur, according to the patient. Establishing a strength and muscle involvement baseline was needed in this case. Muscle tests performed:

Elbow flexion and extension: To confirm that nerve damage is below the elbow.

Radial nerve: Wrist extension (flexor carpi radialis, ulnaris, metatarsophalangeal (MP) extension, thumb MP, and interphalangeal (IP) extension.

Median nerve: pronation, wrist flexion, MP flexion, proximal phalanges (PIP) flexion (flexor digitorum superficialis), distal phalanges (DIP) flexion (flexor digitorum profundus), thumb MP and IP flexion, thumb abduction (abductor longus and brevis tests) and thumb opposition.

Ulnar nerve: Finger abduction and adduction, thumb adduction.

Test Results Revealed the Following:

Wrist extension: Grade 4
Wrist flexion: Grade 3
PIP flexion: Grade 2
DIP flexion: Grade 2
MP flexion: Grade 3
Finger extension: Grade 3+
Thumb (DIP and IP) extension: Grade 3
Thumb abduction: Grade 3
Thumb adduction: Grade 3
Thumb opposition: Grade 2
Thumb PIP flexion: Grade 2
Thumb IP flexion: Grade 2

Grip strength as measured with a hand-held dynamometer was 4 pounds, barely enough to hold a glass of water.

Manual muscle testing was ideal in this instance because there were small muscles involved where the therapist could apply appropriate resistances and easily position the limbs and segments. In addition, specific knowledge was needed to define muscle loss. Grip strength testing could not have provided the important insights gained through individualized muscle testing.

Case 5. Muscle Weakness Following Hip Surgery

The patient is a 78-year-old woman weighing 170 pounds who broke her right hip as a result of a fall from her bicycle. She had surgery to repair the hip 7 months ago and had physical therapy for 5 weeks following the surgery. The patient is reluctant to return to road cycling for fear of falling, so elected to regain her fitness level by training on a stationary cycle. Immediately after beginning her stationary cycling, she found her right leg (affected side) would not perform as well as the left. Her complaint was "lack of push power" on the right and that her leg "wore out" in seconds rather than minutes. Her goal was to cycle vigorously for 30 minutes daily and take a brisk walk every other day.

When the patient's fracture repair was done, a posterior approach that bisects the glutei maximus and medius was done, affecting strength on a more permanent basis. Following surgery she was non–weight-bearing for nearly 3 months and used a walker to ambulate. At month 4 she was permitted toe-touch ambulation and over the past few months has progressed to walking with a single-point cane. Gait observation indicated a shorter stride length on the right and a gluteus medius limp that was masked by the cane. As soon as the patient placed the cane on her arm and attempted to walk unaided, her gluteus medius limp became evident and the short stride on the right became even shorter.

Given the age and sex of the patient and the magnitude of weakness suspected, a manual muscle test was selected for use. In addition, a single limb leg press was used bilaterally to provide side-to-side comparisons and two functional tests were included. Manual muscle testing was done as follows: side-lying for hip abduction and adduction with resistance applied at the ankle, and when she couldn't hold this position, resistance was applied just above the knee, prone-lying for the hip extensors with the knee flexed, with resistance also applied at the knee, and sitting for hip internal and external rotation and the hip flexors. Also tested were the muscles above and below the affected site because it is rare that weakness is present at one segment only. Thus, the core (abdominals, back extensors) and knee flexors and extensors were tested as well. A leg press was used as described and two functional tests chosen: the 30-second chair rise test and the timed stair climb for one flight and the total number of consecutive flights.

Standard procedures were used to obtain manual muscle test grades. Results were as follows:

Abdominals: Grade 3
Back extensors: Grade 4
Hip extensors: Grade 4 left, Grade 2 right
Hip abductors: Grade 4 left, Grade 2 right
Hip adductors: Grade 4 left, Grade 3 right
Internal rotation: Grade 4 left, Grade 4 right
External rotation: Grade 4 left, Grade 3 right
Knee extension: Grade 4 left, Grade 3+ right
Knee flexion: Grade 4 left, Grade 4 right
Unilateral leg press: 140 pounds left, 45 pounds right (optimal: 70 pounds bilaterally)
Chair rises: Without using the chair arms, the patient was able to do one chair rise and this one repetition required multiple attempts.
Stair climb: The patient ascended four flights of stairs total but needed to use the railing and rest momentarily on the landing of the third and fourth flights. She accomplished one flight of 9 stairs up and down in 39 seconds.

This case illustrates the fairly classic scenario of patient discharged long before rehabilitation is complete. Fortunately, the patient had a long exercise history and her current state of weakness and reduced function were unacceptable to her. Thus, she was a prime candidate for a home program of strengthening and endurance work and a community exercise program.

Case 6. Muscle Weakness Following Childbirth

The patient gave birth to her second child 2 years ago. Postpartum exercises were never initiated and she had no history of engaging in any routine physical activity other than childcare. Now she is having difficulty with urine leakage when laughing, coughing, and lifting her toddler. The stress incontinence prompted her to seek help.

Muscles of the pelvic floor and abdomen elongate enormously to accommodate pregnancy and childbirth. In many women, the stretched musculature fails to return to its prepartum strength and length. This pelvic floor/abdominal weakness scenario is especially likely in women who have had multiple births, particularly if they did not perform postpartum exercises.

For this woman, manual muscle testing of the abdominals and pelvic floor was chosen because these muscles are often found to be weak following childbirth. Muscle testing revealed the following.

Bilateral leg lowering test (from 90° of hip flexion toward 0°): Grade 2
Upper abdominals (head and shoulder raise): Grade 2
Pelvic floor (manual test): Grade 3

In summary, childbirth weakened the pelvic floor and abdominal musculature. Even though this weakness is present in nearly all women after delivery, too few are counseled to perform pelvic floor exercises or strengthen abdominals. If the condition persists, urinary incontinence is likely. Standard muscle testing techniques were used to identify weakness.

1. Davies GJ, Wiik K, Ellenbecker T, et al. The shoulder: physical therapy patient management using current evidence. Independent Study Course 16.2.4. Fairfax, VA: American Physical Therapy Association; 2006.
2. Sahrmann SA. Diagnosis and treatment of movement impairment syndromes. New York: Mosby; 2006: 246-260.
3. Steindler A. Kinesiology of the Human Body, ed. 4. Springfield, IL: Charles C Thomas; 1973:459-474.
4. Lunsford BR, Perry J. The standing heel-rise test for ankle plantar flexion: criterion for normal. Phys Ther. 1995;75: 694-698.
5. Jan MH, Chai HM, Lin YF, et al. Effects of age and sex on the results of an ankle plantar-flexor manual muscle test. Phys Ther. 2005;85:1078-1084.

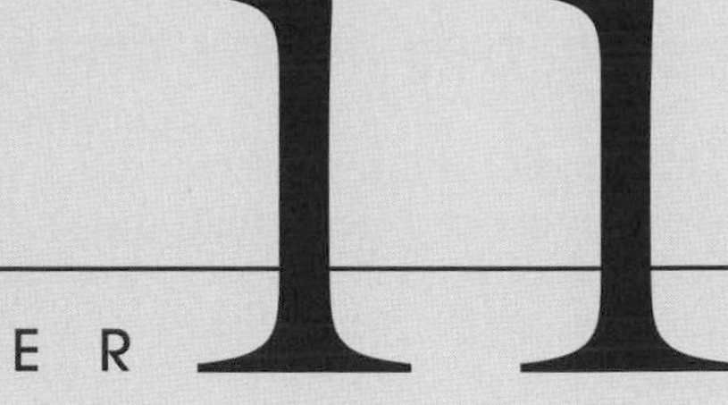

CHAPTER 11

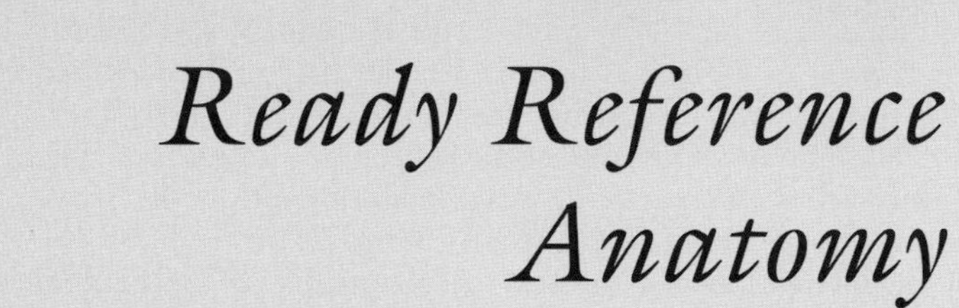

Ready Reference Anatomy

USING THIS READY REFERENCE

This chapter is intended as a quick source of information about muscles—their anatomical description, participation in motions, and innervation. This information is not intended to be comprehensive, and for depth of subject matter the reader is referred to any of the major texts of human anatomy. We relied on the American[1] and British[2] versions of *Gray's Anatomy* as principal references but also used *Sobotta's Atlas*,[3] Clemente,[4] Netter,[5] Hollingshead,[6] Jenkins,[6] Grant,[7] and Moore,[8] among others. The final arbiter in all cases was the 38th edition of *Gray's Anatomy* (British) by Williams et al.[2]

The variations in text descriptions of individual muscles remain exceedingly diverse so at times we have consolidated information to provide abstracted descriptions.

Origins, insertions, descriptions, and functions of individual muscles often are abbreviated but should allow the reader to place the muscle correctly and visualize its most common actions; this in turn may help the reader to recall more detailed anatomy.

Nomina Anatomica nomenclature for the muscles appears in brackets when a more common usage is listed.

The entire *Ready Reference Anatomy* is available on the Evolve site that accompanies this text. Two additional sections are also included, "Part 5. Motions and their Participating Muscles (Motions of the Neck, Trunk, and Limbs)" and "Part 6. Cranial and Peripheral Nerves and the Muscles they Innervate".

Muscle Reference Numbers

Each skeletal muscle in the body has been given an identification (ID), or reference number that is used with that muscle throughout the book. The order of numbering is derived from the regional sequence of muscles used in Part 2 of this reference. The numbering should, however, permit the reader to refer quickly to any one of the summaries or to cross-check information between summaries. In the first part of the Ready Reference section (and also inside the front cover), the muscles are listed in alphabetical order, and this is followed by a list of muscles by region (also inside the back cover). In each muscle test, the participating muscles also are preceded by their assigned identification (reference) number.

A

159 Abductor digiti minimi (hand)
215 Abductor digiti minimi (foot)
224 Abductor hallucis
171 Abductor pollicis brevis
166 Abductor pollicis longus
180 Adductor brevis
225 Adductor hallucis
179 Adductor longus
181 Adductor magnus
173 Adductor pollicis
144 Anconeus
27 Auriculares
201 Articularis genus

B

140 Biceps brachii
192 Biceps femoris
141 Brachialis
143 Brachioradialis
26 Buccinator
120 Bulbospongiosus

C

34 Chondroglossus
116 Coccygeus
139 Coracobrachialis
5 Corrugator supercilii
50 Cricothyroid [Cricothyroideus]
117 Cremaster

D

133 Deltoid [Deltoideus]
23 Depressor anguli oris
24 Depressor labii inferioris
14 Depressor septi
101 Diaphragm
78 Digastric [Digastricus]

E

2 Epicranius
149 Extensor carpi radialis brevis
148 Extensor carpi radialis longus
150 Extensor carpi ulnaris
158 Extensor digiti minimi
154 Extensor digitorum
212 Extensor digitorum brevis
211 Extensor digitorum longus
221 Extensor hallucis longus
155 Extensor indicis
168 Extensor pollicis brevis
167 Extensor pollicis longus

F

151 Flexor carpi radialis
153 Flexor carpi ulnaris
160 Flexor digiti minimi brevis (hand)
216 Flexor digiti minimi brevis (foot)
214 Flexor digitorum brevis
213 Flexor digitorum longus
157 Flexor digitorum profundus
156 Flexor digitorum superficialis
223 Flexor hallucis brevis
222 Flexor hallucis longus
170 Flexor pollicis brevis
169 Flexor pollicis longus

G

205 Gastrocnemius
190 Gemellus inferior
189 Gemellus superior
32 Genioglossus
77 Geniohyoid [Geniohyoideus]
182 Gluteus maximus
183 Gluteus medius
184 Gluteus minimus
178 Gracilis

H

33 Hyoglossus

I

176 Iliacus
66 Iliocostalis cervicis
89 Iliocostalis thoracis
90 Iliocostalis lumborum
41 Inferior pharyngeal constrictor [Constrictor pharyngis inferior]
38 Inferior longitudinal (tongue) [Longitudinalis inferior]
84-87 Infrahyoids (see Sternothyroid, Thyrohyoid, Sternohyoid, Omohyoid)
136 Infraspinatus
102 Intercostales externi
103 Intercostales interni
104 Intercostales intimi
164 Interossei, dorsal (hand) [Interossei dorsales]
219 Interossei, dorsal (foot) [Interossei dorsales]
165 Interossei, palmar or volar [Interossei palmares]
220 Interossei, plantar [Interossei plantares]
69 Interspinales cervicis
97 Interspinales thoracis
98 Interspinales lumborum
70 Intertransversarii cervicis
99 Intertransversarii thoracis
99 Intertransversarii lumborum
121 Ischiocavernosus

L

52 Lateral cricoarytenoid [Cricoarytenoideus lateralis]
30 Lateral pterygoid [Pterygoideus lateralis]
130 Latissimus dorsi
115 Levator ani
17 Levator anguli oris
15 Levator labii superioris
16 Levator labii superioris alaeque nasi
3 Levator palpebrae superioris
127 Levator scapulae
46 Levator veli palatini
107 Levatores costarum
60 Longissimus capitis
64 Longissimus cervicis
91 Longissimus thoracis
74 Longus capitis
79 Longus colli
163 Lumbricales (hand) [Lumbricals]
218 Lumbricales (foot) [Lumbricals]

M

28 Masseter
31 Medial pterygoid [Pterygoideus medialis]
21 Mentalis
42 Middle pharyngeal constrictor [Constrictor pharyngis medius]
94 Multifidi
48 Musculus uvulae
75 Mylohyoid [Mylohyoideus]

N

13 Nasalis

O

54 Oblique arytenoid [Arytenoideus obliquus]
59 Obliquus capitis inferior
58 Obliquus capitis superior
110 Obliquus externus abdominis
11 Obliquus inferior oculi
111 Obliquus internus abdominis
10 Obliquus superior oculi
188 Obturator externus [Obturatorius externus]
187 Obturator internus [Obturatorius internus]
1 Occipitofrontalis
87 Omohyoid [Omohyoideus]
161 Opponens digiti minimi
172 Opponens pollicis
4 Orbicularis oculi
25 Orbicularis oris

P

36 Palatoglossus
49 Palatopharyngeus
162 Palmaris brevis
152 Palmaris longus
177 Pectineus
131 Pectoralis major
129 Pectoralis minor
209 Peroneus brevis
208 Peroneus longus
210 Peroneus tertius
186 Piriformis
207 Plantaris
88 Platysma
202 Popliteus
51 Posterior cricoarytenoid [Cricoarytenoideus posterior]
12 Procerus
147 Pronator quadratus
146 Pronator teres
174 Psoas major

175 Psoas minor
114 Pyramidalis

Q

191 Quadratus femoris
100 Quadratus lumborum
217 Quadratus plantae
196-200 Quadriceps femoris (see Rectus femoris, Vastus intermedius, Vastus medialis longus, Vastus medialis oblique, Vastus lateralis)

R

113 Rectus abdominis
72 Rectus capitis anterior
73 Rectus capitis lateralis
56 Rectus capitis posterior major
57 Rectus capitis posterior minor
196 Rectus femoris
7 Rectus inferior
9 Rectus lateralis
8 Rectus medialis
6 Rectus superior
125 Rhomboid major [Rhomboideus major]
126 Rhomboid minor [Rhomboideus minor]
20 Risorius
71 Rotatores cervicis
96 Rotatores lumborum
95 Rotatores thoracis

S

45 Salpingopharyngeus
195 Sartorius
80 Scalenus anterior
81 Scalenus medius
82 Scalenus posterior
194 Semimembranosus
62 Semispinalis capitis
65 Semispinalis cervicis
93 Semispinalis thoracis
193 Semitendinosus
128 Serratus anterior
109 Serratus posterior inferior
108 Serratus posterior superior
206 Soleus
123 Sphincter ani externus
122 Sphincter urethrae
63 Spinalis capitis
68 Spinalis cervicis
92 Spinalis thoracis
61 Splenius capitis
67 Splenius cervicis
83 Sternocleidomastoid [Sternocleidomastoideus]
86 Sternohyoid [Sternohyoideus]
84 Sternothyroid [Sternothyroideus]
35 Styloglossus
76 Stylohyoid [Stylohyoideus]
44 Stylopharyngeus
132 Subclavius
105 Subcostales
134 Subscapularis
43 Superior pharyngeal constrictor [Constrictor pharyngis superior]
37 Superior longitudinal (tongue) [Longitudinalis superior]
145 Supinator
75-78 Suprahyoids (see Mylohyoid, Stylohyoid, Geniohyoid, Digastric)
135 Supraspinatus

T

29 Temporalis
2 Temporoparietalis
185 Tensor fasciae latae
47 Tensor veli palatini
138 Teres major
137 Teres minor
85 Thyrohyoid [Thyrohyoideus]
55 Thyroarytenoid [Thyroarytenoideus]
203 Tibialis anterior
204 Tibialis posterior
39 Transverse lingual [Transversus linguae]
112 Transversus abdominis
53 Transverse arytenoid [Arytenoideus transversus]
22 Transversus menti
119 Transversus perinei profundus
118 Transversus perinei superficialis
106 Transversus thoracis
124 Trapezius
142 Triceps brachii

U

48 Uvula (see Musculus uvulae)

V

198 Vastus intermedius
199 Vastus medialis longus
200 Vastus medialis oblique
197 Vastus lateralis
40 Vertical lingual [Verticalis linguae]

Z

18 Zygomaticus major
19 Zygomaticus minor

HEAD AND FOREHEAD

1 Occipitofrontalis
2 Temporoparietalis

EYELIDS

3 Levator palpebrae superioris
4 Orbicularis oculi
5 Corrugator supercilii

OCULAR MUSCLES

6 Rectus superior
7 Rectus inferior
8 Rectus medialis
9 Rectus lateralis
10 Obliquus superior
11 Obliquus inferior

NOSE

12 Procerus
13 Nasalis
14 Depressor septi

MOUTH

15 Levator labii superioris
16 Levator labii superioris alaeque nasi
17 Levator anguli oris
18 Zygomaticus major
19 Zygomaticus minor
20 Risorius
21 Mentalis
22 Transversus menti
23 Depressor anguli oris
24 Depressor labii inferioris
25 Orbicularis oris
26 Buccinator

EAR

27 Auriculares

JAW (MASTICATION)

28 Masseter
29 Temporalis
30 Lateral pterygoid
31 Medial pterygoid

TONGUE

32 Genioglossus
33 Hyoglossus
34 Chondroglossus
35 Styloglossus
36 Palatoglossus
37 Superior longitudinal
38 Inferior longitudinal
39 Transverse lingual
40 Vertical lingual

PHARYNX

41 Inferior pharyngeal constrictor
42 Middle pharyngeal constrictor
43 Superior pharyngeal constrictor
44 Stylopharyngeus
45 Salpingopharyngeus
49 Palatopharyngeus (see under *Palate*)

PALATE

46 Levator veli palatini
47 Tensor veli palatini
48 Musculus uvulae
36 Palatoglossus (see under *Tongue*)
49 Palatopharyngeus

LARYNX

50 Cricothyroid
51 Posterior cricoarytenoid
52 Lateral cricoarytenoid
53 Transverse arytenoid
54 Oblique arytenoid
55 Thyroarytenoid

NECK

56 Rectus capitis posterior major
57 Rectus capitis posterior minor
58 Obliquus capitis superior
59 Obliquus capitis inferior
60 Longissimus capitis
61 Splenius capitis
62 Semispinalis capitis
63 Spinalis capitis
64 Longissimus cervicis
65 Semispinalis cervicis
66 Iliocostalis cervicis
67 Splenius cervicis
68 Spinalis cervicis
69 Interspinales cervicis
70 Intertransversarii cervicis
71 Rotatores cervicis
72 Rectus capitis anterior
73 Rectus capitis lateralis
74 Longus capitis
75 Mylohyoid
76 Stylohyoid
77 Geniohyoid
78 Digastricus
79 Longus colli
80 Scalenus anterior
81 Scalenus medius
82 Scalenus posterior
83 Sternocleidomastoid
84 Sternothyroid
85 Thyrohyoid
86 Sternohyoid
87 Omohyoid
88 Platysma

BACK

61 Splenius capitis (see under *Neck*)

67 Splenius cervicis (see under *Neck*)

66 Iliocostalis cervicis (see under *Neck*)

89 Iliocostalis thoracis

90 Iliocostalis lumborum

60 Longissimus capitis (see under *Neck*)

64 Longissimus cervicis (see under *Neck*)

91 Longissimus thoracis

63 Spinalis capitis

68 Spinalis cervicis

92 Spinalis thoracis

62 Semispinalis capitis (see under *Neck*)

65 Semispinalis cervicis (see under *Neck*)

93 Semispinalis thoracis

94 Multifidi

71 Rotatores cervicis (see under *Neck*)

95 Rotatores thoracis

96 Rotatores lumborum

69 Interspinalis cervicis (see under *Neck*)

97 Interspinalis thoracis

98 Interspinalis lumborum

70 Intertransversarii cervicis (see under *Neck*)

99 Intertransversarii thoracis

99 Intertransversarii lumborum

100 Quadratus lumborum

THORAX (RESPIRATION)

101 Diaphragm

102 Intercostales externi

103 Intercostales interni

104 Intercostales intimi

105 Subcostales

106 Transversus thoracis

107 Levatores costarum

108 Serratus posterior superior

109 Serratus posterior inferior

ABDOMEN

110 Obliquus externus abdominis

111 Obliquus internus abdominis

112 Transversus abdominis

113 Rectus abdominis

114 Pyramidalis

PERINEUM

115 Levator ani

116 Coccygeus

117 Cremaster

118 Transversus perinei superficialis

119 Transversus perinei profundus

120 Bulbospongiosus

121 Ischiocavernosus

122 Sphincter urethrae

123 Sphincter ani externus

UPPER EXTREMITY

Shoulder Girdle

124 Trapezius

125 Rhomboid major

126 Rhomboid minor

127 Levator scapulae

128 Serratus anterior

129 Pectoralis minor

Vertebrohumeral

130 Latissimus dorsi

131 Pectoralis major

Shoulder

132 Subclavius

133 Deltoid

134 Subscapularis

135 Supraspinatus

136 Infraspinatus

137 Teres minor

138 Teres major

139 Coracobrachialis

Elbow

140 Biceps brachii

141 Brachialis

142 Triceps brachii

143 Brachioradialis

144 Anconeus

Forearm

145 Supinator

146 Pronator teres

147 Pronator quadratus

140 Biceps brachii (see under *Elbow*)

Wrist

148 Extensor carpi radialis longus

149 Extensor carpi radialis brevis

150 Extensor carpi ulnaris

151 Flexor carpi radialis

152 Palmaris longus

153 Flexor carpi ulnaris

Fingers

154 Extensor digitorum

155 Extensor indicis

156 Flexor digitorum superficialis

157 Flexor digitorum profundus

163 Lumbricales

164 Interossei, dorsal

165 Interossei, palmar

Little Finger and Hypothenar Muscles

158 Extensor digiti minimi

159 Abductor digiti minimi

160 Flexor digiti minimi brevis
161 Opponens digiti minimi
162 Palmaris brevis

Thumb and Thenar Muscles

166 Abductor pollicis longus
167 Extensor pollicis longus
168 Extensor pollicis brevis
169 Flexor pollicis longus
170 Flexor pollicis brevis
171 Abductor pollicis brevis
172 Opponens pollicis
173 Adductor pollicis

LOWER EXTREMITY

Hip and Thigh

174 Psoas major
175 Psoas minor
176 Iliacus
177 Pectineus
178 Gracilis
179 Adductor longus
180 Adductor brevis
181 Adductor magnus
182 Gluteus maximus
183 Gluteus medius
184 Gluteus minimus
185 Tensor fasciae latae
186 Piriformis
187 Obturator internus
188 Obturator externus
189 Gemellus superior
190 Gemellus inferior
191 Quadratus femoris
192 Biceps femoris
193 Semitendinosus
194 Semimembranosus
195 Sartorius

Knee

196-200 Quadriceps femoris
196 Rectus femoris
197 Vastus lateralis
198 Vastus intermedius
199 Vastus medialis longus
200 Vastus medialis oblique
201 Articularis genus
192 Biceps femoris (see under *Hip and Thigh*)
193 Semitendinosus (see under *Hip and Thigh*)
194 Semimembranosus (see under *Hip and Thigh*)
202 Popliteus

Ankle

203 Tibialis anterior
204 Tibialis posterior
205 Gastrocnemius
206 Soleus
207 Plantaris
208 Peroneus longus
209 Peroneus brevis
210 Peroneus tertius

Lesser Toes

211 Extensor digitorum longus
212 Extensor digitorum brevis
213 Flexor digitorum longus
214 Flexor digitorum brevis
215 Abductor digiti minimi
216 Flexor digiti minimi brevis
217 Quadratus plantae
218 Lumbricales
219 Interossei, dorsal
220 Interossei, plantar

Great Toe (Hallux)

221 Extensor hallucis longus
222 Flexor hallucis longus
223 Flexor hallucis brevis
224 Abductor hallucis
225 Adductor hallucis

MUSCLES OF THE FOREHEAD

The Epicranius (Two Muscles)

1 Occipitofrontalis
2 Temporoparietalis

1 OCCIPITOFRONTALIS

Muscle has two parts

Occipital Part (Occipitalis)

Origin:
Occiput (superior nuchal line, lateral ⅔)
Temporal bone (mastoid process)

Insertion:
Galea aponeurotica

Frontal part (Frontalis)

Origin:
Superficial fascia over scalp
No bony attachments
Median fibers continuous with procerus
Intermediate fibers join corrugator supercilii and orbicularis oculi
Lateral fibers also join orbicularis oculi

Insertion:
Galea aponeurotica
Skin of eyebrows and root of nose

Description:
Overlies the cranium from the eyebrows to the superior nuchal line on the occiput. The epicranius consists of the occipitofrontalis with its four thin branches on either side of the head, the broad aponeurosis called the galea aponeurotica, and the temporoparietalis with its two slim branches. The medial margins of the two bellies join above the nose and run together upward and over the forehead.
The galea aponeurotica covers the cranium between the frontal belly and the occipital belly of the epicranius and between the two occipital bellies over the occiput. It is adhered closely to the dermal layers (scalp), which allows the scalp to be moved freely over the cranium.

Function:
Contracting together, both bellies draw the scalp up and back, thus raising the eyebrows (surprise!) and assisting with wrinkling the forehead.
Working alone, the frontal belly raises the eyebrow on the same side.

Innervation:
Facial (VII) nerve
Temporal branches: to frontalis
Posterior auricular branch: to occipitalis

2 TEMPOROPARIETALIS

Origin:
Temporal fascia (superior and anterior to external ear, then fanning out and up over temporal fascia)

Insertion:
Galea aponeurotica (lateral border)
Into skin and temporal fascia somewhere high on lateral side of head

Description:
A thin broad sheet of muscle in two bellies which lie on either side of head. Highly variable. See also description of occipitofrontalis.

Function:
Tightens scalp
Draws back skin over temples
Raises auricula of the ear
In concert with occipitofrontalis, raises the eyebrows, widens the eyes, and wrinkles the skin of the forehead (in expressions of surprise and fright)

Innervation:
Facial (VII) nerve (temporal branches)

MUSCLES OF THE EYELIDS AND EYEBROWS

3 Levator palpebrae superioris
4 Orbicularis oculi
5 Corrugator supercilii

3 LEVATOR PALPEBRAE SUPERIORIS

Origin:
Sphenoid bone (inferior surface of lesser wing)
Roof of orbital cavity

Insertion:
Into several lamellae:
Aponeurosis of the orbital septum
Superior tarsus (a small, thin smooth fiber muscle on the inferior surface of the levator palpebrae and skin of eyelids)
Upper eyelid skin
Sheath of the rectus superior (and with it, blends with the superior fornix of the conjunctiva)

Description:
Thin and flat muscle lying posterior and superior to the orbit. At its origin it is tendinous, broadening out to end in a wide aponeurosis that splits into three lamellae. Connective tissue of the levator fuses with adjoining connective tissue of the rectus superior and this aponeurosis can be traced laterally to a tubercle of the zygomatic bone and medially to the medial palpebral ligament.

Function:
Raises upper eyelid

Innervation:
Oculomotor (III) nerve (superior division)

4 ORBICULARIS OCULI

Muscle has three parts

Origin:
Orbital part
Frontal bone (nasal part)
Maxilla (frontal process in front of lacrimal groove)
Medial palpebral ligament

Palpebral part
Medial palpebral ligament
Frontal bone just in front of and below the palpebral ligament

Lacrimal part
Lacrimal fascia
Lacrimal bone (crest and lateral surface)

Insertion:
Orbital part: The fibers blend with nearby muscles (occipitofrontalis and corrugator supercilii). Some fibers also insert into skin of eyebrow.
Palpebral part: Lateral palpebral raphe
Lacrimal part: Superior and inferior tarsi of the eyelids. Fibers form lateral palpebral raphe.

Description:
Forms a broad thin layer that fills the eyelids (see Figure 7-13) and surrounds the circumference of the orbit but also spreads over the temple and cheek. Orbital fibers form complete ellipses. On the lateral side there are no bony attachments. The upper orbital fiber ellipses blend with the occipitofrontalis and corrugator supercilii muscles. Fibers also insert into the skin of the eyebrow forming a depressor supercilii. Medially some ellipses reach the procerus.
The inferior orbital ellipses blend with the levator labii superioris alaeque nasi, levator labii superioris, and the zygomaticus minor.
The fibers of the palpebral part sweep across the upper and lower eyelids anterior to the orbital septum to form the lateral palpebral raphe. The ciliary bundle is composed of a small group of fibers behind the eyelashes.
The lacrimal part fibers lying behind the lacrimal sac (in the medial corner of the eye) divide into upper and lower slips which insert into the superior and inferior tarsi of the eyelids and the lateral palpebral raphe.

Function:
The orbicularis oculi is the sphincter of the eye.
Orbital part: Although closing the eye is mostly lowering of the upper lid, the lower lid also rises and both are under voluntary control and can work with greater force, as in winking.
Palpebral part: Closes lids in blinking (protective reflex) and for sleep (voluntary).
Lacrimal part: Draws the eyelids and lacrimal canals medially, compressing them against the globe of the eye to receive tears. Also compresses lacrimal sac during blinking.
Entire muscle contraction draws skin of forehead, temple, and cheek toward the medial angle of the eye, tightly closing the eye and displacing the lids medially. The folds formed by this action in later life form "crow's feet." The muscles around the eye are important because they cause blinking, which keeps the eye lubricated and prevents dehydration of the conjunctiva. The muscle also bunches up to protect the eye from excessive light.

Innervation:
Facial (VII) nerve (temporal and zygomatic branches)

5 CORRUGATOR SUPERCILII

Origin:
Frontal bone (superciliary arch, medial end)

Insertion:
Skin (deep surface) of eyebrow over middle of orbital arch

Description:
Fibers of this small muscle lie at the medial end of each eyebrow, deep to the occipitofrontalis and orbicularis oculi muscles with which it often blends.

Function:
Draws eyebrows down and medially, producing vertical wrinkles of the forehead between the eyes (frowning). This action also shields the eyes from bright sun.

Innervation:
Facial (VII) nerve (temporal branch)

OCULAR MUSCLES

6 Rectus superior
7 Rectus inferior
8 Rectus medialis
9 Rectus lateralis
10 Obliquus superior
11 Obliquus inferior

The Extraocular Muscles

There are seven extraocular muscles of the eye: the four recti, the two obliquii, and the levator palpebrae. The recti with the obliquii can move the eyeball in infinite directions, whereas the levator can raise the upper eyelid. In addition, there are superior and inferior tarsal muscles in the upper and lower eyelids; the superior is related to the levator palpebrae superior, whereas the inferior works with the rectus inferior and inferior oblique. The orbicularis oculi also is an extraocular muscle but it is described with the facial muscles.

6-9 THE FOUR RECTI (Figure 11-1)

Rectus Superior, Inferior, Medialis, and Lateralis

Origin:
At the back of the eye, the tendons of the four recti are attached to a common annular tendon. This tendon rings the superior, medial, and inferior margins of the optic foramen and attaches to the sphenoid bone (greater wing). It also adheres to the sheath of the optic nerve. The attachments of the four recti circle the tendon on its medial, superior, and inferior margins. The ring around the optic nerve is completed by a lower fibrous extension (tendon of Zinn), which gives origin to the rectus inferior, part of the rectus medialis, and the lower head of origin of the rectus lateralis. An upper fibrous expansion gives rise to the rectus superior, part of the rectus medialis, and the upper head of the rectus lateralis.

Insertion:
Each of the recti passes anteriorly in the position indicated by its name and inserts via a tendinous expansion into the sclera a short distance behind the cornea.

Description:
From their common origin around the margins of the optic canal these straplike muscles become wider as they pass anteriorly to insert on different points on the sclera (see Figure 11-1) The rectus superior is the smallest and thinnest and inserts on the superoanterior sclera under the orbital roof. The inferior muscle inserts on the inferoanterior sclera just above the orbital floor. The rectus medialis is the broadest of the recti and inserts on the medial scleral wall well in front of the equator. The rectus lateralis, the longest of the recti, courses around the lateral side of the eyeball to insert well forward of the equator.

Function:
The ocular muscles rotate the eyeball in directions that depend on the geometry of their relationships and that can be altered by the eye movements

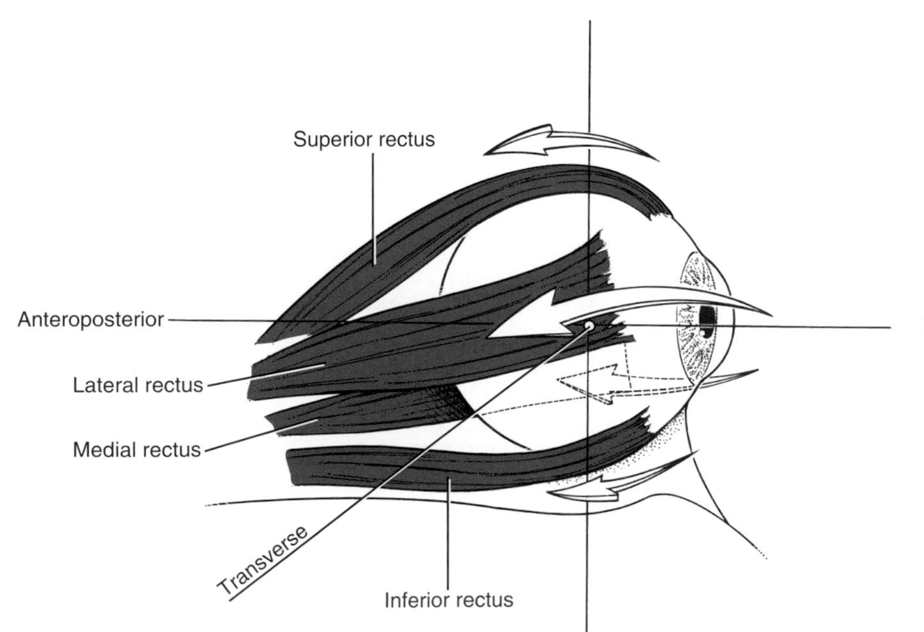

FIGURE 11-1 The four recti, lateral view.

themselves. Eye movements also are accompanied by head motions, which assist with the incredibly complex varieties of stereoscopic vision.

The ocular muscles are not subject to direct study or routine assessment. It is essential to know that a change in the tension of one of the muscles alters the length-tension relationships of all six ocular muscles. It is likely that all six muscles are continuously involved, and consideration of each in isolation is not a functional exercise. The functional relationship between the four recti and the two obliquii may be considered as two differing synergies.

The rectus superior, inferior, and medialis act together as adductors or convergence muscles.

The lateral rectus, together with the two obliquii, act as muscles of abduction or divergence.

Convergence generally is associated with elevation of the visual axis, and divergence with lowering of the visual axis.

Neurologists regularly test the ocular muscles when there is an isolated paralysis which gives greater insight into their functions.[9]

Superior rectus paralysis: Eye turns down and slightly outward. Upward motion is limited.

Medial rectus paralysis: Eyeball turns laterally and cannot deviate medially.

Inferior rectus paralysis: Eyeball deviates upward and somewhat laterally. It cannot be moved downward and the eye is abducted.

Lateral rectus paralysis: The eyeball is turned medially and cannot be abducted.

Inferior oblique paralysis: Eyeball is deviated downward and slightly medially; it cannot be moved upward when in abduction.

Superior oblique paralysis: Here there may be little deviation of the eyeball but downward motion is limited when the eye is adducted. There is no movement toward the midline of the face when looking downward in abduction (intorsion).[9]

Innervation:

Oculomotor (III) nerve: Rectus superior (superior division of III), inferior, and medialis, and obliquus inferior (inferior division of III)

Abducent (VI) nerve: Rectus lateralis

Trochlear (IV) nerve: Obliquus superior

10 OBLIQUUS SUPERIOR OCULI

Origin:

Sphenoid bone (superior and medial to optic canal)

Rectus superior (tendon)

Insertion:

Frontal bone (via a round tendon that inserts through a pulley [a cartilaginous ring called the trochlea] that inserts in the trochlear fovea)

Sclera (behind the equator on the superolateral surface)

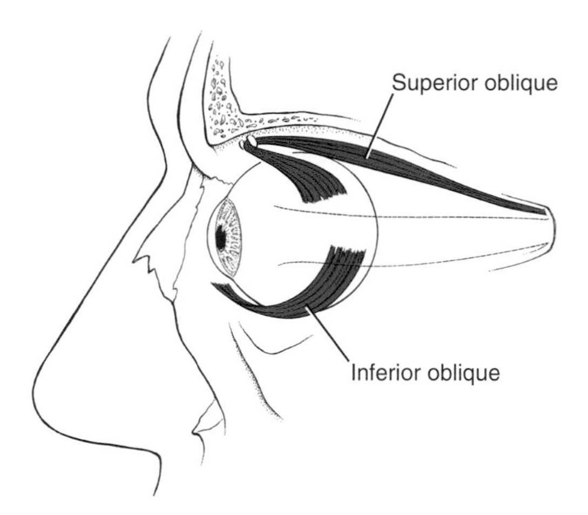

FIGURE 11-2 The oblique extraocular muscles.

Description:

The superior oblique lies superomedially in the orbit (Figure 11-2). It passes forward, ending in the round tendon that loops through the trochlear pulley, which is attached to the trochlear fovea. It then turns abruptly posterolaterally and passes thence to the sclera to end between the rectus superior and the rectus lateralis.

Function:

The superior oblique acts on the eye from above, whereas the inferior oblique acts on the eye directly below; the superior oblique elevates the posterior aspect of the eyeball, and the inferior oblique depresses it. The superior oblique, therefore, rotates the visual axis downward, whereas the inferior oblique rotates it upward, both motions occurring around the transverse axis.

Innervation:

Trochlear (IV) nerve

11 OBLIQUUS INFERIOR OCULI

Origin:

Maxilla (orbital surface, lateral to the lacrimal groove)

Insertion:

Sclera (lateral part) behind the equator of the eyeball between the insertions of the rectus inferior and lateralis and near, but behind, the insertion of the superior oblique

Description:

Located near the anterior margin of the floor of the orbit, it passes laterally under the eyeball between the rectus inferior and the bony orbit. It then bends upward on the lateral side of the eyeball, passing under the rectus lateralis to insert on the sclera beneath that muscle (see Figures 11-1 and 11-2).

Function:
See under *Obliquus superior* (#10).

Innervation:
Oculomotor (III) nerve (inferior division)

MUSCLES OF THE NOSE

12 Procerus
13 Nasalis
14 Depressor septi

12 PROCERUS

Origin:
Nasal bone (dorsum of nose, lower part)
Nasal cartilage (lateral, upper part)

Insertion:
Skin over lower part of forehead between eyebrows
Joins occipitofrontalis

Description:
From its origin over bridge of nose it courses straight upward to blend with frontalis.

Function:
Produces transverse wrinkles over bridge of nose
Draws eyebrows downward

Innervation:
Facial (VII) nerve (buccal branch)

13 NASALIS

Transverse Part (Compressor Nares)

Origin:
Maxilla (above and lateral to incisive fossa)

Insertion:
Aponeurosis over bridge of nose joining with muscle on opposite side

Alar Part (Dilator Nares)

Origin:
Maxilla (above lateral incisor tooth)
Alar cartilage

Insertion:
Ala nasi
Skin at tip of nose

Description:
Muscle has two parts that cover the distal and medial surfaces of the nose. Fibers from each side rise upward and medially, meeting in a narrow aponeurosis near the bridge of the nose.

Function:
Transverse part: Depresses cartilaginous portion of nose and draws alae toward septum
Alar part: Dilates nostrils (during breathing it resists tendency of nares to close from atmospheric pressure).
Noticeable in anger or labored breathing

Innervation:
Facial (VII) nerve (buccal and zygomatic branches)

14 DEPRESSOR SEPTI

Origin:
Maxilla (above and lateral to incisive fossa, i.e., central incisor)

Insertion:
Nasal septum (mobile part) and alar cartilage

Description:
Fibers ascend vertically from central maxillary origin. Muscle lies deep to the superior labial mucous membrane. It often is considered part of the dilator nares (of the nasalis).

Function:
Draws alae of nose downward (constricting nares)

Innervation:
Facial (VII) nerve (buccal and zygomatic branches)

MUSCLES OF THE MOUTH

There are four independent quadrants, each of which has a pars peripheralis which lies along the junction of the red margin of the lip and skin and a pars marginalis which is found in the red margin of the lip (see Figure 7-29). These two parts are supported by fibers from the buccinator and depressor anguli oris (upper lip) and from the buccinator and levator anguli oris (lower lip). These muscles are uniquely developed for speech.

15 Levator labii superioris
16 Levator labii superioris alaeque nasi
17 Levator anguli oris
18 Zygomaticus major
19 Zygomaticus minor
20 Risorius

21 Mentalis
22 Transversus menti
23 Depressor anguli oris
24 Depressor labii inferioris
25 Orbicularis oris
26 Buccinator

15 LEVATOR LABII SUPERIORIS

(Also called quadratus labii superioris)

Origin:
Orbit of eye (inferior margin)
Maxilla
Zygomatic bone

Insertion:
Upper lip

Description:
Converging from a rather broad place of origin on the inferior orbit, the fibers converge and descend into the upper lip between the other levator muscles and the zygomaticus minor.

Function:
Elevates and protracts upper lip

Innervation:
Facial (VII) nerve (buccal branch)

16 LEVATOR LABII SUPERIORIS ALAEQUE NASI

Origin:
Maxilla (frontal process)

Insertion:
Ala of nose
Upper lip

Description:
Muscle fibers descend obliquely lateral and divide into two slips: one to the greater alar cartilage of the nose and one to blend with the levator labii superioris and orbicularis oris (thence to the modiolus)

Function:
Dilates nostrils
Elevates upper lip

Innervation:
Facial (VII) nerve (buccal branch)

17 LEVATOR ANGULI ORIS

Origin:
Maxilla (canine fossa)

Insertion:
Modiolus
Dermal attachment at angle of mouth

Description:
Muscle descends from maxilla, inferolateral to orbit, down to modiolus. It lies partially under the zygomaticus minor.

Function:
Raises angle of mouth and by so doing displays teeth in smiling
Contributes to nasolabial furrow (from side of nose to corner of upper lip). Deepens in sadness and aging.

Innervation:
Facial (VII) nerve (buccal branch)

18 ZYGOMATICUS MAJOR

Origin:
Zygomatic bone (lateral)

Insertion:
Modiolus[10-12]

Description:
Descends obliquely lateral to blend with other modiolar muscles. A small and variable group of superficial fascicles called the malaris are considered part of this muscle.

Function:
Draws angle of mouth lateral and upward (as in laughing)

Innervation:
Facial (VII) nerve (buccal branch)

19 ZYGOMATICUS MINOR

Origin:
Zygomatic bone (malar surface) medial to origin of zygomaticus major

Insertion:
Upper lip; blends with levator labii superioris
Modiolus[10-12]

Commentary on Facial Muscles

The muscles of the face are different from most skeletal muscles in the body because they are cutaneous muscles located in the deep layers of the skin and frequently have no bony attachments. All of them (scalp, eyelids, nose, lips, cheeks, mouth, and auricle) give rise to "expressions" and convey "thought," the most visible of the body language systems (Figure 11-3).

The orbital muscles of the mouth are important for speech, drinking, and ingestion of solid foods.[10-12] Although the buccinator is described in this section, it is not a muscle of expression but does serve an important role in regulating the position of, and action on, food in the mouth.

These muscles are continuously tonic to provide the facial skin with tension; the skin becomes baggy or flabby (resulting in "crow's feet" or "wattles") when it is denervated or in the presence of the atrophic processes associated with aging. There are wide differences in these muscles among individuals and among racial groups, and to deal with such variations craniofacial and plastic surgeons often classify the facial muscles differently (e.g., in single vs. multiple heads) from the system presented here.

Continuous skin tension also gives rise to the gaping wounds that occur with facial lacerations, and surgeons take great care to understand the planes of the muscles to minimize scarring in the repair of such wounds.

The facial muscles all arise from the mesoderm of the second branchial (hyoid) arch. The muscles lie in all parts of the face and head but retain their innervation by the facial (VII) nerve.

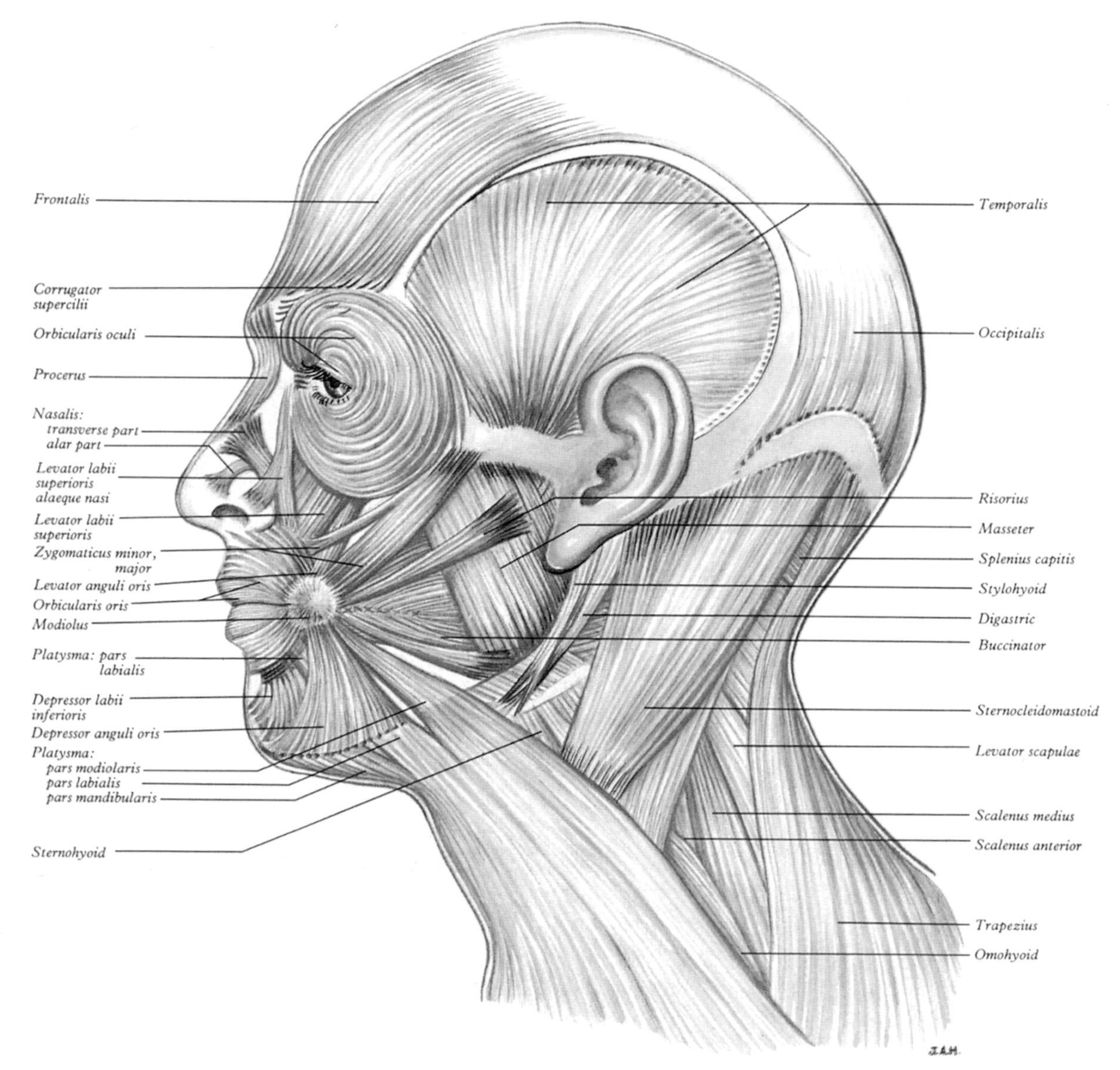

FIGURE 11-3 Muscles of the head and neck (superficial lateral view), including circumorbital, buccolabial, nasal, epicranial, masticatory, and cervical groups. The articular muscles are omitted. Risorius, a variable muscle, here has two fasciculi, of which the lower one is unlabeled. The nature of the modiolus, the modiolar muscles, and their cooperation in facial movement is described in the text. The laminae of the direct labial tractors to both upper and lower lips have been transected to reveal the orbicularis oris underneath. (From Williams PL (ed). *Gray's Anatomy,* 38th ed. London: Churchill Livingstone, 1999.)

Description:
Descends initially with zygomaticus major, then moves medially on top of levator labii superioris, with which it blends.

Function:
Muscle of facial expression (as in sneering, expressions of contempt, and smiling)
Elevates and curls upper lip, exposing the maxillary teeth
Deepens nasolabial furrow

Innervation:
Facial (VII) nerve (buccal branch)

20 RISORIUS

Origin:
Masseteric fascia

Insertion:
Modiolus[10-12]

Description:
This muscle is so highly variable, even when present, it is possibly wrong to classify it as a separate muscle. When present, it passes forward almost horizontally. It may vary from a few fibers to a wide, thin, superficial, fan-shaped sheet. It is often considered the muscle of laughing, but this is equally true of other modiolar muscles.

Function:
When present, retracts angle of mouth

Innervation:
Facial (VII) nerve (buccal branch)

21 MENTALIS

Origin:
Mandible (incisive fossa)

Insertion:
Skin over chin

Description:
Descends medially from its origin just lateral to labial frenulum to center of skin of chin

Function:
Wrinkles skin over chin
Protrudes and raises lower lip (as in sulking or drinking)

Innervation:
Facial (VII) nerve (marginal mandibular branch)

22 TRANSVERSUS MENTI

Origin:
Skin of the chin (laterally)

Insertion:
Skin of the chin
Blends with its contralateral muscle

Description:
As frequently absent as it is present. Very small muscle traverses chin inferiorly and therefore is called the mental sling. Often continuous with depressor anguli oris.

Function:
Depresses angle of mouth; supports skin of chin

Innervation:
Facial (VII) nerve (marginal mandibular branch)

23 DEPRESSOR ANGULI ORIS

Origin:
Mandible (mental tubercle and oblique line)

Insertion:
Modiolus

Description:
Ascends in a curve from its broad origin below tubercle of mandible to a narrow fasciculus into modiolus. Often continuous below with platysma.

Function:
Depresses lower lip and pulls down angle of mouth
Facial expression muscle (as in sadness)

Innervation:
Facial (VII) nerve (marginal mandibular branch)

24 DEPRESSOR LABII INFERIORIS

(Also called quadratus labii inferioris)

Origin:
Mandible (oblique line between symphysis and mental foramen)

Insertion:
Skin and mucosa of lower lip
Modiolus

Description:
Passes upward and medially from a broad origin; then narrows and blends with orbicularis oris and depressor labii inferioris of opposite side

Function:
Draws lower lip down and laterally
Facial expression muscle (sorrow, sadness)

Innervation:
Facial (VII) nerve (marginal mandibular branch)

25 ORBICULARIS ORIS

Origin:
No fascial attachments except the modiolus. This is a composite muscle with contributions from other muscles of the mouth, which form a complex sphincter-like structure, but it is not a true sphincter. Via its incisive components, the muscle attaches to the maxilla (incisivus labii superioris) and mandible (incisivus labii inferioris).

Insertion:
Modiolus
Labial connective tissue

Description[2]*:*
This muscle is not a complete ellipse of muscle surrounding the mouth. The fibers actually form four separate functional quadrants on each side that provide great diversity of oral movements. There is overlapping function among the quadrants (upper, lower, left, and right). The muscle is connected with the maxillae and septum of the nose by lateral and medial accessory muscles.
The incisivus labii superioris is a lateral accessory muscle of the upper lip within the orbicularis oris, and there is a similar accessory muscle, the incisivus labii inferioris, for the lower lip. These muscles have bony attachments to the floor of the maxillary incisive (superior) fossa and the mandibular incisive (inferior) fossa. They arch laterally between the orbicularis fibers on the respective lip and, after passing the buccal angle, insert into the modiolus. The modiolus acts as a force-transmission system to the lips from muscles attached to it.
The orbicularis oris has another accessory muscle, the nasolabialis, which lies medially and connects the upper lip to the nasal septum. (The interval between the contralateral nasolabialis corresponds to the philtrum, the depression on the upper lip beneath the nasal septum.)

Function:
Closes lips
Protrudes lips
Holds lips tight against teeth
Shapes lips for whistling, kissing, sucking, drinking, etc.
Alters shape of lips for speech and musical sounds

Innervation:
Facial (VII) nerve (buccal and marginal mandibular branches)
This innervation is of interest because when one facial nerve is injured distal to the stylomastoid foramen, only half of the orbicularis oris muscle is paralyzed. When this occurs, as in Bell's palsy, the mouth droops and may be drawn to the opposite side.

26 BUCCINATOR

Origin:
Maxilla and mandible (external surfaces of alveolar processes opposite molars)
Pterygomandibular raphe

Insertion:
Modiolus
Submucosa of cheek and lips

Description:
The principal muscle of the cheek is classified as a facial muscle (because of its innervation) despite its role in mastication. The buccinator forms the lateral wall of the oral cavity, lying deep to the other facial muscles and filling the gap between the maxilla and the mandible.

Function:
Compresses cheek against the teeth
Expels air when cheeks are distended (in blowing)
Acts in mastication to control passage of food

Innervation:
Facial (VII) nerve (buccal branch)

EXTRINSIC MUSCLES OF THE EAR

Intrinsic muscles of the ear (six in number) connect one part of the auricle to another and are not accessible or useful for manual testing. The three extrinsic muscles connect the auricle with the skull and scalp.

27 THE AURICULARES (Three Muscles)

Auricularis anterior

Origin:
Anterior fascia in temporal area (lateral edge of epicranial aponeurosis)

Insertion:
Spine of cartilaginous helix of ear

Auricularis superior

Origin:
Temporal fascia

Insertion:
Auricle (cranial surface)

Auriculoris posterior

Origin:
Temporal bone (mastoid process) via a short aponeurosis

Insertion:
Auricle (cranial surface, concha)

Function (All):
Limited function in humans except at parties! The anterior muscle elevates the auricle and moves it forward; the superior muscle elevates the auricle slightly, and the posterior draws it back. Auditory stimuli may evoke minor responses from these muscles.

Innervation:
Facial (VII) nerve (temporal branch to anterior and superior auriculares; posterior auricular branch to posterior auricular muscle)

MUSCLES OF JAW AND MASTICATION

28 Masseter
29 Temporalis
30 Lateral pterygoid
31 Medial pterygoid

28 MASSETER

Muscle has three parts

Superficial part

Origin:
Maxilla (zygomatic process via an aponeurosis)
Zygomatic bone (maxillary process and inferior border of arch)

Insertion:
Mandible (ramus: angle and lower half of lateral surface)

Intermediate part

Origin:
Zygomatic arch (inner surface of anterior ⅔)

Insertion:
Mandible (ramus, central part)

Deep part

Origin:
Zygomatic arch (posterior ⅓ continuous with intermediate part)

Insertion:
Mandible (ramus [superior half] and lateral coronoid process)

Description:
A thick muscle connecting the upper and lower jaws and consisting of three layers that blend anteriorly. The superficial layer descends backward to the angle of the mandible and the lower mandibular ramus. (The middle and deep layers compose the deep part cited in *Nomina Anatomica.*) The muscle is easily palpable and lies under the parotid gland posteriorly; the anterior margin overlies the buccinator.

Function:
Elevates the mandible (occlusion of the teeth in mastication)
Up-and-down biting motion

Innervation:
Trigeminal (V) nerve (mandibular division, masseteric branches)

29 TEMPORALIS

Origin:
Temporal bone (all of temporal fossa)
Temporal fascia (deep surface)

Insertion:
Mandible (coronoid process, medial surface, apex, and anterior border; anterior border of ramus almost to 3rd molar)

Description:
A broad muscle that radiates like a fan on the side of the head from most of the temporal fossa, converging downward to coronoid process of the mandible. The descending fibers converge into a tendon that passes between the zygomatic arch and the cranial wall. The more anterior fibers descend vertically, but the more posterior the fibers the more oblique their course until the most posterior fibers are almost horizontal. Difficult to palpate unless muscle is contracting as in clenching of teeth.

Function:
Elevates mandible to close mouth and approximate teeth (biting motion)
Retracts mandible (posterior fibers)
Participates in lateral grinding motions

Innervation:
Trigeminal (V) nerve (mandibular division, deep temporal branch)

30 LATERAL PTERYGOID

Muscle has two heads

Origin:
Superior head: Sphenoid bone (greater wing, infratemporal crest and surface)
Inferior head: Sphenoid bone (lateral pterygoid plate, lateral surface)

Insertion:
Mandible (condylar neck, pterygoid fossa)
Temporomandibular joint (TMJ) (articular capsule and disc)

Description:
A short, thick muscle with two heads that runs posterolaterally to the mandibular condyle, neck, and disc of the TMJ. The fibers of the upper head are directed downward and laterally, while those of the lower head course horizontally. The muscle lies under the mandibular ramus.

Function:
Protracts mandibular condyle and disc of TMJ forward while the mandibular head rotates on disc (participates in opening of mouth).
The lateral pterygoid, acting with the elevators of the mandible, protrudes the jaw, causing malocclusion of the teeth (i.e., the lower teeth project in front of the upper teeth).
When the lateral and medial pterygoids on the same side act jointly, the mandible and the jaw (chin) rotate to the opposite side (chewing motion).
Assists mouth closure: condyle retracts as muscle lengthens to assist masseter and temporalis.

Innervation:
Trigeminal (V) nerve (mandibular division, nerve to lateral pterygoid)

31 MEDIAL PTERYGOID

Origin:
Sphenoid bone (lateral pterygoid plate)
Palatine bone (grooved surface of pyramidal process)
Maxilla (tuberosity)
Palatine bone (tubercle)

Insertion:
Mandible medial surface of ramus via a strong tendon, reaching as high as mandibular foramen

Description:
This short, thick muscle occupies the position on the inner side of the mandibular ramus, whereas the masseter occupies the outer position. The medial pterygoid is separated by the lateral pterygoid from the mandibular ramus. The deep fibers arise from the palatine bone; the more superficial fibers arise from the maxilla and lie superficial to the lateral pterygoid. The fibers descend posterolaterally to the mandibular ramus.

Function:
Elevates mandible to close jaws (biting).
Protrudes mandible (with lateral pterygoid).
Unilaterally the medial and lateral pterygoids together rotate the mandible forward and to the opposite side. This alternating motion is chewing.
The medial pterygoid and masseter are situated to form a sling that suspends the mandible. This sling is a functional articulation in which the TMJ acts as a guide. As the mouth opens and closes, the mandible moves on a center of rotation established by the sling and the sphenomandibular ligament.

Innervation:
Trigeminal (V) nerve (mandibular division, nerve to medial pterygoid)

MUSCLES OF THE TONGUE

Extrinsic Tongue Muscles

32 Genioglossus
33 Hyoglossus
34 Chondroglossus
35 Styloglossus
36 Palatoglossus

32 GENIOGLOSSUS

Origin:
Mandible (symphysis menti on inner surface of superior mental spine)

Insertion:
Hyoid bone via a thin aponeurosis
Middle pharyngeal constrictor muscle
Undersurface of tongue, whole length mingling with the intrinsic musculature of tongue

Description:
The tongue is separated into lateral halves by the lingual septum, which extends along its full length and inserts inferiorly into the hyoid bone. The extrinsics extend outside the tongue.
The genioglossus is a thin, flat muscle that fans out backward from its mandibular origin, running parallel with and close to the midline. The lower fibers run downward to the hyoid; the median fibers run posteriorly and join the middle constrictor of the pharynx; the superior fibers run upward to insert on the whole length of the underside of the tongue. The muscles of the two sides are blended anteriorly and separated posteriorly by the medial lingual septum (see Figure 7-51).

Function:
Protraction of tongue (tip protrudes beyond mouth)
Depression of central part of tongue

Innervation:
Hypoglossal (XII) nerve, muscular branch

33 HYOGLOSSUS

Origin:
Hyoid bone (side of body and whole length of greater horn)

Insertion:
Side of tongue

Description:
Thin, quadrilateral muscle whose fibers run almost vertically

Function:
Depression and retraction of tongue

Innervation:
Hypoglossal (XII) nerve, muscular branch

34 CHONDROGLOSSUS

Origin:
Hyoid bone (lesser horn, medial side)

Insertion:
Blends with intrinsic muscles on side of tongue

Description:
A very small muscle (about 2 cm long) that is sometimes considered part of the hyoglossus

Function:
Assists in tongue depression

Innervation:
Hypoglossal (XII) nerve, muscular branch

35 STYLOGLOSSUS

Origin:
Temporal bone (styloid process, apex)
Stylomandibular ligament (styloid end)

Insertion:
Muscle divides into two portions before entering side of tongue
Side of tongue near dorsal surface to blend with intrinsics (longitudinal portion)
Overlaps hyoglossus and blends with it (oblique portion)

Description:
Shortest and smallest of extrinsic tongue muscles. The muscle curves down anteriorly and divides into longitudinal and oblique portions. It lies between the internal and external carotid arteries.

Function:
Draws tongue up and backward

Innervation:
Hypoglossal (XII) nerve, muscular branch

36 PALATOGLOSSUS

Origin:
Soft palate (anterior surface)

Insertion:
Side of tongue intermingling with intrinsic muscles

Description:
Technically an extrinsic muscle of the tongue, this muscle is functionally closer to the palate muscles. It is a small fasciculus, narrower in the middle than at its ends. It passes anteroinferiorly and laterally in front of the tonsil to reach the side of the tongue. Along with the mucous membrane covering it, the palatoglossus forms the palatoglossal arch or fold.

Function:
Elevates root of tongue
Closes palatoglossal arch (along with its opposite member) to close the oral cavity from the oropharynx

Innervation:
Vagus (X) nerve (pharyngeal plexus)

Intrinsic Tongue Muscles

37 Superior longitudinal
38 Inferior longitudinal
39 Transverse lingual
40 Vertical lingual

37 SUPERIOR LONGITUDINAL

Attachments and Description:
Oblique and longitudinal fibers run immediately under the mucous membrane on dorsum of tongue.
Arises from submucous fibrous layer near epiglottis and from the median lingual septum. Fibers run anteriorly to the edges of the tongue.

Function and innervation of intrinsics:
See vertical lingual (#40).

38 INFERIOR LONGITUDINAL

Attachments and Description:
Narrow band of fibers close to the inferior lingual surface. Extends from the root to the apex of the tongue. Some fibers connect to hyoid body. Blends with styloglossus anteriorly.

39 TRANSVERSE LINGUAL

Attachments and Description:
Passes laterally across tongue from the median lingual septum to the edges of the tongue. Blends with palatopharyngeus.

40 VERTICAL LINGUAL

Attachments and Description:
Located only at the anterolateral regions and extends from the dorsal to the ventral surfaces of the tongue.

Function of Intrinsics:
These muscles change the shape and contour of the tongue. The longitudinal muscles tend to shorten it. The superior longitudinal also turns the apex and sides upward, making the dorsum concave. The inferior longitudinal pulls the apex and sides downward to make the dorsum convex. The transverse muscle narrows and elongates the tongue. The vertical muscle flattens and widens it.
These almost limitless alterations give the tongue the incredible versatility and precision necessary for speech and swallowing functions.

Innervation of Intrinsics:
Hypoglossal (XII) nerve

MUSCLES OF THE PHARYNX

41 Inferior pharyngeal constrictor
42 Middle pharyngeal constrictor
43 Superior pharyngeal constrictor
44 Stylopharyngeus
45 Salpingopharyngeus
49 Palatopharyngeus (see under *Muscles of the Palate*)

41 INFERIOR PHARYNGEAL CONSTRICTOR

Origin:
Cricoid cartilage (sides)
Thyroid cartilage (oblique line on the side as well as from inferior cornu)

Insertion:
Pharynx (posterior median fibrous raphe, along with its contralateral partner)

Description:
The thickest and largest of the pharyngeal constrictors, the muscle has two parts: the cricopharyngeus and the thyropharyngeus. Both parts spread to join the muscle of the opposite side at the fibrous median raphe. The lowest fibers run horizontally and circle the narrowest part of the pharynx. The other fibers course obliquely upward to overlap the middle constrictor.
During swallowing the cricopharyngeus acts like a sphincter; the thyropharyngeus uses peristaltic action to propel food downward.

Function:
During swallowing all constrictors act as general sphincters and in peristaltic action during swallowing.

Innervation:
Pharyngeal plexus formed by components of vagus (X), accessory (XI), glossopharyngeal (IX), and external laryngeal nerves

42 MIDDLE PHARYNGEAL CONSTRICTOR

Origin:
Hyoid bone (whole length of superior border of lesser and greater cornu) [chondropharyngeal and ceratopharyngeal parts]
Stylohyoid ligament

Insertion:
Pharynx (posterior median fibrous raphe)

Description:
From their origin, the fibers fan out in three directions: the lower ones descend to lie under the inferior constrictor; the medial ones pass transversely, and the superior fibers ascend to overlap the superior constrictor. At its insertion it joins with the muscle from the opposite side.

Function:
Serves as a sphincter and acts during peristaltic functions in deglutition

Innervation:
Pharyngeal plexus formed by components of vagus (X), accessory (XI), and glossopharyngeal (IX) nerves

43 SUPERIOR PHARYNGEAL CONSTRICTOR

Origin (in four parts):
Sphenoid bone (medial pterygoid plate and its hamulus [pterygopharyngeal part])
Pterygomandibular raphe (buccopharyngeal part)
Mandible (mylohyoid line) [mylopharyngeal part]
Side of tongue [glossopharyngeal part]

Insertion:
Median pharyngeal fibrous raphe
Occipital bone (pharyngeal tubercle on basilar part)

Description:
The smallest of the constrictors, the fibers of this muscle curve posteriorly and are elongated by an aponeurosis to reach the occiput. The attachments of this muscle are differentiated as pterygopharyngeal, buccopharyngeal, mylopharyngeal, and glossopharyngeal.
The interval between the superior border of this muscle and the base of the skull is closed by the pharyngobasilar fascia known as the sinus of Morgagni.
A small band of muscle blends with the superior constrictor from the upper surface of the palatine aponeurosis and is called the palatopharyngeal sphincter. This band is visible when the soft palate is elevated; often it is hypertrophied in individuals with cleft palate.

Function:
Acts as a sphincter and has peristaltic functions in swallowing

Innervation:
Pharyngeal plexus (from vagus and accessory)

44 STYLOPHARYNGEUS

Origin:
Temporal bone (styloid process, medial side of base)

Insertion:
Blends with pharyngeal constrictors and palatopharyngeus
Thyroid cartilage (posterior border)

Description:
A long, thin muscle that passes downward along the side of the pharynx and between the superior and middle constrictors to spread out beneath the mucous membrane

Function:
Elevation of upper lateral pharyngeal wall in swallowing

Innervation:
Glossopharyngeal (IX) nerve

45 SALPINGOPHARYNGEUS

Origin:
Auditory (pharyngotympanic) tube (inferior aspect of cartilage near orifice)

Insertion:
Blends with palatopharyngeus

Description:
Small muscle whose fibers pass downward, lateral to the uvula, to blend with fibers of the palatopharyngeus

Function:
Elevates pharynx to move a bolus of food

Innervation:
Pharyngeal plexus

MUSCLES OF THE PALATE

46 Levator veli palatini
47 Tensor veli palatini
48 Musculus uvulae
49 Palatopharyngeus
36 *Palatoglossus* (see under *Muscles of the Tongue*)

46 LEVATOR VELI PALATINI
(Levator Palati)

Origin:
Temporal bone (inferior surface of petrous bone)
Tympanic fascia
Auditory (pharyngotympanic) tube cartilage

Insertion:
Palatine aponeurosis (upper surface, where it blends with opposite muscle at the midline)

Description:
Fibers of this small muscle run downward and medially from the petrous temporal bone to pass above the margin of the superior pharyngeal constrictor and anterior to the salpingopharyngeus. They form a sling for the palatine aponeurosis.

Function:
Elevates soft palate
Retracts soft palate

Innervation:
Pharyngeal plexus

47 TENSOR VELI PALATINI
(Tensor Palati)

Origin:
Sphenoid bone (pterygoid process, scaphoid fossa)
Auditory (pharyngotympanic) tube cartilage
Sphenoid spine (medial part)

Insertion:
Palatine aponeurosis
Palatine bone (horizontal plate)

Description:[13]
This small, thin muscle lies lateral to the levator veli palatini and the auditory tube. It descends vertically between the medial pterygoid plate and the medial pterygoid muscle, converging into a delicate tendon, which turns medially around the pterygoid hamulus.

Function:
Draws soft palate to one side (unilateral)
Tightens soft palate, depressing it and flattening its arch (with its contralateral counterpart)
Opens auditory tube in yawning and swallowing and eases any buildup of air pressure between the nasopharynx and middle ear

Innervation:
Trigeminal (V) nerve (to medial pterygoid)[13]

48 MUSCULUS UVULAE
(Azygos Uvulae)

Origin:
Palatine bones (posterior nasal spine)
Palatine aponeurosis

Insertion:
Uvula (connective tissue and mucous membrane)

Description:
A bilateral muscle, its fibers descend into the uvular mucosa.

Function:
Elevates and retracts uvula to assist with palatopharyngeal closure
Seals nasopharynx (along with levators)

Innervation:
Pharyngeal plexus (X and XI)

49 PALATOPHARYNGEUS
(Pharyngopalatinus)

Origin (by two fasciculi):
Anterior fasciculus:
Soft palate (palatine aponeurosis)
Hard palate (posterior border)
Posterior fasciculus:
Pharyngeal aspect of soft palate (palatine aponeurosis)

Insertion:
Thyroid cartilage (posterior border)
Side of pharynx on an aponeurosis

Description:
Along with its overlying mucosa, it forms the palatopharyngeal arch. It arises by two fasciculi separated by the levator veli palatini, all of which join in the midline with their opposite muscles. The two muscles unite and are joined by the salpingopharyngeus to descend behind the tonsils. The muscle forms an incomplete longitudinal wall on the internal surface of the pharynx.

Function:
Elevates pharynx and pulls it forward, thus shortening it during swallowing. The muscles also narrow the palatopharyngeal arches (fauces).
Depresses soft palate.

Innervation:
Pharyngeal plexus (X and XI)

MUSCLES OF THE LARYNX (Intrinsics)

These muscles are confined to the larynx:

50 Cricothyroid
51 Posterior cricoarytenoid
52 Lateral cricoarytenoid
53 Transverse arytenoid
54 Oblique arytenoid
55 Thyroarytenoid

50 CRICOTHYROID

Origin:
Cricoid cartilage (front and lateral)

Insertion:
Thyroid cartilage (inferior cornu)
Thyroid lamina

Description:
The fibers of this paired muscle are arranged in two groups: a lower oblique group (pars obliqua), which slants posterolaterally to the inferior cornu, and a superior group (pars recta or vertical fibers), which ascends backward to the lamina.

Function:
Regulates tension of vocal folds
Stretches vocal ligaments by raising the cricoid arch, thus increasing tension in the vocal folds

Innervation:
Vagus (X) nerve (external laryngeal branch)

51 POSTERIOR CRICOARYTENOID

Origin:
Cricoid cartilage lamina (broad depression on corresponding half of posterior surface)

Insertion:
Arytenoid cartilage on same side (back of muscular process)

Description:
The fibers of this paired muscle pass cranially and laterally to converge on the back of the arytenoid cartilage on the same side. The lowest fibers are nearly vertical and become oblique and finally almost transverse at the superior border.

Function:
Regulates tension of vocal folds
Opens glottis by rotating arytenoid cartilages laterally and separating (abducting) the vocal folds
Retracts arytenoid cartilages, thereby helping to tense the vocal folds

Innervation:
Vagus (X) nerve (recurrent laryngeal nerve)

52 LATERAL CRICOARYTENOID

Origin:
Cricoid cartilage (cranial border of arch)

Insertion:
Arytenoid cartilage on same side (front of muscular process)

Description:
Fibers run obliquely upward and backward. The muscle is paired.

Function:
Closes glottis by rotating arytenoid cartilages medially, approximating (adducting) the vocal folds for speech

Innervation:
Vagus (X) nerve (recurrent laryngeal branch)

53 TRANSVERSE ARYTENOID

Attachments and Description:
A single muscle (i.e., unpaired) that crosses transversely between the two arytenoid cartilages. Often considered a branch of an arytenoid muscle. It attaches to the back of the muscular process and the adjacent lateral borders of both arytenoid cartilages.

Function:
Approximates (adducts) the arytenoid cartilages, closing the glottis

Innervation:
Vagus (X) nerve (recurrent laryngeal nerve)

54 OBLIQUE ARYTENOID

Origin:
Arytenoid cartilage (back of muscular process)

Insertion:
Arytenoid cartilage on opposite side (apex)

Description:
A pair of muscles lying superficial to the transverse arytenoid. Arrayed as two fasciculi that cross on the posterior midline. Often considered part of an arytenoid muscle. Fibers that continue laterally around the apex of the arytenoid are sometimes termed the aryepiglottic muscle.

Function:
Acts as a sphincter for the laryngeal inlet (by adducting the aryepiglottic folds and approximating the arytenoid cartilages)

Innervation:
Vagus (X) nerve (recurrent laryngeal nerve)

55 THYROARYTENOID

Origin:
Thyroid cartilage (caudal half of angle)
Middle cricothyroid ligament

Insertion:
Arytenoid cartilage (base and anterior surface)
Vocal process (lateral surface)

Description:
The paired muscles lie lateral to the vocal fold, ascending posterolaterally. Many fibers are carried to the aryepiglottic fold.
The lower and deeper fibers, which lie medially, appear to be differentiated as a band inserted into the vocal process of the arytenoid cartilage. This band frequently is called the *vocalis* muscle. It is adherent to the vocal ligament, to which it is lateral and parallel.
Other fibers of this muscle continue as the *thyroepiglotticus* muscle and insert into the epiglottic margin; other fibers that swing along the wall of the sinus to the side of the epiglottis are termed the superior thyroarytenoid and relax the vocal folds.

Function:
Regulates tension of vocal folds.
Draws arytenoid cartilages toward thyroid cartilage, thus shortening and relaxing vocal ligaments.
Rotates the arytenoid cartilages medially to approximate vocal folds.
The vocalis relaxes the posterior vocal folds while the anterior folds remain tense, thus raising the pitch of the voice.
The thyroepiglotticus widens the laryngeal inlet via action on the aryepiglottic folds.
The superior thyroarytenoids relax the vocal cords and aid in closure of the glottis.

Innervation:
Vagus (X) nerve (recurrent laryngeal nerve)

MUSCLES OF THE NECK AND SUBOCCIPITAL TRIANGLE

Capital Extensor Muscles

This group of eight muscles consists of suboccipital muscles extending between the atlas, axis, and skull and large overlapping muscles from the 6th thoracic to the 3rd cervical vertebrae and rising to the skull.

56 Rectus capitis posterior major
57 Rectus capitis posterior minor
58 Obliquus capitis superior
59 Obliquus capitis inferior
60 Longissimus capitis
61 Splenius capitis
62 Semispinalis capitis
63 Spinalis capitis

The capital extensor muscles control the head as an entity separate from the cervical spine.[14] The muscles are paired.

83 Sternocleidomastoid (posterior) (see under *Cervical Spine Flexors*)
124 Trapezius (upper) (see under *Muscles of the Shoulder Girdle*)

56 RECTUS CAPITIS POSTERIOR MAJOR

Origin:
Axis (spinous process)

Insertion:
Occiput (lateral part of inferior nuchal line; surface just inferior to nuchal line)

Description:
Starts as a small tendon and broadens as it rises upward and laterally (review suboccipital triangle in any anatomy text)

Function:
Capital extension
Rotation of head to same side
Lateral bending of head to same side

Innervation:
C1 spinal nerve (suboccipital nerve, dorsal rami)

57 RECTUS CAPITIS POSTERIOR MINOR

Origin:
Atlas (tubercle on posterior arch)

Insertion:
Occiput (medial portion of inferior nuchal line; surface between inferior nuchal line and foramen magnum)

Description:
Begins as a narrow tendon, which broadens into a wide band of muscle as it ascends

Function:
Capital extension

Innervation:
C1 spinal nerve (suboccipital nerve, dorsal rami)

58 OBLIQUUS CAPITIS SUPERIOR

Origin:
Atlas (transverse process, superior surface), where it joins insertion of obliquus capitis inferior

Insertion:
Occiput (between superior and inferior nuchal lines; lies lateral to semispinalis capitis)

Description:
Starts as a narrow muscle and then widens as it rises upward and medially. It is more a postural muscle than a muscle for major motion.

Function:
Capital extension of head on atlas (muscle on both sides)
Lateral bending to same side (muscle on that side)

Innervation:
C1 spinal nerve (suboccipital nerve, dorsal rami)

59 OBLIQUUS CAPITIS INFERIOR

Origin:
Axis (apex of spinous process)

Insertion:
Atlas (transverse process, inferior and dorsal surface)

Description:
Passes laterally and slightly upward. This is the larger of the two obliquii.

Function:
Rotation of head to same side
Lateral bending (muscle on that side)

Innervation:
C1 spinal nerve (suboccipital nerve, dorsal rami)

60 LONGISSIMUS CAPITIS

Origin:
T1-T5 vertebrae (transverse processes)
C4-C7 vertebrae (articular processes)

Insertion:
Temporal bone (mastoid process [posterior margin])

Description:
A muscle with several tendons lying under the splenius cervicis. Sweeps upward and laterally and is considered a continuation of the sacrospinalis.

Function:
Capital extension
Lateral bending and rotation of head to same side

Innervation:
C3-C8 cervical nerves with variations (dorsal rami)

61 SPLENIUS CAPITIS

Origin:
Ligamentum nuchae at C3-C7 vertebrae
C7-T4 vertebrae (spinous processes) with variations

Insertion:
Temporal bone (mastoid process)
Occiput (surface below lateral ⅓ of superior nuchal line)

Description:
Fibers directed upward and laterally as a broad band deep to the rhomboids and trapezius distally and the sternocleidomastoid proximally. It forms the floor of the apex of the posterior triangle of the neck.

Function:
Capital extension
Rotation of head to same side (debated)
Lateral bending of head to same side

Innervation:
C3-C6 cervical nerves with variations (dorsal rami)
C1-C2 (suboccipital and greater occipital nerves off first two dorsal rami)

62 SEMISPINALIS CAPITIS

Origin:
C7 and T1-T6 vertebrae (variable) as series of tendons from tips of transverse processes
C4-C6 vertebrae (articular processes)

Insertion:
Occiput (between superior and inferior nuchal lines)

Description:
Tendons unite to form a broad muscle in the upper posterior neck, which passes vertically upward.

Function:
Capital extension (muscles on both sides)
Rotation of head to opposite side (debated)
Lateral bending of head to same side

Innervation:
C2-T1 spinal nerves (dorsal rami); greater occipital nerve (variable)

63 SPINALIS CAPITIS

Origin:
C5-C7 and T1-T3 vertebrae (variable) (spinous processes)

Insertion:
Occiput (between superior and inferior nuchal lines)

Description:
The smallest and thinnest of the erector spinae, these muscles lie closest to the vertebral column. The spinales are inconstant and are difficult to separate.

Function:
Capital extension

Innervation:
C3-T1 spinal nerves (dorsal rami) (variable)

Cervical Extensor Muscles

This group of eight overlapping cervical muscles arise from the thoracic vertebrae or ribs and insert into the cervical vertebrae. They are responsible for cervical spine extension in contrast to capital (head) extension.

64 Longissimus cervicis
65 Semispinalis cervicis
66 Iliocostalis cervicis
67 Splenius cervicis
68 Spinalis cervicis
69 Interspinales cervicis
70 Intertransversarii cervicis
71 Rotatores cervicis
94 Multifidi (see under *Erector Spinae*)
124 Trapezius (see under *Muscles of the Shoulder Girdle*)
127 Levator scapulae (see under *Muscles of the Shoulder Girdle*)

64 LONGISSIMUS CERVICIS

Origin:
T1-T5 vertebrae (variable) (tips of transverse processes)

Insertion:
C2-C6 vertebrae (posterior tubercles of transverse processes)

Description:
A continuation of the sacrospinalis group, the tendons are long and thin, and the muscle courses upward and slightly medially. The muscles are bilateral.

Function:
Extension of the cervical spine (both muscles)
Lateral bending of cervical spine to same side (one muscle)

Innervation:
C3-T3 spinal nerves (variable) (dorsal rami)

65 SEMISPINALIS CERVICIS

Origin:
T1-T5 vertebrae (variable) (transverse processes)

Insertion:
Axis (C2) to C5 vertebrae (spinous processes)

Description:
A narrow, thick muscle arising from a series of tendons and ascending vertically

Function:
Extension of the cervical spine (both muscles)
Rotation of cervical spine to opposite side (one muscle)
Lateral bending to same side

Innervation:
C2-T5 spinal nerves (dorsal rami) (variable)

66 ILIOCOSTALIS CERVICIS

Origin:
Ribs 3 to 6 (angles); sometimes ribs 1 and 2 also

Insertion:
C4-C6 vertebrae (transverse processes, posterior tubercles)

Description:
Flattened tendons arise from ribs on dorsum of back and become muscular as they rise and turn

medially to insert on cervical vertebrae. The muscle lies lateral to the longissimus cervicis. The iliocostales form the lateral column of the sacrospinalis group.

Function:
Extension of the cervical spine (both muscles)
Lateral bending to same side (one muscle)
Depression of ribs (accessory)

Innervation:
C4-T3 spinal nerves (variable) (dorsal rami)

67 SPLENIUS CERVICIS

Origin:
T3-T6 vertebrae (spinous processes)

Insertion:
C1-C3 vertebrae (variable) (transverse processes, posterior tubercles)

Description:
Narrow tendinous band arises from bone and intraspinous ligaments and forms a broad sheet along with the splenius capitis. This muscle rises upward and laterally under the trapezius and rhomboids and medially to the levator scapulae. The splenii are often absent and are quite variable.

Function:
Extension of the cervical spine (both muscles)
Rotation of cervical spine to same side (one muscle)
Lateral bending to same side (one muscle)
Synergistic with opposite sternocleidomastoid

Innervation:
C4-C8 spinal nerves (variable) (dorsal rami)

68 SPINALIS CERVICIS

Origin:
C6-C7 and sometimes T1-T2 vertebrae (spinous processes)
Ligamentum nuchae (lower part)

Insertion:
Axis (spine)
C2-C3 vertebrae (spinous processes)

Description:
The smallest and thinnest of the erector spinae, it lies closest to the vertebral column. The erector spinae are inconstant and difficult to separate. This muscle is often absent.

Function:
Extension of the cervical spine

Innervation:
C3-C8 spinal nerves (dorsal rami) (variable)

69 INTERSPINALES CERVICIS

Origin and Insertion:
Spinous processes of contiguous cervical vertebrae
Six pairs occur: The first pair runs between the axis and C3; the last pair between C7 and T1.

Description:
One of the smallest and least significant muscles but consists of short, narrow bundles more evident in cervical spine than at lower levels.

Function:
Extension of the cervical spine (weak)

Innervation:
C3-C8 spinal nerves (dorsal rami) (variable)

70 INTERTRANSVERSARII CERVICIS

Origin and Insertion:
Both anterior and posterior pairs occur at each segment. The anterior muscles interconnect the anterior tubercles of contiguous transverse processes and are innervated by the ventral primary rami. The posterior muscles interconnect the posterior tubercles of contiguous transverse processes and are innervated by the dorsal primary rami.

Description:
These muscles are small paired fasciculi that lie between the transverse processes of contiguous vertebrae. The cervicis is the most developed of this group which includes the anterior intertransversarii cervicis, the posterior intertransversarii cervicis, a thoracic group, and a medial and lateral lumbar group.

Function:
Extension of spine (muscles on both sides)
Lateral bending to same side (muscles on one side)

Innervation:
Anterior cervicis: C3-C8 spinal nerves (ventral rami)
Posterior cervicis: C3-C8 spinal nerves (dorsal rami)

71 ROTATORES CERVICIS

(See *Rotatores thoracis*)

Origin:
Transverse process of one cervical vertebra

Insertion:
Base of spine of next highest vertebra

Description:
The rotatores cervicis lies deep to the multifidus and cannot be readily separated from it. Both muscles are irregular and not functionally significant at the cervical level.

Function:
Extension of the cervical spine (assist)
Rotation of spine to opposite side

Innervation:
C3-C8 spinal nerves (dorsal rami)

Muscles of Capital Flexion

The primary capital flexors are the short recti that lie between the atlas and the skull and the longus capitis. Reinforcing these muscles are the suprahyoid muscles from the mandibular area.

72 Rectus capitis anterior
73 Rectus capitis lateralis
74 Longus capitis

Suprahyoids

75 Mylohyoid
76 Stylohyoid
77 Geniohyoid
78 Digastric

72 RECTUS CAPITIS ANTERIOR

Origin:
Atlas (C1) (transverse process and anterior surface of lateral mass)

Insertion:
Occiput (inferior surface of basilar part)

Description:
Short, flat muscle found immediately behind longus capitis. Upward trajectory is vertical and slightly medial.

Function:
Capital flexion
Stabilization of atlanto-occipital joint

Innervation:
C1-C2 spinal nerves (ventral rami)

73 RECTUS CAPITIS LATERALIS

Origin:
Atlas (C1) (transverse process, upper surface)

Insertion:
Occiput (jugular process)

Description:
Short, flat muscle; courses upward and laterally

Function:
Lateral bending of head to same side (obliquity of muscle)
Assists head rotation
Stabilizes atlanto-occipital joint (assists)
Capital flexion

Innervation:
C1-C2 spinal nerves (ventral rami)

74 LONGUS CAPITIS

Origin:
C3-C6 vertebrae (transverse processes, anterior tubercles)

Insertion:
Occiput (inferior basilar part)

Description:
Starting as four tendinous slips, muscle merges and becomes broader and thicker as it rises, converging medially toward its contralateral counterpart.

Function:
Capital flexion
Rotation of head to same side (muscle of one side)

Innervation:
C1-C3 spinal nerves (ventral rami)

75 MYLOHYOID

Origin:
Mandible (whole length of mylohyoid line from symphysis in front to last molar behind)

Insertion:
Hyoid bone (body, superior surface)
Mylohyoid raphe (from symphysis menti of mandible to hyoid bone)

Description:
Flat triangular muscle; the muscles from the two sides form a floor for the cavity of the mouth.

Function:
Raises hyoid bone and tongue for swallowing
Depresses the mandible when hyoid bone fixed
Capital flexion (weak accessory)

Innervation:
Trigeminal (V) nerve (mylohyoid branch of inferior alveolar nerve off mandibular division)

76 STYLOHYOID

Origin:
Temporal bone, styloid process (posterolateral surface)

Insertion:
Hyoid bone (body at junction with greater horn)

Description:
Slim muscle passes downward and forward and is perforated by digastric near its distal attachment. Muscle occasionally is absent.

Function:
Hyoid bone drawn upward and backward (in swallowing)
Capital flexion (weak accessory)
Assists in opening mouth (depression of mandible)
Participation in mastication and speech (roles not clear)

Innervation:
Facial (VII) nerve (posterior trunk, stylohyoid branch)

77 GENIOHYOID

Origin:
Mandible (symphysis menti, inferior mental spine)

Insertion:
Hyoid bone (body, anterior surface)

Description:
Narrow muscle lying superficial to the mylohyoid, it runs backward and somewhat downward. It is in contact (or may fuse) with its contralateral counterpart at the midline.

Function:
Elevation and protraction of hyoid bone
Capital flexion (weak accessory)
Assists in depressing mandible

Innervation:
C1 spinal nerve via hypoglossal (XII) nerve

78 DIGASTRIC

Origin:
Posterior belly: temporal bone (mastoid notch)
Anterior belly: mandible (digastric fossa)

Insertion:
Intermediate tendon and from there to hyoid bone via a fibrous sling

Description:
Consists of two bellies united by a rounded intermediate tendon. Lies below the mandible and extends as a sling from the mastoid to the symphysis menti, perforating the stylohyoid, where the two bellies are joined by the intermediate tendon.
Electromyography (EMG) data show that the two bilateral muscles always work together.[15]

Function:
Mandibular depression (muscles on both sides)
Elevation of hyoid bone (in swallowing)
Anterior belly: draws hyoid forward
Posterior belly: draws hyoid backward
Capital flexion (weak synergist)

Innervation:
Anterior belly: trigeminal (V) nerve (mylohyoid branch of inferior alveolar nerve)
Posterior belly: facial (VII) nerve, digastric branch

Cervical Spine Flexors

The primary cervical spine flexors are the longus colli (a prevertebral mass), the three scalene muscles, and the sternocleidomastoid. Superficial accessory muscles are the infrahyoid muscles and the platysma.

79 Longus colli
80 Scalenus anterior
81 Scalenus medius
82 Scalenus posterior
83 Sternocleidomastoid
88 Platysma

Infrahyoids:

84 Sternothyroid
85 Thyrohyoid
86 Sternohyoid
87 Omohyoid

79 LONGUS COLLI

Three heads
Superior oblique

Origin:
C3-C5 vertebrae (anterior tubercles of transverse processes)

Insertion:
Atlas (tubercle on anterior arch)

Inferior oblique

Origin:
T1-T3 vertebrae (variable) (anterior bodies)

Insertion:
C5-C6 vertebrae (anterior tubercles of transverse processes)

Vertical portion

Origin:
T1-T3 and C5-C7 vertebrae (anterolateral bodies) (variable)

Insertion:
C2-C4 vertebrae (anterior bodies)

Description:
Situated on the anterior surface of the vertebral column from the thoracic spine rising to the cervical vertebrae. It is cylindrical and tapers at each end.

Function:
Cervical flexion (weak)
Cervical rotation to opposite side (inferior oblique head)
Lateral bending (superior and inferior oblique heads) (debatable)

Innervation:
C2-C6 spinal nerves (ventral rami)

The Scalenes

These muscles are highly variable in their specific anatomy, and this possibly leads to disputes about minor functions. Though not described here, a fourth scalene muscle, the scalenus minimus (of no functional significance), runs, when present, from C7 to the 1st rib.

80 SCALENUS ANTERIOR

Origin:
C3-C6 vertebrae (anterior tubercles of transverse processes)

Insertion:
1st rib (scalene tubercle on inner border and ridge on upper surface)

Description:
Lying deep at the side of the neck under the sternocleidomastoid, it descends vertically. Attachments are highly variable.

A fourth scalene (scalenus minimus) is occasionally associated with the cervical pleura and runs from C7 to the 1st rib.

Function:
Flexion of cervical spine (both muscles)
Elevation of 1st rib in inspiration
Rotation of cervical spine to same side
Lateral bending of neck to same side

Innervation:
C4-C6 cervical nerves (ventral rami)

81 SCALENUS MEDIUS

Origin:
C2-C7 (posterior tubercles of transverse processes)
Atlas (sometimes)

Insertion:
1st rib (widely over superior surface)

Description:
Longest and largest of the scalenes. Descends vertically alongside of vertebrae.

Function:
Cervical flexion (weak)
Lateral bending of cervical spine to same side
Elevation of 1st rib in inspiration
Cervical rotation to same side

Innervation:
C3-C8 cervical nerves (ventral rami)

82 SCALENUS POSTERIOR

Origin:
C4-C6 vertebrae (variable; posterior tubercles of transverse processes)

Insertion:
2nd rib (outer surface)

Description:
Smallest and deepest lying of the scalene muscles. Attachments are highly variable. Often not separable from scalenus medius.

Function:
Cervical flexion (weak)
Elevation of 2nd rib in inspiration
Lateral bending of cervical spine to same side (accessory)
Cervical spine rotation to same side

Innervation:
C6-C8 cervical nerves (ventral rami)

83 STERNOCLEIDOMASTOID

Origin:
Sternal (medial) head: sternum (manubrium, ventral surface)
Clavicular (lateral) head: clavicle (superior and anterior surface of medial ⅓)

Insertion:
Temporal bone (mastoid process, lateral surface)
Occiput (lateral half of superior nuchal line)

Description:
The two heads of origin gradually merge in the neck as the muscle rises upward laterally and posteriorly. Their oblique (lateral to medial) course across the sides of the neck is a very prominent feature of surface anatomy.

Function:
Flexion of cervical spine (both muscles)
Lateral bending of cervical spine to same side
Rotation of head to opposite side
Capital extension (posterior fibers)
Raises sternum in forced inspiration

Innervation:
Accessory (XI) nerve (spinal part)
C2-C3 (sometimes C4) cervical nerves (ventral rami)

84 STERNOTHYROID

Origin:
Sternum (manubrium, posterior surface)
1st rib (cartilage)

Insertion:
Thyroid cartilage (oblique line)

Description:
A deep-lying, somewhat broad muscle rising vertically and slightly laterally just lateral to the thyroid gland.

Function:
Cervical flexion (weak)
Draws larynx down after swallowing or vocalization
Depression of hyoid, mandible, and tongue (after elevation)

Innervation:
C1-C3 cervical nerves (branch of ansa cervicalis)

85 THYROHYOID

Origin:
Thyroid cartilage (oblique line)

Insertion:
Hyoid bone (inferior border of greater horn)

Description:
Appears as an upward extension of Sternothyroid. It is a small rectangular muscle lateral to the thyroid cartilage.

Function:
Cervical flexion (This small muscle is attached to mobile structures and its role in cervical flexion seems unlikely as a functional entity.)
Draws hyoid bone downward
Elevates larynx and thyroid cartilage

Innervation:
Hypoglossal (XII) and branches of C1 spinal nerve (which run in hypoglossal nerve)

86 STERNOHYOID

Origin:
Clavicle (medial end, posterior surface)
Sternum (manubrium, posterior)
Sternoclavicular ligament

Insertion:
Hyoid bone (body, lower border)

Description:
Thin strap muscle that ascends slightly medially from clavicle to hyoid bone

Function:
Cervical flexion (weak)
Depresses hyoid bone after swallowing

Innervation:
Hypoglossal (XII) nerve
C1-C3 cervical nerves (branches of ansa cervicalis)

87 OMOHYOID

Has two bellies
Inferior belly

Origin:
Scapula (superior margin to variable extent; subscapular notch)
Superior transverse ligament

Insertion:
Intermediate tendon of omohyoid under sternocleidomastoid
Clavicle by fibrous expansion

Superior belly

Origin:
Intermediate tendon of omohyoid

Insertion:
Hyoid bone (lower border of body)

Description:
Muscle consists of two fleshy bellies united at an angle by a central tendon. The inferior belly is a narrow band that courses forward and slightly upward across the lower front of the neck. The superior belly rises vertically and lateral to the sternohyoid.

Function:
Depression of hyoid after elevation
Cervical flexion
No EMG data to support function

Innervation:
Hypoglossal (XII) (ansa cervicalis) via C1 (branches from ansa cervicalis) and C2-C3 cervical nerves

88 PLATYSMA

Origin:
Fascia covering upper pectoralis major and deltoid

Insertion:
Mandible (below the oblique line)
Modiolus[10-12]
Skin and subcutaneous tissue of lower lip and face
Contralateral muscles join at midline

Description:
A broad sheet of muscle, it rises from the shoulder, crosses the clavicle, and rises obliquely upward and medially to the side of the neck.
The muscle is very variable.

Function:
Draws lower lip downward and backward (expression of surprise or horror) and assists with jaw opening.
Cervical flexion (weak). Electromyogram shows great activity in extreme effort and in sudden deep inspiration.[16]
Can pull skin up from clavicular region, increasing diameter of neck. Wrinkles skin of nuchal area obliquely, thereby decreasing concavity of neck.
Forced inspiration.
Platysma is not a very functional muscle.

Innervation:
Facial (VII) nerve (cervical branch)

MUSCLES OF THE TRUNK

Deep Muscles of the Back

These muscles consist of groups of serially arranged muscles ranging from the occiput to the sacrum. There are four subgroups plus the quadratus lumborum.

In this section readers will note that the cervical portions of each muscle group are not included. These muscles are described as part of the neck muscles because their functions involve capital and cervical motions. They are, however, mentioned in the identification of each group for a complete overview.
Splenius (in neck only)
Erector spinae
Transversospinalis group
Interspinal-intertransverse group
Quadratus lumborum

Erector Spinae

The muscles of this group cover a large area of the back, extending laterally from the vertebral column to the angle of the ribs and vertically from the sacrum to the occiput. This large musculotendinous mass is covered by the serratus posterior inferior and thoracodorsal fascia below the rhomboid and splenius muscles above. The erector spinae vary in size and composition at different levels.
Sacral region: Strong, dense, tendinous sheet, narrow at base (common tendon)
Lumbar region: Expands into thick muscular mass (palpable); visible surface contour on lateral side
Thoracic region: Muscle mass much thinner than that found in lumbar region; surface groove along lateral border follows costal angles until covered by scapula

Common Tendon of Erector Spinae
This is the origin of the broad thick tendon as described in Grant[7]
Sacrum (median and lateral crests, anterior surface of the tendon of erector spinae; L1-L5 and T12 vertebrae (spinous processes); supraspinous, sacrotuberous, and sacroiliac ligaments; iliac crests (inner aspect of dorsal part).
From the common tendon the muscles rise to form a large mass that is divided in the upper lumbar region into three longitudinal columns based on their areas of attachment in the thoracic and cervical regions.

Lateral Column of Muscle

66 Iliocostalis cervicis (see *Muscles of the Neck*)
89 Iliocostalis thoracis
90 Iliocostalis lumborum

Intermediate Column of Muscle

60 Longissimus capitis (see *Muscles of the Neck*)

64 Longissimus cervicis (see *Muscles of the Neck*)

91 Longissimus thoracis

Medial Column of Muscle

63 Spinalis capitis (see *Muscles of the Neck*)

68 Spinalis cervicis (see *Muscles of the Neck*)

92 Spinalis thoracis

The Iliocostalis Column (Lateral)

66 Iliocostalis cervicis (see *Muscles of the Neck*)

89 ILIOCOSTALIS THORACIS

Origin:
Ribs 12 to 7 (upper borders at angles)

Insertion:
Ribs 1 to 6 (at angles)
C7 (transverse process, dorsum)

Innervation:
T1-T12 spinal nerves

90 ILIOCOSTALIS LUMBORUM

Origin:
Common tendon of erector spinae (anterior surface)
Thoracolumbar fascia
Iliac crest (external lip)
Sacrum (posterior surface)

Insertion:
Lumbar vertebrae (all) (transverse processes)
Ribs 5 or 6 to 12 (angles on inferior border)

Description (all iliocostales):
This is the most lateral column of the erector spinae. The lumbar portion of this muscle is the largest, and it subdivides as it ascends.

Function:
Extension of spine
Lateral bending of spine (muscles on one side)
Depression of ribs (lumborum)
Elevation of pelvis

Innervation:
L1-L5 spinal nerves, dorsal rami (variable)

Longissimus Column (Intermediate)

91 LONGISSIMUS THORACIS

Origin:
Thoracolumbar fascia
L1-L5 vertebrae (transverse and accessory processes)

Insertion:
T1-T12 vertebrae (transverse processes)
Ribs 2 to 12 (between tubercles and angles)

Description (all longissimi):
These are the intermediate erector spinae. They lie between the iliocostales (laterally) and the spinales (medially). The fibers of the longissimus are inseparable from those of the iliocostales until the upper lumbar region.

Function (longissimus thoracis):
Extension of the spine
Lateral bending of spine to same side (muscles on one side)
Depression of ribs

Innervation:
T1-L1 spinal nerves (dorsal rami)

Spinalis Column (Medial)

92 SPINALIS THORACIS

Origin:
T11-T12 and L1-L2 vertebrae (spinous processes)

Insertion:
T1-T4 or through T8 vertebrae (spinous processes)

Description:
The smallest and thinnest of the erector spinae, they lie closest to the vertebral column. The spinales are inconstant and difficult to separate.

Function:
Extension of spine

Innervation:
T1-T12 (variable) dorsal rami

Transversospinales Group

Muscles of this group lie deep to the erector spinae, filling the concave region between the spinous and transverse processes of the vertebrae. They ascend obliquely and medially from the vertebral transverse processes to adjacent and sometimes more remote vertebrae. A span over four to six vertebrae is not uncommon.

62 Semispinalis capitis (see *Muscles of the Neck*)
65 Semispinalis cervicis (see *Muscles of the Neck*)
93 Semispinalis thoracis
94 Multifidi
71 Rotatores cervicis (see *Muscles of the Neck*)
95 Rotatores thoracis
96 Rotatores lumborum

93 SEMISPINALIS THORACIS

Origin:
T6-T10 vertebrae (transverse processes)

Insertion:
C6-T4 vertebrae (spinous processes)

Description:
This group is found only in the thoracic and cervical regions, extending to the head. They lie deep to the spinalis and longissimus columns of the erector spinae.

Function:
Extension of thoracic spine

Innervation:
T1-T12 spinal nerves (dorsal rami) variable

94 MULTIFIDI

Origin:
Sacrum (posterior, as low as the S4 foramen)
Aponeurosis of erector spinae
Ilium (posterior superior iliac spine) and adjacent crest
Sacroiliac ligaments (posterior)
L1-L5 vertebrae (mamillary processes)
T1-T12 vertebrae (transverse processes)
C4-C7 vertebrae (articular processes)

Insertion:
A higher vertebra (spinous process): Most superficial fibers run to the 3rd or 4th vertebra above; middle fibers run to the 2nd or 3rd above; deep fibers run between contiguous vertebrae.

Description:
These muscles fill the grooves on both sides of the spinous processes of the vertebrae from the sacrum to the middle cervical vertebrae (or may rise as high as C1). They lie deep to the erector spinae in the lumbar region and deep to the semispinales above. Each fasciculus ascends obliquely, traversing over two to four vertebrae as it moves toward the midline to insert in the spinous process of a higher vertebra.

Function:
Extension of spine
Lateral bending of spine (muscle on one side)
Rotation to opposite side

Innervation:
Spinal nerves (whole length of spine), segmentally (dorsal rami)

The Rotatores

The rotatores are the deepest muscles of the transversospinales group, lying as 11 pairs of very short muscles beneath the multifidi. The fibers run obliquely upward and medially or almost horizontal. They may cross more than one vertebra on their ascending course, but most commonly they proceed to the next higher one. Found along the entire length of the vertebral column, they are distinguishable as developed muscles only in the thoracic area.

95 ROTATORES THORACIS

Origin:
T1 to T12 vertebrae (transverse processes)

Insertion:
Vertebra above (lamina)

Description:
There are 11 pairs of these small muscles. Adjacent muscles start from the posterior transverse process of one vertebra and rise to attach to the lower body and lamina of the next higher vertebra.

Function:
Extension of thoracic spine
Rotation to opposite side

Innervation:
T1-T12 spinal nerves (dorsal rami)

96 ROTATORES LUMBORUM

The rotatores are highly variable and irregular in these regions.

Description:
This muscle lies deep to the multifidi and cannot be readily separated from the deepest fibers of the multifidi. Pattern is similar to that of the thoracis.

Function:
Extension of spine
Rotation of spine to opposite side

Innervation:
L1-L5 spinal nerves (dorsal rami) (highly variable)

Interspinal-Intertransverse Group

- **69** Interspinalis cervicis (see *Muscles of the Neck*)
- **70** Intertransversarii cervicis, anterior and posterior (see *Muscles of the Neck*)
- **97** Interspinalis thoracis
- **98** Interspinalis lumborum
- **99** Intertransversarii thoracis
- **99** Intertransversarii lumborum, medial and lateral

The Interspinales and Intertransversarii

The short, paired muscles in the interspinales group pass segmentally from the spinous processes (superior surface) of one vertebra to the inferior surface of the next on either side of the interspinous ligament. They are most highly developed in the cervical region, and quite irregular in distribution in the thoracic and lumbar spines.

The intertransversarii are small fasciculi lying between the transverse processes of contiguous vertebrae. They are most developed in the cervical spine. The cervical muscles have both anterior and posterior parts; the lumbar muscles have medial and lateral fibers. The thoracic muscles are single without divisions as seen in the other spine areas and are not constant.

97 INTERSPINALES THORACIS

Origin and Insertion:
Between spinous processes of contiguous vertebrae
Three pairs are reasonably constant: (1) between the 1st and 2nd thoracic vertebrae; (2) between the 2nd and 3rd thoracic vertebrae (variable); (3) between the 11th and 12th thoracic vertebrae

Function:
Extension of spine

Innervation:
T1-T3; T11-T12 (irregular) spinal nerves (dorsal rami)

98 INTERSPINALES LUMBORUM

Origin:
There are four pairs lying between the five lumbar vertebrae. Fasciculi run from the spinous process (superior) of L2-L5.

Insertion:
To inferior surfaces of spinous processes of the vertebra above the vertebra of origin.

Function:
Extension of spine

Innervation:
L1-L4 spinal nerves (dorsal rami), variable

99 INTERTRANSVERSARII THORACIS AND LUMBORUM

Intertransversarii thoracis

Origin:
T11-L1 (transverse processes, superior surfaces)

Insertion:
T10-T12 (transverse processes, inferior surfaces)

Function:
Extension of spine (muscles on both sides)
Lateral bending to same side (muscles on one side)
Rotation to opposite side

Innervation:
T1-T12, L1-L5 spinal nerves (dorsal rami)

Intertransversarii lumborum

Origin:
L2-S1 vertebrae (accessory and costal processes)

Insertion:
Vertebra above the vertebra of origin (mamillary processes, costal processes, inferior surfaces, transverse processes, inferior surfaces)

Function:
Lateral bending of lumbar spine
Postural control
Extension of the spine
Stabilization of adjacent vertebrae

Innervation:
Lumbar and sacral spinal nerves (dorsal and ventral rami)

100 QUADRATUS LUMBORUM

Origin:
Ilium (crest, inner lip)
Iliolumbar ligament

Insertion:
12th rib (lower border)
L1-L4 vertebrae (apices of transverse processes)
T12 vertebral body (occasionally)

Description:
An irregular quadrilateral muscle located against the posterior (dorsal) abdominal wall, this muscle is encased by layers of the thoracolumbar fascia. It fills the space between the 12th rib and the iliac crest. Its fibers run obliquely upward and medially from the iliac crest to the inferior border of the 12th rib and transverse processes of the lumbar vertebrae. The muscle is variable in size and occurrence.

Function:
Elevation of pelvis (weak in contrast to lateral abdominals)
Extension of lumbar spine (muscles on both sides)
Inspiration (via stabilization of lower attachments of diaphragm)
Fixation of lower portions of diaphragm for prolonged vocalization which needs sustained expiration.
Lateral bending of lumbar spine to same side (pelvis fixed)
Fixation and depression of 12th rib

Innervation:
T12-L3 spinal nerves (ventral rami)

Muscles of the Thorax for Respiration

101 Diaphragm
102 Intercostales externi
103 Intercostales interni
104 Intercostales intimi
105 Subcostales
106 Transversus thoracis
107 Levatores costarum
108 Serratus posterior superior
109 Serratus posterior inferior

101 DIAPHRAGM

Origin:
Muscle fibers take origin from the circumference of the thoracic outlet in three groups:
Sternal: Xiphoid (posterior surface)
Costal: Ribs 7 to 12 (bilaterally; inner surfaces of the cartilage and the deep surfaces on each side)
Lumbar: L1-L3 vertebrae (from the medial and lateral arcuate ligaments (also called lumbocostal arches) and from bodies of the vertebrae by two muscular crura)

Insertion:
Central tendon (trifoliate-shaped) of diaphragm immediately below the pericardium and blending with it. The central tendon has no bony attachments. It has three divisions called leaflets (because of its clover leaf pattern) in an otherwise continuous sheet of muscle, which affords the muscle great strength.

Description:
This half-dome–shaped muscle of contractile and fibrous structure forms the floor of the thorax (convex upper surface) and the roof of the abdomen (concave inferior surface). (Figure 11-4).

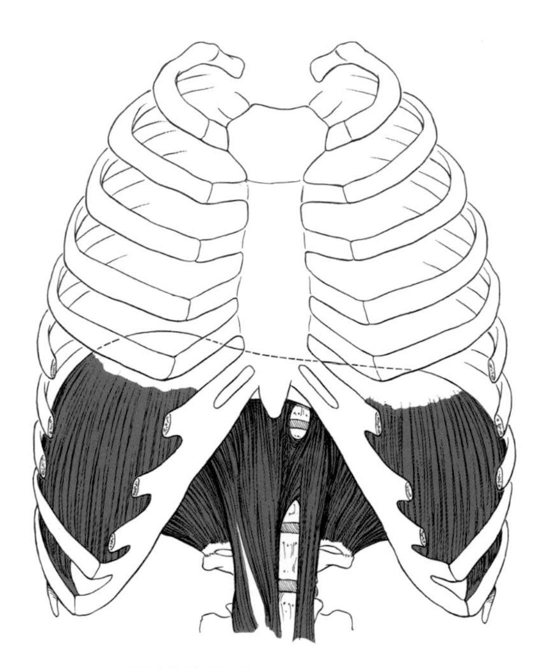

FIGURE 11-4 The diaphragm.

The diaphragm is muscular on the periphery and its central area is tendinous. It closes the opening of the thoracic outlet and forms a convex floor for the thoracic cavity. The muscle is flatter centrally than at the periphery and higher on the right (reaching rib 5) than on the left (reaching rib 6). From the peak on each side, the diaphragm abruptly descends to its costal and vertebral attachments. This descending slope is much more precipitous and longer posteriorly.

Function:
Inspiration: Contraction of the diaphragm with the lower ribs fixed draws the central tendon downward and forward during inspiration. This increases the vertical thoracic dimensions and pushes the abdominal viscera downward. It also decreases the pressure within the thoracic cavity, forcing air into the lungs through the open glottis by the higher pressure of the atmospheric air.
These events occur along with intercostal muscle action, which elevates the ribs, sternum, and vertebrae, increasing the anteroposterior and transverse thoracic dimensions for the inspiratory effort.
The diaphragm adds power to expulsive efforts: lifting heavy loads, sneezing, coughing, laughing, parturition, and evacuation of bladder and bowels. These activities are preceded by deep inspiration.
Expiration: Passive relaxation allows the half-dome to ascend, thus decreasing thoracic cavity volume and increasing its pressure.

Innervation:
Phrenic nerve, C4 (with contributions from C3 and C5)

The Intercostals

The intercostal muscles are slim layers of muscle and tendon occupying each of the intercostal spaces; the externals are the most superficial, the internals come next, and deepest are the intimi.

102 EXTERNAL INTERCOSTALS
(Intercostales Externi)

There are 11 pairs of muscles

Origin:
Ribs 1 to 11 (lower borders and costal tubercles)
Superior costotransverse ligaments

Insertion:
Ribs 2 to 12 (upper border of rib below)
Aponeurotic external intercostal membrane
Sternum (via aponeurosis)

Description:
There are 11 of these muscles on each side of the chest. Each arises from the inferior margin of one rib and inserts on the superior margin of the rib below. They extend in the intercostal spaces from the tubercles of the ribs dorsally to the cartilages of the ribs ventrally.
The muscle fibers run obliquely inferolaterally on the dorsal thorax; they run inferomedially and somewhat ventrally on the anterior thorax (down and toward the sternum).
The externi are the thickest of the three intercostal muscles. In appearance they may seem to be continuations of the external oblique abdominal muscles.

Function:
The muscles of respiration are highly coordinated between abdominal and thoracic processes with the diaphragm being the major muscle of inspiration, accounting for about ⅔ of vital capacity. The external intercostals are more active in inspiration than expiration but work closely with the internal intercostals to stiffen the chest wall, preventing paradoxical motion during descent of the diaphragm.
Elevation of ribs in inspiration. There are data to support this claim for the upper four or five muscles, but the more dorsal and lateral fibers of the same muscles also are active in early expiration. It is possible that the activity of the intercostals during respiration varies with the depth of breathing.[17]
Depression of the ribs in expiration (supporting data sparse).
Rotation of thoracic spine to opposite side (unilateral).
Stabilization of rib cage.

Innervation:
T1-T11 intercostal nerves (ventral rami)
These nerves are numbered sequentially according to interspace (e.g., the 5th intercostal nerve innervates muscle occupying the 5th intercostal space between the 5th and 6th ribs).

103 INTERNAL INTERCOSTALS
(Intercostales Interni)

Origin:
Ribs 1 to 11 (ridge on inner surface, then passing down and toward spine)
Costal cartilage of same rib
Sternum (anterior)
Upper border and costal cartilage of rib below
Internal intercostal membrane (aponeurosis)

Insertion:
Ribs 2 to 12 (upper border of next rib below)

Description:
There are 11 pairs of these muscles. They extend from the sternal end of the ribs anteriorly to the angle of the ribs posteriorly. The fibers run obliquely downward but at a 90° angle to the external intercostals.

Function:
Not as strong as the external intercostals.
Elevation of ribs in inspiration. This may be true at least for the 1st to 5th muscles. The more lateral muscle fibers run more obliquely inferior and posterior and are most active in expiration.[17]
Stabilization of rib cage.

Innervation:
T1-T11 intercostal nerves (ventral rami)

104 INTERCOSTALES INTIMI

Origin:
Costal groove of rib above the rib of insertion. Found in lower costal interspaces when present, but no consistent evidence in upper five to six interspaces.

Insertion:
Upper margin of the rib below the rib of origin. Found in lower costal interspaces.

Description:
There is dispute about whether this is a separate muscle or just a part of the internal intercostals. It is a thin sheet lying deep to the internal

intercostals, but arguments in favor of a separate muscle are not convincing. If they are separate, there may be five to six pairs, with no consistent presence in the upper costal interspaces. Considered insignificant.

Function:
Presumed to be identical to intercostales interni.

Innervation:
T1-T11 intercostal nerves (ventral rami) (inconsistent)

105 SUBCOSTALES

Origin:
Lower ribs (variable) on inner surface near angle

Insertion:
Inner surface of two or three ribs below rib of origin

Description:
Lying on the dorsal thoracic wall, these muscles are discretely developed only in the lower thorax. Fibers run in the same direction as those of the intercostales interni.

Function:
Draws adjacent ribs together or depresses ribs (no supporting data)

Innervation:
T7-T11 intercostal nerves (ventral rami)

106 TRANSVERSE THORACIS

Origin:
Sternum (caudal ⅓; xiphoid, posterior surface)
Ribs 3 to 6 (costal cartilages, inner side)

Insertion:
Ribs 2 to 5 (costal cartilages, caudal borders)

Description:
A thin plane on the inner surface of the anterior wall of the thorax. The fibers pass obliquely up and laterally, diverging more as they insert. The lowest fibers are horizontal and are continuous with the transversus abdominis. The highest fibers are almost vertical. Attachments vary from side to side in the same person and among different people.

Function:
Draws ribs downward; narrows chest
Active in forced expiration

Innervation:
T2-T11 intercostal nerves (ventral rami)

107 LEVATORES COSTARUM

There are 12 pairs of muscles

Origin:
C7 and T1-T11 vertebrae (transverse processes)

Insertion:
Rib immediately below rib of origin (upper margin, outer edge between angle and tubercle)

Description:
There are 12 pairs of these muscles on either side of the thorax on its posterior wall. Fibers run obliquely inferolaterally, like those of the external intercostal muscles. The most inferior fibers divide into two fasciculi, one of which inserts as described; the other descends to the 2nd rib below its origin.

Function:
Elevation of ribs in inspiration (disputed)
Lateral bending of spine

Innervation:
T1-T11 intercostal nerves and sometimes C8 (dorsal rami)

108 SERRATUS POSTERIOR SUPERIOR

Origin:
C7 and T1-T3 vertebrae (spinous processes)
Ligamentum nuchae
Supraspinous ligaments

Insertion:
Ribs 2 to 5 (upper borders, lateral to angles)

Description:
Muscle lies on the upper dorsal thorax, over the erector spinae and under the rhomboids. Fibers run inferolaterally.

Function:
Elevates upper ribs (debated)
Presumably increases thoracic volume (function uncertain)

Innervation:
T2-T5 spinal nerves (ventral rami)

109 SERRATUS POSTERIOR INFERIOR

Origin:
T11-T12 and L1-L2 vertebrae (spinous processes via thoracolumbar fascia)
Supraspinous ligaments

Insertion:
Ribs 9 to 12 (inferior borders, lateral to angles)

Description:
A thin muscle, composed of four digitations, lying at the border between the thoracic and lumbar regions. Fibers ascend laterally. It is much broader than the serratus posterior superior and lies four ribs below it. It lies over the erector spinae and under the latissimus dorsi.[4] The muscle may have fewer than four digitations or may be absent.

Function:
Depresses lower ribs and moves them dorsally
Has an uncertain role in respiration

Innervation:
T9-T12 spinal nerves (ventral rami)

Muscles of the Abdomen

Anterolateral Walls

110 Obliquus externus abdominis
111 Obliquus internus abdominis
112 Transversus abdominis
113 Rectus abdominis
114 Pyramidalis

110 OBLIQUUS EXTERNUS ABDOMINIS

Origin:
Ribs 5 to 12 (by digitations that attach to the external and inferior surfaces and alternate with digitations of the serratus anterior and latissimus dorsi)

Insertion:
Iliac crest (anterior half of outer lip)
Iliac fascia
Aponeurosis from the prominence of 9th costal cartilage to anterior superior iliac spine (ASIS); aponeuroses from both sides meet at the linea alba

Description:
The largest and most superficial flat, thin muscle of the abdomen curves around the anterior and lateral walls. Its muscular fibers lie on the lateral wall, whereas its aponeurosis traverses the anterior wall in front of the rectus abdominis, meeting its opposite number to form the linea alba. The digitations form an oblique line that runs down and backward. The linea alba extends from the xiphoid process to the symphysis pubis.
The upper (superior) five digitations increase in size as they descend and alternate with the corresponding digitations of the serratus anterior. The distal three digitations decrease in size as they descend and alternate with digitations of the latissimus dorsi. The superior fibers travel inferomedially; the posterior fibers pass more vertically.

Function:
Flexion of trunk (bilateral muscles)
Tilts pelvis posteriorly
Elevates pelvis (unilateral)
Rotation of trunk to opposite side (unilateral)
Lateral bending of trunk (unilateral)
Support and compression of abdominal viscera, counteracting effect of gravity on abdominal contents
Assists defecation, micturition, emesis, and parturition (i.e., expulsion of contents of abdominal viscera and air from lungs)
Important accessory muscle of forced expiration (during expiration it forces the viscera upward to elevate the diaphragm)

Innervation:
T7-T12 spinal nerves (ventral rami)

111 OBLIQUUS INTERNUS ABDOMINIS

Origin:
Thoracolumbar fascia
Inguinal ligament (lateral ⅔ of upper aspect)
Iliac crest (anterior ⅔ of intermediate line)

Insertion:
Ribs 9 to 12 (inferior borders and cartilages by digitations that appear continuous with internal intercostals)
Aponeurosis that splits at the lateral border of the rectus abdominis to encircle the muscle and reunite at the linea alba
Cartilages of ribs 7 to 9 (via an aponeurosis)
Pubis (crest and pecten pubis) from tendinous sheath of transverse abdominis

Description:
This muscle is smaller and thinner than the external oblique under which it lies in the lateral and ventral abdominal wall. The fibers from the iliac crest pass upward and medially to ribs 9 to 12 and the aponeurosis; the more lateral the fibers, the more they run toward the vertical. The lowest fibers pass almost horizontally on the lower abdomen.

Function:
Flexion of spine (bilateral)
Lateral bending of spine (unilateral)
Rotation of trunk to same side (unilateral)
Increases abdominal pressure to assist in defecation and other expulsive actions
Forces viscera upward during expiration to elevate diaphragm
Elevation of pelvis

Innervation:
T7-T12 spinal nerves (ventral rami)
L1 spinal nerve (iliohypogastric and ilioinguinal branches) (ventral rami)

112 TRANSVERSE ABDOMINIS

Origin:
Inguinal ligament (lateral ⅓)
Iliac crest (anterior ⅔ of inner lip)
Thoracolumbar fascia (between iliac crest and 12th rib)
Ribs 7 to 12 (costal cartilages)

Insertion:
Pubis (crest and pecten pubis) via aponeurosis along with aponeurosis of the internal oblique to form the falx inguinalis
Linea alba (upper and middle fibers pass medially to blend with the posterior layer of the broad aponeurosis encircling the rectus abdominis)

Description:
The innermost of the flat abdominal muscles, the transversus abdominis lies under the internal oblique. Its name derives from the direction of its fibers, which pass horizontally across the lateral abdomen to an aponeurosis and the linea alba. The length of the fibers varies considerably depending on the insertion site, the most inferior to the pubis being the longest. At its origin on ribs 7 to 12, the muscle interdigitates with similar diaphragmatic digitations separated by a narrow raphe.

Function:
Constricts (flattens) abdomen, compressing the abdominal viscera and assisting in expelling their contents
Forced expiration

Innervation:
T7-T12 spinal nerves (ventral rami)
L1 spinal nerve (iliohypogastric and ilioinguinal branches) (ventral rami)

113 RECTUS ABDOMINIS

Origin:
By two tendons inferiorly:
Lateral: pubis (tubercle on crest and pecten pubis)
Medial: ligaments covering front of symphysis pubis

Insertion:
Ribs 5 to 7 (costal cartilages by three fascicles of differing size)
Sternum (xiphoid process, costoxiphoid ligaments)

Description:
A long muscular strap extending from the ventral lower sternum to the pubis. Its vertical fibers lie centrally along the abdomen, each separated from its contralateral partner by the linea alba. The muscle is interrupted (but not all the way through) by three (or more) fibrous bands called the *tendinous intersections,* which pass transversely across the muscle in a zigzag fashion. The most superior intersection generally is at the level of the xiphoid; the lowest is at the level of the umbilicus, and the second intersection is midway between the two. These are readily visible on bodybuilders or others with well-developed musculature.

Function:
Flexion of spine (draws symphysis and sternum toward each other)
Posterior tilt of pelvis
With other abdominal muscles, compresses abdominal contents

Innervation:
T7-T12 spinal nerves (ventral rami)
T7 innervates fibers above the superior tendinous intersection; T8 innervates fibers between the superior and middle intersections; T9 innervates fibers between the middle and distal intersections.

114 PYRAMIDALIS

Origin:
Pubis (front of body and symphysis via ligamentous fibers)

Insertion:
Linea alba (midway between umbilicus and pubis)

Description:
A small triangular muscle located in the extreme distal portion of the abdominal wall and lying anterior to the lower rectus abdominis. Its origin on the pubis is wide, and it narrows as it rises to a pointed insertion. The muscle varies considerably from side to side, and may be present or absent.

Function:
Tenses the linea alba

Innervation:
T12 spinal nerve (subcostal nerve) (ventral ramus)

Muscles of the Perineum

115 Levator ani
116 Coccygeus

117 Cremaster
118 Transversus perinei superficialis
119 Transversus perinei profundus
120 Bulbospongiosus
121 Ischiocavernosus
122 Sphincter urethrae
123 Sphincter ani externus

115 LEVATOR ANI (Pubococcygeus, Puborectalis, Iliococcygeus)

Origin:
Pubococcygeus part: Pubis (inner surface of superior ramus)
Coccyx (anterior)
Blends with longitudinal rectus muscle and fascia
Puborectal is part: Same origin as pubococcygeus but splits off to join its opposite member, along with sphincter externus, to form an anorectal sling
Iliococcygeus part: Ischium (inner surface of spine)
Obturator fascia

Insertion:
Coccyx (last two segments)
Anococcygeal raphe
Sphincter ani externus

Description:
A part of the pelvic diaphragm, this broad, thin sheet of muscle unites with its contralateral partner to form a complete pelvic floor. Anteriorly it is attached to the pubis lateral to the symphysis, posteriorly to the ischial spine, and between these to the obturator fascia. The fibers course medially with varying obliquity.
There are links to the sphincter urethrae, to the prostate as the levator prostatae, to the pubovaginalis walls of the vagina in the female, and to the perineal body and rectum in both men and women. In animals these parts are attached to caudal vertebrae and control tail motions. Loss of a tail in humans leaves these muscles to form a stronger pelvic floor.

Function:
Constriction of rectum and vagina contributing to continence; they must relax to permit expulsion.
Along with the coccygei, the levator forms a muscular pelvic diaphragm that supports the pelvic viscera and opposes sudden increases in intra-abdominal pressure, as in forced expiration, or the Valsalva maneuver.

Innervation:
S2-S3 spinal nerves (pudendal nerve) (ventral rami) and nerves from sacral plexus

116 COCCYGEUS

Origin:
Ischium (spine and pelvic surface)
Sacrospinous ligament

Insertion:
Coccyx (lateral margins)
Sacrum (last or 5th segment, side)

Description:
The paired muscle lies posterior and superior to the levator ani and contiguous with it in the same plane. The muscle occasionally is absent. It is considered the pelvic aspect of the sacrospinous ligament.

Function:
The coccygei pull the coccyx forward and support it after it has been pushed back for defecation or parturition.
With the levatores ani and piriformis, compresses the posterior pelvic cavity and outlet in women ("the birth canal").

Innervation:
S3-S4 spinal nerves (pudendal plexus) (ventral rami)

117 CREMASTER

Origin:
Lateral part: Inguinal ligament (continuous with internal oblique and occasionally from transverse abdominis). Technically this is an abdominal muscle.
Medial part: Pubis (crest, tubercle, and falx inguinalis). This part is inconstant.

Insertion:
Pubis (tubercle and crest)
Sheath of rectus abdominis and transversus abdominis

Description:
Consists of loose fasciculi lying along the spermatic cord and held together by areolar tissue to form the cremasteric fascia around the cord and testis. Often said to be continuous with the internal oblique abdominal muscle or with the transversus abdominis. After passage through the superficial inguinal ring, the muscle spreads into loops of varying lengths over the spermatic cord.
Although the muscle fibers are striated, this is not usually a voluntary muscle. Stimulation of the skin on the medial thigh evokes a reflex response, the cremasteric reflex.
Found as a vestige in women.

Function:
Elevation of testis toward superficial inguinal ring
Thermoregulation of testes by adjusting position

Innervation:
L1-L2 spinal nerves (genitofemoral nerve) (ventral rami)

118 TRANSVERSUS PERINEI SUPERFICIALIS

Origin:
Ischial tuberosity (inner and anterior part)

Insertion:
Perineal body (a centrally placed, modiolar-like structure on which perineal muscles and fascia converge)
Tendon of perineum

Description:
A narrow slip of muscle in both the male and female perineum, it courses almost transversely across the perineal area in front of the anus. It is joined on the perineal body by the muscle from the opposite side. The muscle is sometimes absent, poorly developed, or may be doubled.

Function:
Bilateral action serves to fix the centrally located perineal body.
Support of pelvic viscera.

Innervation:
S2-S4 spinal nerves (pudendal nerve) (ventral rami)

119 TRANSVERSUS PERINEI PROFUNDUS

Origin:
Ischium (ramus, medial aspect)

Insertion:
Male: Perineal body
Female: Vagina (side); perineal body

Description:
Small deep muscle with similar structure and function in both male and female. The bilateral muscles meet at the midline on the perineal body. This muscle is in the same plane as the sphincter urethrae, and together they form most of the bulk of the urogenital diaphragm. (Together they used to be called the constrictor urethrae.) Together, the two muscles "tether" the perineal body.

Function:
Fixation of perineal body
Supports pelvic viscera

Innervation:
S2-S4 spinal nerves (pudendal nerve) (ventral rami)

120 BULBOSPONGIOSUS

Formerly called:
Male: Bulbocavernosus; accelerator urinae
Female: Sphincter vaginae

In the Female

Origin:
Perineal body
Blending with sphincter ani externus and median raphe
Fascia of urogenital diaphragm

Insertion:
Corpora cavernosus clitoridis

Description:
Surrounds the orifice of the vagina and covers the lateral parts of the vestibular bulb. The fibers run anteriorly on each side of the vagina and send a slip to cover the clitoral body.

Function:
Arrests micturition; helps to empty urethra after bladder empties
Constriction of vaginal orifice
Constriction of deep dorsal vein of clitoris by anterior fibers, contributing to erection of clitoris

Innervation:
S2-S4 spinal nerves (pudendal nerve) (ventral rami)

In the Male

Origin:
Perineal body
Median raphe over bulb of penis

Insertion:
Urogenital diaphragm (inferior fascia)
Aponeurosis over corpus spongiosum penis
Body of penis anterior to ischiocavernosus
Tendinous expansion over dorsal vessels of penis

Description:
Located in the midline of the perineum anterior to the anus and consisting of two symmetrical parts united by a tendinous raphe. Its fibers divide like the halves of a feather. The posterior fibers disperse on the inferior fascia of the urogenital diaphragm; the middle fibers encircle the penile bulb and the corpus spongiosum and form a strong aponeurosis with fibers from the opposite side; and the anterior fibers spread out over the corpora cavernosa.

Function:
Empties urethra at end of micturition (is capable of arresting urination).
Middle fibers assist in penis erection by compressing the bulbar erectile tissue; anterior fibers assist by constricting the deep dorsal vein.
Contracts repeatedly in ejaculation.

Innervation:
S2-S4 spinal nerves (pudendal nerve) (ventral rami)

121 ISCHIOCAVERNOSUS

In the Female

Origin:
Ischium (tuberosity [inner surface] and ramus)
Crus clitoridis (surface)

Insertion:
Aponeurosis inserting into sides and inferior surface of crus clitoridis

Description:
Covers the unattached surface of crus clitoridis. Muscle is smaller than the male counterpart.

Function:
Compresses crus clitoridis, retarding venous return and thus assisting erection

Innervation:
S2-S4 spinal nerves (pudendal)

In the Male

Origin:
Ischium (tuberosity, medial aspect dorsal to crus penis and ischial rami)

Insertion:
Aponeurosis into the sides and undersurface of the body of the penis

Description:
The muscle is paired and covers the crus of the penis.

Function:
Compression of crus penis, maintaining erection by retarding return of blood through the veins

Innervation:
S2-S4 spinal nerves (pudendal nerve, perineal branch) (ventral rami)

122 SPHINCTER URETHRAE

In the Female

Origin:
Pubis (inferior ramus on each side)
Transverse perineal ligament and fascia

Insertion:
Surrounds lower urethra, neck of bladder; sends fibers to wall of vagina.
Blends with fibers from opposite muscle to urethra.
Perineal membrane (posterior edge)

Description:
Has both superior and inferior fibers. The inferior fibers arise on the pubis and course across the pubic arch in front of the urethra to circle around it. The superior fibers merge into the smooth muscle of the bladder.

Function:
Constricts urethra, particularly when the bladder contains fluid.
It is relaxed during micturition but contracts to expel remaining urine after micturition.

Innervation:
Pudendal nucleus (Onuf's nucleus)
S2-S4 spinal nerves (pudendal nerve) (ventral rami)

In the Male

Origin:
Ischiopubic ramus (superior fibers)
Transverse perineal ligament (inferior fibers)

Insertion:
Perineal body (converges with muscles from other side)

Description:
Surrounds entire length of membranous portion of urethra and is enclosed in the urogenital diaphragm fascia

Function:
Compression of urethra (bilateral action)
Active in ejaculation
Relaxes during micturition but contracts to expel last of urine

Innervation:
Pudendal nerve nucleus (Onuf's nucleus)
S2-S4 spinal nerves (ventral rami)

123 SPHINCTER ANI EXTERNUS

Origin:
Skin surrounding margin of anus
Coccyx (via anococcygeal ligament)

Insertion:
Perineal body
Blends with other muscles in area

Description:
Surrounds entire anal canal and is adherent to skin. Consists of three parts, all skeletal muscle:
1. *Subcutaneous:* Around lower anal canal; fibers course horizontally beneath the skin at the anal orifice. Some fibers join perineal body and others the anococcygeal ligament.
2. *Superficial:* Surrounds the lower part of the internal sphincter; attaches to both the perineal body and coccyx (via the terminal coccygeal ligament, the only bony attachment of the muscle).
3. *Deep part:* Thick band around the upper internal sphincter with fibers blending with the puborectalis of the levator ani and fascia.

Function:
Keeps anal orifice closed. It is always in a state of tonic contraction and has no antagonist. Muscle relaxes during defecation, allowing orifice to open. The muscle can be voluntarily contracted to close the orifice more tightly as in forced expiration or the Valsalva maneuver.

Innervation:
S2-S3 spinal nerves (pudendal nerve, inferior rectal branch) (ventral rami)
S4 spinal nerve (perineal branch)

MUSCLES OF THE UPPER EXTREMITY
(Shoulder Girdle, Elbow, Forearm, Wrist, Fingers, Thumb)

Muscles of the Shoulder Girdle Acting on the Scapula

124 Trapezius
125 Rhomboid major
126 Rhomboid minor
127 Levator scapulae
128 Serratus anterior
129 Pectoralis minor

124 TRAPEZIUS

A paired muscle

Origin:
Upper:
Occiput (external protuberance and medial ⅓ of superior nuchal line)
Ligamentum nuchae
C7 vertebra (spinous process)
Middle:
T1-T5 vertebrae (spinous processes)
Supraspinous ligaments
Lower:
T6-T12 vertebrae (spinous processes)
Supraspinous ligaments

Insertion:
Upper:
Clavicle (posterior surface, lateral ⅓)
Middle:
Scapula (medial margin of acromion; spine of scapula and crest of its superior lip)
Lower:
Scapula (spine: tubercle at lateral apex and aponeurosis at root of spine)

Description:
A flat, triangular muscle lying over the posterior neck, shoulder, and upper thorax. The upper trapezius fibers course down and laterally from the occiput; the middle fibers are horizontal; and the lower fibers move upward and laterally from the vertebrae to the scapular spine. The name of the muscle is derived from the shape of the muscle with its contralateral partner: a diamond-shaped quadrilateral figure, or trapezoid.

Function:
All: Stabilizes scapula during movements of the arm.
Upper and Lower:
Rotation of the scapula so glenoid faces up (inferior angle moves laterally and forward)
Upper:
Elevation of scapula and shoulder ("shrugging") (with levator scapulae)
Rotation of head to opposite side (one)
Capital extension (both)
Cervical extension (both)
Middle:
Scapular adduction (retraction) (with rhomboids)
Lower:
Scapular adduction, depression, and upward rotation

Innervation:
Accessory (XI) nerve (upper and middle)
While the accessory nerve provides the major motor supply to the trapezius, there also is some supply from the cervical plexus (C3-C4) and this may be the primary supply of the lower fibers with contributions from the accessory nerve.[18]

125 RHOMBOID MAJOR
(Rhomboideus Major)

Origin:
T2-T5 vertebrae (spinous processes)
Supraspinous ligaments

Insertion:
Scapula (medial [vertebral] border between root of spine above and inferior angle below)

Description:
Fibers of the muscle run slightly inferolaterally between the thoracic spine and the vertebral border of the scapula.

Function:
Scapular adduction
Downward rotation of scapula (glenoid faces down)
Scapular elevation

Innervation:
C5 dorsal scapular nerve

126 RHOMBOID MINOR

Origin:
C7-T1 vertebrae (spinous processes)
Ligamentum nuchae (lower)

Insertion:
Scapula (root of spine on medial [vertebral] border)

Description:
Lies just superior to rhomboid major, and its fibers run parallel with the larger muscle.

Function:
Scapular adduction
Scapular downward rotation (glenoid faces down)
Scapular elevation

Innervation:
C5 dorsal scapular nerve

127 LEVATOR SCAPULAE

Origin:
C1-C4 vertebrae (transverse processes and posterior tubercles)

Insertion:
Scapula (vertebral border between superior angle and root of scapular spine)

Description:
Lies on the dorsolateral neck and descends deep to the sternocleidomastoid on the floor of the posterior triangle of the neck. Its vertebral attachments vary considerably.

Function:
Elevates and adducts scapula
Scapular downward rotation (glenoid faces down)
Lateral bending of cervical spine to same side (one)
Cervical rotation to same side (one)
Cervical extension (both assist)

Innervation:
C3-C4 spinal nerves (ventral rami)
C5 dorsal scapular nerve (to lower fibers) (ventral rami)

128 SERRATUS ANTERIOR

Origin:
Ribs 1 to 8 (often 9 and 10 also) by digitations (superior and outer surfaces). Each digitation (except first) arises from a single rib. The 1st digitation arises from the 1st and 2nd ribs. All others arise from a single rib and fascia covering the intervening intercostals.
Aponeurosis of intercostal muscles.

Insertion:
Scapula (ventral surface of whole vertebral border)
First digitation: Superior angle of scapula on anterior aspect
Second and third digitations: Anterior (costal) surface of whole vertebral border
Fourth to eighth digitations: Inferior angle of scapula (costal surface)

Description:
This large sheet of muscle curves posteriorly around the thorax from its origin on the lateral side of the ribs, passing under the scapula to attach to its vertebral border.

Function:
Scapular abduction
Upward rotation of the scapula (glenoid faces up)
Medial border of scapula drawn anteriorly close to the thoracic wall (preventing "winging")

Functional Relationships:
The serratus works with the trapezius in a force couple to rotate the scapula upward (glenoid up), allowing the arm to be elevated fully (150° to 180°). Three component forces act around a

center of rotation located in the center of the scapula: (1) upward pull on the acromial end of the spine of the scapula by the upper trapezius; (2) downward pull on the base of the spine of the scapula by the lower trapezius; (3) lateral and anterior pull on the inferior angle by the inferior fibers of the serratus.[19-21]

The reader is referred to comprehensive texts on kinesiology for further detail.

Innervation:
C5-C7 long thoracic nerve

129 PECTORALIS MINOR

Origin:
Ribs 3 to 5 and sometimes 2 to 4 (upper and outer surfaces near the costal cartilages)
Aponeurosis of intercostal muscles

Insertion:
Scapula (coracoid process, medial border, and superior surface)

Description:
This muscle, broader at its origins, lies on the upper thorax directly under the pectoralis major. It forms part of the anterior wall of the axilla (along with the pectoralis major). The fibers pass upward and laterally and converge in a flat tendon.

Function:
Scapular protraction (abduction): scapula moves forward around the chest wall. Works here with serratus anterior.
Elevation of ribs in forced inspiration when scapula is fixed by the levator scapulae

Innervation:
C5-T1 medial and lateral pectoral nerves

Vertebrohumeral Muscles

130 Latissimus dorsi
131 Pectoralis major

130 LATISSIMUS DORSI

Origin:
T6-T12 vertebrae (spinous processes)
L1-L5 and sacral vertebrae (spinous processes by way of the thoracolumbar fascia)
Ribs 9 to 12 (interdigitates with the external abdominal oblique)
Ilium (posterior ⅓ of iliac crest)
Supraspinous ligament

Insertion:
Humerus (intertubercular groove, floor, distal)
Deep fascia of arm

Description:
A broad sheet of muscle that covers the lumbar and lower portion of the posterior thorax. From this wide origin, the muscle fibers converge on the proximal humerus. The superior fibers are almost horizontal, passing over the inferior angle of the scapula, whereas the lowest fibers are almost vertical. As the muscle approaches its tendinous insertion, the fibers from the upper and lower portions fold on themselves so that the superior fibers are attached inferiorly in the intertubercular groove; similarly, the sacral and lumbar fibers become more superior.

Function:
Extension, adduction, and internal rotation of shoulder.
Hyperextension of spine (muscles on both sides), as in lifting.
The muscle is most powerful in overhead activities (such as swimming [downstroke] and climbing), crutch walking (elevation of trunk to arms, i.e., shoulder depression), or swinging.[22]
Adducts raised arm against resistance (with pectoralis major and teres major).
It is very active in strong expiration, as in coughing and sneezing, and in deep inspiration.
Elevation of pelvis with arms fixed.

Innervation:
C6-C8 Thoracodorsal nerve (ventral rami)

131 PECTORALIS MAJOR

Origin:
Clavicular (upper) portion:
Clavicle (sternal half of anterior surface)
Sternocostal portion:
Sternum (half of the anterior surface down to level of 6th rib)
Ribs (cartilage of all true ribs except rib 1 and sometimes rib 7)
Aponeurosis of obliquus externus abdominis

Insertion:
Humerus (intertubercular sulcus, lateral border via a bilaminar tendon)

Description:
This muscle is a large, thick, fan-shaped muscle covering the anterior and superior surfaces of the thorax. The pectoralis major forms part of the anterior wall of the axilla (the anterior axillary fold, conspicuous in abduction). The muscle is

divided into two portions that converge toward the axilla.
The clavicular fibers pass downward and laterally toward the humeral insertion. The sternocostal fibers pass horizontally from midsternum and upward and laterally from the rib attachments. The lower fibers rise almost vertically toward the axilla. Both parts unite in a common tendon of insertion to the humerus.

Function:
Adduction of shoulder (glenohumeral) joint (whole muscle, proximal attachment fixed)
Internal rotation of shoulder
Elevation of thorax in forced inspiration (with both upper extremities fixed)
Clavicular fibers:
Internal rotation of shoulder
Flexion of shoulder
Horizontal shoulder adduction
Sternocostal fibers:
Horizontal shoulder adduction
Extension of shoulder
Draws trunk upward and forward in climbing

Innervation:
Clavicular fibers: C5-C7 lateral pectoral nerve
Sternocostal fibers: C6-T1 medial and lateral pectoral nerves

Scapulohumeral Muscles

There are six shoulder muscles, which extend from the scapula to the humerus. Also included here are the subclavius and the coracobrachialis.

132 Subclavius
133 Deltoid
134 Subscapularis
135 Supraspinatus
136 Infraspinatus
137 Teres minor
138 Teres major
139 Coracobrachialis

All act on the shoulder (glenohumeral) joint. The largest of the muscles (deltoid) also attaches to the clavicle and overlies the remaining muscles.

132 SUBCLAVIUS

Origin:
Rib 1 and its cartilage (at their junction)

Insertion:
Clavicle (inferior surface, groove in middle ⅓)

Description:
A small elongated muscle lying under the clavicle between it and the 1st rib. The fibers run upward and laterally following the contour of the clavicle.

Function:
Shoulder depression (assist)
Depresses and moves clavicle forward, thus stabilizing it during shoulder motion

Innervation:
C5-C6 (nerve to subclavius off brachial plexus) (ventral rami)

133 DELTOID

Origin:
Anterior fibers: Clavicle (shaft: anterior border and superior surface of lateral ⅓)
Middle fibers: Scapula (acromion, lateral margin, and superior surface)
Posterior fibers: Scapula (spine on lower lip of posterior border)

Insertion:
Humerus (deltoid tuberosity on lateral midshaft via humeral tendon)

Description:
This large multipennate, triangular muscle covers the shoulder anteriorly, posteriorly, and laterally. From a wide origin on the scapula and clavicle, all fibers converge on the humeral insertion, where it gives off an expansion to the deep fascia of the arm. The anterior fibers descend obliquely backward and laterally; the middle fibers descend vertically; the posterior fibers descend obliquely forward and laterally.

Function:
Abduction of shoulder (glenohumeral joint): primarily the acromial middle fibers. The anterior and posterior fibers in this motion stabilize the limb in its cantilever position.
Flexion and internal rotation of shoulder (anterior fibers).
Extension and external rotation: posterior fibers.
The deltoid tends to displace the humeral head upward.
Shoulder horizontal abduction (posterior fibers).
Shoulder horizontal adduction (anterior fibers).

Innervation:
C5-C6 axillary nerve (ventral rami)

134 SUBSCAPULARIS

Origin:
Scapula (subscapular fossa and groove along axillary margin)
Aponeurosis separating this muscle from the teres major and triceps brachii (long head)
Tendinous laminae

Insertion:
Humerus (lesser tubercle)
Capsule of glenohumeral joint (anterior)

Description:
This is one of the rotator cuff muscles. It is a large triangular muscle that fills the subscapular fossa of the scapula. The tendon of insertion is separated from the scapular neck by a large bursa, which is really a protrusion of the synovial lining of the joint. Variations are rare.

Function:
Internal rotation of shoulder joint
Stabilization of glenohumeral joint by humeral depression (keeps humeral head in glenoid fossa)

Innervation:
C5-C6 subscapular nerves (upper and lower)

135 SUPRASPINATUS

Origin:
Scapula (supraspinous fossa, medial ⅔)
Supraspinatus fascia

Insertion:
Humerus (greater tubercle, highest facet)
Articular capsule of glenohumeral joint

Description:
This is one of the four rotator cuff muscles. Occupying all of the supraspinous fossa, the muscle fibers converge to form a flat tendon that crosses above the glenohumeral joint (beneath the acromion) on its way to a humeral insertion. This tendon is the most commonly ruptured element of the rotator cuff mechanism around the joint.

Function:
Maintains humeral head in glenoid fossa (with other rotator cuff muscles)
Abduction of shoulder
External rotation of shoulder

Innervation:
C5-C6 suprascapular nerve

136 INFRASPINATUS

Origin:
Scapula (fills most of infraspinous fossa, rises from medial ⅔)
Infraspinous fascia

Insertion:
Humerus (greater tubercle, middle facet)

Description:
Occupies most of the infraspinous fossa. The muscle fibers converge to form the tendon of insertion, which glides over the lateral border of the scapular spine and then passes across the posterior aspect of the articular capsule to insert on the humerus. This is the third of the rotator cuff muscles.

Function:
Stabilizes shoulder joint by depressing humeral head in glenoid fossa
External rotation of shoulder

Innervation:
C5-C6 suprascapular nerve

137 TERES MINOR

Origin:
Scapula (proximal ⅔ of flat surface on dorsal aspect of axillary border)
Aponeurotic laminae (two such), one of which separates it from the teres major, the other from the infraspinatus

Insertion:
Humerus (greater tubercle, most inferior facet, upper fibers)
Humerus (shaft: below the lowest facet, lower fibers)
Capsule of glenohumeral joint (posterior)

Description:
A somewhat cylindrical and elongated muscle, the teres minor ascends laterally and upward from its origin to form a tendon that inserts on the greater tubercle of the humerus. It lies inferior to the infraspinatus, and its fibers lie parallel with that muscle. It is one of the rotator cuff muscles.

Function:
Maintains humeral head in glenoid fossa, thus stabilizing the shoulder joint
External rotation of shoulder
Adduction of shoulder (weak)

Innervation:
C5-C6 axillary nerve

138 TERES MAJOR

Origin:
Scapula (dorsal surface near the inferior scapular angle on its lateral margin)
Fibrous septa between this muscle and the teres minor and infraspinatus

Insertion:
Humerus (intertubercular sulcus, medial lip)

Description:
The teres major is a flattened but thick muscle that ascends laterally and upward to the humerus. Its tendon lies behind that of the latissimus dorsi, and they generally unite for a short distance.

Function:
Internal rotation of shoulder
Adduction and extension of shoulder
Extension of shoulder from a flexed position

Innervation:
C5-C6 subscapular nerve (lower)

139 CORACOBRACHIALIS

Origin:
Scapula, coracoid process (apex)
Intermuscular septum

Insertion:
Humerus (midway along medial border of shaft)

Description:
The smallest of the muscles of the arm, it lies along the upper medial portion of the arm, appearing as a small rounded ridge. The muscle fibers lie along the axis of the humerus. The origin on the coracoid process is in common with the tendon of the biceps brachii (short head).

Function:
Flexion of arm
Adduction of shoulder

Innervation:
C5-C7 musculocutaneous nerve

Muscles Acting on the Elbow

140 Biceps brachii
141 Brachialis
142 Triceps brachii
143 Brachioradialis
144 Anconeus

140 BICEPS BRACHII

Origin:
Short head
Scapula (apex of coracoid process)
Long head
Capsule of glenohumeral joint and glenoid labrum
Scapula (supraglenoid tubercle at apex of glenoid cavity)

Insertion:
Radius (radial tuberosity on posterior rough surface)
Broad bicipital aponeurosis fusing with deep fascia over forearm flexors

Description:
Long muscle on the anterior surface of the arm consisting of two heads. The tendon of origin of the short head is thick and flat; the tendon of the long head is long and narrow, curving up, over and down the humeral head before giving way to the muscle belly. The muscle fibers of both heads lie fairly parallel to the axis of the humerus. The heads can be readily separated except for the distal portion near the elbow joint, where they join before ending in a flat tendon.
The distal tendon spirals so that its anterior surface becomes lateral at the point of insertion.
Both the short head and the coracobrachialis arise from the coracoid apex. The muscle flexes the elbow most forcefully when the forearm is in supination. It is attached, via the bicipital aponeurosis, to the posterior border of the ulna, the distal end of which is drawn medially in supination.

Function:
Both heads:
Flexion of elbow
Supination of forearm (powerful)
Long head: Stabilizes and depresses humeral head in glenoid fossa during deltoid activity.

Innervation:
C5-C6 musculocutaneous nerve

141 BRACHIALIS

Origin:
Humerus (shaft: distal ½ of anterior surface)
Intermuscular septa (medial ½)

Insertion:
Ulna (ulnar tuberosity and rough surface of coronoid process, anterior aspect)
Anterior ligament of elbow joint
Bicipital aponeurosis (occasionally)

Description:
Positioned over the distal half of the front of the humerus and the anterior aspect of the elbow joint. It may be divided into several parts or may be fused with nearby muscles.
The C7 innervation by the radial nerve is to the lateral part of the muscle and is not large.

Function:
Flexion of elbow, forearm supinated or pronated.

Innervation:
C5-C6 musculocutaneous nerve
C7 radial nerve[23]

142 TRICEPS BRACHII

Has three heads

Origin:
Long head:
Scapula (infraglenoid tuberosity)
Blends above with capsule of glenohumeral joint
Lateral head:
Humerus (shaft: oblique ridge on posterior surface)
Lateral intermuscular septum
Medial head:
Humerus (shaft: entire posterior surface distal to radial groove down almost to trochlea)
Medial and lateral intermuscular septa
Humerus (medial border)

Insertion:
Three heads join in a common tendon
Ulna (olecranon process, proximal posterior surface)
Antebrachial fascia
Capsule of elbow joint

Description:
Located along the entire dorsal aspect of the arm in the extensor compartment. It is a large muscle arising in three heads: long, lateral, and medial. All heads join in a common tendon of insertion, which begins at the midpoint of the muscle. A fourth head is not uncommon.

Function:
Extension of elbow
Long and lateral heads: Especially active in resisted extension, otherwise minimally active[24]
Long head: Extension and adduction of shoulder (assist)
Medial head: Active in all forms of extension

Innervation:
C6-C8 radial nerve (ventral rami)

143 BRACHIORADIALIS

Origin:
Humerus (lateral supracondylar ridge, proximal ⅔)
Lateral intermuscular septum (anterior)

Insertion:
Radius (lateral side of shaft just proximal to styloid process)

Description:
The most superficial muscle on the radial side of the forearm, it forms the lateral side of the cubital fossa. It has a rather thin belly, which descends to the midforearm, where its long flat tendon begins and continues to the distal radius. The brachioradialis often is fused proximally with the brachialis. Its tendon may be divided and the muscle may be absent (rarely).
This is a flexor muscle despite its innervation by an "extensor" nerve.

Function:
Flexion of elbow
Note: This muscle evolved with the extensor muscles and is innervated by the radial nerve, but its action is that of a forearm flexor. Muscle is less active when the forearm is fully supinated because it crosses the joint laterally rather than anteriorly. It works most efficiently when the forearm is in some pronation.

Innervation:
C5-C6 radial nerve (C7 innervation sometimes cited)

144 ANCONEUS

Origin:
Humerus (lateral epicondyle, posterior surface)
Capsule of elbow joint

Insertion:
Ulna (olecranon, lateral aspect, and posterior surface of upper ¼ of shaft)

Description:
A small triangular muscle on the dorsum of the elbow whose fibers descend medially a short distance to their ulnar insertion. Considered a continuation of the triceps and often blended with it.

Function:
Elbow extension (assist)

Innervation:
C6-C8 radial nerve

Muscles Acting on the Forearm

145 Supinator
140 Biceps brachii (see *Muscles Acting on the Elbow*)
146 Pronator teres
147 Pronator quadratus

145 SUPINATOR

Origin:
Humerus (lateral epicondyle)
Radial collateral ligament of elbow joint
Annular ligament of radioulnar joint
Ulna (dorsal surface of shaft, supinator crest)
Aponeurosis of supinator

Insertion:
Radius (tuberosity and oblique line; shaft: lateral surface of proximal ⅓)

Description:
Broad muscle whose fibers form two planes that curve around the upper radius. The two planes arise together from the epicondyle: the superficial plane from the tendon and the deep plane from the muscle fibers. This muscle is subject to considerable variation.

Function:
Supination of forearm

Innervation:
C6-C7 radial nerve (posterior interosseous branch)

146 PRONATOR TERES

Has two heads

Origin:
Humeral head (superficial and larger head):
Shaft proximal to medial epicondyle
Common tendon of origin of forearm flexor muscles
Intermuscular septum
Antebrachial fascia
Ulnar head (deep head):
Coronoid process, medial side
Joins tendon of humeral head

Insertion:
Radius (shaft: lateral surface of middle)

Description:
The humeral head is much larger; the thin ulnar head joins its companion at an acute angle, and together they pass obliquely across the forearm to end in a flat tendon of insertion near the radius. The lateral border of the ulnar head is the medial limit of the cubital fossa, which lies just anterior to the elbow joint. The pronator teres is less active than the pronator quadratus.[25]

Function:
Pronation of forearm
Elbow flexion (accessory)

Innervation:
C6-C7 median nerve

147 PRONATOR QUADRATUS

Origin:
Ulna (shaft: oblique ridge, anterior and medial surfaces of distal ¼)
Aponeurosis over middle ⅓ of the muscle

Insertion:
Radius (shaft: anterior surface of distal ¼; deeper fibers to a narrow triangular area above ulnar notch)

Description:
This small, flat quadrilateral muscle passes across the anterior aspect of the distal ulna to the distal radius. Its fibers are quite horizontal. The pronator quadratus is the main pronator of the forearm, being joined by the pronator teres only in rapid or strong motions.[25]

Function:
Pronation of forearm

Innervation:
C7-C8 median nerve (anterior interosseous branch)

Muscles Acting at the Wrist

148 Extensor carpi radialis longus
149 Extensor carpi radialis brevis
150 Extensor carpi ulnaris
151 Flexor carpi radialis
152 Palmaris longus
153 Flexor carpi ulnaris

148 EXTENSOR CARPI RADIALIS LONGUS

Origin:
Humerus (distal ⅓ of lateral supracondylar ridge)
Lateral intermuscular septum
Common extensor tendon

Insertion:
2nd metacarpal (dorsal surface of base on radial side). Occasionally slips to 1st and 3rd metacarpals.

Description:
Descends lateral to brachioradialis. Muscle fibers end at midforearm in a flat tendon, which descends along the lateral radius.

Function:
Extension and radial deviation of wrist
Synergist for finger flexion by stabilization of wrist
Elbow flexion (accessory)

Innervation:
C6-C7 radial nerve (lateral muscular branch)

149 EXTENSOR CARPI RADIALIS BREVIS

Origin:
Humerus (lateral epicondyle via common extensor tendon)
Radial collateral ligament of elbow joint
Aponeurotic sheath and intermuscular septa

Insertion:
3rd metacarpal (dorsal surface of base on radial side distal to styloid process)
Slips sent to 2nd metacarpal base

Description:
This short, thick muscle lies partially under the extensor carpi radialis longus in the upper forearm. Its muscle fibers end well above the wrist in a flattened tendon, which descends alongside the extensor carpi radialis longus tendon to the wrist.

Function:
Extension of wrist
Radial deviation of wrist (weak)
Finger flexion synergist (by stabilizing the wrist)

Innervation:
C7-C8 radial nerve (posterior interosseous branch)

150 EXTENSOR CARPI ULNARIS

Origin:
Humerus (lateral epicondyle via common extensor tendon)
Ulna (posterior border by an aponeurosis common to flexor carpi ulnaris and flexor digitorum profundus)
Overlying fascia

Insertion:
5th metacarpal (tubercle on ulnar side of base)

Description:
Muscle fibers descend on the dorsal ulnar side of the forearm and join a tendon located in the distal ⅓ of the forearm that is the most medial tendon on the dorsum of the hand. This tendon can be palpated lateral to the groove found just over the ulna's posterior border.

Function:
Extension of wrist
Ulnar deviation (adduction) of wrist

Innervation:
C7-C8 radial nerve (posterior interosseous branch)

151 FLEXOR CARPI RADIALIS

Origin:
Humerus (medial epicondyle by common flexor tendon)
Intermuscular septa
Antebrachial fascia

Insertion:
2nd and 3rd metacarpals (base, palmar surface)

Description:
A slender aponeurotic muscle at its origin, it descends in the forearm between the pronator teres and the palmaris longus. It increases in size as it descends to end in a tendon about halfway down the forearm.

Function:
Flexion of wrist
Radial deviation (abduction) of wrist
Extends fingers (tenodesis action)
Flexion of elbow (weak assist)
Pronation of forearm (weak assist)

Innervation:
C6-C7 median nerve

152 PALMARIS LONGUS

Origin:
Humerus (medial epicondyle via common flexor tendon)
Intermuscular septa and deep fascia

Insertion:
Flexor retinaculum
Palmar aponeurosis
Slip sent frequently to the short thumb muscles

Description:
A slim fusiform muscle, it ends in a long tendon midway in the forearm. Muscle is quite variable and frequently is absent.

Function:
Tension of palmar fascia (anchor for palmar fascia and skin)
Flexion of wrist (weak or questionable)
Flexion of elbow (weak or questionable)
Abduction of thumb

Innervation:
C7-C8 median nerve

153 FLEXOR CARPI ULNARIS

Has two heads

Origin:
Humeral head:
Humerus (medial epicondyle via common flexor tendon)
Ulnar head:
Ulna (olecranon, medial border and shaft: upper ⅔ of posterior border via an aponeurosis)
Intermuscular septum

Insertion:
Pisiform bone
Hamate bone
5th metacarpal (occasionally 4th)
Flexor retinaculum

Description:
This is the most ulnar-lying of the flexors in the forearm. The humeral head is small in contrast to the extensive origin of the ulnar head. The two heads are connected by a tendinous arch under which the ulnar nerve descends. The muscle fibers end in a tendon that forms along the anterolateral border of the muscle's distal half.

Function:
Flexion of wrist
Ulnar deviation (adduction) of wrist
Flexion of elbow (assist)

Innervation:
C7-T1 ulnar nerve

Muscles Acting on the Fingers (Figure 11-5 and Figure 11-6)

154 Extensor digitorum
155 Extensor indicis
156 Flexor digitorum superficialis
157 Flexor digitorum profundus

154 EXTENSOR DIGITORUM

Origin:
Humerus (lateral epicondyle via common extensor tendon)

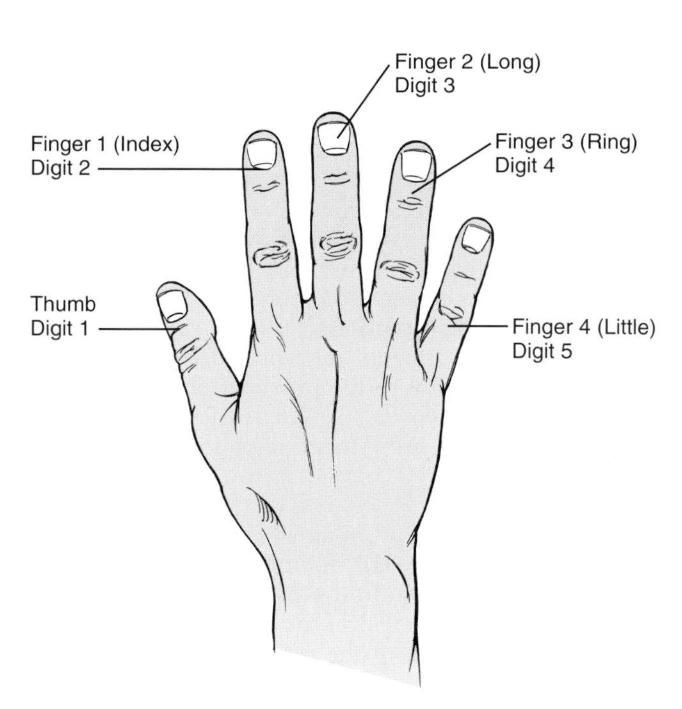

FIGURE 11-5 Fingers and digits of the hand.

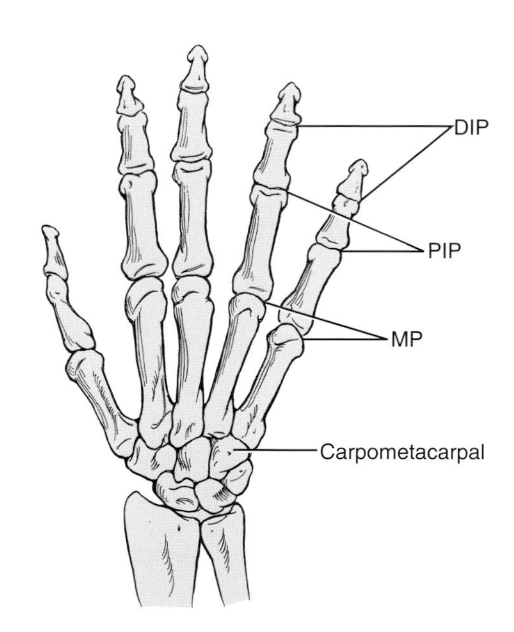

FIGURE 11-6 The bones and joints of the hand.

Intermuscular septa
Antebrachial fascia

Insertion:
Digits 2 to 5: Divides distally into four tendons that insert into the digital expansion over the proximal and middle phalanges.
Intermediate slips: To middle phalanges
Lateral slips: Distal phalanges (dorsum of base of digits 2 to 5)

Description:
The extensor digitorum is the only extensor of the metacarpophalangeal (MP) joints. The muscle divides above the wrist into four distinct tendons, which traverse (with the extensor indicis) a tunnel under the extensor retinaculum in a common sheath. Over the dorsum of the hand the four tendons diverge, one to each finger. The tendon to the index finger is accompanied by the extensor indicis tendon.
The digital attachments are achieved by a fibrous expansion dorsal to the proximal phalanges. All of the digital extensors, as well as the lumbricales and interossei, are integral to this mechanism.

Function:
Extension of MP and proximal (PIP) and distal interphalangeal (DIP) joints, digits 2 to 5.
Extensor digitorum can extend any and all joints over which it passes via the dorsal expansion
Independent action of the extensor digitorum:
Hyperextends MP joint (proximal phalanges) by displacing dorsal expansion proximally
Extends IP joints (middle and distal phalanges) when MP joints are slightly flexed by intrinsics
Wrist extension (accessory)
Abduction of ring, index, and little fingers with extension but no such action on the middle finger

Innervation:
C7-C8 radial nerve, posterior interosseous branch

155 EXTENSOR INDICIS

Origin:
Ulna (posterior surface of shaft below origin of extensor pollicis longus)
Interosseous membrane

Insertion:
Index finger (2nd digit) (extensor hood)

Description:
Arises just below the extensor pollicis longus and travels adjacent with it down to the level of the wrist. After passing under the extensor retinaculum near the head of the 2nd metacarpal, it joins with the index tendon of the extensor digitorum on its ulnar side and then inserts into the extensor hood of the 2nd digit.

Function:
Extension of MP joint of index finger
Extension of IP joints (with intrinsics)
Adduction of index finger (accessory)
Wrist extension (accessory)

Innervation:
C7-C8 radial nerve, posterior interosseous branch

156 FLEXOR DIGITORUM SUPERFICIALIS

Has two heads

Origin:
Humeral-ulnar head:
Humerus (medial epicondyle via the common flexor tendon)
Ulnar collateral ligament of elbow joint
Ulna (coronoid process, medial side)
Intermuscular septa
Radial head:
Radius (oblique line on anterior surface of shaft)

Insertion:
From four tendons arranged in two pairs:
Superficial pair: Long and ring fingers (sides of middle phalanges)
Deep pair: Index and little fingers (sides of middle phalanges)

Description:
Lies deep to the other forearm flexors but is the largest superficial flexor. The muscle separates into two planes of fibers, superficial and deep. The superficial plane (joined by radial head) divides into two tendons for digits 3 and 5. The deep plane fibers divide and join the tendons to digits 2 and 5. This can be remembered by touching the tips of the little and index fingers (deep) together underneath the ring and middle fingers (superficial).
The four tendons sweep under the flexor retinaculum arranged in pairs (for the long and ring fingers, and for the index and little fingers). The tendons diverge again in the palm, and at the base of the proximal phalanges each divides into two slips to permit passage of the flexor digitorum profundus to each finger. The slips reunite and then divide again for a final time to insert on both sides of each middle phalanx.
The radial head may be absent.

Function:
Flexion of PIP joints of digits 2 to 5
Flexion of MP joints of digits 2 to 5 (assist)
Flexion of wrist (accessory, especially in forceful grasp)

Innervation:
C8-T1 median nerve

157 FLEXOR DIGITORUM PROFUNDUS

Origin:
Ulna (shaft: upper ¾ of anterior and medial surfaces; also coronoid process, medial side via an aponeurosis)
Interosseous membrane (ulnar half)

Insertion:
Ends in four tendons:
Digits 2 to 5 (distal phalanges, palmar surface and base). Index finger tendon is distinct in its course.

Description:
Lying deep to the superficial flexors, the profundus is located on the ulnar side of the forearm. The muscle fibers end in four tendons below the midforearm; the tendons pass into the hand under the transverse carpal ligament. The tendon for the index finger remains distinct, but the tendons for the other fingers are intertwined and connected to tendinous slips down into the palm.
After passing through the tendons of the flexor digitorum superficialis they move to their insertions on each distal phalanx. The four lumbrical muscles arise from the profundus tendons in the palm.
The profundus, like the superficialis, can flex any or all joints over which it passes, but it is the only muscle that can flex the DIP joints.

Function:
Flexion of DIP joints of digits 2 to 5
Flexion of MP and PIP joints of digits 2 to 5 (assist)
Flexion of wrist (accessory)

Innervation:
C8-T1 median nerve (anterior interosseous nerve) for digits 2 and 3
C8-T1 ulnar nerve for digits 4 and 5

Muscles Acting on the Little Finger (and Hypothenar Muscles)

158 Extensor digiti minimi
159 Abductor digiti minimi
160 Flexor digiti minimi brevis
161 Opponens digiti minimi
162 Palmaris brevis

158 EXTENSOR DIGITI MINIMI

Origin:
Common extensor tendon
Intermuscular septa
Antebrachial fascia

Insertion:
Digit 5 via extensor hood on the radial side, as a separate long tendon to the little finger. From its origin in the forearm the long tendon passes under the extensor retinaculum at the wrist. The tendon divides into two slips: one joining the extensor digitorum to the 5th digit. All three tendons then join the extensor hood, which covers the dorsum of the proximal phalanx.

Description:
A slim extensor muscle that lies medial to the extensor digitorum and usually is associated with that muscle. It descends in the forearm (between the extensor digitorum and the extensor carpi ulnaris), passes under the extensor retinaculum at the wrist in its own compartment, and then divides into two tendons. The lateral tendon joins directly with the tendon of the extensor digitorum; all three join the extensor expansion, and all insert on the middle phalanx of digit 5. The extensor digiti minimi can extend any of the joints of digit 5 via the dorsal digital expansion.

Function:
Extension of MP, IP, and DIP joints of digit 5 (little finger)
Wrist extension (accessory)
Abduction of digit 5 (accessory)

Innervation:
C7-C8 radial nerve (posterior interosseous branch)

159 ABDUCTOR DIGITI MINIMI

Origin:
Pisiform bone (often passes a slip to 5th metacarpal)
Tendon of flexor carpi ulnaris
Pisohamate ligament

Insertion:
5th digit (proximal phalanx, base on ulnar side)
Into dorsal digital expansion of extensor digiti minimi

Description:
Located on the ulnar border of the palm

Function:
Abduction of 5th digit away from ring finger
Flexion of proximal phalanx of 5th digit at the MP joint
Opposition of 5th digit (assist)

Innervation:
C8-T1 ulnar nerve (deep branch)

160 FLEXOR DIGITI MINIMI BREVIS

Origin:
Hamate bone (hamulus or “hook”)
Flexor retinaculum (palmar surface along with abductor digiti minimi)

Insertion:
5th digit (proximal phalanx, base on ulnar side along with abductor digiti minimi)

Description:
This short flexor of the little finger lies in the same plane as the abductor digiti minimi on its radial side. The muscle may be absent or fused with the abductor.

Function:
Flexion of little finger at the MP joint
Opposition of 5th digit (assist)

Innervation:
C8-T1 ulnar nerve (deep branch)

161 OPPONENS DIGITI MINIMI

Origin:
Hamate (hamulus, often called "hook")
Flexor retinaculum

Insertion:
5th metacarpal (entire length of ulnar margin)

Description:
A triangular muscle lying deep to the abductor and the flexor. It commonly is blended with its neighbors.

Function:
Opposition of little finger to thumb (abduction, flexion, and lateral rotation, deepening the palmar hollow)

Innervation:
C8-T1 ulnar nerve (deep branch)

162 PALMARIS BREVIS

Origin:
Flexor retinaculum and palmar aponeurosis

Insertion:
Skin on ulnar border of palm (hypothenar eminence)

Description:
A thin superficial muscle whose fibers run directly laterally across the hypothenar eminence

Function:
Draws the skin of the ulnar side of the hand toward the palm. This deepens the hollow of the hand and seems to increase the height of the hypothenar eminence, possibly assisting in grasp.

Innervation:
C8-T1 ulnar nerve (superficial branch)

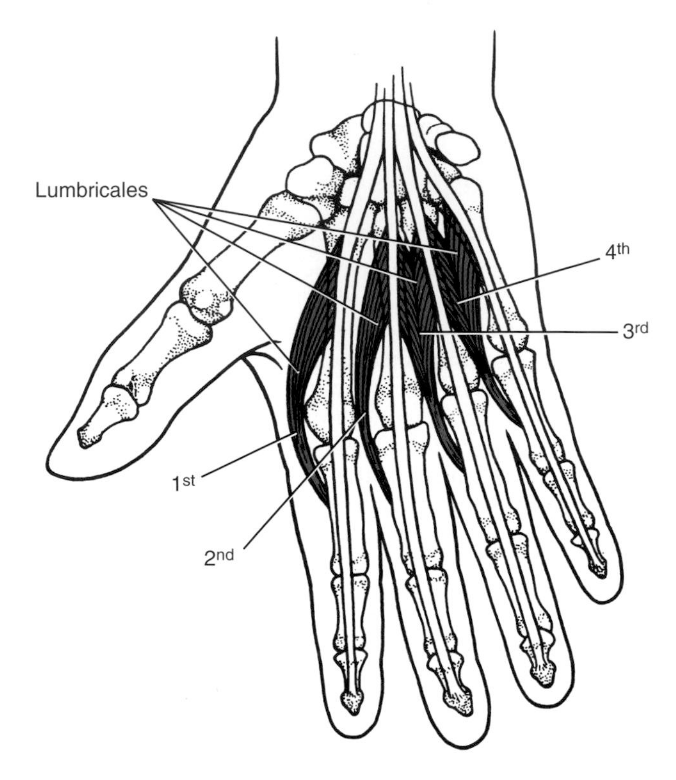

FIGURE 11-7 The lumbricales, palmar view.

Intrinsic Muscles of the Hand

163 Lumbricales
164 Interossei, dorsal
165 Interossei, palmar

163 LUMBRICALES (Figure 11-7)

Origin:
Flexor digitorum profundus tendons:
1st Lumbrical: Index finger (digit 2) arises by single head from the radial side, palmar surface
2nd Lumbrical: Long (middle) finger (digit 3), radial side, palmar surface
3rd Lumbrical: Long and ring fingers (digits 3 and 4) by double heads from adjacent sides of tendons of flexor digitorum profundus
4th Lumbrical: Ring and little fingers (digits 4 and 5), adjacent sides of tendon

Insertion:
Extensor digitorum expansion:
Each muscle extends distally to the radial side of its corresponding digit and attaches to the dorsal digital expansion:
1st Lumbrical: To index finger (digit 2)
2nd Lumbrical: To long (middle) finger (digit 3)
3rd Lumbrical: To ring finger (digit 4)
4th Lumbrical: To little finger (digit 5)

Description:
These four small muscles arise from the tendon of the flexor digitorum profundus over the metacarpals. They may be unipennate or bipennate. They extend to the middle phalanges of digits 2 to 5 (fingers 1 to 4), where they join the dorsal extensor hood on the radial side of each digit (see Figure 11-7). Essentially, they link the flexor to the extension tendon systems in the hand. The exact attachments are quite variable. This gives rise to complexity of movement and differences in description.[26]

Function:
Flexion of MP joints (proximal phalanges) of digits 2 to 5 and simultaneous extension of the PIP and DIP joints
Opposition of digit 5 (4th lumbrical)

Innervation:
1st and 2nd Lumbricales: C8-T1 median nerve
3rd and 4th Lumbricales: C8-T1 ulnar nerve
Note: The 3rd lumbrical may receive innervation from both the ulnar and median nerves or all from the median.

164 DORSAL INTEROSSEI (Figure 11-8)

These are four bipennate muscles

Origin:
Each muscle arises by two heads from adjacent sides of the metacarpals between which each lies.

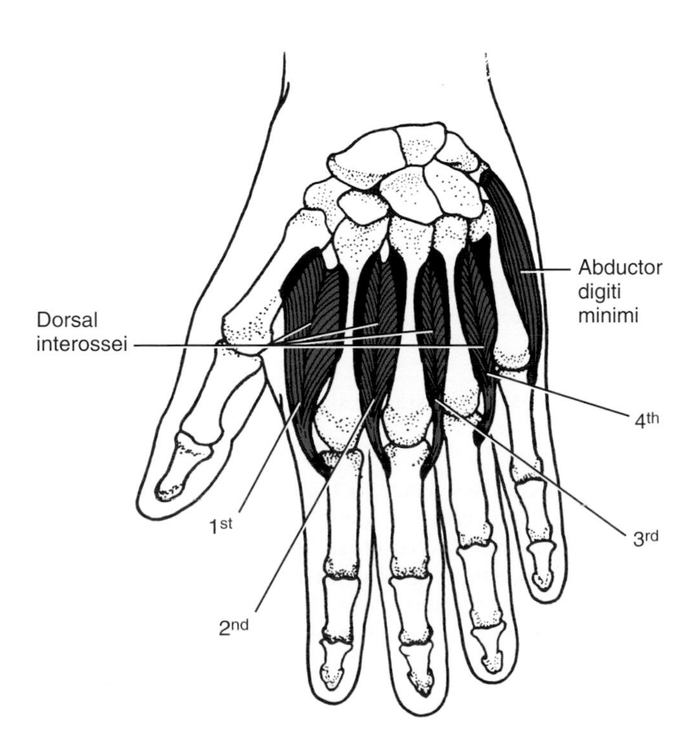

FIGURE 11-8 The dorsal interossei.

1st Dorsal: (also called abductor indicis): Between thumb and index fingers
2nd Dorsal: Between index and long fingers
3rd Dorsal: Between long and ring fingers
4th Dorsal: Between ring and little fingers

Insertion:
All: Dorsal extensor expansion.
Proximal phalanges (bases)
1st Dorsal: Index finger (radial side)
2nd Dorsal: Long finger (radial side)
3rd Dorsal: Long finger (ulnar side)
4th Dorsal: Ring finger (ulnar side)

Description:
This group comprises four bipennate muscles (see Figure 11-8). In general, they originate via two heads from the adjacent metacarpal but more so from the metacarpal of the digit where they will insert distally. They insert into the bases of the proximal phalanges and dorsal expansions.

Function:
Abduction of fingers away from an axis drawn through the center of the long (middle) finger
Flexion of fingers at MP joints (assist)
Extension of fingers at IP joints (assist)
Thumb adduction (assist)

Innervation:
C8-T1 ulnar nerve (deep branch)

165 PALMAR (VOLAR) INTEROSSEI

There are three palmar interossei muscles (a 4th muscle is described) (Figure 11-9).

Origin:
Metacarpal bones 2, 4, and 5. These muscles lie on the palmar surface of the metacarpals rather than between them. There is no palmar interosseous on the long finger.
1st Palmar: 2nd metacarpal (ulnar side)
2nd Palmar: 4th metacarpal (radial side)
3rd Palmar: 5th metacarpal (radial side)

Insertion:
All: Dorsal expansion
Proximal phalanges
1st Palmar: Index finger (ulnar side)
2nd Palmar: Ring finger (radial side)
3rd Palmar: Little finger (radial side)

Description:
The palmar interossei are smaller than their dorsal counterparts. They are found on the palmar surface of the hand at the metacarpal bones. There are three very distinct volar interossei

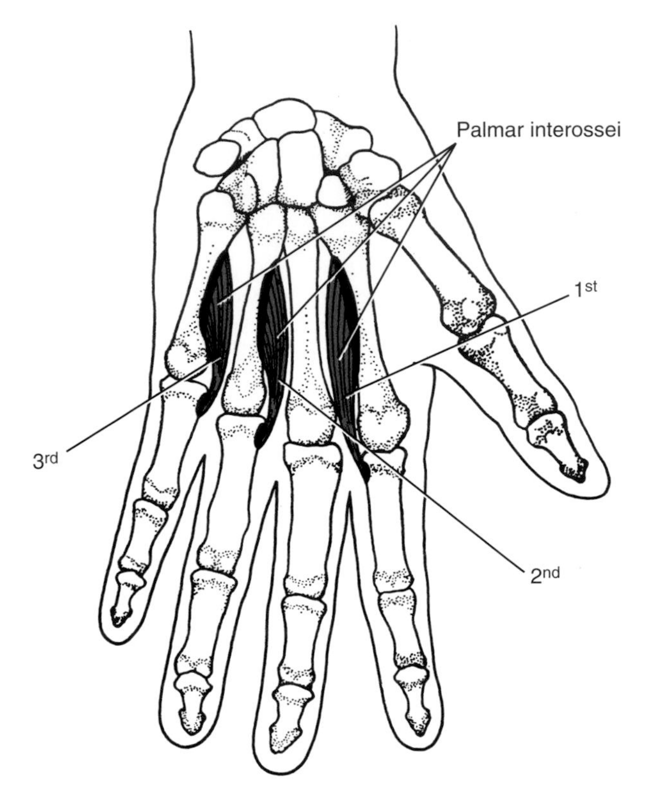

FIGURE 11-9 The palmar (volar) interossei.

(see Figure 11-9), and some authors describe a 4th interosseus, to which they give the number 1 for its attachment on the thumb. When this is found as a discrete muscle, the other palmar interossei become numbers 2, 3, and 4, respectively. When the thumb interosseus exists it is on the ulnar side of the metacarpal and proximal phalanx. Some authors (including us) consider the interosseus of the thumb part of the adductor pollicis.

The middle finger has no interosseous muscle.

Function:
Adduction of fingers (index, ring, and little) toward an axis drawn through the center of the long finger
Flexion of MP joints (assist)
Extension of IP joints (assist)
Opposition of digit 5 (3rd interosseus)

Innervation:
C8-T1 ulnar nerve (deep branch)

Muscles Acting on the Thumb

166 Abductor pollicis longus
167 Extensor pollicis longus
168 Extensor pollicis brevis
169 Flexor pollicis longus
171 Abductor pollicis brevis
172 Opponens pollicis
170 Flexor pollicis brevis
173 Adductor pollicis

166 ABDUCTOR POLLICIS LONGUS

Origin:
Ulna (posterior surface of shaft)
Radius (middle ⅓ of posterior surface of shaft)
Interosseous membrane

Insertion:
1st metacarpal bone (radial side of base)
Trapezium bone

Description:
Lies immediately below the supinator and sometimes is fused with that muscle. Traverses obliquely down and lateral to end in a tendon at the wrist. The tendon passes through a groove on the lateral side of the distal radius along with the tendon of the extensor pollicis brevis. Its tendon is commonly split; one slip attaches to the radial side of the 1st metacarpal and the other to the trapezium.[27]

Function:
Abduction and extension of thumb at carpometacarpal (CMC) joint
Extension of thumb at CMC joint (in concert with thumb extensors)
Radial deviation of wrist (assist)
Wrist flexion (weak)

Innervation:
C7-C8 radial nerve (posterior interosseous branch)

167 EXTENSOR POLLICIS LONGUS

Origin:
Ulna (posterolateral surface of middle shaft)
Interosseous membrane

Insertion:
Thumb (base of distal phalanx, dorsal side)

Description:
The muscle rises distal to the abductor pollicis longus and courses down and lateral into a tendon over the distal radius, which lies in a narrow oblique groove on the dorsal radius. It descends obliquely over the tendons of the carpal extensors. It separates from the extensor pollicis brevis and can be seen during thumb extension as the ulnar margin of a triangular depression called the *anatomical snuff box*. This is a larger muscle than the extensor pollicis brevis.

Function:
Extension of the thumb at all joints:
Distal phalanx (alone)
MP and CMC joints (along with extensor pollicis brevis and abductor pollicis longus)
Radial deviation of wrist (accessory)

Innervation:
C7-C8 radial nerve (posterior interosseous branch)

168 EXTENSOR POLLICIS BREVIS

Origin:
Radius (posterior surface of shaft)
Interosseous membrane

Insertion:
Thumb (proximal phalanx base on dorsal surface)
Attachment to distal phalanx via tendon of extensor pollicis longus is common.[27]

Description:
Arises distal and lies medial to the abductor pollicis longus and descends with it so that the tendons of the two muscles pass through the same groove on the lateral side of the distal radius. During its descent it wraps itself around a bony fulcrum (Lister's tubercle), which alters the line of pull from forearm to thumb.
The muscle often is connected with the abductor or may be absent. Its tendon forms the radial margin of the "snuff box."

Function:
Extension of MP joint of thumb
Extension and abduction of 1st CMC joint of thumb
Radial deviation of wrist (accessory)

Innervation:
C7-C8 radial nerve (posterior interosseous branch)

169 FLEXOR POLLICIS LONGUS

Origin:
Radius (grooved anterior surface of middle of shaft)
Interosseous membrane
Ulna (coronoid process), variable
Humerus (medial epicondyle), variable[28]

Insertion:
Thumb (base of distal phalanx, palmar surface)

Description:
Descends on the radial side of the forearm in the same plane as, but lateral to, the flexor digitorum profundus

Function:
Flexion of IP joint of thumb
Flexion of the MP and CMC joints of thumb (accessory)
Flexion of wrist (accessory)

Innervation:
C7-C8 median nerve (anterior interosseous branch)

170 FLEXOR POLLICIS BREVIS

Has two heads

Origin:
Superficial head:
Flexor retinaculum (distal border)
Trapezium bone (tubercle)
Deep head:
Trapezoid bone
Capitate bone
Palmar ligaments of distal row of carpal bones

Insertion:
Pollex (both heads: proximal phalanx, base on radial side)

Description:
The superficial head runs more laterally and accompanies the flexor pollicis longus. Its tendon of insertion contains the radial sesamoid bone at a point where it unites with the tendon of the deep head. The deep head is sometimes absent. Of the thenar muscles, only the abductor pollicis brevis consistently joins the dorsal extensor expansion of the thumb.

Function:
Flexion of the MP and CMC joints of the thumb
Opposition of thumb (assist)

Innervation:
Superficial head: C8-T1 median nerve (lateral branch)
Deep head: C8-T1 ulnar nerve (deep branch)

171 ABDUCTOR POLLICIS BREVIS

Origin:
Flexor retinaculum
Scaphoid bone (tubercle)
Trapezium bone (tubercle)
Tendon of abductor pollicis longus

Insertion:
Thumb (proximal phalanx, radial side of base)
Dorsal extensor expansion of thumb

Description:
The most superficial muscle on the radial side of the thenar eminence

Function:
Abduction at CMC and MP joints (in a plane 90° from the palm)
Opposition of thumb (assist)
Extension of IP joint (assist)

Innervation:
C8-T1 median nerve

172 OPPONENS POLLICIS

Origin:
Trapezium bone (tubercle)
Flexor retinaculum

Insertion:
1st metacarpal bone (along entire length of radial [lateral] side of shaft)

Description:
A small triangular muscle lying deep to the abductor

Function:
Flexion of CMC joint medially across the palm
Abduction of CMC joint
Medial rotation of CMC joint
These motions occur simultaneously in the motion called opposition, which brings the thumb into contact with any of the other fingers on their palmar digital aspect (pads)

Innervation:
C8-T1 median nerve
C8-T1 ulnar nerve[29-31] (terminal branch)

173 ADDUCTOR POLLICIS

Rises from two heads

Origin:
Oblique head:
Capitate bone
2nd and 3rd metacarpal bones (bases)
Palmar carpal ligaments
Tendon sheath of flexor carpi radialis
Flexor retinaculum (small slip)
Unites with tendon of transverse head
Transverse head:
3rd metacarpal bone (distal ⅔ of palmar surface)
Converges with oblique head and with 1st palmar interosseous

Insertion (both heads):
Thumb (base, proximal phalanx on ulnar side)
Extensor retinaculum (on its medial side) of the thumb

Description:
The muscle lies deep on the palmar side of the hand and has two heads, which vary in their comparative sizes. Both heads arise from the 3rd metacarpal and insert into both sides of the proximal phalanx,[7] or, as more frequently cited, the medial side of the proximal phalanx. The two heads are divided by the radial artery and the extent of their convergence also is variable.

Function:
Adduction of CMC joint of thumb (approximates the thumb to the palm)
Adduction and flexion of MP joint (assist)

Innervation:
C8-T1 ulnar nerve (deep branch)

MUSCLES OF THE LOWER EXTREMITY
(Knee, Ankle, Toes, Hallux)

Muscles of the Hip

174 Psoas major
175 Psoas minor
176 Iliacus
177 Pectineus
178 Gracilis
179 Adductor longus
180 Adductor brevis
181 Adductor magnus
182 Gluteus maximus
183 Gluteus medius
184 Gluteus minimus
185 Tensor fasciae latae
186 Piriformis
187 Obturator internus
188 Obturator externus
189 Gemellus superior
190 Gemellus inferior
191 Quadratus femoris
192 Biceps femoris (long head and short heads)
193 Semitendinosus
194 Semimembranosus
195 Sartorius

174 PSOAS MAJOR

Origin:
L1-L5 vertebrae (transverse processes, inferior border)
T12-L5 vertebral bodies and intervertebral discs between them (by five digitations)
Tendinous arches across the lumbar vertebral bodies

Insertion:
Femur (lesser trochanter)

Description:
A long muscle lying next to the lumbar spine, its fibers descend downward and laterally. It decreases in size as it descends along the pelvic brim. It passes anterior to the hip joint and joins in a tendon with the iliacus to insert on the lesser trochanter.
The iliopsoas muscle is a compound muscle consisting of the iliacus and the psoas major, which join in a common tendon of insertion on the lesser trochanter of the femur.
The roots from the lumbar plexus enter the muscle directly and are contained within the muscle; the root branches move out and away from its borders.

Function:
Hip flexion with origin fixed[32]
Trunk flexion (sit-up) with insertion fixed
(These two functions occur in conjunction with the iliacus)
Hip external (lateral) rotation
Flexion of lumbar spine (muscles on both sides)
Lateral bending of lumbar spine to same side (muscle on one side)

Innervation:
L2-L4 (lumbar plexus) spinal nerves (ventral rami)
L1 also cited

175 PSOAS MINOR

Origin:
T12-L1 vertebral bodies (sides) and the intervertebral disc between them

Insertion:
Pecten pubis (i.e., pectineal line)
Ilium (iliopectineal eminence and linea terminalis of inner surface of the pelvis)
Iliac fascia

Description:
Lying anterior to the psoas major, this is a long thin muscle whose belly lies entirely within the abdomen along its posterior wall, but its long flat tendon descends to the ilium. The muscle frequently is absent.
The pecten pubis, or pectineal line, is the distal end of the iliopectineal line, which in turn is a segment of the linea terminalis. These three segments together form the anterior part of the pelvic brim.

Function:
Flexion of trunk and lumbar spine

Innervation:
L1 spinal nerve

176 ILIACUS

Origin:
Ilium (superior ⅔ of iliac fossa)
Iliac crest (inner lip)
Anterior sacroiliac and iliolumbar ligaments
Sacrum (lateral)

Insertion:
Femur (lesser trochanter via insertion on tendon of the psoas major and shaft below lesser trochanter)

Description:
A broad flat muscle, it fills the iliac fossa and descends along the fossa, converging laterally with the tendon of the psoas major. The iliacus, acting alone in contraction on a fixed femur, results in flexion of the pelvis on the femur (an anterior tilt termed "symphysis down") of the pelvis. This leads to increased lumbar extension (lordosis).

Function:
Hip flexion
Flexes pelvis on femur

Innervation:
L2-L3 femoral nerve

177 PECTINEUS

Origin:
Pecten pubis (between iliopectineal eminence and pubic tubercle)
Anterior fascia

Insertion:
Femur (shaft: on a line from lesser trochanter to linea aspera)

Description:
A flat muscle forming part of the wall of the femoral triangle in the upper medial aspect of the thigh. It descends posteriorly and laterally on the medial thigh.

Function:
Hip adduction
Hip flexion (accessory)

Innervation:
L2-L3 femoral nerve
L3 accessory obturator nerve (when present)

178 GRACILIS

Origin:
Pubis (inferior ramus near symphysis via aponeurosis)
Ischial ramus

Insertion:
Tibia (medial surface of shaft below tibial condyle)
Pes anserina
Deep fascia of leg

Description:
Lies most superficially on the medial thigh as a thin and broad muscle that tapers and narrows distally. The fibers are directed vertically and join a tendon that curves around the medial condyle of the femur and then around the medial condyle of the tibia. Its tendon is one of three (along with those of the sartorius and semitendinosus) that unite to form the pes anserinus.

Function:
Hip adduction
Knee flexion
Internal (medial) rotation of knee (accessory)

Innervation:
L2-L3 obturator nerve (anterior division) (ventral rami)

179 ADDUCTOR LONGUS

Origin:
Pubis (anterior at the angle where the crest meets the symphysis)

Insertion:
Femur (by an aponeurosis on the middle ⅓ of the linea aspera on its medial lip)

Description:
The most anterior of the adductor muscles arises in a narrow tendon and widens into a broad muscle belly as it descends backward and laterally to insert on the femur.
As part of their function, the hip adductors are not frequently called upon for strenuous activity, but they are capable of such. They play a major synergistic role in the complexity of gait and in some postural activities, but are relatively quiescent in quiet standing.

Function:
Hip adduction
Hip flexion (accessory)
Hip rotation (depends on position of thigh)[29]
Hip external (lateral) rotation (when hip is in extension; accessory)

Innervation:
L2 or L3-L4 obturator nerve (anterior division)

180 ADDUCTOR BREVIS

Origin:
Pubis (inferior ramus and body, external aspect)

Insertion:
Femur (along a line from the lesser trochanter to the proximal ⅓ of medial lip of the linea aspera via an aponeurosis)

Description:
The muscle lies under the pectineus and adductor longus with its fibers coursing laterally and posteriorly as it broadens and descends.

Function:
Hip adduction
Hip flexion

Innervation:
L2-L3 or L4 obturator nerve (posterior division)

181 ADDUCTOR MAGNUS

Origin:
Pubis (inferior ramus)
Ischium (inferior ramus; ischial tuberosity, inferior and lateral aspect)

Insertion:
Femur (whole length of linea aspera and medial supracondylar line by an aponeurosis; adductor tubercle on medial condyle via a rounded tendon; the rounded tendon attaches to the medial supracondylar line by a fibrous expansion)

Description:
The largest of the adductor group, this muscle is located on the medial thigh and appears as three distinct bundles. The superior fibers from the pubic ramus are short and horizontal. The medial fibers move down and laterally. The most distal bundle descends almost vertically to a tendon on the distal ⅓ of the thigh.
Occasionally the fibers that arise from the ramus of the pubis are inserted into a line from the greater trochanter to the linea aspera and seem to form a distinct separate muscle. When this occurs the muscle is called the adductor minimis.

The innervation of the adductor magnus comes from the anterior divisions of the lumbar plexus suggesting a primitive flexor action for the muscle.

Function:
Hip adduction
Hip extension (inferior fibers)
Hip flexion (superior fibers; weak)
The role of the adductor magnus in rotation of the hip is dependent on the position of the thigh.[33]

Innervation:
Superior and middle fibers: L2-L4 obturator nerve (posterior division)
Inferior fibers: L2-L4 sciatic nerve (tibial division)

182 GLUTEUS MAXIMUS

Origin:
Ilium (posterior gluteal line and crest)
Sacrum (dorsal surface)
Coccyx (lateral surface)
Erector spinae aponeurosis
Sacrotuberous ligament
Aponeurosis of gluteus medius

Insertion:
Iliotibial tract of fascia lata
Femur (gluteal tuberosity)

Description:
The maximus is the largest and most superficial of the gluteal muscles, forming the prominence of the buttocks. The fibers descend laterally, inserting widely on the thick tendinous iliotibial tract.

Function:
Hip extension (powerful)
Hip external (lateral) rotation
Hip abduction (upper fibers)
Hip adduction (lower fibers)
Through its insertion into the iliotibial band it stabilizes the knee

Innervation:
L5-S2 inferior gluteal nerve

183 GLUTEUS MEDIUS

Origin:
Ilium (outer surface between the iliac crest and the posterior gluteal line)
Gluteal aponeurosis

Insertion:
Femur (greater trochanter, oblique ridge on lateral surface)

Description:
The posterior fibers of the medius lie deep to the maximus; its anterior ⅔ is covered by fascia (gluteal aponeurosis). It lies on the outer surface of the pelvis.
The gluteus medius helps to maintain erect posture in walking. During single-limb stance when the swing limb is raised from the ground, all body weight is placed on the opposite (stance) limb, which should result in a noted sagging of the pelvis of the swing limb. The action of the gluteus medius on the stance limb prevents such a tilt or sag. When the gluteus medius is weak, the trunk tilts (lateral lean) to the weak side with each step in an attempt to maintain balance (this is the deliberate compensation for the positive Trendelenburg sign). It is called a *Gluteus medius sign* or gait.
The uncompensated positive Trendelenburg results in a pelvic drop of the contralateral side. This is the so-called Trendelenburg gait.

Function:
Hip abduction (in all positions)
Hip internal rotation (anterior fibers)
Hip external (lateral) rotation (posterior fibers)
Hip flexion (anterior fibers) and hip extension (posterior fibers) as accessory functions

Innervation:
L4-S1 superior gluteal nerve (inferior branch)

184 GLUTEUS MINIMUS

Origin:
Ilium (outer surface between the anterior and inferior gluteal lines; also from margin of the greater sciatic notch).

Insertion:
Femur (greater trochanter, anterior border)
Expansion to capsule of hip joint

Description:
The minimus is the smallest of the gluteal muscles and lies immediately under the medius. Its fibers pass obliquely lateral and down, forming a fan-shaped muscle that converges on the great femoral trochanter.

Function:
Hip abduction
Hip internal (medial) rotation

Innervation:
L4-S1 superior gluteal nerve (superior branch)

185 TENSOR FASCIAE LATAE

Origin:
Ilium (iliac crest; anterior part of outer lip; anterior superior iliac spine [ASIS])
Fascia lata (deep surface)

Insertion:
Iliotibial tract (both layers)

Description:
The tensor descends between and is attached to the deep and superficial layers of the iliotibial band.
The smallish muscle belly is highly variable in length. The muscle lies superficially on the border between the anterior and lateral thigh. Functions at the knee that have been attributed to the tensor could not be confirmed in EMG studies; indeed, there was no electrical activity in the tensor during knee motions.[34-36]

Function:
Hip flexion
Hip internal (medial) rotation
Knee flexion (accessory via iliotibial band) once the knee is flexed beyond 30° (no confirmation)
Knee extension with external rotation (no confirmation)
Knee external (lateral) rotation (assist) (no confirmation)

Innervation:
L4-S1 superior gluteal nerve (inferior branch)

186 PIRIFORMIS

Origin:
Sacrum (via three digitations attached between the 1st and 4th anterior sacral foramina)
Ilium (gluteal surface near posterior inferior iliac spine
Capsule of sacroiliac joint
Sacrotuberous ligament (pelvic surface)

Insertion:
Femur (greater trochanter, superior border of medial aspect)

Description:
Runs parallel to the posterior margin of the gluteus medius posterior to the hip joint. It lies against the posterior wall on the interior of the pelvis. The broad muscle belly narrows to exit through the greater sciatic foramen and converge on the greater trochanter. The insertion tendon often is partly blended with the common tendon of the obturator internus and gemelli.

Function:
Hip external (lateral) rotation
Abducts the flexed hip (assist) (muscle probably too small to do much of this)

Innervation:
S1-S2 spinal nerves (nerve to piriformis)

187 OBTURATOR INTERNUS

Origin:
Pelvis (obturator foramen, around most of its margin; from pelvic brim to greater sciatic foramen above and obturator foramen below)
Ischium (ramus)
Pubis (inferior ramus)
Obturator membrane (pelvic surface)
Obturator fascia

Insertion:
Femur (greater trochanter, medial surface proximal to the trochanteric fossa)
Tendon fuses with gemelli

Description:
Muscle lies internal in the osteoligamentous pelvis and also external behind the hip joint. The fibers converge toward the lesser sciatic foramen and hook around the body of the ischium, which acts as a pulley; it exits the pelvis via the lesser sciatic foramen, crosses the capsule of the hip joint, and proceeds to the greater trochanter.

Function:
Hip external (lateral) rotation
Abduction of flexed hip (assist)

Innervation:
L5-S1 nerve to obturator internus off lumbosacral plexus

188 OBTURATOR EXTERNUS

Origin:
Pubic ramus
Ischial ramus
Obturator foramen (margin)
Obturator membrane (medial ⅔ of outer surface)

Insertion:
Femur (trochanteric fossa)

Description:
This flat, triangular muscle covers the external aspect of the anterior pelvic wall from a very broad origin on the medial margin of the obturator foramen. Its fibers pass posteriorly and laterally in

a spiral to a tendon that passes behind the femoral neck to insert in the trochanteric fossa.
This muscle, along with the other small lateral rotators, may serve more postural functions (such as stability) than prime movement. They maintain the integrity of hip joint actions.

Function:
Hip external (lateral) rotation
Hip adduction (assist)

Innervation:
L3-L4 obturator nerve (posterior branch)

189 GEMELLUS SUPERIOR

Origin:
Ischial spine (gluteal surface)

Insertion:
Femur (greater trochanter, medial surface)

Description:
Muscle lies in parallel with and superior to the tendon of obturator internus, which it joins. This is the smaller of the two gemelli and may be absent.

Function:
Hip external (lateral) rotation
Hip abduction with hip flexed (accessory)

Innervation:
L5-S1 nerve to obturator internus (off lumbar plexus)

190 GEMELLUS INFERIOR

Origin:
Ischium (tuberosity, superior surface)

Insertion:
Femur (greater trochanter, medial surface)

Description:
This small muscle parallels and joins the tendon of the obturator internus on its inferior side. The two gemelli may be considered adjunct to the obturator internus.

Function:
Hip external (lateral) rotation
Hip abduction with hip flexed (weak assist)

Innervation:
L5-S1 nerve to quadratus femoris (off lumbar plexus)

191 QUADRATUS FEMORIS

Origin:
Ischium (tuberosity, upper external border)

Insertion:
Femur (quadrate tubercle on posterior aspect)

Description:
This flat quadrilateral muscle lies between the gemellus inferior and the adductor magnus. Its fibers pass almost horizontally, posterior to the hip joint and femoral neck.

Function:
Hip external (lateral) rotation

Innervation:
L5-S1 nerve to quadratus femoris (off lumbar plexus)

192 BICEPS FEMORIS

Origin:
Long head:
Ischium (tuberosity, inferior and medial aspects, in common with tendon of semitendinosus)
Sacrotuberous ligament
Short head:
Femur (linea aspera, entire length of lateral lip; lateral supracondylar line)
Lateral intermuscular septum

Insertion:
Aponeurosis of long head distally. The short head inserts into the deep surface of this aponeurosis to form the "lateral hamstring tendon."
Fibula (head, lateral aspect via main portion of lateral hamstring tendon)
Tibia (lateral condyle via lamina from lateral hamstring tendon)[37]
Fascia on lateral leg

Description:
This lateral hamstring muscle is a two-head muscle on the posterolateral thigh. Its long head is a two-joint muscle. The muscle fibers of the long head descend laterally, ending in an aponeurosis that covers the posterior surface of the muscle. Fibers from the short head also converge into the same aponeurosis, which narrows into the lateral hamstring tendon of insertion. At the insertion the tendon divides into two slips to embrace the fibular collateral ligament. The short head is sometimes absent.
The different nerve supply, tibial division for the long head and common peroneal division for the short head, reflects both flexor and extensor muscle derivations.

The biceps femoris as a posterior femoral muscle flexes the knee and extends the hip (from a stooped posture) against gravity. When the hip is extended, this muscle is an external rotator of the hip. When the knee is flexed, the biceps is an external rotator of the knee. When at any time the body's center of gravity moves forward of the transverse axis of the hip joint, the biceps femoris contracts.

Function:
Knee flexion (only the short head is a pure knee flexor)
Knee external rotation
Hip extension and external rotation (long head)

Innervation:
Long head: L5-S2 sciatic nerve (tibial division)
Short head: L5-S2 sciatic nerve (common peroneal division)

193 SEMITENDINOSUS

Origin:
Ischium (tuberosity, inferior medial aspect)
Aponeurosis to share tendon with biceps femoris (long head)
Pes anserina

Insertion:
Tibia (shaft on proximal medial side)
Deep fascia of leg

Description:
A muscle on the posteromedial thigh known for its long, round tendon, which extends from midthigh to the tibia. The semitendinosus unites with the tendons of the sartorius and the gracilis to form a flattened aponeurosis called the *pes anserinus.*

Function:
Knee flexion
Knee internal rotation
Hip extension
Hip internal rotation (accessory)

Innervation:
L5-S2 sciatic nerve (tibial division)

194 SEMIMEMBRANOSUS

Origin:
Ischium (tuberosity, superior and lateral facets)
Complex proximal tendon along with fibers from biceps femoris and semitendinosus

Insertion:
Tibia (tubercle on medial condyle)
Oblique popliteal ligament of knee joint
Aponeurosis over distal part of muscle to form tendon of insertion

Description:
The semimembranosus is the larger of the two medial hamstrings. Its name derives from its flat, membranous tendon of origin that partially envelops the anterior surface of the upper portion of the biceps femoris and semitendinosus. Its fibers descend from midthigh to a distal aponeurosis, which narrows into a short, thick tendon before inserting on the tibia. The semitendinosus is superficial to the semimembranosus throughout its extent.

Function:
Knee flexion
Knee internal rotation
Hip extension
Hip internal rotation (accessory)

Innervation:
L5-S2 sciatic nerve (tibial division)

195 SARTORIUS

Origin:
Ilium (ASIS; notch below ASIS)

Insertion:
Tibia (proximal medial surface of the shaft distal to the tibial condyle)
Aponeurosis
Capsule of knee joint

Description:
The longest muscle in the body, its parallel fibers form a narrow, thin muscle. It descends obliquely from lateral to medial to just above the knee, where it turns abruptly downward and passes posterior to the medial condyle of the femur. It expands into a broad aponeurosis before inserting on the medial surface of the tibia. The sartorius is the most superficial of the anterior thigh muscles and occasionally is absent. It forms the lateral border of the femoral triangle.

Function:
Hip external rotation, abduction, and flexion
Knee flexion
Knee internal rotation
Assists in "tailor sitting"

Innervation:
L2-L3 femoral nerve (two branches usually)

Muscles of the Knee

196-200 Quadriceps femoris
201 Articularis genus

192 Biceps femoris (see *Muscles of the Hip*)
193 Semitendinosus (see *Muscles of the Hip*)
194 Semimembranosus (see *Muscles of the Hip*)
202 Popliteus

196-200 QUADRICEPS FEMORIS

This muscular mass on the anterior thigh has five component muscles (or heads), which together make this the most powerful muscle group in the human body. The five components are the great extensors of the knee.

196 Rectus femoris
197 Vastus lateralis
198 Vastus intermedius
199 Vastus medialis longus
200 Vastus medialis oblique

196 RECTUS FEMORIS

Origin:
Arises by two tendons, which conjoin to form an aponeurosis from which the muscle fibers arise:
Ilium (anterior inferior iliac spine)
Acetabulum (groove above posterior rim and superior margin of labrum)
Capsule of hip joint

Insertion:
Patella (base; from an aponeurosis which gradually narrows into a tendon which inserts into the center portion of the quadriceps tendon, thence into the ligamentum patellae to a final insertion on the tibial tuberosity)

Description:
This most anterior of the quadriceps lies 6° medial to the axis of the femur. Its superficial fibers are bipennate, but the deep fibers are parallel. It traverses a vertical course down the thigh. It is a two-joint muscle, crossing both the hip and knee, whereas the vasti are one-joint muscles crossing only the knee.

197 VASTUS LATERALIS

Origin:
Femur (linea aspera, lateral lip; greater trochanter, anterior and inferior borders; proximal intertrochanteric line; gluteal tuberosity)
Lateral intermuscular septum

Insertion:
Patella, into an underlying aponeurosis over the deep surface of the muscle, which narrows and attaches to the lateral border of the quadriceps tendon; to a lateral expansion, which blends with the capsule of the knee and the iliotibial tract.
The quadriceps tendon joins the ligamentum patellae to insert into the tibial tuberosity.

Description:
The lateralis is the largest of the quadriceps group and, as its name suggests, it forms the bulk of the lateral thigh musculature. It arises via a broad aponeurosis lateral to the femur. Its fibers run at an angle of 17° to the axis of the femur. It descends to the thigh under the iliotibial band. It is the muscle of choice for biopsy in the lower extremity.

198 VASTUS INTERMEDIUS

Origin:
Femur (anterior and lateral surfaces of upper ⅔ of shaft)
Lateral intermuscular septum (lower part)

Insertion:
Patella (base: into an anterior aponeurosis of muscle which attaches to the middle part of the deep layer of the quadriceps tendon, and then into the ligamentum patellae to insert into the tibial tuberosity)

Description:
The deepest of the quadriceps muscles, this muscle lies under the rectus femoris, the vastus medialis, and the vastus lateralis. It often appears inseparable from the medialis. It almost completely surrounds the proximal ⅔ of the shaft of the femur. A small muscle, the articularis genus, occasionally is distinguishable from the intermedius, but more commonly it is part of the intermedius.

199 VASTUS MEDIALIS LONGUS[38,39]

Origin:
Femur (intertrochanteric line, lower half; linea aspera, medial lip, proximal portion)
Tendons of adductors longus and magnus
Medial intermuscular septum

Insertion:
Patella, via an aponeurosis into the superior medial margin of the quadriceps tendon, thence to the ligamentum patellae and insertion into the tibial tuberosity

Description:
The fibers of this muscle course upward at an angle of 15° to 18° to the longitudinal axis of the femur.

200 VASTUS MEDIALIS OBLIQUE[38,39]

Origin:
Femur (linea aspera, medial lip, distal portion; medial supracondylar line, proximal portion)
Tendon of adductor magnus
Medial intermuscular septum

Insertion:
Patella:
Into the medial quadriceps tendon and along medial margin of the patella
Expansion aponeurosis to the capsule of the knee joint
Tibial tuberosity via ligamentum patellae

Description:
The fibers of this muscle run at an angle of 50° to 55° to the longitudinal axis of the femur. The muscle appears to bulge quickly with training and to atrophy with disuse before the other quadriceps show changes. This is deceiving because the medialis oblique has the most sparse and thinnest fascial investment, making changes in it more obvious to observation.

Insertion (all):
The tendons of the five heads unite at the distal thigh to form a common strong tendon (quadriceps tendon) that inserts into the proximal margin of the patella. Fibers continue across the anterior surface to become the patellar tendon (ligamentum patellae), which inserts into the tuberosity of the tibia.

Function (all):
Knee extension (none of the heads functions independently)
Hip flexion (by rectus femoris, which crosses the hip joint)

Innervation (all):
L2-L4 femoral nerve

201 ARTICULARIS GENUS

Origin:
Femur (shaft, lower anterior surface)

Insertion:
Knee joint (synovial membrane, upper part)

Description:
This small muscle is mostly distinct but also it may be inseparable from the vastus intermedius

Function:
Retracts the synovial membrane during knee extension, purportedly preventing this membrane from being entrapped between the patella and the femur

Innervation:
L2-L4 femoral nerve

202 POPLITEUS

Origin:
Capsule of knee joint (by a strong tendon to lateral condyle of the femur)
Femur (lateral condyle, popliteal groove on anterior surface)
Arcuate popliteal ligament
Lateral meniscus of knee joint[40]

Insertion:
Tibia (posterior triangular surface above soleal line)
Tendinous expansion of muscle

Description:
Sweeps across the upper leg from lateral to medial just below the knee. Forms the lower floor of the popliteal fossa. It is believed to protect the lateral meniscus from a crush injury during external rotation of the femur and flexion of the knee.[40]

Function:
Knee flexion
Knee internal rotation (proximal attachment fixed)
Hip external rotation (tibia fixed)

Innervation:
L4-S1 tibial nerve (high branch)

Muscles of the Ankle

203 Tibialis anterior
204 Tibialis posterior
205 Gastrocnemius
206 Soleus
207 Plantaris
208 Peroneus longus
209 Peroneus brevis
210 Peroneus tertius

203 TIBIALIS ANTERIOR

Origin:
Tibia (lateral condyle and proximal ⅔ of lateral surface)
Interosseous membrane
Deep surface of crural fascia
Intermuscular septum

Insertion:
1st (medial) cuneiform bone (on medial and plantar surfaces)
1st metatarsal bone (base)

Description:
Located on the lateral aspect of the tibia, the muscle has a thick belly proximally but is tendinous distally. The fibers drop vertically and end in a prominent tendon on the anterior surface of the lower leg. Muscle is contained in the most medial compartments of the extensor retinacula.

Function:
Ankle dorsiflexion (talocrural joint)
Foot inversion and adduction (supination) at subtalar and midtarsal joints
Supports medial-longitudinal arch of foot in walking

Innervation:
L4-L5 (often S1) deep peroneal nerve

204 TIBIALIS POSTERIOR

Origin:
Tibia (proximal ⅔ of posterior lateral shaft)
Fibula (proximal ⅔ of posterior medial shaft and head)
Interosseous membrane (entire posterior surface except lower portion where flexor hallucis longus originates)
Deep transverse fascia and intermuscular septa

Insertion:
Navicular bone (tuberosity)
Cuneiform bones (media, intermediate, lateral)
Cuboid (slip)
2nd, 3rd, and 4th metatarsals (bases) (variable)

Description:
Most deeply placed of the flexor group, high on the posterior leg, this muscle is overlapped by both the flexor hallucis longus and the flexor digitorum longus. It rises by two narrow heads and descends centrally on the leg, forming its distal tendon in the distal ¼. This tendon passes behind the medial malleolus (with the flexor digitorum longus), enters the foot on the plantar surface (where it contains a sesamoid bone), and then divides to its several insertions.
During weight bearing the tibialis posterior assists in arch support and distribution of weight on the foot to maintain balance.

Function:
Foot inversion
Ankle plantar flexion (accessory)

Innervation:
L4-L5 (sometimes S1) tibial nerve (low branches)

205 GASTROCNEMIUS

Rises via two heads

Origin:
Medial head:
Femur (medial condyle, depression on upper posterior part; popliteal surface adjacent to medial condyle)
Capsule of knee joint
Aponeurosis
Lateral head:
Femur (lateral condyle and posterior surface of shaft above lateral condyle; lower supracondylar line)
Capsule of knee joint
Aponeurosis

Insertion:
Calcaneus (via tendo calcaneus into middle posterior surface). Fibers of tendon rotate 90° such that those associated with gastrocnemius are attached more laterally on the calcaneus.

Description:
The most superficial of the calf muscles, it gives the characteristic contour to the calf. It is a two-joint muscle with two heads arising from the condyles of the femur and descending to the calcaneus. The medial head is the larger, and its fibers extend further distally before spreading into a tendinous expansion, as does the lateral head. The two heads join as the aponeurosis narrows and form the tendo calcaneus. The belly of the muscle extends to about midcalf (the medial head is the longer) before inserting into the aponeurosis.

Function:
Ankle plantar flexion
Knee flexion (accessory)
Foot eversion

Innervation:
S1-S2 tibial nerve

206 SOLEUS

Origin:
Fibula (head, posterior surface; shaft: proximal ⅓ on posterior surface)
Tibia (soleal line and middle ⅓ of medial side of shaft)
Fibrous arch between tibia and fibula
Aponeurosis (anterior aspect)

Insertion:
Aponeurosis over posterior surface of muscle, which, with tendon of gastrocnemius, thickens to become the tendo calcaneus

Calcaneus (posterior surface via tendo calcaneus along with gastrocnemius)[41]
Tendinous raphe in midline of muscle

Description:
This is a one-joint muscle, the largest of the triceps surae. It is broad and flat and lies just under the gastrocnemius. Its anterior attachment is a wide aponeurosis, and most of its fibers course obliquely to the descending tendon on its posterior side. Below midcalf the soleus is wider than the tendon of the gastrocnemius and on both sides. It is, thereby, accessible for biopsy and electrophysiological studies.
The soleus is constantly active in quiet stance. It responds to the forward center of mass to prevent the body from falling forward.

Function:
Ankle plantar flexion
Foot inversion

Innervation:
S1-S2 tibial nerve

207 PLANTARIS

Origin:
Femur (supracondylar line, lateral)
Oblique popliteal ligament of knee joint

Insertion:
Tendo calcaneus (medial border) to calcaneum
Plantar aponeurosis

Description:
This small fusiform muscle lies between the gastrocnemius and the soleus. It is sometimes absent; at other times it is doubled. Its short belly is followed by a long slender tendon of insertion along the medial border of the tendo calcaneus and inserts with it on the posterior calcaneum.
Plantaris is somewhat like palmaris longus in the hand and is of little function in humans.[41]

Function:
Ankle plantar flexion (assist)
Knee flexion (weak accessory)

Innervation:
S1-S2 tibial nerve (high branches)

208 PERONEUS LONGUS

Origin:
Fibula (head and upper ⅔ of lateral shaft)
Tibia (lateral condyle, occasionally)
Deep crural fascia and intermuscular septa

Insertion:
1st metatarsal (lateral plantar side of base)
1st (medial) cuneiform (lateral plantar aspect)
2nd metatarsal (occasionally by a slip)

Description:
Muscle is found proximally on the fibular side of the leg where it is superficial to the peroneus brevis. The belly ends in a long tendon that passes behind the lateral malleolus (with the brevis) and then runs obliquely forward lateral to the calcaneus and crosses the plantar aspect of the foot to reach the 1st metatarsal and medial cuneiform.
It maintains concavity of foot (along with brevis) during toe-off and tiptoeing.

Function:
Foot eversion
Ankle plantar flexion (assist)
Depression of 1st metatarsal
Support of longitudinal and transverse arches

Innervation:
L5-S1 superficial peroneal nerve

209 PERONEUS BREVIS

Origin:
Fibula (shaft: distal ⅔ of lateral surface)
Intermuscular septa

Insertion:
5th metatarsal (tuberosity on lateral surface of base)

Description:
The peroneus brevis lies deep to the longus and is the shorter and smaller muscle of the two. The belly fibers descend vertically to end in a tendon, which courses (with the longus) behind the lateral malleolus (the pair of muscles share a synovial sheath). It bends forward on the lateral side of the calcaneus, passing forward to the 5th metatarsal.

Function:
Foot eversion
Ankle plantar flexion (accessory)

Innervation:
L5-S1 superficial peroneal nerve

210 PERONEUS TERTIUS

Origin:
Fibula (distal ⅓ of medial surface)
Interosseous membrane (anterior)
Intermuscular septum

Insertion:
5th metatarsal (dorsal surface of base; shaft: medial aspect)

Description:
This muscle is considered part of the extensor digitorum longus (i.e., the 5th tendon). The muscle descends on the lateral leg, diving under the extensor retinaculum in the same passage as the extensor digitorum longus, to insert on the 5th metatarsal. Muscle varies greatly.

Function:
Ankle dorsiflexion
Foot eversion (accessory)

Innervation:
L5-S1 deep peroneal nerve

Muscles Acting on the Toes

211 Extensor digitorum longus
212 Extensor digitorum brevis
213 Flexor digitorum longus
214 Flexor digitorum brevis
215 Abductor digiti minimi
216 Flexor digiti minimi brevis
217 Quadratus plantae (flexor digitorum accessorius)
218 Lumbricales
219 Interossei, dorsal (foot)
220 Interossei, plantar

211 EXTENSOR DIGITORUM LONGUS

Origin:
Tibia (lateral condyle on lateral side)
Fibula (shaft: upper ¾ of medial surface)
Interosseous membrane (anterior surface)
Deep crural fascia and intermuscular septum

Insertion:
Tendon of insertion divides into four tendon slips to dorsum of foot that form an expansion over each toe:
Toes 2 to 5:
Middle phalanges (PIP joints) of the four lesser toes (intermediate slip to dorsum of base of each)
Distal phalanges (two lateral slips to dorsum of base of each)

Description:
Muscle lies in the lateral aspect of the anterior leg. It descends lateral to the tibialis anterior, and its distal tendon accompanies the tendon of the peroneus tertius before dividing. It is attached in the manner of the extensor digitorum of the hand.

Function:
MP extension of four lesser toes
PIP and DIP extension (assist) of four lesser toes
Ankle dorsiflexion (accessory)
Foot eversion (accessory)

Innervation:
L5-S1 deep peroneal nerve

212 EXTENSOR DIGITORUM BREVIS

Origin:
Calcaneus (superior proximal surface anterolateral to the calcaneal sulcus)
Lateral talocalcaneal ligament
Extensor retinaculum (inferior)

Insertion:
Ends in four tendons:
(1) Hallux (proximal phalanx). This tendon is the largest and most medial. It frequently is described as a separate muscle, the extensor hallucis brevis.
(2, 3, 4) Three tendons join the tendon of extensor digitorum longus (lateral surfaces).

Description:
The muscle passes medially and distally across the dorsum of the foot to end in four tendons, one to the hallux and three to toes 2, 3, and 4. Varies considerably.

Function:
Hallux (great toe): MP extension
Toes 2 to 4: MP extension
Toes 2 to 4: IP extension (assist)

Innervation:
L5-S1 deep peroneal nerve, lateral terminal branch

213 FLEXOR DIGITORUM LONGUS

Origin:
Tibia (shaft: posterior surface of middle ⅔)
Fascia covering tibialis posterior

Insertion:
Toes 2 to 5 (distal phalanges: base, plantar surface)

Description:
Muscle lies deep on the tibial side of the leg and increases in size as it descends. The tendon of insertion extends almost the entire length of the muscle and is joined in the sole of the foot by the tendon of the quadratus plantae. It finally

divides into four slips, which insert into the four lateral toes.

Function:
Toes 2 to 5: MP, PIP, and DIP flexion
Ankle plantar flexion (accessory)
Foot inversion (accessory)

Innervation:
L5-S2 tibial nerve

214 FLEXOR DIGITORUM BREVIS

Origin:
Calcaneus (tuberosity, medial process)
Intermuscular septa (adjacent)
Plantar aponeurosis (central part)

Insertion:
Toes 2 to 5 (by four tendons to middle phalanges, both sides)

Description:
This muscle is located in the middle of the sole of the foot immediately above the plantar aponeurosis. It divides into four tendons, one for each of the four lesser toes. At the base of the proximal phalanx each is divided into two slips, which encircle the tendon of the flexor digitorum longus. The tendons divide a second time and insert onto both sides of the middle phalanges. The pattern of insertion is the same as the tendons of the flexor digitorum superficialis in the hand.

Function:
Toes 2 to 5 MP and PIP flexion

Innervation:
S1-S2 medial plantar nerve

215 ABDUCTOR DIGITI MINIMI (Foot)

Origin:
Calcaneus (tuberosity, medial and lateral processes)
Plantar aponeurosis and intermuscular septum

Insertion:
Toe 5 (base of proximal phalanx, lateral aspect)
Insertion is in common with flexor digiti minimi brevis

Description:
Lies along the lateral border of the foot and inserts in common with the flexor digiti minimi brevis. Its insertion on the lateral side of the base of the 5th toe makes it as much a flexor as an abductor.

Function:
Toe 5 abduction
Toe 5 MP flexion

Innervation:
S1-S3 lateral plantar nerve

216 FLEXOR DIGITI MINIMI BREVIS

Origin:
5th metatarsal (base, plantar surface)
Sheath of peroneus longus

Insertion:
Toe 5 (proximal phalanx, lateral aspect of base)

Description:
Muscle lies superficial to the 5th metatarsal and looks like an interosseous muscle. Sometimes fibers are inserted into the lateral distal half of the 5th metatarsal, and these have been described as a distinct muscle called the opponens digiti minimi.

Function:
Toe 5 MP flexion

Innervation:
S2-S3 lateral plantar nerve (superficial branch)

217 QUADRATUS PLANTAE
(Flexor Digitorum Accessorius)

Rises via two heads

Origin:
Lateral head:
Calcaneus (lateral border distal to lateral process of tuberosity)
Long plantar ligament
Medial head:
Calcaneus (medial concave surface)
Long plantar ligament (medial border)

Insertion:
Tendon of flexor digitorum longus (lateral margin) may fuse with long flexor tendon.[42]

Description:
This muscle is sometimes known as the flexor digitorum accessorius, or just flexor accessorius.
The medial head is larger, whereas the lateral head is more tendinous. They rise from either side of the calcaneus, pass medially, and join in an acute angle at midfoot, to end in the lateral margin of the tendon of the flexor digitorum longus. Muscle may be absent.

Function:
Toes 2 to 5 DIP flexion (in synergy with the flexor digitorum longus)

Innervation:
S1-S3 lateral plantar nerve

218 LUMBRICALES (Foot)

These are four small muscles considered accessories to the flexor digitorum longus.

Origin:
1st Lumbrical: Originates by a single head from the medial side of the tendon of the flexor digitorum longus bound for toe 2.
2nd, 3rd, and 4th Lumbricales: Originate by double heads from adjacent sides of tendons of the flexor digitorum longus bound for toes 3, 4, and 5.

Insertion (all):
Toes 2 to 5 (proximal phalanges and dorsal expansions of the tendons of extensor digitorum longus)

Description:
The lumbricales are four small muscles intrinsic to the foot. They are numbered from the medial (hallux) side of the foot so that the 1st lumbrical goes to toe 2 and the 4th lumbrical goes to toe 5.

Function:
Toes 2 to 5: MP flexion
Toes 2 to 5: PIP and DIP extension (assist)

Innervation:
1st Lumbrical: L5-S1 medial plantar nerve
2nd, 3rd, and 4th Lumbricales: S2-S3 lateral plantar nerve, deep branch

219 DORSAL INTEROSSEI (Foot)

There are four dorsal interossei

Origin:
Metatarsal bones (each head arises from the adjacent sides of the metatarsal bones between which it lies)

Insertion:
1st Dorsal: Toe 2 proximal phalanx, medial side of base
2nd Dorsal: Toe 2 proximal phalanx, lateral side of base
3rd Dorsal: Toe 3 proximal phalanx, lateral side of base
4th Dorsal: Toe 4 proximal phalanx, lateral side of base
All: Tendons of extensor digitorum longus via dorsal digital expansion

Description:
The dorsal interossei are four bipennate muscles, each arising by two heads. They are similar to the interossei of the hand except that their action is considered relative to the midline of the 2nd digit (the longitudinal axis of the foot). The muscles are innervated by the lateral plantar nerve, deep branch, except for the 4th dorsal muscle which lies in the 4th interosseous space; it is supplied by the superficial branch of the same nerve.

Function:
Toes 2 to 4: abduction from longitudinal axis of foot, which lines up through toe 2
Toes 2 to 4: MP flexion (accessory)
Toes 2 to 4: IP extension (possibly)

Innervation:
1st, 2nd, and 3rd Dorsals: S2-S3 lateral plantar nerve, deep branch
4th Dorsal: S2-S3 lateral plantar nerve, superficial branch (1st dorsal also may receive a slip from the deep peroneal, medial branch; the 2nd dorsal may receive a slip from the deep peroneal, lateral branch)

220 PLANTAR INTEROSSEI

Origin:
3rd, 4th, and 5th metatarsal bones (bases and medial sides)

Insertion:
Proximal phalanges of same toe (bases and medial sides)
Dorsal digital expansion

Description:
These are three muscles that lie along the plantar surface of the metatarsals rather than between them. Each connects with only one metatarsal. As with the dorsal interossei, the muscles are innervated by the deep branch of the lateral plantar nerve except for the 3rd plantar muscle, which lies in the 4th interosseous space and is innervated by the superficial branch of the same nerve.

Function:
Toes 3, 4, and 5: Adduction (toward the axis of toe 2)
MP flexion
IP extension (assist)

Innervation:
1st and 2nd Plantars: S2-S3 lateral plantar nerve (deep branch)
3rd Plantar: S2-S3 lateral plantar nerve (superficial branch)

Muscles Acting on the Great Toe

221 Extensor hallucis longus
222 Flexor hallucis longus
223 Flexor hallucis brevis
224 Abductor hallucis
225 Adductor hallucis

221 EXTENSOR HALLUCIS LONGUS

Origin:
Fibula (shaft: medial aspect of middle half)
Interosseous membrane

Insertion:
Hallux (base of distal phalanx, dorsal surface)
Expansion to base of proximal phalanx of hallux

Description:
This thin muscle travels lateral to medial as it descends in the leg between and largely covered by the tibialis anterior and the extensor digitorum longus. Its tendon does not emerge superficially until it reaches the distal ⅓ of the leg. It may be joined with the extensor digitorum longus.

Function:
Hallux: MP and IP extension
Ankle dorsiflexion (accessory)
Foot inversion (accessory)

Innervation:
L5 deep peroneal nerve
L4-S1 also cited

222 FLEXOR HALLUCIS LONGUS

Origin:
Fibula (shaft: inferior ⅔ of posterior surface)
Interosseous membrane
Posterior crural intermuscular septum
Fascia over tibialis posterior

Insertion:
Hallux (distal phalanx at base on plantar surface)
Slip to tendon of flexor digitorum longus

Description:
This muscle lies deep in the lateral side of the leg. Its fibers pass obliquely down via a long tendon that runs along the whole length of its posterior surface and then crosses over the distal end of the tibia, talus, and the inferior surface of the calcaneus. It then runs forward on the sole of the foot to the distal phalanx of the hallux.

Function:
Hallux IP flexion
Hallux MP flexion (accessory)
Ankle plantar flexion and foot inversion (accessory)

Innervation:
L5-S2 tibial nerve (low branches)

223 FLEXOR HALLUCIS BREVIS

Origin:
Lateral part:
Cuboid (medial part of plantar surface)
Cuneiform (lateral)
Medial part:
Tendon of tibialis posterior
Medial intermuscular septum

Insertion:
Hallux: sides of base of proximal phalanx
The medial part blends with the abductor hallucis
The lateral part blends with adductor hallucis

Description:
One of the muscles of the third layer (of four layers) of plantar muscles. It is located adjacent to the plantar surface of the 1st metatarsal.

Function:
Hallux abduction (away from toe 2)
Hallux MP flexion

Innervation:
S1-S2 medial plantar nerve

224 ABDUCTOR HALLUCIS

Origin:
Flexor retinaculum
Calcaneus (tuberosity, medial process)
Plantar aponeurosis and intermuscular septum

Insertion:
Hallux (base of proximal phalanx, medial side)
Medial sesamoid of hallux
Joins tendon of flexor hallucis brevis

Description:
This muscle lies along the medial border of the foot. Its tendon attaches distally to the medial tendon of the flexor hallucis brevis and they insert together on the hallux.
When fibers from the muscle are attached to the first metatarsal, it can be considered an opponens hallucis.

Function:
Hallux abduction (away from toe 2)
Hallux MP flexion (accessory)

Innervation:
S1-S2 medial plantar nerve

225 ADDUCTOR HALLUCIS

Arises from two heads

Origin:
Oblique head
2nd, 3rd, and 4th metatarsals (bases)
Sheath of peroneus longus tendon

Transverse Head
Toes 3 to 5: Plantar metatarsophalangeal ligaments
Deep transverse metatarsal ligaments between toes

Insertion:
Oblique:
Hallux (base of proximal phalanx, lateral aspect)
Lateral sesamoid bone of hallux
Blends with flexor hallucis brevis

Transverse:
Proximal phalanx of hallux (debated)
Lateral sesamoid of hallux

Description:
The two heads are unequal in size, the oblique being the larger and more muscular. It is located in the third layer of plantar muscles. The oblique head crosses the foot from center to medial on a long oblique axis; the transverse head courses transversely across the metatarsophalangeal joints.

Function:
Hallux adduction (toward toe 2)
Hallux MP flexion (accessory)
Support of transverse metatarsal arch

Innervation:
S2-S3 lateral plantar nerve, deep branch

THE MOTOR NERVE ROOTS AND THE MUSCLES THEY INNERVATE

In this portion of the Ready Reference chapter, the spinal roots for the axial and trunk skeletal muscles are outlined, along with the muscles innervated by each root. There are many variations of these innervation patterns, but this text presents a consensus derived from classic anatomy and neurology texts.

The muscles are presented here as originating from the dorsal or ventral primary rami. Each muscle is always preceded by its reference number for cross-reference. Named peripheral nerves for individual muscles are listed in parentheses (e.g., thoracodorsal) after the muscle. The specific muscle or part is in brackets.

The spinal nerves arise in the spinal cord and exit from it via the intervertebral foramina. There are 31 pairs: cervical (8), thoracic (12), lumbar (5), sacral (5), and coccygeal (1). These innervations are especially variable.

Each spinal nerve has two roots that unite to form the nerve: the *ventral root* (motor), which exits the cord from the ventral (anterior) horn, and the *dorsal root* (sensory), which enters the cord from the dorsal (posterior) horn. This text will address only the motor roots.

Each motor root divides into two parts:

1. Primary ventral rami (Figure 11-10)

The ventral rami supply the ventral and lateral trunk muscles and all limb muscles. The cervical, lumbar, and sacral ventral rami merge near their origin to form plexuses. The thoracic ventral rami remain individual and are distributed segmentally.

2. Primary dorsal rami

The dorsal rami supply the muscles of the dorsal neck and trunk. The dorsal primary rami do not join any of the plexuses.

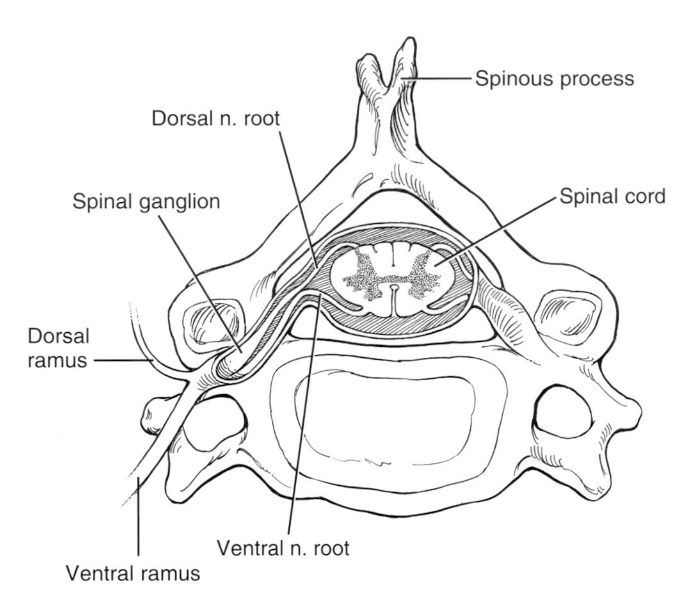

FIGURE 11-10 Rami of spinal nerves.

The major plexuses formed by the cervical, lumbar, and sacral nerves are as follows:

Cervical plexus (ventral primary rami of C1-C4 and connecting cranial nerves)
Brachial plexus (ventral primary rami of C5-T1 and connections from C4 and T2
Lumbosacral plexus (ventral primary rami of lumbar, sacral, pudendal, and coccygeal nerves)
Lumbar plexus (ventral primary rami of L1-L4 and communication from T12)
Sacral plexus (ventral primary rami of L4-L5 and S1-S3)
Pudendal plexus (ventral primary rami of S2-S4)
Coccygeal plexus (S4-S5)

THE CERVICAL ROOTS AND NERVES

C1

Ventral Primary Ramus

72 Rectus capitis anterior
73 Rectus capitis lateralis
74 Longus capitis
77 Geniohyoid
84 Sternothyroid
85 Thyrohyoid
86 Sternohyoid
87 Omohyoid

Dorsal Primary Ramus (of C1)

56 Rectus capitis posterior major
57 Rectus capitis posterior minor
58 Obliquus capitis superior
59 Obliquus capitis inferior

C2

Ventral Primary Ramus

72 Rectus capitis anterior
73 Rectus capitis lateralis
74 Longus capitis
79 Longus colli

83 Sternocleidomastoid
84 Sternothyroid
86 Sternohyoid
87 Omohyoid

Dorsal Primary Ramus[2,3]

60 Longissimus capitis
62 Semispinalis capitis
65 Semispinalis cervicis
94 Multifidi

C3

Ventral Primary Ramus

70 Intertransversarii cervicis
74 Longus capitis
79 Longus colli
84 Sternothyroid
86 Sternohyoid
87 Omohyoid
127 Levator scapulae (dorsal scapular)
81 Scalenus medius
83 Sternocleidomastoid
101 Diaphragm (C4)
124 Trapezius

Dorsal Primary Ramus (of C3)

60 Longissimus capitis
61 Splenius capitis
62 Semispinalis capitis
63 Spinalis capitis
64 Longissimus cervicis
65 Semispinalis cervicis
68 Spinalis cervicis
69 Interspinales cervicis
70 Intertransversarii cervicis [posterior]
71 Rotatores cervicis
94 Multifidi

C4

Ventral Primary Ramus

79 Longus colli
70 Intertransversarii cervicis [anterior]
127 Levator scapulae (dorsal scapular)
80 Scalenus anterior
81 Scalenus medius
101 Diaphragm (phrenic)

Dorsal Primary Ramus

61 Splenius capitis
62 Semispinalis capitis
63 Spinalis capitis
64 Longissimus cervicis
65 Semispinalis cervicis
66 Iliocostalis cervicis
67 Splenius cervicis
68 Spinalis cervicis
69 Interspinalis cervicis
70 Intertransversarii cervicis [posterior]
71 Rotatores cervicis
94 Multifidi

C5

Ventral Primary Ramus

79 Longus colli
70 Intertransversarii cervicis (anterior)
80 Scalenus anterior
81 Scalenus medius
132 Subclavius (nerve to subclavius)
101 Diaphragm
127 Levator scapulae (dorsal scapular)
125 Rhomboid major (dorsal scapular)
126 Rhomboid minor (dorsal scapular)
128 Serratus anterior (long thoracic)
129 Pectoralis minor (medial and lateral pectoral)
131 Pectoralis major [clavicular head] (lateral pectoral)

135 Supraspinatus (suprascapular)
136 Infraspinatus (suprascapular)
134 Subscapularis (subscapular, upper and lower)
138 Teres major (subscapular, lower)
133 Deltoid (axillary)
137 Teres minor (axillary)
139 Coracobrachialis (musculocutaneous)
140 Biceps brachii (musculocutaneous)
141 Brachialis (musculocutaneous)
143 Brachioradialis (radial)

Dorsal Primary Ramus (of C5)

60 Longissimus capitis
61 Splenius capitis
62 Semispinalis capitis
63 Spinalis capitis
64 Longissimus cervicis
65 Semispinalis cervicis
66 Iliocostalis cervicis
67 Splenius cervicis
68 Spinalis cervicis
69 Interspinalis cervicis
70 Intertransversarii cervicis [posterior]
72 Rotatores cervicis
94 Multifidi

C6

Ventral Primary Ramus

79 Longus colli
70 Intertransversarii cervicis [anterior]
80 Scalenus anterior
81 Scalenus medius
82 Scalenus posterior
130 Latissimus dorsi (thoracodorsal)
132 Subclavius (nerve to subclavius)
128 Serratus anterior (long thoracic)
131 Pectoralis major [clavicular head] (lateral pectoral), [sternocostal head] (medial and lateral pectorals)
129 Pectoralis minor (medial and lateral pectorals)
136 Infraspinatus (suprascapular)
135 Supraspinatus (suprascapular)
134 Subscapularis (subscapular, upper and lower)
138 Teres major (subscapular, lower)
133 Deltoid (axillary)
137 Teres minor (axillary)
139 Coracobrachialis (musculocutaneous)
140 Biceps brachii (musculocutaneous)
141 Brachialis (musculocutaneous)
142 Triceps brachii (radial)
143 Brachioradialis (radial)
144 Anconeus (radial)
145 Supinator (radial)
148 Extensor carpi radialis longus (radial)
146 Pronator teres (median)
151 Flexor carpi radialis (median)

Dorsal Primary Ramus (of C6)

60 Longissimus capitis
61 Splenius capitis
62 Semispinalis capitis
63 Spinalis capitis
64 Longissimus cervicis
65 Semispinalis cervicis
66 Iliocostalis cervicis
67 Splenius cervicis
68 Spinalis cervicis
69 Interspinales cervicis
70 Intertransversarii cervicis [posterior]
71 Rotatores cervicis
93 Multifidi

C7

Ventral Primary Ramus

70 Intertransversarii cervicis [anterior]
81 Scalenus medius
82 Scalenus posterior
128 Serratus anterior (long thoracic)
130 Latissimus dorsi (thoracodorsal)

131 Pectoralis major, sternocostal head (medial and lateral pectorals)

129 Pectoralis minor (medial and lateral pectorals)

139 Coracobrachialis (musculocutaneous)

141 Brachialis (radial)

142 Triceps brachii (radial)

144 Anconeus (radial)

145 Supinator (radial)

148 Extensor carpi radialis longus (radial)

149 Extensor carpi radialis brevis (radial)

150 Extensor carpi ulnaris (radial)

154 Extensor digitorum (radial)

155 Extensor indicis (radial)

158 Extensor digiti minimi (radial)

166 Abductor pollicis longus (radial)

167 Extensor pollicis longus (radial)

168 Extensor pollicis brevis (radial)

146 Pronator teres (median)

147 Pronator quadratus (median)

151 Flexor carpi radialis (median)

152 Palmaris longus (median)

153 Flexor carpi ulnaris (median)

169 Flexor pollicis longus (median)

Dorsal Primary Ramus (of C7)

60 Longissimus capitis

62 Semispinalis capitis

63 Spinalis capitis

64 Longissimus cervicis

65 Semispinalis cervicis

66 Iliocostalis cervicis

67 Splenius cervicis

68 Spinalis cervicis

69 Interspinales cervicis

70 Intertransversarii cervicis [posterior]

71 Rotatores cervicis

94 Multifidi

C8

Ventral Primary Ramus

70 Intertransversarii cervicis [anterior]

81 Scalenus medius

82 Scalenus posterior

130 Latissimus dorsi (thoracodorsal)

131 Pectoralis major, sternocostal (lateral and medial pectorals)

129 Pectoralis minor (medial and lateral pectorals)

142 Triceps brachii (radial)

144 Anconeus (radial)

149 Extensor carpi radialis brevis (radial)

150 Extensor carpi ulnaris (radial)

154 Extensor digitorum (radial)

155 Extensor indicis (radial)

158 Extensor digiti minimi (radial)

166 Abductor pollicis longus (radial)

167 Extensor pollicis longus (radial)

168 Extensor pollicis brevis (radial)

147 Pronator quadratus (median) (C8)

152 Palmaris longus (median)

156 Flexor digitorum superficialis (median)

157 Flexor digitorum profundus, digits 2 and 3 (median)

163 Lumbricales, 1st and 2nd (median)

169 Flexor pollicis longus (median)

170 Flexor pollicis brevis, superficial head (median)

171 Abductor pollicis brevis (median)

172 Opponens pollicis (median, ulnar)

170 Flexor pollicis brevis, deep head (ulnar)

173 Adductor pollicis (ulnar)

153 Flexor carpi ulnaris (ulnar)

157 Flexor digitorum profundus, digits 4 and 5 (ulnar)

163 Lumbricales, 3rd and 4th (ulnar)

164 Interossei, dorsal (ulnar)

165 Interossei, palmar (ulnar)

159 Abductor digiti minimi (ulnar)

161 Opponens digiti minimi (ulnar)

160 Flexor digiti minimi brevis (ulnar)

162 Palmaris brevis (ulnar)

Dorsal Primary Ramus (of C8)

60 Longissimus capitis

62 Semispinalis capitis

63 Spinalis capitis

64 Longissimus cervicis

65 Semispinalis cervicis

66 Iliocostalis cervicis (variable)

67 Splenius cervicis

68 Spinalis cervicis (variable)

69 Interspinales cervicis

70 Intertransversarii cervicis [posterior]

71 Rotatores cervicis

94 Multifidi

THE THORACIC ROOTS AND NERVES

There are 12 pairs of thoracic nerves arising from the ventral primary rami: T1 to T11 are called the *intercostals* and T12 is called the *subcostal nerve*. These nerves are not part of a plexus. T1 and T2 innervate the upper extremity as well as the thorax; T3-T6 innervate only the thoracic muscles; the lower thoracic nerves innervate the thoracic and abdominal muscles.

T1

Ventral Primary Ramus

107 Levatores costarum

102 Intercostales externi

103 Intercostales interni

104 Intercostales intimi

131 Pectoralis major [sternocostal head] (medial and lateral pectoral)

129 Pectoralis minor (medial and lateral pectorals)

147 Pronator quadratus (median)

156 Flexor digitorum superficialis (median)

157 Flexor digitorum profundus, digits 2 and 3 (median)

163 Lumbricales, 1st and 2nd (median)

170 Flexor pollicis brevis [superficial head] (median)

171 Abductor pollicis brevis (median)

172 Opponens pollicis (median and ulnar)

153 Flexor carpi ulnaris (ulnar)

157 Flexor digitorum profundus, digits 4 and 5 (ulnar)

159 Abductor digiti minimi (ulnar)

160 Flexor digiti minimi brevis (ulnar)

161 Opponens digiti minimi (ulnar)

162 Palmaris brevis (ulnar)

163 Lumbricales, 3rd and 4th (ulnar)

164 Interossei, dorsal (ulnar)

165 Interossei, palmar (ulnar)

170 Flexor pollicis brevis [deep head] (ulnar)

173 Adductor pollicis (ulnar)

Dorsal Primary Ramus (of T1)

62 Semispinalis capitis

65 Semispinalis cervicis

93 Semispinalis thoracis

64 Longissimus cervicis

91 Longissimus thoracis

63 Spinalis capitis (highly variable)

92 Spinalis thoracis

89 Iliocostalis thoracis

66 Iliocostalis cervicis (variable)

94 Multifidi

99 Intertransversarii thoracis

95 Rotatores thoracis

97 Interspinales thoracis

T2

Ventral Primary Ramus

107 Levatores costarum

102 Intercostales externi

103 Intercostales interni

104 Intercostales intimi

108 Serratus posterior superior

106 Transversus thoracis

Dorsal Primary Ramus (of T2)

65 Semispinales cervicis (variable)
93 Semispinalis thoracis
64 Longissimus cervicis
91 Longissimus thoracis
92 Spinalis thoracis
66 Iliocostalis cervicis (variable)
89 Iliocostalis thoracis
94 Multifidi
95 Rotatores thoracis
97 Interspinales thoracis
99 Intertransversarii thoracis

T3

Ventral Primary Ramus

107 Levatores costarum
102 Intercostales externi
103 Intercostales interni
104 Intercostales intimi
108 Serratus posterior superior
106 Transversus thoracis

Dorsal Primary Ramus

93 Semispinalis thoracis
64 Longissimus cervicis (variable)
65 Semispinalis cervicis
91 Longissimus thoracis
92 Spinalis thoracis
66 Iliocostalis cervicis
89 Iliocostalis thoracis
94 Multifidi
95 Rotatores thoracis
97 Interspinales thoracis
99 Intertransversarii thoracis

T4, T5, T6

Ventral Primary Ramus

107 Levatores costarum
102 Intercostales externi
103 Intercostales interni
104 Intercostales intimi
106 Transversus thoracis
108 Serratus posterior superior (to T5)

Dorsal Primary Ramus

65 Semispinalis cervicis
89 Iliocostalis thoracis
93 Semispinalis thoracis
91 Longissimus thoracis
92 Spinalis thoracis
94 Multifidi
95 Rotatores thoracis
99 Intertransversarii thoracis

T7

Ventral Primary Ramus

107 Levatores costarum
103 Intercostales interni
102 Intercostales externi
104 Intercostales intimi
105 Subcostales
106 Transversus thoracis
110 Obliquus externus abdominis
111 Obliquus internus abdominis
112 Transversus abdominis
113 Rectus abdominis

Dorsal Primary Ramus

93 Semispinalis thoracis
91 Longissimus thoracis
92 Spinalis thoracis
89 Iliocostalis thoracis
94 Multifidi
95 Rotatores thoracis
99 Intertransversarii thoracis

T8

Ventral Primary Ramus

107 Levatores costarum
103 Intercostales interni
102 Intercostales externi
104 Intercostales intimi
105 Subcostales
106 Transversus thoracis
110 Obliquus externus abdominis
111 Obliquus internus abdominis
112 Transversus abdominis
113 Rectus abdominis

Dorsal Primary Ramus

93 Semispinalis thoracis
91 Longissimus thoracis
92 Spinalis thoracis
89 Iliocostalis thoracis
94 Multifidi
95 Rotatores thoracis
99 Intertransversarii thoracis

T9, T10, T11

Ventral Primary Ramus

107 Levatores costarum
103 Intercostales interni
102 Intercostales externi
104 Intercostales intimi
105 Subcostales
106 Transversus thoracis
109 Serratus posterior inferior
110 Obliquus externus abdominis
111 Obliquus internus abdominis
112 Transversus abdominis
113 Rectus abdominis

Dorsal Primary Ramus

93 Semispinalis thoracis
91 Longissimus thoracis
92 Spinalis thoracis
89 Iliocostalis thoracis
94 Multifidi
95 Rotatores thoracis
97 Interspinales thoracis
99 Intertransversarii thoracis

T12

Ventral Primary Ramus

100 Quadratus lumborum
112 Transversus abdominis
109 Serratus posterior inferior
110 Obliquus externus abdominis
111 Obliquus internus abdominis
113 Rectus abdominis
114 Pyramidalis

Dorsal Primary Ramus

93 Semispinalis thoracis
91 Longissimus thoracis
92 Spinalis thoracis
89 Iliocostalis thoracis
94 Multifidi
95 Rotatores thoracis
97 Interspinales thoracis
99 Intertransversarii thoracis

THE LUMBAR ROOTS AND NERVES

The lumbar plexus is formed by the first four lumbar nerves and a communicating branch from T12. The fourth lumbar nerve gives its largest part to the lumbar plexus and a smaller part to the sacral plexus. The fifth lumbar nerve and the small segment of the fourth lumbar nerve form the lumbosacral trunk, which is part of the sacral plexus.

L1

Ventral Primary Ramus

100 Quadratus lumborum
175 Psoas minor
112 Transversus abdominis

111 Obliquus internus abdominis
117 Cremaster (genitofemoral)

Dorsal Primary Ramus

90 Iliocostalis lumborum
91 Longissimus thoracis
96 Rotatores lumborum
94 Multifidi
98 Interspinales lumborum
99 Intertransversarii lumborum

L2

Ventral Primary Ramus

100 Quadratus lumborum
174 Psoas major
176 Iliacus
117 Cremaster (genitofemoral)
177 Pectineus (femoral)
178 Gracilis (obturator)
179 Adductor longus (obturator)
180 Adductor brevis (obturator)
181 Adductor magnus
Superior and middle fibers (obturator)
Inferior fibers (sciatic, tibial)
195 Sartorius (femoral)
196-200 Quadriceps femoris (femoral)
196 Rectus femoris
197 Vastus intermedius
198 Vastus lateralis
199 Vastus medialis longus
200 Vastus medialis obliquus
201 Articularis genus (femoral)

Dorsal Primary Ramus

90 Iliocostalis lumborum (variable)
96 Rotatores lumborum
94 Multifidi
98 Interspinales lumborum
99 Intertransversarii lumborum

L3

Ventral Primary Ramus

100 Quadratus lumborum
174 Psoas major
176 Iliacus (femoral)
177 Pectineus (femoral)
178 Gracilis (obturator)
179 Adductor longus (obturator)
180 Adductor brevis (obturator)
181 Adductor magnus, superior and medial fibers (obturator)
Inferior fibers (sciatic, tibial)
188 Obturator externus (obturator)
195 Sartorius (femoral)
196-200 Quadriceps femoris (femoral)
196 Rectus femoris
197 Vastus intermedius
198 Vastus lateralis
199 Vastus medialis longus
200 Vastus medialis obliquus
201 Articularis genus (femoral)

Dorsal Primary Ramus

90 Iliocostalis lumborum
96 Rotatores lumborum
94 Multifidi
98 Interspinales lumborum
99 Intertransversarii lumborum

L4

Ventral Primary Ramus

175 Psoas major
179 Adductor longus (obturator)
181 Adductor magnus
Superior and middle fibers (obturator)
Lower fibers (sciatic, tibial)
183 Gluteus medius (superior gluteal)
184 Gluteus minimus (superior gluteal)
185 Tensor fasciae latae (superior gluteal)
188 Obturator externus (obturator)

195-200 Quadriceps femoris (femoral)
196 Rectus femoris
197 Vastus lateralis
198 Vastus intermedius
199 Vastus medialis longus
200 Vastus medialis obliquus
201 Articularis genus (femoral)
202 Popliteus (tibial)
203 Tibialis anterior (deep peroneal)
204 Tibialis posterior (tibial)

Dorsal Primary Ramus

90 Iliocostalis lumborum
96 Rotatores lumborum
94 Multifidi
98 Interspinales lumborum
99 Intertransversarii lumborum

L5

Ventral Primary Ramus

182 Gluteus maximus (inferior gluteal)
183 Gluteus medius (superior gluteal)
184 Gluteus minimus (superior gluteal)
185 Tensor fasciae latae (superior gluteal)
187 Obturator internus (nerve to obturator internus)
189 Gemellus superior (nerve to obturator internus)
190 Gemellus inferior (nerve to quadratus femoris)
191 Quadratus femoris (nerve to quadratus femoris)
192 Biceps femoris
Short head (sciatic, common peroneal)
Long head (sciatic, tibial)
194 Semimembranosus (sciatic, tibial)
193 Semitendinosus (sciatic, tibial)
202 Popliteus (tibial)
204 Tibialis posterior (tibial)
213 Flexor digitorum longus (tibial)
222 Flexor hallucis longus (tibial)
203 Tibialis anterior (deep peroneal)
210 Peroneus tertius (deep peroneal)
211 Extensor digitorum longus (deep peroneal)
212 Extensor digitorum brevis (deep peroneal)
221 Extensor hallucis longus (deep peroneal)
208 Peroneus longus (superficial peroneal)
209 Peroneus brevis (superficial peroneal)
218 Lumbricales, 1st [foot] (medial plantar)

Dorsal Primary Ramus

90 Iliocostalis lumborum
96 Rotatores lumborum
94 Multifidi
99 Intertransversarii lumborum

THE LUMBOSACRAL ROOTS AND NERVES

The intermingling of the ventral primary rami of the lumbar, sacral, and coccygeal nerves is known as the lumbosacral plexus. There is uncertainty about any motor innervation from the dorsal primary rami below S3. The nerves branching off this plexus supply the lower extremity in part and also the perineum and coccygeal areas via the pudendal and coccygeal plexuses.

S1

Ventral Primary Ramus

182 Gluteus maximus (inferior gluteal)
183 Gluteus medius (superior gluteal)
184 Gluteus minimus (superior gluteal)
185 Tensor fasciae latae (superior gluteal)
186 Piriformis (nerve to piriformis)
187 Obturator internus (nerve to obturator internus)
189 Gemellus superior (nerve to obturator internus)
190 Gemellus inferior (nerve to quadratus femoris)
191 Quadratus femoris (nerve to quadratus femoris)
192 Biceps femoris
Short head (sciatic, common peroneal nerve)
Long head (sciatic, tibial nerve)
194 Semimembranosus (sciatic, tibial division)
193 Semitendinosus (sciatic, tibial division)
205 Gastrocnemius (tibial)

207 Plantaris (tibial)

202 Popliteus (tibial)

204 Tibialis posterior (tibial)

206 Soleus (tibial)

213 Flexor digitorum longus (tibial)

222 Flexor hallucis longus (tibial)

223 Flexor hallucis brevis (tibial)

203 Tibialis anterior (deep peroneal [often])

210 Peroneus tertius (deep peroneal)

211 Extensor digitorum longus (deep peroneal)

212 Extensor digitorum brevis (deep peroneal)

208 Peroneus longus (superficial peroneal)

209 Peroneus brevis (superficial peroneal)

215 Abductor digiti minimi (lateral plantar)

217 Quadratus plantae [flexor digitorum accessorius] (lateral plantar)

214 Flexor digitorum brevis (medial plantar)

224 Abductor hallucis (medial plantar)

218 Lumbricales, 1st [foot] (medial plantar)

Dorsal Primary Rami

94 Multifidi

99 Intertransversarii lumborum

S2

Ventral Primary Ramus

182 Gluteus maximus (inferior gluteal)

186 Piriformis (nerve to piriformis)

192 Biceps femoris

Short head (sciatic, common peroneal nerve)

Long head (sciatic, tibial nerve)

194 Semimembranosus (sciatic, tibial division)

193 Semitendinosus (sciatic, tibial division)

205 Gastrocnemius (tibial)

206 Soleus (tibial)

207 Plantaris (tibial)

213 Flexor digitorum longus (tibial)

222 Flexor hallucis longus (tibial)

214 Flexor digitorum brevis (medial plantar)

224 Abductor hallucis (medial plantar)

217 Quadratus plantae [flexor digitorum accessorius] (lateral plantar)

215 Abductor digiti minimi (lateral plantar)

216 Flexor digiti minimi brevis [foot] (lateral plantar)

225 Adductor hallucis (lateral plantar)

218 Lumbricales 2nd, 3rd, and 4th [foot] (lateral plantar)

219 Interossei, dorsal (lateral plantar)

220 Interossei, plantar (lateral plantar)

115 Levator ani (pudendal)

118 Transversus perinei superficialis (pudendal)

119 Transversus perinei profundus (pudendal)

120 Bulbocavernosus (pudendal)

121 Ischiocavernosus (pudendal)

122 Sphincter urethrae (pudendal)

123 Sphincter ani externus (pudendal)

Dorsal Primary Rami

94 Multifidi

S3

Ventral Primary Ramus

217 Quadratus plantae [flexor digitorum accessorius] (lateral plantar)

215 Abductor digiti minimi (lateral plantar)

216 Flexor digiti minimi brevis [foot] (lateral plantar)

225 Adductor hallucis (lateral plantar)

218 Lumbricales 2nd, 3rd, and 4th [foot] (lateral plantar)

219 Interossei, dorsal (lateral plantar)

220 Interossei, plantar (lateral plantar)

115 Levator ani (pudendal)

116 Coccygeus (pudendal)

118 Transversus perinei superficialis (pudendal)

119 Transversus perinei profundus (pudendal)

120 Bulbocavernosus (pudendal)

121 Ischiocavernosus (pudendal)

122 Sphincter urethrae (pudendal)

123 Sphincter ani externus (pudendal)

S4 AND S5

Ventral Primary Ramus

116 Coccygeus (to S4, pudendal)

123 Sphincter ani externus (to S4, perineal)

118 Transversus perinei superficialis (to S4, pudendal)

119 Transversus perinei profundus (to S4, pudendal)

120 Bulbocavernosus (to S4, pudendal)

121 Ischiocavernosus (to S4, pudendal)

122 Sphincter urethrae (to S4, pudendal)

123 Sphincter ani externus (to S4, perineal)

REFERENCES

1. Clemente CD. Gray's Anatomy. 30th (American) ed. Philadelphia: Lea & Febiger; 1985.
2. Williams PL. Gray's Anatomy. 38th (British) ed. London: Churchill-Livingstone; 1995.
3. Figge FHJ. Sobotta's Atlas of Human Anatomy. vol. 1. *Atlas of Bones, Joints and Muscles*, 8th English ed. New York: Hafner; 1968.
4. Clemente CD. Anatomy: A Regional Atlas of the Human Body. Baltimore: Urban & Schwarzenberg; 1998.
5. Netter FH, Colacino S. Atlas of Human Anatomy. Summit, NJ: Ciba-Geigy, 1998.
6. Jenkins DB. Hollingshead's Functional Anatomy of the Limbs and Back. Philadelphia: WB Saunders; 1998.
7. Grant JCB. An Atlas of Anatomy. 10th ed. Baltimore: Lippincott Williams & Wilkins; 1999.
8. Moore KL. Clinically Oriented Anatomy. 3rd ed. Baltimore: Williams & Wilkins; 1992.
9. Haerer AF. DeJong's The Neurological Examination. 5th ed. Philadelphia: JB Lippincott; 1992.
10. DuBrul EL. Sicher and DuBrul's Oral Anatomy. 8th ed. St Louis: Ishiyaku EuroAmerica; 1990.
11. Nairn RI. The circumoral musculature: structure and function. Br Dent J. 1975;138:49-56.
12. Lightoller GH. Facial muscles: the modiolus and muscles surrounding the rima oris with remarks about the panniculus adiposus. J Anat. 1925;60:1-85.
13. Keller JT, Saunders MC, Van Loveren H, et al. Neuroanatomical considerations of palatal muscles: tensor and levator palatini. Cleft Palate J. 1984;21:70-75.
14. Perry J, Nickel VL. Total cervical-spine fusion for neck paralysis. J Bone Joint Surg [Am]. 1959;41:37-60.
15. Moyers RE. Electromyographic analysis of certain muscles involved in temporomandibular movement. Am J Orthodont. 1950;36:481-515.
16. DeSousa OM. Estudoelectromiografico do m. platysma. Folio Clin Biol. 1964;33:42-52.
17. Jones DS, Beargie RJ, Pauly JE. An electromyographic study of some muscles of costal respiration in man. Anat Rec. 1953;117:17-24.
18. Soo KC, Guiloff RF, Pauly JE. Innervation of the trapezius muscle: a study in patients undergoing neck dissections. Head Neck. 1990;12:488-495.
19. Basmajian JV. Muscles Alive. 2nd ed. Baltimore: Williams & Wilkins; 1967.
20. Sodeberg GL. Kinesiology: Application to Pathologic Motion. Baltimore: Williams & Wilkins; 1997.
21. Doody SG, Freedman L, Waterland JC. Shoulder movements during abduction in the scapular plane. Arch Phys Med Rehabil. 1970;10:595-604.
22. Perry J. Muscle control of the shoulder. In Rowe CR, ed. The Shoulder. New York: Churchill-Livingstone; 1988:17-34.
23. Ip M, Chang KS. A study of the radial supply of the human brachialis muscle. Anat Rec. 1968;162:363-371.
24. Basmajian JV, DeLuca CJ. Muscles Alive. 5th ed. Baltimore: Williams & Wilkins; 1985.
25. Basmajian JV, Travill AA. Electromyography of the pronator muscles of the forearm. Anat Rec. 1961;139:45-49.
26. Flatt AE. *Kinesiology of the Hand.* Am Acad Orthop Surg Instructional Course Lectures XVIII. St. Louis: CV Mosby; 1961.
27. Muller T. Variations in the abductor pollicis longus and extensor pollicis brevis in the South African Bantu. South Afr J Lab Clin Med. 1959;5:56-62.
28. Martin BF. The annular ligament of the superior radioulnar joint. J Anat. 1958;92:473-482.
29. Day MH, Napier JR. The two heads of the flexor pollicis brevis. J Anat. 1961;95:123-130.
30. Harness D, Sekales E, Chaco J. The double motor innervation of the opponens pollicis: an electromyographic study. J Anat. 1974;117:329-331.
31. Forrest WJ. Motor innervation of human thenar and hypothenar muscles in 25 hands: a study combining EMG and percutaneous nerve stimulation. Can J Surg. 1967;10: 196-199.
32. McKibben B. Action of the iliopsoas muscle in the newborn. J Bone Joint Surg [Br]. 1968;50:161-165.
33. DeSousa OM, Vitti M. Estudio electeromiografica de los musculos adductores largo y mayor. Arch Mex Anat. 1966; 7:52-53.
34. Janda V, Stara V. The role of thigh adductors in movement patterns of the hip and knee joint. Courier. 1965;15:1-3.
35. Kaplan EB. The iliotibial tract. Clinical and morphological significance. J Bone Joint Surg [Am]. 1958;40:817-831.
36. Pare EB, Stern JT, Schwartz JM. Functional differentiation within the tensor fasciae latae. J Bone Joint Surg [Am]. 1981;63:1457-1471.
37. Sneath R. Insertion of the biceps femoris. J Anat. 1955; 89:550-553.
38. Lieb FJ, Perry J. Quadriceps function: an anatomical and mechanical study using amputated limbs. J Bone Joint Surg [Am]. 1968;50:1535-1548.
39. Lieb FJ, Perry J. Quadriceps function: an electromyographic study under isometric conditions. J Bone Joint Surg [Am]. 1971;53:749-758.
40. Last RJ. The popliteus muscle and the lateral meniscus. J Bone Joint Surg [Br]. 1950;32:93-99.
41. Cummins EJ, Anson BJ, Carr BW, et al. Structure of the calcaneal tendon (of Achilles) in relation to orthopedic surgery; with additional observations of the plantaris muscle. Surg Gynecol Obstet. 1946;83:107-116.
42. Lewis OJ. The comparative morphology of m. flexor accessorius and the associated flexor tendons. J Anat. 1962;96: 321-333.

Other Readings

Smith R, Nyquist-Battie C, Clark M, et al. Anatomical characteristics of the upper serratus anterior: cadaver dissection. J Orthop Sports Phys Ther. 2003;33:449-454.

INDEX

Page numbers followed by "f" indicate figures, "t" indicate tables, and "b" indicate boxes.

C

D

E

F

G

H

I

J

K

L

M

N

O

P

Q

R

S

T

U

V

W

Z